Thoracic Surgical Oncology

Thoracic Surgical Oncology

Edward J. Beattie, M.D.
Professor
Department of Surgery
Mount Sinai School of Medicine
of the City University of New York
Chief
Division of Thoracic Surgery
Department of Surgery
Director
Kriser Lung Cancer Center
Beth Israel Medical Center
New York, New York

Norman D. Bloom, M.D.
Clinical Professor
Department of Surgery
New York Medical College
Valhalla, New York
Chief
Division of Surgical Oncology
Department of Surgery
Metropolitan Hospital Center
New York, New York

James C. Harvey, M.D.
Attending Surgeon
Department of Surgery
Beth Israel Medical Center
New York, New York

Illustrations by Hugh Thomas

Churchill Livingstone
New York, Edinburgh, London, Melbourne, Tokyo

Library of Congress Cataloging-in-Publication Data
Beattie, Edward J., (date)
Thoracic surgical oncology / Edward J. Beattie, Norman D. Bloom, James C. Harvey ; illustrations by Hugh Thomas.
p. cm.
Includes bibliographical references and index.
ISBN 0-443-08589-7
1. Chest—Cancer—Surgery. I. Bloom, Norman D. II. Harvey, James C. III. Title.
[DNLM: 1. Surgery, Operative—methods. 2. Surgery, Operative--methods—atlases. 3. Thoracic Neoplasms—surgery. 4. Thoracic Neoplasms—surgery—atlases. WF 980 B369t]
RD667.B43 1992
616.99 ' 494059—dc20
DNLM/DLC
for Library of Congress 92-20056
CIP

Distributed in the United Kingdom by Churchill Livingstone, Robert Stevenson House, 1–3 Baxter's Place, Leith Walk, Edinburgh EH1 3AF, and by associated companies, branches, and representatives throughout the world.

Accurate indications, adverse reactions, and dosage schedules for drugs are provided in this book, but it is possible that they may change. The reader is urged to review the package information data of the manufacturers of the medications mentioned.

The Publishers have made every effort to trace the copyright holders for borrowed material. If they have inadvertently overlooked any, they will be pleased to make the necessary arrangements at the first opportunity.

Acquisitions Editor: *Avé McCracken*
Assistant Editor: *Nancy Terry*
Copy Editor: *David Terry*
Production Designer: *Patricia McFadden*
Production Supervisor: *Sharon Tuder*

Printed in the United States of America

First published in 1992 7 6 5 4 3 2 1

To Nicole Beattie

Without her industry and word processor
this volume would have appeared much later.

Edward J. Beattie, M.D.
Norman D. Bloom, M.D.
James C. Harvey, M.D.

Contributors

C. Frederick Kittle, M.D.

Professor, Department of Cardiovascular-Thoracic Surgery, Rush Medical College of Rush University; Senior Attending Physician and Director, Section of Thoracic Surgery, Department of Surgery, Rush-Presbyterian-St. Luke's Medical Center, Chicago, Illinois

Juliana Pisch, M.D.

Assistant Professor, Department of Radiation Oncology, Mount Sinai School of Medicine of the City University of New York; Attending Radiologist, Department of Radiology, Beth Israel Medical Center, New York, New York

Preface

Currently we are experiencing a national disaster in the incidence of lung cancer; 168,000 new cases are reported annually in the United States, with an anticipated mortality of almost 90 percent. New cases of esophageal carcinoma number 10,600 a year and are equally lethal.

The high incidence and high mortality of these diseases signal an ever increasing need for a multidisciplinary approach to treatment. However, this demand occurs at a time when there is a shortage of well-trained thoracic surgical oncologists. It is not uncommon for a patient with lung cancer to be seen by a medical oncologist, chest physician, and radiation oncologist and a treatment plan established for a "nonoperable cancer" without the consultation of a thoracic surgical oncologist.

In the care of the patient there must be cooperative concern, not rivalry, among specialists. Constant effort must be made to better our means of diagnosis, staging, and treatment. It is our contention that cooperative multidisciplinary effort can prolong useful life for many cancer patients. It is our hope that this text substantiates how this may be achieved.

In Chapter 1, C. Frederick Kittle, an outstanding surgical historian, traces the significant developments in the history of thoracic surgery. Chapter 2 outlines critical aspects of anatomy and surgical pathology. Chapter 3 is devoted to the lung. Treatment results are based primarily on our team's published papers. Text sections on diagnosis, staging, and principles of management are followed by a surgical atlas. Here, we believe, the drawings of Hugh Thomas excel. For ease in following a surgical procedure, text description of each step is coupled with the appropriate drawing.

Throughout the atlas, we have chosen to demonstrate a simple and safe form of operation. Any surgical procedure can have successful variations. However, to present numerous ways of operating can prove confusing and undermine the text's instructional value. The surgical trainee may not recognize the basic principles underlying all surgery and may not learn a standard safe technique. By distilling our experience into the most efficient methods, we have tried to provide a surgical guide equally useful to both the trainee and experienced surgeon.

In Chapter 4, James C. Harvey uses the same format established in the previous chapter to cover tumors of the esophagus. In Chapters 5 through 9, Norman D. Bloom discusses surgical oncology of the mediastinum; chest wall and thoracic outlet; spine; and the heart, great vessels, and diaphragm.

The final chapter comprises illustrative cases. For these patients, whose cancers ranged from simple to complex, it was possible to achieve unexpectedly good results. We cite their case studies as a reminder that oncologists and patients alike should maintain hope. None of us can tell in advance which of our patients will do well and which will do poorly. Statistics and survival curves are not meaningful for a particular patient, whose outcome is either cure or no cure. Consequently it is important to prolong an individual's useful life in the hope that some day that individual may live to be cured. As the approach is aggressive, we must constantly be alert and strive to make the treatment safer. We are driven by our failures. While great progress has been made, the goal is to increase the amount of good done through better research and development, better clinical research, and better clinical care.

We hope our effort will be of interest not only to thoracic surgeons but also to chest physicians, medical oncologists, and radiation oncologists. But most especially we hope it will improve the care of our thoracic cancer patients.

Edward J. Beattie, M.D.

Acknowledgments

The authors were very fortunate to have Hugh Thomas lend his artwork to the text. Hugh is a true artist, whose eye captures the essence of an operative scene.

Our publishers and editors deserve special thanks and commendation for their forbearance. We presume most books are not finished precisely on schedule. We do appreciate the faith exhibited by Robert Hurley and Avé McCracken. Nancy Terry's editing we feel was spectacular.

The extra effort and uncomplaining support by our administrative assistant, Elena Horohoe, was a necessary ingredient for the production of this book.

We wish to thank the staff of the Beth Israel Medical Center Library, especially Dorothy Schwartz, Ellen Poisson, and Patricia Gallagher. Their assistance was invaluable.

David Kriser began supporting our multidisciplinary lung cancer effort two decades ago at the Memorial Sloan-Kettering Cancer Center. His continuing interest established the Kriser Lung Cancer Center at Beth Israel Medical Center in 1985.

This book reflects the multidisciplinary approach to thoracic oncology that has been developing for the past twenty-five years at three institutions with which I have been associated: the Memorial Sloan-Kettering Cancer Center, the Jackson Memorial Hospital in conjunction with the University of Miami School of Medicine, and the Kriser Lung Cancer Center in conjunction with Beth Israel Medical Center. The following table acknowledges some of the individuals who have been part of our team:

	MSKCC 1966–1983	JMH/UM 1983–1985	KLCC/BIMC 1985–Present
Surgery	Nael Martini Manjit Bains Patricia McCormack	Richard Thurer	James Harvey
Radio- therapy	Basil Hilaris Dattatreyudo Nori	Juan Fayos Jae Ho Kim	Juliana Pisch Bhadrassain Vikram
Medical Oncology	Robert Golbey Richard Gralla Robert Wittes	Kasi Sridhar	Stephen Malamud
Chest Medicine	Charles LaMonte	Phillip Rubin	Raymond Keller Patricia Villamena

Edward J. Beattie, M.D.

Contents

1

History of Thoracic Surgical Oncology

C. Frederick Kittle

"Only the man who is familiar with art and science of the past is competent to aid in its progress in the future."
—Theodor Billroth

Gertrude Stein said it better: "Let me recite what history teaches: history teaches."

The history of thoracic oncology is concerned chiefly with surgical efforts in malignancies of the esophagus and lung. Operations on the chest wall and mediastinum also evolved but are less important because of their lesser frequency. Oncology is essentially a modern concept—bringing together a multimodality approach of surgery, radiation, chemotherapy, and other disciplines, enhancing each individual effort. Most malignancies of the thorax are surgical targets, best cured by extirpation, although extensive disease and some neoplasms are nonsurgical problems.

PULMONARY RESECTION

EARLY EFFORTS

Because of the prevalence of tuberculosis and other pulmonary infections, early surgical efforts at pulmonary resection began with procedures for treating empyema, tuberculosis, and lung abscess. The technical problems of open pneumothorax, hemorrhage, bronchial closure, and infection complicated thoracic operations and were present for many years before acceptable solutions were developed.

Before the twentieth century lung cancer was a rare disease—it is a disease of the twentieth century and mankind's internal and external environmental pollution. Slightly more than a century ago Rokitansky (1849) stated: "Thus, primitive cancer of the salivary glands, or of the small intestine, very seldom occurs, of the lungs or of the spleen scarcely ever."[1] This is in contrast to its present incidence; bronchogenic carcinoma is the most common cause of death by cancer.

The earliest known lung cancers, in retrospect since they were not clearly identified, were observed among Schneeberg miners in the Black Forest region of Germany. Mining began in this region in 1410 and, over the years, provided silver, copper, iron, cobalt, arsenic, and uranium. It was recognized early that these miners had severe and often fatal pulmonary disorders because of their occupation. The fatal Mala Metallorum was well known to Paracelsus (1531) and Agricola (1556).

However, it was not until 1879 that Haerting and Hesse, physicians to the miners in this area, described an incidence of 75 percent of all deaths due to pulmonary tumors, mistakenly interpreted as lymphosarcomas. Although their interpretation of the pathology was incorrect, their epidemiologic conclusion was unequivocal.[2] The first clinical report of primary lung cancer is that by Bayle in 1810[3]; he described a 72-year-old man with a mass in the hilum of the left lung and metastatic spread to the lymph nodes, liver, and subcutaneous tissue.

In 1912 Adler, in his monograph on lung cancer, emphasized the rarity of this tumor when he could find only 374 instances in a search of the world literature.[4] Tuberculosis, which was very common, was thought to be the cause of lung cancer, a concept stressed by the famous American pathologist Ewing in the several editions of his *Neoplastic Diseases: A Treatise on Tumors*.[5]

Surgical attempts at lung resection began late and moved slowly. Like other surgical procedures, the early lung resections were done because of trauma. Rolandini, in 1499, is generally credited with the first. His patient had sustained a chest wound, which he described: "I found a portion of the lung issued between two ribs; . . . it was not possible to reduce it. The compression exercised by the ribs retained its nutriment from it, and it was so mortified that worms had developed in it."[6] Rolandini transected the extruded portion and packed the wound open. In the seventeenth century similar accounts were related by Fabricus[7] and Tulpius.[8] In 1786, when faced with the same problem, Bell introduced a new technique: he applied a ligature to remove the protruding lung.[3] As recently as 1898 Murphy stated that if he were going to do a lobectomy he would first exteriorize the lung and then amputate it in a second procedure.[10]

In the early nineteenth century the American surgeon Antony resected part of the chest wall and the underlying lung (Fig. 1-1), because of an infection after an accident, removing "all the disorganized parenchyma of the lung" and establishing his claim for performing an early chest wall and lung resection.[11] Concern about this procedure was expressed by Dieffenbach: ". . . such opera-

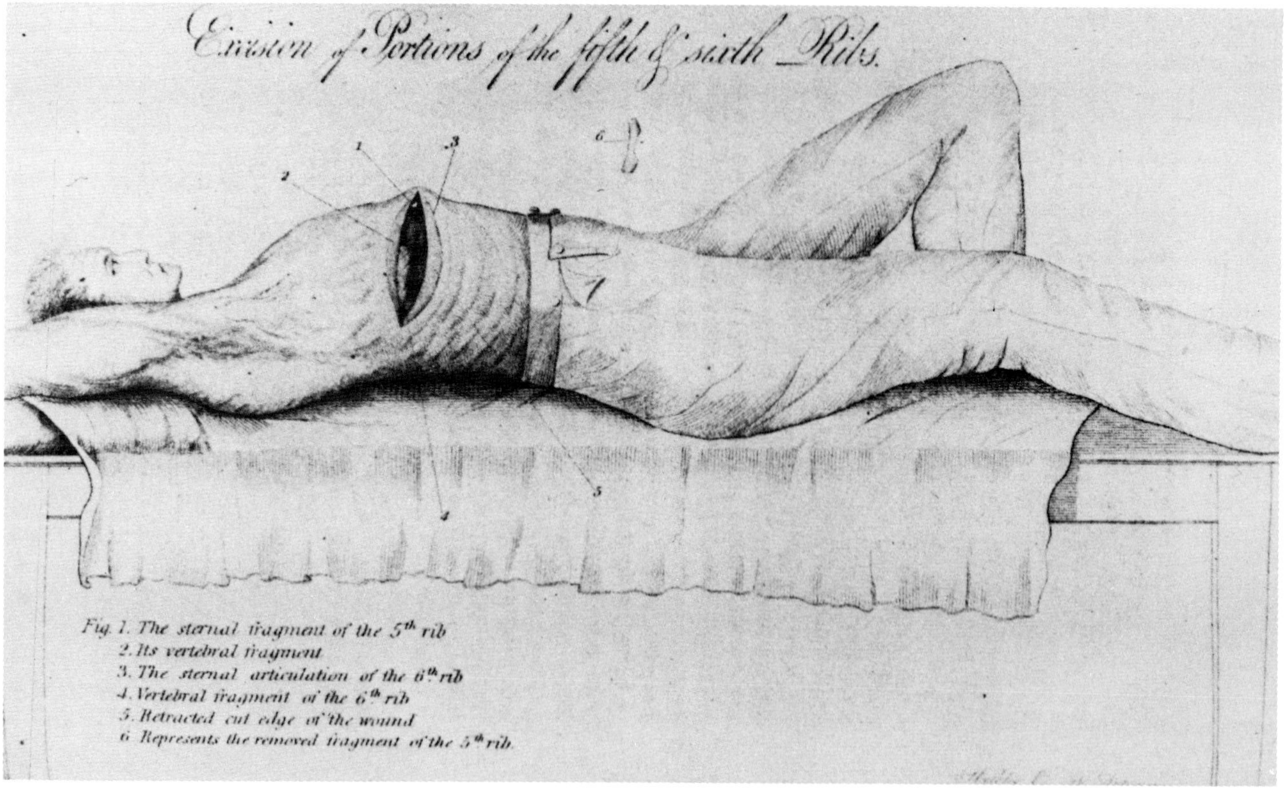

Fig. 1-1. Seventeen-year-old male operated on by Antony on March 3, 1821. He had fallen from a horse several years previously and had developed an "extensive abscess . . . about this carious bone." Portions of the fifth and sixth ribs and the underlying lung were removed (1823).

tions are too greatly out of harmony with all physiology and give the beautiful art of healing the appearance of cruel destructive mechanics."[12]

Kroenlein similarly did a resection of the lung together with the chest wall for a sarcoma in 1884[13]; the patient was still well 2 years later. Numerous other chest wall resections followed. The first lung resection for tumor was performed in 1861 by Pean, who described removing part of a patient's lung by using cautery.[14]

In 1881 Block reported performing experimental pulmonary resections in rabbits and established that pneumonectomy had a low mortality and that it could be tolerated by the animals postoperatively.[15]

Other experimental studies followed, some involving the technique of first prolapsing (exteriorizing) the lung and then later excising it by ligation, a method endorsed later by Murphy[10] and used as recently as 1927 by Whittemore.[16] In the 1880s, the ligation method was used by Schmid[17] in dogs and pigs; his experimental work was verified by Gluck[18] and Biondi.[19] The conclusions of these early investigators were well stated by Biondi in his prediction: "It is to be hoped that in the not too distant future this operation . . . will find its useful application in man, and on the day when the first lung is removed and the first tubercular patient is cured, humanity will triumph over one of its most terrible enemies."[20]

Despite the encouraging results of these experiments, the only surgeon to attempt lung resection in a human was Block, who operated on a relative for tuberculosis. He did a bilateral apical resection with fatal results; this disturbed the surgeon so much that he later committed suicide. Fifty-five years would pass until the results of these experiments would become realized as regards lung cancer.

These early experiments stimulated sporadic attempts at lung resection, chiefly for tuberculosis. The first successful operation was by the French surgeon Tuffier in 1891.[21] He too, had worked on lung resection in the laboratory and, on the basis of these experiences, decided to attempt operation clinically. He entered the thorax anteriorly through the second interspace; "passing my finger behind the apex of the lung I was able to seize it with a special instrument which did no damage to the friable tissue. I could now draw it through the opening in the pleura." He identified the diseased portion and resected it by using a circumferential suture. The patient did well and eight days later climbed two flights of stairs to be presented at the

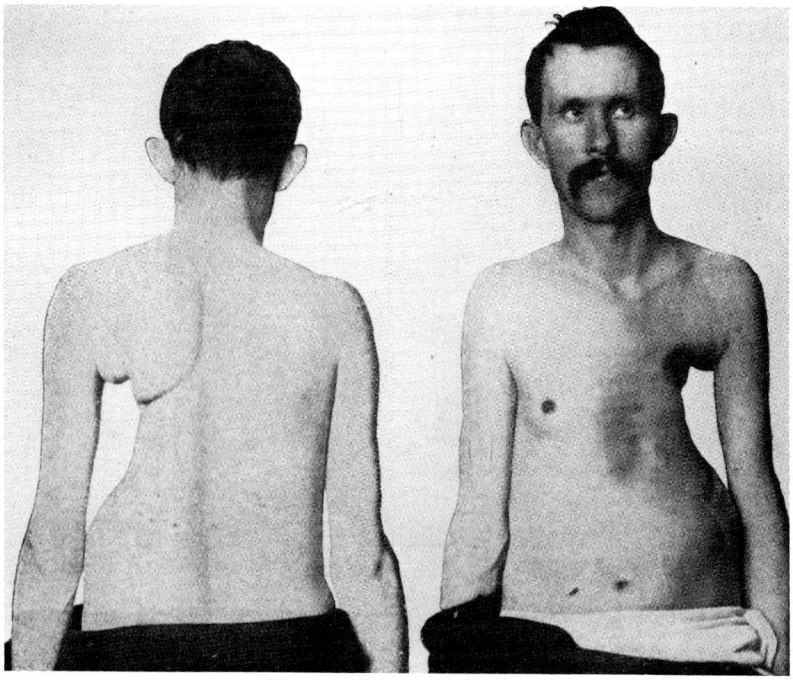

Fig. 1-2. Postoperative photograph of the first pneumonectomy patient. MacEwen operated on him in 1895 for empyema and abscess. In addition to the empyema, he found a large pulmonary abscess and widespread tuberculosis. The entire lung was removed piecemeal; a four-rib thoracoplasty was done 1 month later (1906).

Society of Surgeons of Paris! Other successes were reported by Quincke[22] and Murphy.[10] A successful lobectomy was done by Heidenhain in 1901 in a patient with multiple abscesses secondary to bronchiectasis.[23] The cavities were drained initially and the lobe removed at a second procedure.

These successes were followed by the first pneumonectomy, done by MacEwen in 1895.[24] This patient was operated on for empyema, with the intent of drainage, but MacEwen found the entire lung involved by abscesses. All of the diseased lung was removed, and the wound was packed open. One month later thoracoplasty was done, and the recovery was uneventful (Fig. 1-2). Forty-five years later the patient was fully active and returned for a hernia repair!

HISTORIC DETERRENTS TO PULMONARY SURGERY

PREVENTION OF PNEUMOTHORAX

The chief deterrent to pulmonary surgery at this time, and also the source of much confusion, was the problem of pneumothorax and the inability of surgeons to deal with it satisfactorily. Although Vesalius had fully described the use of an endotracheal tube in maintaining ventilation in animals (1543) (Fig. 1-3), Snow[25] described its use in administering chloroform in rabbits (in 1858, marking the first endotracheal administration of anesthesia in animals), and it was employed successfully in man by Trendelenburg (1869).[26] For many years there was considerable resistance to its use. Initially the endotracheal tube, or tracheal tube, as it was first called, was inserted via a tracheotomy; however, in 1880 MacEwen showed that it could be inserted transorally and used this route for chloroform anesthesia.[27]

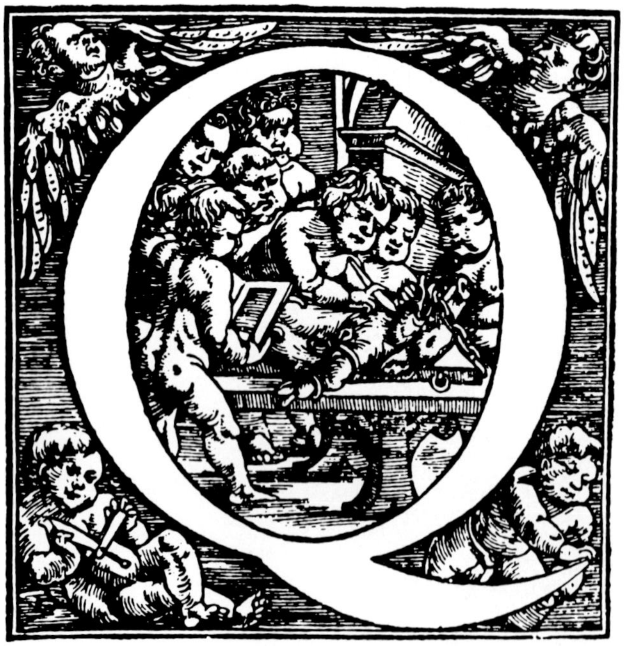

Fig. 1-3. Initial Q from Vesalius's *Fabrica* (1543) showing preliminary tracheotomy before insertion of a tube for ventilation.

Further assistance in entering the pleural cavity came with the gradual development of a device to insufflate air into the lungs to maintain ventilation. Such a method was used as early as 1869 in the United States by Truehead, according to Matas.[28] An apparatus consisting of a hand bellows was designed by Fell for artificial respiration, but this required insertion of a tube through a tracheotomy or a face mask. O'Dwyer modified the technique for intubating the larynx, thus eliminating the tracheotomy and providing a simple but effective device[29] (Fig. 1-4).

The French surgeons Tuffier and Hallion (1896)[30] inserted a long tube connected to a bellows into a dog's larynx for artificial respiration during thoracotomy. Their experiments impressed the American surgeon Matas,[30] although the results were essentially ignored by others. Matas recognized the value of this concept for thoracic surgery, and in 1899 wrote, "The procedure that promises the most benefit is . . . rhythmic maintenance of artificial respiration by a tube in the glottis directly connected with a bellows."[31] With insight and clarity he continued[31]:

> Like other discoveries, it is not only elementary in its simplicity, but the fundamental ideas involved in this important suggestion have been lying idle before the eyes of the profession for years.
>
> It is curious that surgeons should have failed to apply for so long a time the suggestions of the physiological laboratory, where the bellows and tracheal tubes have been in constant use from the days of Magendie (1783–1855) to the present, in practicing artificial respiration on animals.

Parham, one of his colleagues, heeded these suggestions and used this method in 1898 to resect successfully a chest wall sarcoma.[32]

Further attention to insufflation anesthesia was provided by Barthelemy and Dufour in France (1907)[33] and by the experimental work of Meltzer and Auer in the United States (1909)[34]; Meltzer and Auer had previously described oral intubation methods (1905). These techniques were soon ap-

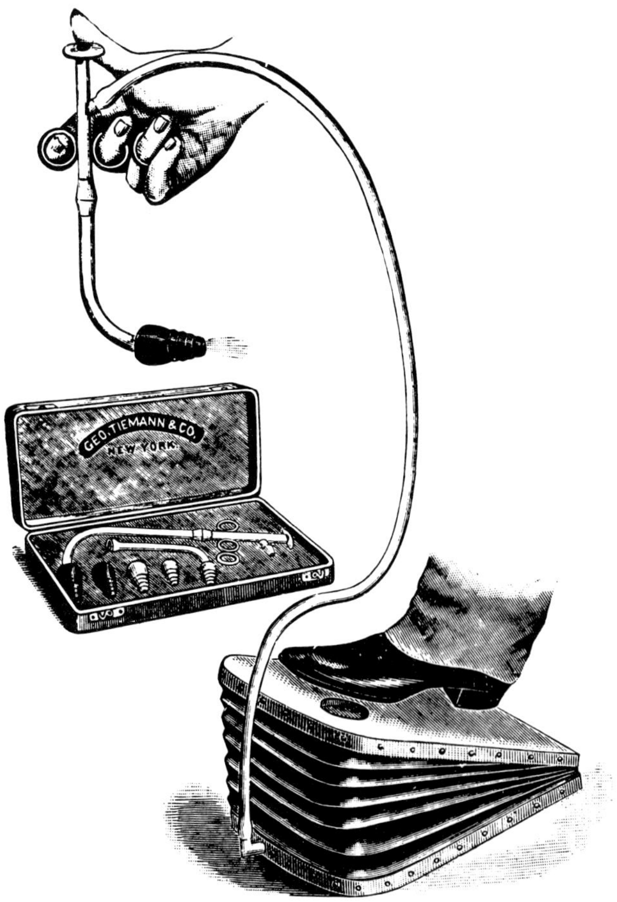

Fig. 1-4. The original Fell-O'Dwyer apparatus for lung insufflation. Note the foot bellows and the various sizes of cannulas for laryngeal intubation. This device was used in the United States in the late 1890s.

plied clinically by Eggers (1910), Peck (1912),[35] and many others using different anesthetic agents. Jackson's perfection of the laryngoscope in 1895, initially introduced by Kirstein in 1895,[36] allowed direct visualization of the larynx and contributed much to the success of endotracheal intubation.

In Germany Kuehn recommended cocainization of the larynx as an aid to intubation; his book in 1911 described many of the techniques used today.[37]

However, all was not clear sailing in attempts to find a safe anesthetic method for opening the pleural cavity. Sometimes advances are held back by researchers who are equally convinced that another method is much better—and so it was in this instance. The German surgeon von Mikulicz had realized the importance of differential pressures in ventilation and assigned his pupil Sauerbruch, soon to be even more famous than the teacher, to this problem. Their reasoning was simple: the lungs could not deflate, even after the thoracic cavity had been opened, if they were within a negative pressure chamber. Let the patient's head be outside the chamber, but keep the chamber containing the thorax at subatmospheric pressure.[38] Working first with animals (Fig. 1-5), Sauerbruch developed first a cuirass-type chamber, next a larger box to accommodate the entire body except the head (Fig. 1-6), and finally, for human surgery, a large pressure chamber sufficient to accommodate patient, surgeon, and assistants (Fig. 1-7).[39,40] An antechamber was at-

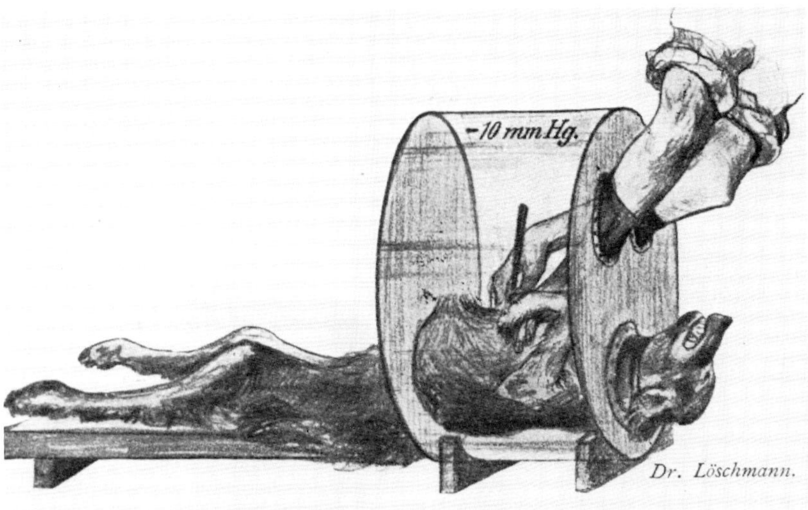

Fig. 1-5. Cuirass type of negative-pressure chamber developed by Sauerbruch of Breslau, Germany (1904).

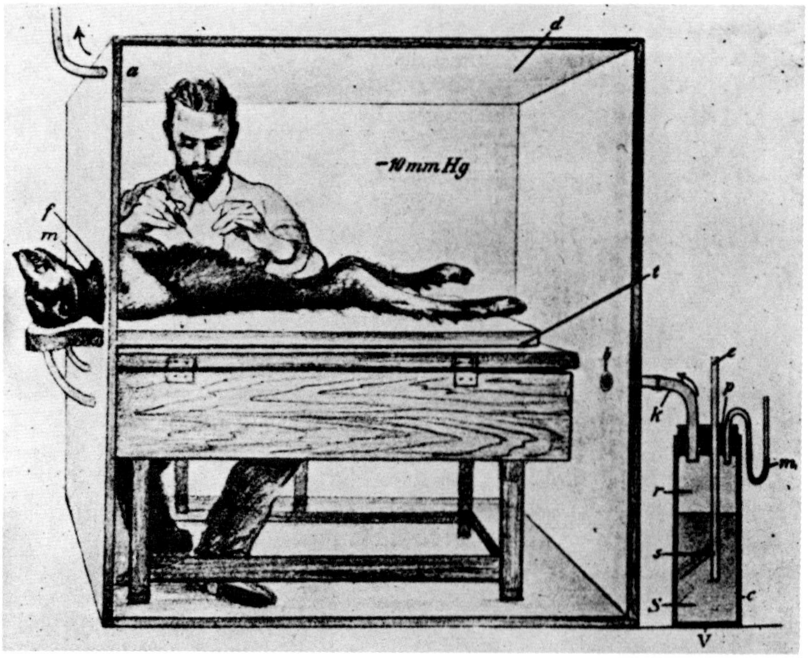

Fig. 1-6. A larger negative pressure chamber, the "pneumatic chamber," developed by Sauerbruch to contain both the surgeon and the body of the experimental animal (1904).

tached so that people could enter and leave without altering the negative pressure. Sauerbruch, because of his fame and importance, excited interest in and loyalty to his ideas throughout Europe and among the Americans who visited or studied with him.

Sauerbruch's chamber found quick use throughout Europe, in Berlin, Cologne, Vienna, St. Petersburg, and elsewhere, but it reached its ultimate development in New York. Meyer was convinced of the superiority of this method of anesthesia over positive-pressure endotracheal anesthesia and built several chambers, first for experimental use at the Rockefeller Institute and finally at the Lenox Hill Hospital (previously the German Hospital). The last of these devices, the Universal Negative Pressure Chamber (Fig. 1-8), could accommodate 15 people! In Boston Robinson (1910) was firmly opposed to endotracheal intubation: " . . . reminded by the throat specialist of the difficulty in introducing and maintaining instrumentation within the deep trachea, I look with grave doubts on the application of this method to the human."[41] Accordingly, he developed a positive-pressure chamber, sealed around the patient's head to maintain lung expansion. The many problems of the negative-pressure and the positive-pressure chambers, related devices, and experiences with intrathoracic wounds in World War I quickly resulted in the disappearance of these chambers.

These excursions from the orderly development of endotracheal intubation and positive-pressure ventilation were unfortunate and retarded the progress of thoracic surgery.

COMPLICATIONS OF SURGERY TO HILAR STRUCTURES

For many years the hilar structures were a technical problem, with hemorrhage and bronchopleural fistula being common complications. Initially a mass ligature was used around the entire hilum, allowing the distal lung tissue to become necrotic and slough away. Dissection with individual clamping and ligation of the hilar structures was not considered feasible by the surgeons despite the use (and success) of this technique in the laboratory. The experimental results with pulmonary resection surpassed clinical results for many years.

Lobectomies and pneumonectomies, generally using the cautery, did continue with a modicum of success. In 1929 Brunn established a technique for one-stage lobectomy, which reduced the mortality rate to more acceptable levels.[42] Only a few

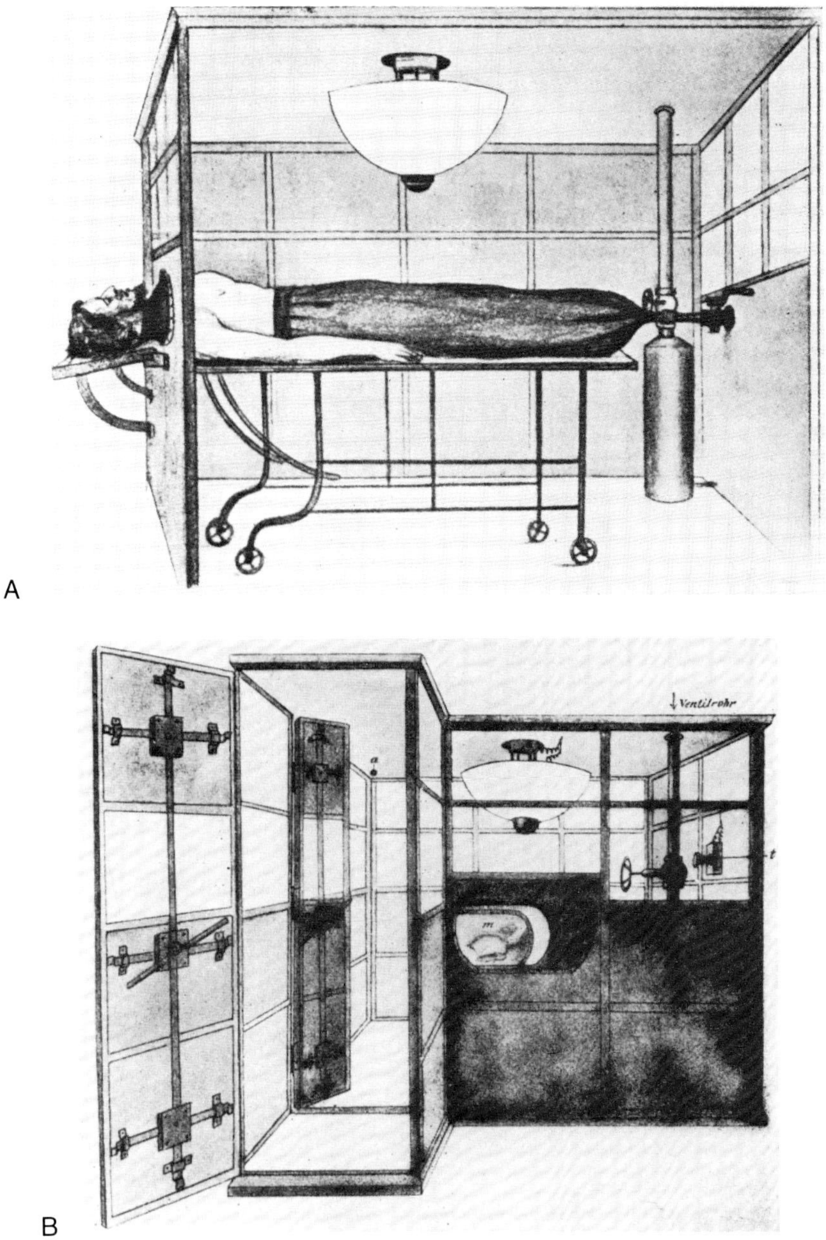

Fig. 1-7. Two different negative-pressure chambers used at University Hospital in Breslau. **(A)** Position of patient in chamber. **(B)** Antechamber used to enter and leave during the operation.

resections were attempted for carcinoma (Fig. 1-9). In 1922 in Germany, Hinz did a pneumonectomy for carcinoma, but the patient died on the third postoperative day.[44] Several years later (1930) Churchill operated on a patient with a carcinoma and planned to do a pneumonectomy by the usual mass ligation technique.[45] However, because the tumor was so close to the hilum, it was necessary to dissect the vessels individually. The vessels were satisfactorily managed, but, recalling Sauerbruch's warning about the dangers of mediastinal emphysema, Churchill did not close the bronchus but drained it by an intrapleural tube. This patient died of bronchopneumonia on the third postoperative day. Finally, two successful cases of pneumonectomy, although for benign disease, were reported by Nissen (1931)[46] and Haight (1934).[47]

The development of an anatomic dissection of hilar structures was slow. The first description of

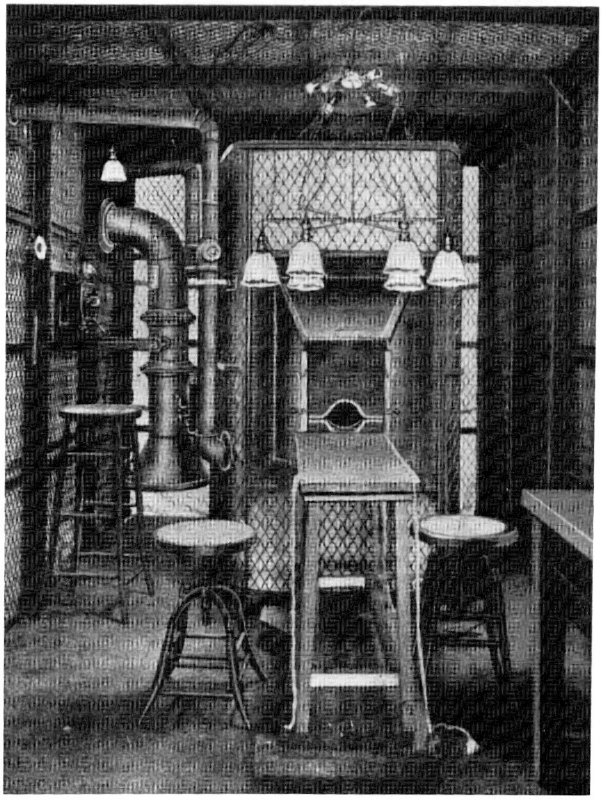

Fig. 1-8. Inside view of Meyer's negative- and positive-pressure chamber. This shows the anesthetist's room kept at positive pressure. The European chambers were made for either positive or negative pressure, but not both. The chambers used by Willy Meyer in his experiments and clinical operations were constructed by his brother John, an engineer. This device was used at the Rockefeller Institute, the Jefferson Medical College (for a demonstration before the American Surgical Association), and finally the German Hospital in New York (now the Lenox Hill Hospital).

deliberate dissection of the hilar structures was in 1912 by the English surgeon Davies, who resected a right lower lobe for carcinoma using essentially the same technique as today.[48] Unfortunately the patient died one week postoperatively. Speed seemed paramount in operations, and accordingly in 1932 Shenstone and Janes developed a special snare to control the hilar vessels and provide hemostasis during lobectomy.[49] In the same year Churchill described individual dissection and ligation in a patient undergoing lobectomy for carcinoma.[45] In 1935 Young detailed his procedure for individual isolation of the vessels and separate management of the bronchus for upper lobectomy. No further specific mention was made of individual-vessel dissection and ligation until the article in 1940 by Kent and Blades for the procedure of lower lobectomy.[50]

Various attempts were also made to obliterate the pleural space to prevent pneumothorax during dissection. These generally involved the introduction of an irritating substance such as talc (Alexander), an extrapleural plombage (Sauerbruch), or abrasion with a gauze (Churchill).[45] Only after the pleural space had been obliterated could it be entered. Thoracic operations were complicated. The mortality rate of lobectomy for bronchiectasis approximated 50 percent in the 1930s.

SUCCESSFUL PNEUMONECTOMY FOR CARCINOMA

Then at the 1933 meeting of the American Association for Thoracic Surgery, Graham (Fig. 1-10) presented an account of the first successful pneumonectomy for cancer of the lung.[51] The patient was a 48-year-old physician, and Graham intended to do a lobectomy. At operation (April 15, 1933) the tumor (Fig. 1-11) was found near the hilum and a pneumonectomy was required. Hilar structures were secured by mass ligation, and the lung was removed with cautery. The bronchus was closed with catgut after cauterization of the bronchial mucosa; the pulmonary artery was ligated with catgut. Radon seeds were implanted. Endotracheal anesthesia was used.

Fearing infection in the pleural cavity, Graham elected to do a thoracoplasty removing the third through the ninth ribs. Subsequently the patient underwent resection of the first and second ribs and several drainage procedures for postoperative empyema. The pathology report showed squamous cell carcinoma with metastases to the regional nodes.

The patient survived for 30 years after his operation, continued to smoke, and, like MacEwen's patient, outlived his surgeon—who also continued to smoke and died of inoperable lung cancer.

The enthusiasm of Graham and his success with this patient were a great stimulus. As stated so eloquently by Brock[52]:

> Those of us who were struggling with the surgery of bronchial carcinoma in the early 1930's remember only too well the apparent hopelessness of the problem facing the surgeon. Then, like a great light, shone out the report of Graham's success in removing the whole lung in a case of cancer. The news of this travelled rapidly throughout the world. . . . It was not only one case; it was the leaven that stimulated and invigorated the whole field of lung surgery.

TABLE 119.—RADICAL OPERATIONS FOR CARCINOMA OF THE LUNG. (CASES COLLECTED BY CARLSON AND BALLON.[1,2])

Surgeon.	Publication.	Operation.	Results.	Cause of death.
1. Sauerbruch	Chir. der Brustorgane, vol. **1**, p. 849, 1920	Resection of lung	Died in 5 days	Pneumonia.
2. Sauerbruch	Chir. der Brustorgane, vol. **1**, p. 849, 1920	Lobectomy, left lower	Alive 5 yrs.	
3. Sauerbruch	Chir. der Brustorgane, vol. **1**, p. 849, 1920	Excision of tumor	Died in 5 days	Pneumonia.
4. Sauerbruch	Chir. der Brustorgane, vol. **1**, p. 849, 1920	Resection of lung and diaphragm	Lived 3 yrs., not followed further.	
5. Sauerbruch	Zentralbl. f. Chir., vol. **53**, p. 852, 1926	Lobectomy?	Successful (follow up?).	
6. Heidenhain	Quoted by Sauerbruch	Resection, bronchiectasis (carcinoma present)	Died in 2 mos.	Other causes.
7. Kümmel	Quoted by Sauerbruch and Payr	Pneumectomy	Died in 7 days	?
8. Rotter	Quoted by Sauerbruch	Resection	Died in 3 mos.	Pneumonia.
9. Payr	Arch. f. klin. Chir., vol. **133**, p. 700, 1924	Resection of lung and chest wall	Died in 5 mos.	Recurrence?
10. Brunn	Arch. Surg., vol. **12**, p. 406, 1926	Cautery pneumectomy	Seen 5 mos. after operation.	
11. Brunn	Arch. Surg., vol. **12**, p. 406, 1926	Cautery pneumectomy	Died	Pneumothorax.
12. Sato	Deutsch. Ztschr. f. Chir., vol. **207**, p. 424, 1928	Lobectomy	Recurrence in 50 days; reoperation	Died in shock after second operation.
13. Hinz	Quoted by Sato and Divis:	Left pneumectomy	Died on third day	(?) Died suddenly.
14. Walzel	Der Chirurgie, vol. **1**, p. 113, 1928	Resection of lobe and separation from aorta	No evidence of recurrence in : ½ mos.	
15. Lilienthal	Surg. Clin. North America, vol. **9**, p. 551, 1929	Lobectomy	Died on ninth day	Bronchopneumonia; collapse of right middle lobe.
16. Mirizzi	Semana med., vol. **36**, p. :69, 19_9	Lobectomy	Died on sixth day	Fibrinopurulent pleurisy and fibrinopurulent pericarditis.
17. Sussi	Gazz. internaz. med. chir., vol. **39**, p. 221, 1931	Resection close to hilus	Died on third day	Pneumonia, both lower lobes.
18. Harrington	Surg., Gynec. and Obst., vol. **52**, p. 417, 1931	Partial lobectomy	Lived less than 1 yr.	Recurrence.
19. Harrington	Surg., Gynec. and Obst., vol. **52**, p. 417, 1931	Partial lobectomy	Lived less than 1 yr.	Recurrence.
20. Harrington	Surg., Gynec. and Obst., vol. **52**, p. 417, 1931	Partial lobectomy?	Died on seventh day	Cerebral embolism.
21. Archibald	Ballon *et al.*: Jour. Thoracic Surg., vol. **1**, p. 525, 1932	Lobectomy	Died on fourth day	Septicemia.
22. Eloesser	Jour. Thoracic Surg., vol. **1**, vol. 485, 1932	Lobectomy	Died in 11 days	Hemorrhage.
23. Churchill	15th Annual Meet., Am. Assn. Thoracic Surg., Ann Arbor, Mich., 1932	Lobectomy*	Died on third day	Bronchopneumonia.
24. Churchill	15th Annual Meet., Am. Assn. Thoracic Surg., Ann Arbor, Mich., 1932	Lobectomy	Recovery (4 mos.).	
25. Edwards	Brit. Med. Jour., vol. i, p. 827, 1932	Resection of lung	Free of symptoms 2 yrs.	
26. Edwards	Brit. Med. Jour., vol. i, p. 827, 1932	Lobectomy (right middle)	Free of symptoms 13 mos.	
27. Nissen	Arch. f. klin. Chir., vol. **170**, p. 118, 1932	Extrapleural type of lobectomy	Operation successful.	
28. Allen and Smith	Surg., Gynec. and Obst., vol. **55**, p. 151, 1932	Lobectomy	Alive after 2 yrs.	
29. Graham	Unpublished data	Cautery pneumectomy, roentgenray and radium implants	J. B., No. 32527; died in 3 mos.	Carcinoma of lung, with metastases.
30. Graham	Unpublished data	Cautery pneumectomy, roentgenray and radium pack	C. T., No. 19396; died in 24 days	Carcinoma of lung, with metastases.
31. Graham	Unpublished data	Cautery pneumectomy, roentgenray	J. M., No. 10143; died first day	Carcinoma of lung, with metastases (cerebral embolus).
32. Graham	Unpublished data	Cautery pneumectomy and roentgen-ray	A. M., No. 20183; died in 11 mos.	? (No necropsy.)
33. Graham	Unpublished data	Cautery pneumectomy	C. S., No. 17222; died in 37 days	? (No necropsy.)
34. Graham	Unpublished data	Cautery pneumectomy	J. W., No. 5536; died in 25 days	? (No necropsy.)
35. Graham	Unpublished data	Cautery pneumectomy and roentgen-ray	A. K., No. 957; died in 60+ days	? (No necropsy.)

[1] Carcinoma of the Lung, Jour. Thoracic Surg., vol. **2**, p. 323, 1933.
[2] For additional cases see references by Graham, E. A., and Singer, J. J.: Jour. Am. Med. Assn., vol. **101**, p. 1371, 1933; Haight, C.: Surg., Gynec. and Obst., vol. **58**, p. 768, 1934.

(834)

Fig. 1-9. Table listing previous cases of operations for carcinoma of the lung. Note the cautery pneumonectomies done by Graham prior to his successful procedure. (From Graham et al.,[43] with permission.)

Five more pneumonectomies were done in 1933, four for cancer and one for benign disease. The Canadian surgeon Archibald did a successful left pneumonectomy in a patient with a sarcoma on July 7, 1933, a few months after Graham and several weeks before another successful pneumonectomy by Rienhoff on July 24. This was in a young girl with a benign tumor of the left bronchus. Several weeks later he operated on an adult with a carcinoma.

In both patients Rienhoff used preoperative pneumothorax 2 weeks preoperatively to accustom the patients to breathing with only one lung. He entered the pleural cavity through an anterior third interspace incision, performed individual dissection and ligation/suture of the hilar struc-

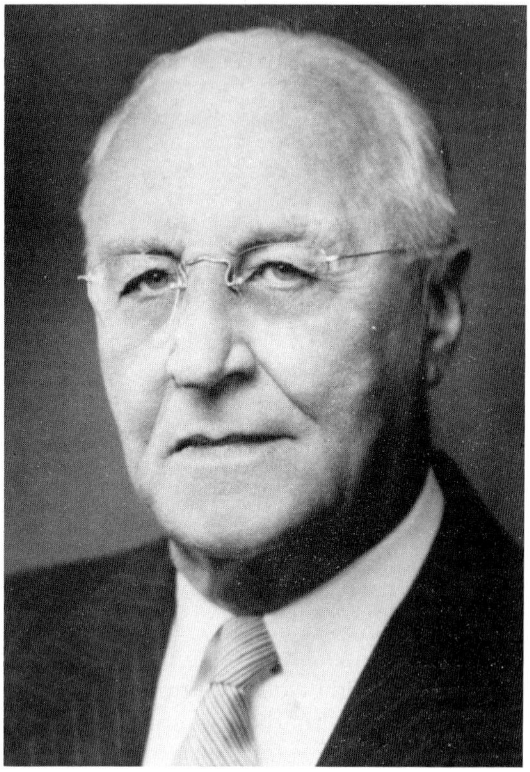

Fig. 1-10. Ewarts A. Graham (1883–1957), who did the first successful pneumonectomy for carcinoma of the lung in 1933. Although he was an early author with Wynder (1951) proving the link between smoking and carcinoma of the lung, he continued throughout life to smoke and died of inoperable lung cancer.

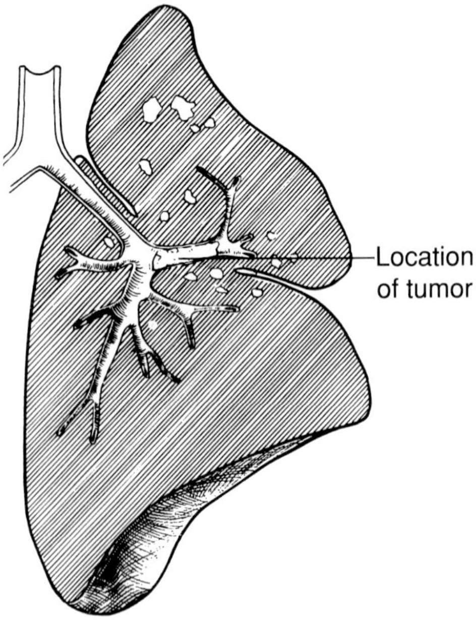

Fig. 1-11. Sketch of the left lung removed by Graham in 1933. Note the location of the tumor near the bifurcation of the bronchus and the numerous small abscesses throughout the lung, particularly the upper lobe.

tures, and did not drain the pleural space postoperatively. As regards management of the chest after pneumonectomy, Rienhoff wrote[53]:

> It is not necessary to perform a thoracoplasty at the same time as a pneumonectomy, because the remaining lung will, in uninfected clean cases, obliterate the ensuing dead space. To prevent infection, mass ligatures and cauterization of the bronchus should be abandoned. Individual ligation of the vessels and the minimal amount of injury to the bronchus in suturing permits primary healing of the bronchial mucous membrane.

He did cover the bronchial stump with mediastinal pleura.

Later in 1933 Freedlander did a left pneumonectomy for cancer, although the patient died after a thoracoplasty done 3 weeks following the initial procedure.[45] Lastly, in that same year, Alexander reported a left pneumonectomy for carcinoma.[45] All these initial pneumonectomies were on the left; the first successful right pneumonectomy was done by Overholt in 1934.[45]

The improved techniques used by Rienhoff and Archibald, in contrast to those used in the first three pneumonectomies (those by Nissen, Haight, and Graham), are essentially those used today and properly distinguish these two surgeons as the fathers of modern pneumonectomy.

An important monograph, *On the Technique of Pneumonectomy in Man*, was written by the Swedish surgeon Crafoord in 1938 on the basis of his experiences with 16 patients.[54] He recommended individual dissection and ligation of the hilar vessels, closure of the bronchial stump by invagination, covering of the bronchial stump with pleura, and the use of a fifth-rib subperiosteal incision. Perhaps his most important suggestion, for which he credits his chief, Giertz, was the use of a mechanical positive-pressure ventilator, a spiropulsator, for endotracheal anesthesia. He packed the mainstem bronchus on the side to be resected with a gauze sponge to prevent its ventilation during operation. Removal of the hilar lymph nodes was stressed in patients with malignancy.

A dictum of pneumonectomy for carcinoma soon developed. In 1933 Graham and Singer wrote[51]:

> Just as experience with carcinoma in other parts of the body has taught that the number of cures is,

> in general, directly proportional to the extent of radical removal, so it may be inferred, perhaps, that if the entire lung is removed the patient will have less chance of a recurrence than if only one lobe or a smaller portion is removed.

This concept was reinforced by others. In 1939 Ochsner and DeBakey declared, "Treatment of pulmonary malignancy consists of total extirpation of the involved lung and removal of mediastinal lymph nodes. Lobectomy and mass ligation of the hilar structures are condemned. . . "[55] Rienhoff was equally emphatic: "Surgical measures short of total pneumonectomy are not efficacious."[56]

LUNG CONSERVATION

It was soon noted, however, that pneumonectomy resulted in an appreciable mortality and morbidity rate from cardiac failure and pulmonary insufficiency. Enthusiasm for removal of the entire lung gradually waned, and lobectomy was shown to be as effective as pneumonectomy in many instances. The concept of "lung conservation" evolved, and lobectomy has been followed by segmentectomy and even wedge resection in appropriate patients with carcinoma of the lung. Segmentectomy was initiated and fortified in 1939 by Churchill and Belsey, who applied segmental resection to various problems and wrote, "It is suggested that the bronchopulmonary segment may replace the lobe as the surgical unit of the lung."[57]

In recent years the technical aspects of pulmonary resection have been further refined by stapling devices, originally developed by the Russians, for the bronchus and lung. The flexible fiberoptic bronchoscope has helped greatly in earlier detection of lung cancer and postoperative care. Staging methods have enabled a much better description of the operative pathology. The laser finds application in the palliation of endobronchial obstruction. Photodynamic therapy deserves further exploration. Lastly, multimodality cooperative techniques have offered better survival rates than previously and suggest exciting new vistas for the future.

ESOPHAGEAL RESECTION

More than 2,000 years ago the dysphagia of esophageal carcinoma was described by the Chinese. Scattered accounts of esophageal tumors appeared throughout the centuries: Galen in the second century referred to fleshy growths causing obstruction to the gullet: Avicenna in the tenth century mentioned tumors as a cause of dysphagia. The earliest surgical procedures on the esophagus were done to remove foreign bodies and abscesses; later attempts were made to dilate the esophagus for stricture. These efforts led to familiarity with esophagotomy, primarily in the cervical region.

Carcinoma of the esophagus has been treated surgically only in recent times (Table 1-1). Its late diagnosis, the technical problems of pneumothorax and anastomotic leaks, and the pessimism associated with esophageal resection were best expressed by Turner (1936) when he quoted John Ruskin: "There is a time and a way when things, all things, can be done; none shorter, none smoother. For all noble things, the time is long and the way is rude.[58]

On the basis of clinical and pathologic observations of cervical carcinoma, Billroth (1871) did experiments on dogs, removing segments of their cervical esophagus.[59] As a result he believed that the procedure could be done in humans. Cancer of the cervical esophagus did not spread to the lymphatics and could therefore be resected and cured. His plan was to excise the cervical esophagus, dilate the lower esophagus, and, at some time in the future, mobilize the remaining esophagus into the neck, expecting healing to be similar to that for external urethrotomy. Several animal experiments had proved the feasibility of this hypothesis.

EARLY EFFORTS

The first esophageal resection was performed by Czerny, a former assistant of Billroth, in 1877.[60] As he wrote, "In a case of annular carcinoma of the esophagus which caused a stricture that would not admit an esophageal sound, I resected a piece 6 cm. of the entire wall of the esophagus. The lower end of the esophagus was sewn into the neck." The patient, a 51-year-old woman, survived for more than a year before dying of tumor recurrence.

By 1885 there had been nine reported resections for esophageal cancer, chiefly by German surgeons. At least five of these patients died in the immediate postoperative period, but several survived for a year and some were able to swallow. In 1886 von Mikulicz described resection of the cervical esophagus with esophageal reconstruction by a skin tube in the neck, enabling the patient to swallow. The patient died of tumor recurrence 11 months later. In 1894 the Swiss surgeon Bircher suggested that a skin tube from the neck and tho-

Table 1-1. Historical Developments in Esophageal Carcinoma

Year	Surgeon	Development
1871	Billroth	Experiments in dogs with resection of cervical esophagus.
1877	Czerny	Resected cervical esophagus for carcinoma, leaving cervical esophagostomy. Patient lived for 15 months.
1886	von Mikulicz	Successful resection of cervical esophageal carcinoma; patient lived for 15 months. Fed through distal esophageal opening.
1895	Biondi	Esophagogastrostomy in dogs transpleurally.
1901	Dobromysslow	Successful intrathoracic resection and esophageal anastomosis in dogs.
1904	Wullstein	Used jejunum for antethoracic esophageal reconstruction.
1905	Beck	Described gastric tube from greater curvature.
1907	Sauerbruch	Extensive animal experiments with use of button for anastomosis.
1907	Bircher	Two patients operated on with antethoracic skin tube for reconstruction.
1907	Roux	First successful use of jejunum for antethoracic esophagus.
1908	Voelcker	First successful resection of cardia and esophagus for carcinoma with transabdominal esophagogastrostomy.
1911	Kelling	Used transverse colon for antethoracic esophagus.
1911	Vulliet	Same method as Kelling in cadavers.
1912	Jianu	Independently developed same method as Beck.
1912	Ropke	Successful use of Beck-Jianu tube in humans.
1913	Zaaijer	Successful resection of carcinoma of cardia through combined abdominothoracic approach.
1913	Torek	First successful transthoracic excision of esophageal carcinoma. Patient lived 13 years postoperatively.
1913	Denk	"Blunt" esophagectomy described.
1920	Kirschner	Suggested intrathoracic esophagogastrostomy rather than colon or other interpositions.
1922	Hedblom	Successful abdominothoracic resection of carcinoma of cardia.
1923	Roith	Antethoracic reconstruction of esophagus by using right colon.
1933	Ohsawa	Reported eleven successful resections of carcinoma of esophagus and/or cardia.
1937	Marshall	First successful instance of intrathoracic esophagogastrostomy for cancer.
1938	Adams	First transthoracic esophagogastrotomy for esophageal carcinoma.

rax be fashioned and subsequently joined to the stomach.[61] He attempted the procedure without success, but Payr's reconstruction by this method in 1917 did succeed.[62]

Various types of esophagoplasty were tried to enable the patient to swallow and avoid the use of external feeding through the gastrostomy or esophagostomy. Wullstein recommended use of the jejunum (1904), Lexer (1908) combined skin and jejunum, and Herzen (1908) successfully finished a "staged Roux operation" 3 years before its description by Roux (1908).[63–66] Most of these were done more frequently for stricture (Fig. 1-12) since carcinoma resection was still infrequent.

Use of the greater curvature of the stomach to make a tube was described by Beck and Carrel (1905),[67] although Beck did not use this clinically. It was subsequently used by Jianu (1914)[68] as well as others, and has recently been revived by Gavalu. This tube has been placed subcutaneously, beneath the pectoral muscles, and intrapleurally.

The use of colon as a replacement of the esopha-

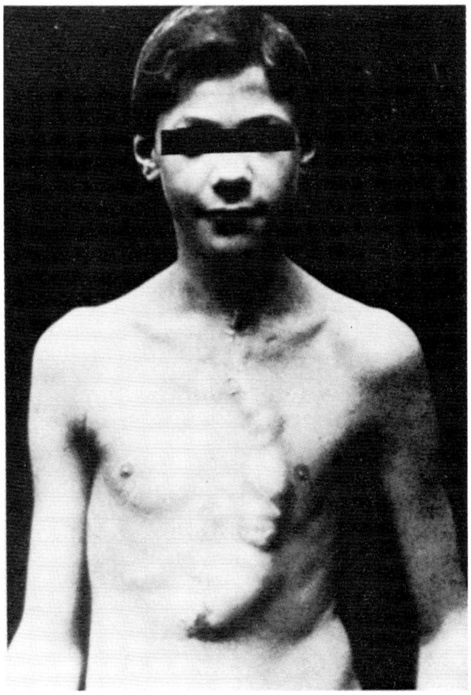

Fig. 1-12. Photograph of an 11-year-old boy with lye stricture and reconstruction by Roux-en-Y loop[66] (Roux, 1907).

gus was mentioned by Kelling in 1911; he attempted without success to place the transverse colon subcutaneously for a cancer of the mid-esophagus.[69] His suggestion was to use a peristaltic portion of colon and to do the operation in two stages. In the same year Vulliet recommended the use of the left colon in an antiperistaltic manner.

In 1895 an Italian surgeon, Biondi, first suggested that the stomach be pulled upward into the chest and anastomosed to the esophagus after resection: " . . . there are cases of cancer of the lower part of the esophagus in which esophago-gastrotomy might be tried."[70] Although he deserves credit for this suggestion, his article fails to describe any clinical experiences. An unsuccessful attempt was made by von Mikulicz in 1896 to resect the thoracic esophagus, suturing the diaphragmatic pleura to the parietal pleura to avoid pneumothorax.[45] Further anecdotal reports can be found during this period without any appreciable successes or substantial advances. Of interest is the description by Dobromysslow in 1901 of the first successful intrathoracic resection and anastomosis.[71] After raising a large skin flap based posteriorly from the sixth to the tenth ribs, he resected 3 to 4 cm of esophagus, reanastomosed the ends, and sutured the skin flap around the anastomosis. No details of long-term follow-up were given.

Approaching the esophagus through the posterior mediastinum to avoid a pneumothorax was recommended by Demoulin (1888)[72] and Bryant (1895),[45] although it was not used clinically. Subsequently considerable debate ensued over the better approach to the thoracic esophagus—the right or the left side. Transdiaphragmatic esophagogastrostomy was proposed in 1903 by Gosset, although he did not do the operation.[73] Further experimentation occurred with development of Sauerbruch's negative-pressure chamber. Sauerbruch found that use of the Murphy button gave the best results in dogs for anastomosing the esophagus to the stomach without any clinical successes.

"Blind" or "blunt" esophagectomy was first described in 1913 by Denk, who mobilized the esophagus with either his finger or a stripper similar to the Mayo vein stripper.[74] By this method he avoided entering the pleural cavity. He advised restoration of esophageal continuity by a skin tube at a later date.

By 1900 the Germans were preeminent in surgery, particularly regarding the esophagus. The *Handbuch der Praktischen Chirurgie* (1899) expressed their pessimism about operating on esophageal cancer[45]:

> . . . surgeons are not justified at present in undertaking resection of the thoracic portion of the esophagus when it is the site of a carcinoma—the more so because they cannot perform an adequately radical operation since the diagnosis is seldom or never made early enough for it to do any good.

This attitude persisted for many years.

TOREK'S LANDMARK ESOPHAGECTOMY

Then, in 1913, the greatest impetus to esophageal cancer surgery came with a report by Torek.[75] He operated on a 67-year-old woman who had an extensive carcinoma of the mid-esophagus. The procedure entailed entering the chest through a seventh intercostal space incision, with transection posteriorly of the seventh through fourth ribs. The aorta was mobilized after division of several of the intercostal branches to free the esophagus at this level. Torek attempted to preserve the vagus nerves since it was believed that division of the vagi in the upper thorax would cause instant death by cardiac collapse. The esophagus was adherent to the left mainstem bronchus, which was cut longitudinally during dissection and then repaired. After its mobilization the esophagus was divided distally slightly above the diaphragm and invaginated. Proximally the esophagus was brought through a cervical incision at the anterior border of the sternocleidomastoid muscle. The esophagus was transected above the tumor, tunneled under the skin to the second intercostal space anteriorly, and sutured to the skin (esophagostomy).

The operation lasted 1 hour and 45 minutes. It was done by using endotracheal anesthesia and the Meltzer-Auer apparatus, unusual at this time, and was administered by the soon to be famous thoracic surgeon, Eggers. The squamous cell carcinoma had not grown through the wall at any point; the resected specimen did not contain any lymph nodes.

The patient had a gastrostomy preoperatively, and on the eighth postoperative day the esophagostomy and gastrostomy were connected by a rubber tube (Fig. 1-13). He lived in good health for 13 years. As Torek stated: "I succeeded in demonstrating the feasibility of resection of the middle portion of the oesophagus for carcinoma."[75] Despite the success of the "rubber esophagus," Torek believed that a tube of the greater curvature of the stomach placed subcutaneously would be the best method of esophagoplasty.

From 1913 into the 1930s many transthoracic esophageal resections were attempted, generally with high mortality rates due to anesthetic problems and leaking anastomoses.[76,77] The first successful resection of a carcinoma of the cardia was by Zaaijer (1913) by a staged procedure.[78] Some surgeons (Hedblom and Zaaijer) advocated a preliminary thoracoplasty to prevent the extent of the frequent empyema.[79]

Numerous other attempts with various modifications occurred in the next several decades (Fig. 1-14). There were discussions about right thoracotomy versus the left-sided approach and the best method of restoring continuity, either externally, subcutaneously, or internally, and with what structure. Fischer[80] and Starr[81] both described

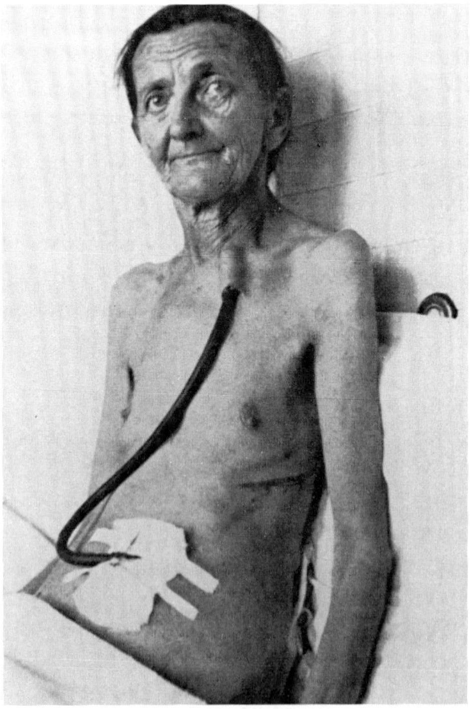

Fig. 1-13. Sixty-seven-year-old patient operated on by Torek in 1913 for carcinoma of thoracic esophagus. Until that time surgeons believed that transection of both vagi would be fatal. The external rubber tube worked so well that no esophageal reconstruction was attempted. The patient survived in good health for 13 years.

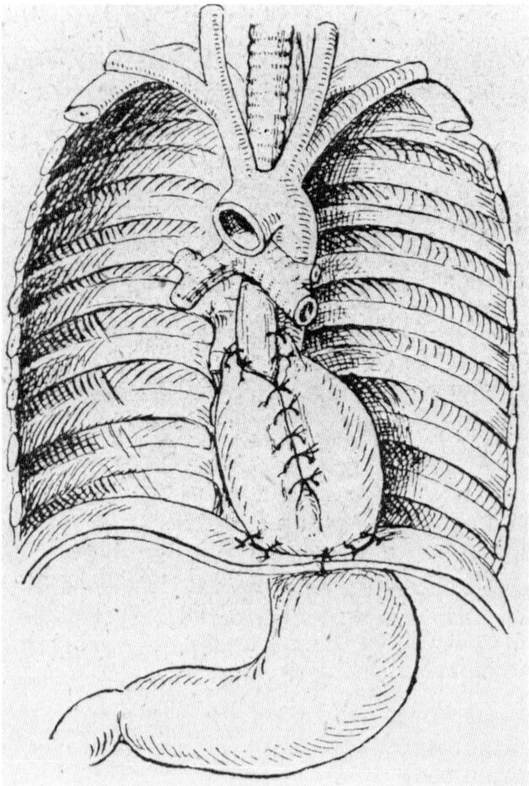

Fig. 1-14. Technique described by Kirschner in 1920 based on experimental studies in dogs for resection of the lower esophagus and cardia. Although he had no clinical successes, this is essentially the procedure done today. He thought this preferable to the use of a colon or jejunal interposition.

mobilization of the stomach and thoracic esophagogastrectomy as a desirable technique without clinical successes. In 1933 Turner[58] reaffirmed interest in the "blunt" esophagectomy as proposed originally by Denk,[74] restoring continuity at a later time by an antethoracic skin tube as described by Rovsing (1926).[82] His patient survived for many months.

An article by the Japanese surgeon Ohsawa in 1933 received scant attention from the world for many years.[83] He reported 25 operations for cancer of the cardia and esophagus, with 11 cures (Table 1-2). Ohsawa advocated "free thoracotomy" and believed that " . . . an apparatus for differential pressure is not only unnecessary, but actually a hindrance."[83]

MARSHALL'S ESOPHAGOGASTRECTOMY

Credit must be given to Marshall (1937) for the first esophagogastrectomy performed in the United States.[84] The proximal stomach and lower esophagus were resected, and the distal stomach was mobilized into the chest. "The stump of the esophagus was then transplanted into the anterior wall of the stomach through an incision placed several cm. below the point of division of the stomach. The anastomosis was completed by an inner mucosal layer of interlocking catgut, reinforced by several stitches of silk."[84] The tumor was an adenocarcinoma with lymph node metastases. Although the patient had a wound disruption postoperatively, she survived for more than a year.

Table 1-2. List of 68 Transthoracic Operations and Diseases and Their Classifications Published by Ohsawa in 1933

Procedure or Disease	Number
Procedure	
Free thoracotomy	20
Free thoracolaparotomy or free laparothoracotomy	17
Free transdiaphragmatic thoracolaparotomy	19
Posterior mediastinal approach	7
Anterior mediastinal approach	2
Transdiaphragmatic thoracotomy	1
Transdiaphragmatic extrapleural approach	1
Extrapleural-abdominal approach	1
Total	68
Disease	
Carcinoma of the thoracic part and of the cardiac part of the esophagus	49
Carcinoma of the upper segment of the stomach	3
Myoma	1
Idiopatic dilatation	7
Foreign body	1
Spastic disease	1
Oesophagitis	2
Elongatio oesophagi	2
Sarcoma of the mediastinum	2
Total	68

(From Ohsawa,[83] with permission.)

Obviously there was an increasing interest in carcinoma of the cardia and esophagus. Further efforts and enthusiasm were kindled at the American Association of Thoracic Surgery meeting in April 1938, when Adams and Phemister reported their successful resection of the cardia and lower esophagus with esophagogastrostomy (Fig. 1-15) for a squamous cell carcinoma with lymph node metastasis.[85] They entered the pleural cavity by resecting the eighth rib and did not use endotracheal anesthesia, agreeing with the concept of Ohsawa and several others by stating that "most intrathoracic operations may be performed, and some with greater ease, under simple mask gas-oxygen inhalation anesthesia."[85] Their operation for esophageal carcinoma was done 6 months after the one for a carcinoma of the cardia described by Marshall. Despite the involved lymph node, this patient survived for more then 10 years postoperatively.

Many other surgeons soon reported their efforts in resecting the esophagus, with varying degrees of success. Gradually the problems of anastomotic leaks decreased; direct anastomosis of the stomach and the esophagus rather than an external connection was accepted; and more extensive esophageal resections were attempted by using skin, jejunum, or some part of the colon to restore continuity. Whether a right or left thoracotomy was the better approach to resection of the lower esophagus prompted discussions with Phemister (1942) and Churchill and Sweet (1942) advocating the left while Ochsner (1942) and Lewis (1946) recommended the right.[86–90]

Use of the Roux jejunal loop after resection of the upper esophagus was reported with successful results by Rienhoff (1946).[91] Previously Kelling (1911) had discussed use of the transverse colon in an antethoracic location in a 45-year-old patient with a carcinoma of the mid-esophagus[69] and Vulliet (1911), working with cadavers, had suggested the left colon.[91] Roith (1923) detailed the use of the right colon as an antethoracic esophagus.[92] How-

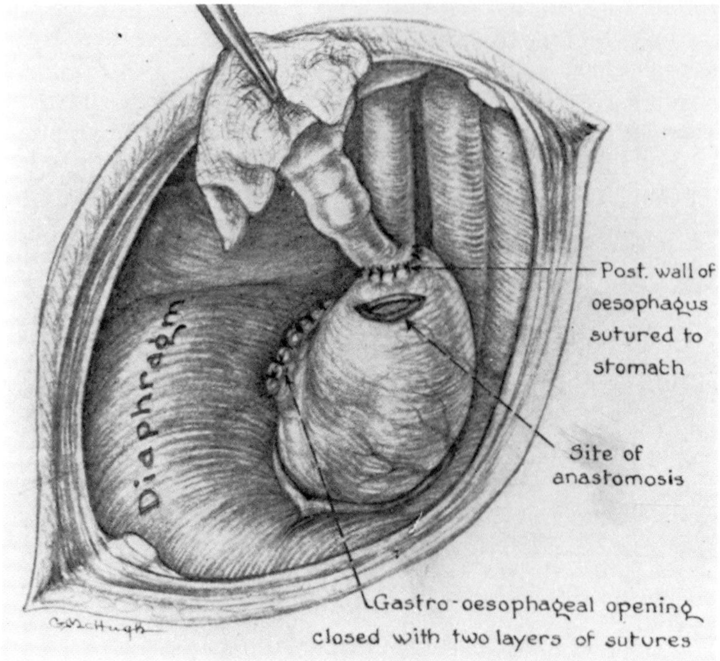

Fig. 1-15. Operative diagram of the first transthoracic esophageal resection for carcinoma in the United States by Adams and Phemister in 1938.[85]

ever, it was several decades before the use of the colon was accepted with any frequency.[93,94] In 1954 Sweet described his encouraging results and operative techniques in 303 resections among 450 patients with carcinoma of the esophagus.[95] In the same year Nakayama described the value of an abdominothoracic incision with transection of the costal arch anteriorly, an approach endorsed by Garlock and Klein.[96,97]

In recent years the attack on esophageal carcinoma has centered on technical refinements in reducing anastomotic leaks postoperatively—assisted by the mechanical stapling devices—and by many studies designed to evaluate the use of chemotherapy and/or radiation preoperatively.

REFERENCES

1. Rokitansky K: A Manual of Pathologic Anatomy. p. 258, Vol. 1. Sydenham Society, London, 1849
2. Haerting GH, Hesse W: Der Lungenkrebs, die Bergkrankheit in den Schneeberger Gruben. Vrtjschr Gerlichti Med 30:296 and 31:102, 1879
3. Bayle GH: Recherches sur la Phthisie Pulmonaire. p. 24, 34. Gabon, Paris, 1810
4. Adler I: Primary Malignant Growths of the Lungs and Bronchi. Longmans, New York, 1912
5. Ewing J: Neoplastic Diseases: A Treatise on Tumors. 3rd Ed. p. 851. WB Saunders, Philadelphia, 1928 (see also 4th Ed, 1940)
6. Rolandini: Surgery of the Chest. p. 85. John Wright, Bristol, 1896
7. Fabricus H: Observationem et curationem chirurgicarum centuria. apud M Merianum, Francofurti, 1627
8. Tulping N: Observationes medicae. apud L Elzevirium, Amstelredami, 1652
9. Bell R: Case report in Duncan's Medical Commentaries for December 11, 1786; cited in Hochberg LA: Thoracic Surgery before the 20th Century. p. 173. Vantage Press, New York, 1960
10. Murphy JB: Oration in surgery. JAMA 31:356, 1898
11. Antony M: Case of extensive caries of the fifth and sixth ribs, and disorganization of the greater part of the right lobe of lungs, with a description of the operation for the same. Philos J Med Phys Sci 6:108, 1823
12. Dieffenbach JF: Die Operative Chirurgie. F A Brockhaus, Leipzig, 1845–1848
13. Kroenlein: Ueber Lungenchirurgie. Berling Klin Wochenschr 21:129, 1884
14. Pean J: Chirurgie des poumons. Discussion. Assoc Ranc Chir Proc Verb (Paris) 9:72, 1895
15. Block MH: Experimentelles zur Lungenresection. Dtsch Med 7:634, 1881
16. Whittemore W: The treatment of such cases of chronic suppurative bronchiectasis as are limited to one lobe of the lung. Ann Surg 86:219, 1927

17. Schmid H: Experimentelle Studien ueber partielle Lungenresection Gegen draineren Comiter Drainage. Berlin Med Ges 51:757, 1881
18. Gluck T: Experimenteller beitrag zur frage der lungenextirpatien. Berlin Klin Wchnschr 18:645, 1881
19. Biondi D: Estirpazione polmone. Contribuzione sperimantale. Gior Int Sci Med (n s) 6:759, 1882
20. Biondi D: Estirpazione del polmone. Contribuzione sperimentale. Gior Int Sci Med (n s) 5:417, 1883
21. Tuffier T: De la resection du sommet du poumon. Semin Med 2:202, 1891
22. Quincke H: Zur operativen Behandlung der Lungenabscesse. Berlin Klin Wochenschr 24:337, 1887
23. Heidenhain H: Ausgedehnte Lungenresection wegen zahlreicher eiternder Bronchiectasien inneinen Unterlappen. Verh Dtsch Ges Chir 30:636, 1901. In Demoulin MA: Cancer de la portion thoracique de l'oesophage. Extirpation du neoplasme la voie mediastinale posterior droite, combine a une incision cervicale. Bull Mem Soc Paris 29:122, 1903
24. MacEwen W: The Cavendish lecture on some points in the surgery of the lung. Br Med J 2:1, 1906
25. Snow J: On chloroform and other anesthetics: their action and administration. John Churchill, London, 1858
26. Trendelenburg F: Beitraege zur den Operationen an den Luftwegen. Tamponnade der Trachea. Arch Klin Chir 12:121, 1871
27. MacEwen W: Clinical observations on the introduction of tracheal tubes by the mouth instead of performing tracheotomy or laryngotomy. Br Med J 2:122 and 163, 1880
28. Matas R: Intralaryngeal insufflation for the relief of acute surgical pneumothorax. Its history and methods with a description of the latest devices for this purpose. JAMA 34:1468, 1900
29. O'Dwyer J: Fifty cases of croup in private practice treated by intubation of the larynx, with a description of the method and of the dangers incident thereto. Med Rec 32:557, 1887
30. Tuffier and Hallion: Operations intrathoraciques avec respiration artificielle par insufflation. C R Soc Biol 48:951, 1896
31. Matas R: On the management of acute traumatic pneumothorax. Ann Surg 29:409, 1899
32. Parham FW: Thoracic resection for tumors growing from the bony wall of the chest. Tr South S A 11:223, 1898
33. Barthélemy and Dufour: L'anesthésie dans la chirurgie de la face. Presse Med 15:475, 1907
34. Meltzer SJ, Auer J: Continuous respiration without respiratory movements. J Exp Med 11:622, 1909
35. Peck CH: Intratracheal insufflation anaesthesia (Meltzer-Auer). Observations on a series of 216 anesthesias with the Elsberg apparatus. Ann Surg 56:192, 1912
36. Kirstein A: Autoskopie dies Larynx und der Trachea. Berlin Klin Wochenschr 32:476, 1895
37. Kuehn F: Die perorale Intubation; ein Leitfaden zur Erlernung und Ausfuehrung der Methode mit reicher Kasuistik. Karger, Berlin, 1911
38. von Mikulicz J: Ein Fall von Resection des Carcinomatosen Oesophagus mit Plastischen Ersatz des excirdirten Stuckes. Prag Med Wochenschr 11:03, 1886
39. Sauerbruch F: Zur Pathologie des offenen Pneumothorax und die Grundlagen meines Verfahrens zu seiner Ausschaltung. Mitt Grenz Med Chir 13:399, 1904
40. Sauerbruch F: Experimentelle Beitraege zur Oesophagus-Chirurgie. Verh Dtsch Ges Chir 34:140, 1905
41. Robinson S: The surgery of bronchiectasis. Including a report of five complete resections of the lower lobe of the lung with one death. Surg Gynecol Obstet 24:192, 1917
42. Brunn H: Surgical principles underlying one stage lobectomy. Arch Surg 18:490, 1929
43. Graham EA, Singer JJ, Ballon: Surgical Diseases of the Chest. p. 834. Lea & Febiger, Philadelphia, 1935
44. Hinz R: Totale Exstirpation der linken Lunge wegen Bronchialcarcinom. Arch Klin Chir 124:104, 1923
45. Meade R: A History of Thoracic Surgery. p. 94. Charles C Thomas, Springfield, 1961
46. Nissen R: Exstirpation eines gansen Lungenflugels. Zentralbl. Chir 47:3005, 1931
47. Haight C: Total removal of the left lung for bronchiectasis. Surg Gynecol Obstet 78:768, 1934
48. Davies HM: Recent advances in the surgery of the lung and pleura. Br J Surg 1:228, 1913
49. Shenstone NS, Janes RM: Experience in pulmonary lobectomy. Can Med Assoc J 27:138, 1932
50. Kent EM, Blades B: Surgical anatomy of pulmonary lobes. J Thorac Surg 12:18, 1942
51. Graham EA, Singer JJ: Successful removal of an entire lung for carcinoma of the bronchus. JAMA 101:1371, 1933
52. Brewer L III: The first pneumonectomy. Historical notes. J Thorac Cardiovasc Surg 88:810, 1984
53. Rienhoff WF Jr: Pneumonectomy. A preliminary report of the operative technique in two successful cases. Bull Johns Hopkins Hosp 53:390, 1933
54. Crafoord C: On the technique of pneumonectomy in man. Acta Chir Scand 81(suppl. 54):1, 1938
55. Ochsner A, DeBakey M: Primary pulmonary malignancy. Treatment by total pneumonectomy. Analysis of 79 collected cases and presentation of 7 personal cases. Surg Gynecol Obstet 68:435, 1939
56. Rienhoff WF Jr: The present status of the surgical

treatment of primary carcinoma of the lung. JAMA 126:1123, 1944
57. Churchill ED, Belsey R: Segmental pneumonectomy in bronchiectasis. The lingula segment of the left upper lobe. Ann Surg 109:481, 1939
58. Turner G: Excision of the thoracic oesophagus for carcinomas with construction of an extrathoracic gullet. Lancet ii:1315, 1933
59. Billroth T: Ueber die Resection des Oesophagus. Arch Klin Chir 13:65, 1871
60. Czerny: Neue Operationen. Zentralbl Chir 4:433, 1877
61. Bircher E: Ein Beitrag zur plastichen Bildung eines neuen Oesophagus. Zentralbl Chir 34:1479, 1907
62. Payr: Fall von antethorakalen Oesophagoplastik. Munch Med Wochenschr 64:783, 1917
63. Wullstein L: Ueber antethorakale Oesophagojejunostomie und operationen nach gliechem Prinzip. Dtsche Med Wochenschr 30:734, 1904
64. Lexer: Vollstaendiger Ersatz der Speiseroehre. Munch Med Wochenschr 58:1548, 1911
65. Herzen: Ein Modification der Roux'schen Oesophagojejunogastrotomie. Zentralbl Chir 35:210, 1908
66. Roux C: L'Esophago-jejuno-gastromie, nouvelle operation pour retrecissement Infranchisable de l'Oesophage. Semin Med 27:37, 1907
67. Beck C, Carrell A: Demonstration of specimens illustrating a method of formation of a prethoracic esophagus. Ill Med J 7:463, 1905 (See also Surg Gynecol Obstet 20:170, 1915)
68. Jianu A: Ueber Oesophagoplastic. Dtsch Chir 131:397, 1914
69. Kelling: Oesophagoplastik mit Hilfe des Quercolon. Zentralbl Chir 38:1212, 1911
70. Biondi D: Experimental intrathoracic esophagogastrostomy. Policlinico, suppl. 964, 1895
71. Dobromyssloff: Ein Fall von transpleuraler Oesophagectomie ein Brustabschnitte. Zentralbl Chir xx:1, 1901
72. Demoulin MA: Cancer de la portion thoracique de l'oesophage. Extirpation du neoplasme la voie mediastinale posterior droite, combine a une incision cervicale. Bull Mem Soc Chir Paris 29:122, 1903
73. Gosset A: De l'oesophago-gastrostomie transdiaphragmatique. Rev Chir 28:694, 1903
74. Denk W: Zur Radikaloperation des Oesphaguskarzinoms. Zentralbl Chir 40:1065, 1913
75. Torek F: The first successful case of resection of the thoracic portion of the oesophagus for carcinoma. Surg Gynecol Obstet 16:614, 1913 (See also Ann Surg 81:697, 1925)
76. Meyer W: Resection of the cardia for carcinoma. Ann Surg 62:693, 1915
77. Lilienthal H: Carcinoma of the thoracic oesophagus: successful resection. Ann Surg 74:116, 1921
78. Zaaijer JH: Erfolgreiche Transpleurale Resektion eines Cardiacarcinoms. Beitr Klin Chir 83:419, 1913
79. Hedblom C: Combined transpleural and transperitoneal resection of the thoracic esophagus and cardia for carcinoma. Surg Gynecol Obstet 35:284, 1922
80. Fischer H: Surgical treatment of the esophagus. Arch Surg 6:256, 1923
81. Starr FNG: Letter to H Fischer. Arch Surg 16:246, 1926
82. Rovsing T: The technique of my method of antethoracic oesophagoplasty. Surg Gynecol Obstet 43:781, 1926
83. Ohsawa T: The surgery of the oesophagus. Jpn Chir 10:604, 1933
84. Marshall SF: Carcinoma of the esophagus: successful resection of lower end of esophagus with reestablishment of esophageal gastric continuity. Surg Clin N Am 18:643, 1938
85. Adams WE, Phemister DB: Carcinoma of the lower thoracic esophagus. Report of a successful resection and esophagogastrostomy. J Thorac Surg 7:621, 1937–1938
86. Phemister DB: Discussion. Ann Surg 115:91, 1942
87. Churchill ED, Sweet RE: Transthoracic resection of tumors of the stomach and esophagus. Ann Surg 115:897, 1942
88. Ochsner A: Discussion. Ann Surg 115:91, 1942
89. Lewis I: The surgical treatment of carcinoma of the oesophagus with special reference to the new operation for growths in the middle third. Br J Surg 34:18, 1946
90. Rienhoff WF Jr: Intrathoracic esophagojejunostomy for lesions of the upper third of the esophagus. South Med J 39:928, 1946
91. Vulliet: De l'oesophagoplastie et de ses diverse modifications. Semin Med 31:529, 1911
92. Roith O: Die einzeitige antethorakale Oesophagaplastik aus dem Dickdarm. Dtsch Zentralbl Chir 183:419, 1923–1924
93. Orsoni P, Toupet A: Utilization du colon. Descendent et de la partie gauche du colon transverse pour l'oesophagoplastic prethoracique. Presse Med 58:804, 1950 (See also J Chir 67:491, 1951)
94. Goligher JC, Robin IG: Use of the left colon for reconstruction of pharynx and oesophagus after pharyngectomy. Br J Surg 42:283, 1954
95. Sweet RH: Late results of surgical treatment of carcinoma of the esophagus. JAMA 155:422, 1954
96. Nakayama K: Die Ergebnisse der chirurgischen Behandlung des Oesophaguscarcinoms. Chirurg 28:241, 1957
97. Garlock J, Klein SH: Surgical treatment of carcinoma of the esophagus and cardia. Analysis of 457 cases. Ann Surg 139:91, 1954

2

Surgical Pathology of the Chest

ANATOMY

THE LUNGS

The respiratory apparatus consists of the tracheobronchial tree, which subdivides into lobes, bronchopulmonary segments, subsegments, and ultimately the basic functional unit of the lung, the alveolus. The main airways are lined by a pseudostratified columnar ciliated epithelium. Present in this mucosa are mucus cells, neuroendocrine cells, basal cells, brush cells, migrating lymphocytes, and mast cells. Ciliated cells lining the tracheobronchial tree have 200 to 300 cilia per cell. The cilia beat 20 times per minute in a low-viscosity layer beneath the surface mucus. The cilia have a slight hook on the end, and they beat effectively with a straight-arm cephalic stroke with a curling return. The mucus layer is very critical for their satisfactory function. Injury of the cilia layer may be caused by drying, infection, and inhaled irritants. Distally, the mucous layer becomes discontinuous and the pseudostratified columnar epithelium, with its ciliated ends, terminates. The mucosa becomes cuboidal in the bronchioles. Clara cells are nonciliated and exist among the ciliated cells in the mainstem bronchus. They are most numerous in the terminal bronchioles.[1] Their function is unknown, but postulated roles include secretion of material that regulates bronchomotor tone.

There are approximately 300 million alveoli in the adult human lung. Each alveolus is polyhydral with one side open. When the alveoli distend on inspiration, they expand in such a fashion that they do not obstruct pulmonary capillary vessels in the walls of the alveoli. The diameter of the expanded alveolus is approximately 250 μm. The alveolus is lined mostly with type 1 pneumocytes. Also present in the alveolar lining are type II pneumocytes, which are smaller than the type I pneumocytes but double in number. Surfactant essential to lowering the surface tension for lung expansion is produced by the type II pneumocytes.

If the alveolar lining is damaged, the repair tends to consist of cuboidal lining cells. Between the alveoli there are numerous other cells and compounds of considerable importance, such as the macrophages and lymphocytes, which produce immunoglobulins and lymphokines. Some 5 million macrophages per hour migrate upward and are expectorated from the trachea.

THE VASCULAR SYSTEM

The major blood flow to the lungs is by the pulmonary arteries, which end in the pulmonary capillaries in the intra-alveolar septa. The oxygenated blood returns to the heart via the pulmonary venous system. There are also important collateral communications between the pulmonary arteries and pulmonary veins proximal to capillaries at the level of the bronchopulmonary segments. The pulmonary veins in the lung drain to the periphery of the bronchopulmonary segments, and they then run in the intersegmental planes to the hila of the segments, where they unite to form the superior and inferior pulmonary veins, which drain into the left atrium. The location of these intersegmental veins is an important landmark for identification of the boundaries of the bronchopulmonary segments.

Nerves accompany the bronchi and the blood vessels. There are branches from the phrenic and vagus nerves that produce autonomic nervous system control. The nerves are essential for the involuntary cough reflex. Along with the nerves, there are neuroepithelial chemoreceptors and stretch receptors that initiate the Hering-Breuer reflex. Juxtacapillary receptors in the alveoli are sensitive to changes in pulmonary venous pressure.

The lung, like the liver, has a dual blood supply. The right and left lungs may have one or two bronchial arteries, which are normally branches from the intercostal arteries. The bronchial systemic arteries accompany and are the major source of nutrition for the bronchi. Bronchial veins drain the bronchial vascular system and carry blood into the azygos and hemiazygos venous systems. Consequently, obstruction of either the bronchial system or the pulmonary artery system will not cause gangrene of the lung; both systems would have to be obstructed for that to occur. Most tumors involving the bronchi receive their nutrition via the bronchial vascular system. Direct infusion of bronchial tumors by injection of chemotherapeutic compounds into bronchial vessels has been advocated.

THE LYMPH SYSTEM

The lymphocytes form an important scavenging system in the lung. There are no lymphatics in the alveoli. The lymph vessels start at the central acinar area and in the interlobular septa. The lymphatics accompany the blood vessels to the hilum of the lung and communicate freely from lung to lung. The lymphatics pass the lymph nodes as they run cephalad. The lymphatics on the left side join the thoracic duct, which arches into the neck and enters posterior to the venous system at the junction of the left subclavian vein and the internal jugular vein. The lymphatics of the right side move cephalad via the right lymphatic duct system, which is considerably smaller than the thoracic duct. This vessel enters the venous system in the right neck posterior to the veins at the junction of the subclavian vein and internal jugular vein. There are communications between these systems, which explains why lung cancers invading mediastinal lymph nodes can cross to the contralateral side of the mediastinum.

The lung has another system of cleansing via the cilia and the cough, either reflexly or voluntarily. By means of the mucous layer and the cilia, foreign bodies and debris can be moved cephalad by the ciliary action until irritation of the bronchi and trachea produces a cough, leading to expectoration of debris.

PATHOLOGY

MALIGNANT EPITHELIAL TUMORS

Lung cancer is classified as so-called non-small cell lung carcinoma or small cell carcinoma[1] (Table 2-1). The exact proportion of non-small cell and small cell cases is reported variously but approximately 75 to 85 percent of lung cancer is non-small cell and some 15 to 25 percent is small cell.

The classification of cancer by cell is complicated by a mixture of cell types. The more diligently the pathologist examines the tumor, the greater the chance that other cell types may be found. Most of the time the classification of a tumor is based on the predominant cell type. In certain situations it is better to report the mixed cellularity of the tumors. A large cell tumor that also contains evidence of a small cell component has a worse prognosis secondary to detection of its small cell elements.

In the patient with suspected primary lung cancer, clearly one of the first things that the physician must obtain is a satisfactory biopsy or sample

Table 2-1. World Health Organization Histologic Classification of Malignant Epithelial Tumors of the Lung (1981)

1. Squamous cell carcinoma (epidermoid carcinoma)
   Variant:
   a. Spindle cell (squamous) carcinoma
2. Small cell carcinoma
   a. Oat cell carcinoma
   b. Intermediate cell type
   c. Combined oat cell carcinoma
3. Adenocarcinoma
   a. Acinar adenocarcinoma
   b. Papillary adenocarcinoma
   c. Bronchioloalveolar carcinoma
   d. Solid carcinoma with mucus formation
4. Large cell carcinoma
   Variant:
   a. Giant cell carcinoma
   b. Clear cell carcinoma
5. Adenosquamous carcinoma
6. Carcinoid tumor
7. Bronchial gland carcinomas
   a. Adenoid cystic carcinoma
   b. Mucoepidermoid carcinoma
   c. Others
8. Others

(From World Health Organization,[2] with permission.)

of the tumor involved so that the pathologist can establish the proper diagnosis.

Non-small cell lung carcinomas and small cell lung carcinomas tend to behave differently. Surgical excision has been the chief means of cure in the former, and chemotherapy plus radiotherapy without surgical excision have been standard care in the latter, although we shall show that this is changing somewhat. Ideally we would like a better way to determine tumor virulence and curability. Flow cytometry seems helpful in that increase in DNA seems more unfavorable. Recent studies with the presence of the K-*ras* gene in adenocarinomas also seem to identify a less favorable group.

However, the most important factor in treatment and survival that has had the most attention in recent years is the *correct staging* of the tumor.

NON-SMALL CELL CARCINOMA

Adenocarcinoma

At present in the United States adenocarcinoma is the most common non-small cell lung carcinoma. Characteristically, the adenocarcinomas are glandular cancers. They are recognized by their mucin production and the formation of tubular or papillary structures. The World Health Organization classification recognizes four subtypes, namely, adenocarcinoma (acinar, tubular), papillary, bronchioloalveolar, and solid. The intercellular mucin is visualized by special stains, such as periodic acid-Schiff, alcian blue, and muci-carmine, as droplets or vacuoles. Since many other kinds of adenocarcinoma tumors originate outside the thorax, it may be difficult to be certain that the adenocarcinoma in the chest is a primary rather than a metastatic tumor. Pathologic expertise and careful study of the patient may be necessary before the tumor's primary status can be determined. Occasionally, primary pulmonary adenocarcinoma simulates colonic carcinoma if it has signet ring cells. Some of the cells resemble Clara cells or type II pneumocytes.

Adenocarcinomas tend to develop in peripheral sites in the lung. They frequently contain scarring. At times it is very difficult to tell whether the adenocarcinoma has developed in a scar and is a true "scar cancer" or whether the lung scar is secondary to tumor growth. Frequently this matter is resolved only by serial chest x-rays showing that a scar had been present for some time and a tumor developed within the scar. Certainly scars in the lung that have been present for some time do represent a hazard to the patient. They are a risk factor, and we believe that chronic lung scars should be monitored by annual chest x-rays for the same reason that smokers of cigarettes over the age of 45 should be given annual chest x-rays.

A subtype of adenocarcinoma is the so-called bronchioloalveolar carcinoma. In this type of cancer the tumor grows along the alveolar septa and may leave the alveolar architecture quite intact. This tumor is often multifocal, either developing throughout the involved lobe or spreading to other lobes of the lung. Bronchioloalveolar carcinoma, if it is definitely diagnosed, is a primary tumor of the lung, as distinct from the other adenocarcinomas. It may produce a considerable amount of mucin and in general has a less favorable prognosis. The non-mucin-producing form of bronchioloalveolar carcinoma is more likely to consist of the Clara cells or type III pneumocytes.

Squamous Cell Carcinoma

In our experience squamous cell carcinoma currently is less common than adenocarcinoma, representing some 30 to 40 percent of non-small cell carcinomas. Squamous cell carcinoma tends to be located in a more central position in the lung, and frequently it is in a main or lobar bronchus. More often the upper lobes are involved. Occasionally small in situ squamous cell carcinomas can be detected by desquamated cancer cells in the sputum but will not be visible in a standard chest x-ray. These early forms of tumor are quite curable, even though they tend to be recurrent. In fact, all patients cured of lung cancers are at risk for the development of new lung cancers.

Central squamous cell tumors are more likely to produce symptoms of bronchial obstruction, pneumonia, and bleeding than are peripheral adenocarcinoma tumors, which tend to be more silent coin lesions, at least initially. Occasionally squamous cell carcinomas have a malignant spindle cell appearance and may look somewhat like a sarcoma. The presence of keratin in the tumor is a relatively reliable indicator that the tumor cell is squamous cell carcinoma. Microscopically the presence of intercellular bridges is also an indication of squamous cell carcinoma.

Large Cell Carcinomas

The rarest of the non-small cell lung cancers are the large cell carcinomas; these represent approximately 10 percent of the non-small cell lung cancers. The large cell carcinomas examined by electron microscopy reveal evidence of squamous glandular or neuroendocrine differentiation or a combination of these, and thus seem to be a collection of poorly differentiated epithelial tumors. This matter is currently under debate. It is especially important to have a large enough biopsy or piece of tissue for the pathologist to examine to be certain about the diagnosis of a large cell carcinoma. The World Health Organization has recognized two subgroups of large cell carcinoma, namely, giant cell carcinoma, which usually occurs in heavy smokers, and clear cell carcinoma. Large cell carcinomas are characterized by rapid growth and carcinoembryonic antigen (CEA) is often present. It may be difficult to distinguish these from metastatic tumors.

SMALL CELL CARCINOMA

Small cell carcinomas of the lung are subdivided in the World Health Organization classification as oat cell carcinoma, intermediate cell type, or combined small cell carcinoma. It is not clear that these subdivisions have any important clinical prognostic features. The small cell carcinomas generally are centrally located. They tend to grow rapidly and to disseminate early. They are sensitive to radiation therapy and chemotherapy, but long-term survival of patients is limited.

Paraneoplastic syndromes are particularly common. The most common of these syndromes is a myasthenic syndrome caused by an antibody that interferes with acetylcholine production and transmission across synapses. This has been called the Lambert-Eaton myasthenic syndrome and has been found in as many as 65 percent of these tumors.

Peptide hormones are also produced by small cell carcinomas. The inappropriate production of antidiuretic hormone can be the most troublesome. This can occur in about one-third of the patients and is often severe, with hyponatremia and hypoosmolality due to loss of urinary sodium in 5 to 10 percent of the patients.

Adrenocorticotropic hormone (ACTH) can be produced, and this gives rise to glucose intolerance and frequently severe hypocalcemic alkalosis. Calcitonin can produce hypercalcemia, which can be quite difficult to treat. Growth hormone can also be produced.

In the pathologic examination of these tumors, the important feature aside from their small size is the fact that their arrangement resembles a spread of oats. Electron microscopy studies of these tumors reveal neuroendocrine granules. These vary from 50 to 200 nm in diameter but average about 100 nm. Immunohistochemistry has been used in an attempt to distinguish more accurately between small cell and non-small cell carcinomas, but a completely satisfactory marker has not been found, and usually a panel of antibodies is used.

CARCINOID TUMORS

Carcinoid tumors (bronchial carcinoids) are neuroendocrine tumors that are histologically similar to those seen in the gastrointestinal tract. Usually they are centrally located in the tracheobronchial tree, but they can be peripheral. Formerly they were called bronchial adenomas, but this term should not be used for bronchial carcinoids since they behave as malignant tumors. Their degree of malignancy is less than that of carcinoma of the lung, but they do metastasize. Bronchial carcinoids are relatively rare, representing only 1 to 2 percent of all the primary lung tumors.

One of their important features is that they tend to occur in a younger population than carcinoma of the lung, and they may occur in young children. Their cause is unknown, but it is unrelated to cigarette smoking or to any other known toxic agent. In general the symptoms are those of airway obstruction, since they tend to occur in bronchi and even the trachea. If they become ulcerated, they may produce hemoptysis as a presenting complaint. These tumors can be quite vascular, and the hemoptysis can be severe. Because of this possible vascularity, the thoracic surgeon has to exercise caution in the biopsy of these tumors. The carcinoid syndrome occurs in only 5 percent of these patients.

If the bronchial carcinoid tumor is less than 3.0 cm in diameter without metastasis to regional lymph nodes, the 5-year survival rate is 90 to 95 percent. However, if it is more than 3.0 cm in diameter, with metastasis to regional lymph nodes, the curability decreases to 60 percent. It is therefore important to remember that even in younger patients and children, airway obstruction must always be investigated and diagnosed accurately. Failure to diagnose the presence of a bronchial carcinoid can be a serious omission. Radiation therapy is usually added to surgical treatment when lymph node metastases have occurred. In our experience, these tumors have not been particularly sensitive to chemotherapy.

ADENOSQUAMOUS CARCINOMA

It has been stated already that lung carcinomas are frequently of mixed cell types. A classification is reserved for the diagnosis of adenosquamous carcinoma, when both squamous and glandular aspects are seen on light microscopy and are consistently present in most of the tumor. This situation is rare, and the tumor tends to behave like an adenocarcinoma. In consequence, the treatment and handling of these lesions are not different.

BRONCHIAL GLAND CARCINOMAS

Adenoid Cystic Carcinoma

In the older literature the adenoid cystic carcinoma was also referred to as a cylindroma. This tumor occurs in both sexes and is a tumor of middle age. Most of the tumors occur in the main bronchi, and they may extend into the trachea. They tend to be slow-growing tumors. Since they have a tendency to submucosal and perineural spread, it is difficult to treat these tumors effectively with an adequate surgical margin. Therefore, they may recur locally after a period of years. When they occur in the tracheobronchial tree, metastasis is uncommon but can occur. These tumors should be treated with relatively wide local excision and with preservation of as much lung tissue as possible. They tend not to be sensitive to radiotherapy or chemotherapy.

Mucoepidermoid Carcinomas

Mucoepidermoid carcinomas can also involve the tracheobronchial tree. They tend to be more malignant than the bronchial carcinoids and the adenoid cystic carcinomas. They behave more like the common carcinomas of the lung. Mucoepidermoid tumors contain glandular and squamous elements. The low-grade tumors with little atypia or few mitoses rarely metastasize and resection is usually curative. In the high-grade tumors metastasis to lymph nodes can occur. They may be confused with the adenosquamous variety of lung cancer, but more usually develop in relationship to the major tracheobronchial tree. Their surgical treatment is the same as that of lung carcinomas.

BENIGN EPITHELIAL TUMORS

In our experience these are the most common of the benign tumors of the lung. In a tumor registry of 8,000 lung cancers we found that incidence of benign lung tumors to be less than 1.0 percent. The overwhelming majority of these tumors are either chondromas or so-called hamartomas. They are connective tissue tumors, and by definition a hamartoma is a disorganized proliferation of the connective and epithelial tissues normally present in the lung.[3] Another definition has been an overgrowth of normal tissue that seems to serve no useful purpose. These tumors are rare in childhood, but usually appear in adults and continue to grow. Most of the lesions are asymptomatic and are peripheral. The problem is to differentiate these from malignant carcinomas. Usually they present as "coin lesions" that must be excised before the correct diagnosis can be established. Only a small percentage occur in major airways, where they might ultimately cause symptoms by airway obstruction.

Any of the tissues present in the lung can theoretically produce benign tumors. These are rare but do occur. The thoracic surgeon should be alert to this possibility since any kind of tumor can occur. Since benign tumors exist, it is important that they be diagnosed. It is equally important that unduly destructive surgical procedures not be carried out for benign tumors.

MALIGNANT NONEPITHELIAL TUMORS

MISCELLANEOUS SARCOMAS

Sarcomas arising in the lungs as primary tumors[4] are extremely rare. They usually come from smooth muscle or fibrous tissue. The problem is to differentiate them from metastatic sarcomas. If no primary sarcoma can be found elsewhere, this rare diagnosis is considered. It is distinguished by the fact that it is a solitary lesion whereas most metastatic sarcomas tend to be multiple. They should be treated with surgical excision.

HEMANGIOPERICYTOMA

Hemangiopericytomas presumably arise from pericytes. They occur in a mean age group that is slightly younger than that for lung cancers. Like all tumors, they may be central or peripheral, large or small, and difficult to diagnose.

The tumors lack a true capsule. Their malignant potential is best recognized by their size rather than the microscopic picture. Those that reach a dimension of more than 8.0 cm seem to have greater malignant potential. Usually their malignant behavior is based on their growth and invasion in the chest rather than on distant metastases, but distant metastases can occur. If possible, the tumors should be completely excised. They usually originate in one site but may have multiple origins in the chest. They can be difficult to distinguish from localized fibrous mesotheliomas.

KAPOSI'S SARCOMA

The origin of Kaposi's sarcoma is still debated, but it seems that its malignant cells arrive from the endothelium in either lymphatics or blood vessels. It used to be an excessively rare tumor, but with the advent of the acquired immunodeficiency syndrome (AIDS) it is now common. Most of the Kaposi's sarcomas formerly started in the skin, but we now see primary Kaposi's sarcoma in the lung. When this tumor occurs in the lungs of AIDS patients, it is important primarily for diagnostic purposes since these patients are very poor candidates for resectional surgery of the lung. If possible, we prefer to make a diagnosis by needle biopsies and transbronchial needle biopsies rather than thoracotomies.

LYMPHOMAS

Most lymphomas in the lung are secondary metastatic involvement. Lymphomas confined to the lung are very rare. In the rare instances we have seen, they have usually required excision for diagnosis, but then, depending on the cell type, they have required chemotherapy and/or radiotherapy.

METASTATIC MALIGNANT TUMORS

Malignant tumors from almost any place in the body can metastasize to the lungs. Malignant tumors that occur in the peritoneal cavity will usually first appear as metastases in the liver if they invade the portal venous drainage. If these liver metastases continue to grow and the venous drainage of the liver is invaded, these tumors have direct access to the systemic venous circulation and hence to the lungs.

There are abdominal tumors that, because of their location, can enter the systemic venous system directly. These include tumors in the lower rectum, where the drainage via the hemorrhoidal veins is systemic. The kidneys have direct access to the inferior vena cava. Any of the malignant tumors of the abdomen can reach the lungs.

Malignant tumors elsewhere in the body can travel to the lungs via the systemic venous system. The exception to this seems to be tumors in the brain, which, even though they are aggressive malignant tumors growing inside the skull, ordinarily do not metastasize to lungs. In similar fashion most of the tumors of the head and neck region have a tendency to grow locally and recur locally before entering the bloodstream and metastasizing to lungs.

It is not possible to calculate the exact number of tumors that metastasize only to the lungs. Usually when lung metastases occur, they tend to be multiple rather than single. Sarcomas that metastasize to the lungs tend to cause their ill effects by growing locally. The symptoms are determined by where they grow. If they grow peripherally they may invade the pleural cavity. If so, pleural or bloody pleural effusions containing tumor cells may result. The tumor may obliterate the pleural space and grow directly into the chest wall. As the sarcomas grow, they can invade the pulmonary venous drainage and have access for return to the left atrium, pass through the heart, and develop systemic metastases. The majority of the tumors go where most of the blood flows. Tumors leaving the chest have a predilection to end up in the brain, skeleton, or liver. Sarcomas tend not to involve the thoracic lymphatic system.

The carcinoma metastases into the lungs, however, have a predilection to spread to hilar and mediastinal lymph nodes. They also can enlarge and cause symptoms dependent upon their location. They also can cause malignant pleural effusions, invade the chest wall, and invade blood vessels and hence metastasize outside the chest.

PLEURAL TUMORS—MESOTHELIOMA

Most pleural tumors are metastatic. The most common primary malignant tumor of the pleura is mesothelioma. Since the 1960s it has been known to be caused by asbestos fibers, particularly crocidolite and amosite. The fiber size is important. Diameters less than 0.25 μm and lengths over 5 μm are the sizes associated with mesothelioma. Whether such fibers other than those from asbestos can cause mesotheliomas is not certain. It is thought that about 7 percent of patients with asbestos exposure develop mesothelioma. Asbestos workers who smoke cigarettes have high incidences of lung carcinoma.

The typical picture of mesothelioma is that of a painful pleural effusion, which frequently is bloody. Mesotheliomas are difficult to diagnose by cytologic examination, and open pleural biopsies or biopsies with adequate tissue are needed for pathologic examination. Mesotheliomas can be benign, but it is not possible to establish the diagnosis of benign mesotheliomas by needle biopsies, and so open biopsies with sufficient tissue are required.

The microscopic picture of mesothelioma varies from the epithelial type to a spindle cell sarcomatous type and may be mixed. Regardless, few patients survive for more than 2 years after diagnosis.

REFERENCES

1. Corrin B (ed): The Lungs. Churchill Livingston, New York, 1990
2. World Health Organization: Histological Typing of Lung Tumours. 2nd Ed. World Health Organization, Geneva, 1981
3. Shah JP, Choudhry KV, Huvos AG et al: Hamartoma of the Lung. Surg Obstet Gynecol 136:406, 1973
4. Martini N, Hajdu S, Beattie EJ: Primary sarcoma of the lung. J Thorac & Cardiovasc Surg 61:33, 1971

3

Lung

Lung cancer is the most disastrous of all the current cancers in the United States. This is true in most of the world where cigarettes are commonly smoked and where populations have a life expectancy into the seventh decade.[1] In 1990 it was projected that there would be 158,000 new lung cancer patients in the United States and that 143,000 would die of their disease. This is a mortality rate of 90 percent. There is a great feeling of pessimism among most physicians in the United States concerning the curability of lung cancer. This grim picture was well described by Doll and Peto, who reported an update of an earlier review[2] at the Union Internationale Contre le Carcinome meeting in Hamburg, Germany, in August 1990, on the epidemiology of cigarette smoking. There were 5.5 billion persons alive in the world in 1990. If the current smoking habits and the present deaths from cigarette smoking remained unchanged to the year 2010, Doll and Peto predicted that one-half billion individuals now living would die as a result of smoking cigarettes.[2] In addition to fatal lung cancers, this statistic includes morbidity from cardiovascular diseases and other complications of cigarette smoking. Because of the general pessimism about early detection and cure of lung cancer, our national health experts have switched their emphasis to prevention by cessation of cigarette smoking.

ETIOLOGY

It is well accepted that approximately 86 percent of the lung cancer found annually in the United States is secondary to the smoking of cigarettes.[3] Smoking one pack of 20 cigarettes per day for 20 years puts the individual at high risk for the future development of lung cancer. The rapid growth of cigarette smoking in the United States began with cigarette smoking by males in World War I. It was aggravated by the free cigarettes and increased smoking by the military in World War II and continued in the Korean and Vietnam conflicts. Published data from the British Armed Forces show that the military, with cheap and readily available tobacco and alcohol, had two and one-half times the death rate from disease compared with civilian populations of the same age.[4]

The relationship between cigarette smoking and lung cancer was proposed and reported by Evarts Graham and Ernst Wynder in 1950.[5] Their study was received with skepticism by the tobacco industry. Only in recent times have the tobacco companies stopped insisting that there is no relationship. In 1969 the U.S. Surgeon General's statement that "cigarette smoking may be hazardous to your health" was required to be printed on all packs of cigarettes. This ruling has been beneficial to the tobacco companies in that smokers now are alerted to the fact that they smoke at their own risk. Unfortunately, this has not deterred a relatively large number of women from starting to smoke cigarettes. The disastrous result is that since 1988 more American women die of lung cancer than of any other cancer.

In the current incidence of lung cancer in the United States men outnumber women 2 : 1, and it is clear that "women who smoke like men die like men who smoke." With the increased publicity about the dangers of cigarette smoking, the number of smokers in the United States has fallen to less than 30 percent. Still, millions of Americans do smoke cigarettes, and there is a large population at risk.

The role of air pollution is indicted by the public. However, in epidemiologic studies Wynder has found that cigarette smoking is 50 times more important as a cause of lung cancer than the polluted environment of our cities.[6] It is known that individuals who are exposed to a combination of carcinogens, such as asbestos workers and uranium miners who smoke cigarettes, have a very high incidence of lung cancer. Hammond et al. have shown that if the risk of lung cancer in the population at large is 1, the risk of lung cancer in a nonsmoking asbestos worker is 5.[7] The risk of lung cancer in a cigarette smoker not exposed to asbestos is 10. The worst of all is the smoking asbestos worker, who has a risk of 50. Individuals who work in uranium mines and who are smokers have an even higher risk of lung cancer than asbestos workers who smoke. In areas of the country with a high concentration of radon gas nonsmoking individuals have an increased risk of lung cancer over normal controls.

The role of passive smoking in the production of lung cancer in nonsmokers is not entirely clear but is probably important. In a Japanese study, the epidemiologist Hirayama at the National Cancer Center Hospital in Tokyo reported that there was a distinct increase in lung cancer in nonsmoking wives whose husbands are heavy smokers.[8] This might be related to the fact that Japanese homes are small and therefore passive smoking would have a major effect from a higher concentration of tobacco smoke. In the United States, where homes are larger and many offices are air conditioned, the significance of passive smoking is not clear. Janerich et al. studied the effects of exposure to household smoking on children and adolescents.[9] One hundred ninety-one nonsmokers with lung cancer were compared with nonsmokers without lung cancer. This calculation measured the number of years of exposure to cigarette smoke upon the child or adolescent, and this number of years was multiplied by the number of persons smoking in that household. This gave a figure that was identified as smoker-years of exposure. The authors found that exposure to 25 or more smoker-years in childhood and adolescence doubled the risk of lung cancer. Only 15 percent of the controls had this much exposure. The authors found that exposure to spousal smoking (one-third of the household exposure) did not increase the risk for lung cancer. Passive smoking in the workplace also did not increase the risk of lung cancer. Their conclusion was that household smoking seems injurious to young persons.

Currently in the United States it is generally thought that cigarettes with low tar, low nicotine, and filtered tips are less harmful to health. Since cigarette smoking is a nicotine addiction and smokers smoke for the nicotine effect, one must smoke harder and longer or smoke more cigarettes to get the same nicotine effect. Although the number of smokers has decreased, the number of cigarettes sold in the United States has risen disproportionately because of this "weakening" of the cigarette.[10] Approximately one-third of the cigarettes produced by U.S. tobacco companies are for export. These exported cigarettes are nonfilter and are higher in nicotine and tar than cigarettes produced for domestic consumption. The rest of the world is disinclined to pay more for a cigarette low in nicotine content. At present, the highest incidence of lung cancer in the world is found in the male population of Scotland. The highest incidence in women is also found in Scotland. U.S. men rank third in the world, and U.S. women rank eleventh.[1]

EARLY DETECTION OF LUNG CANCER

The mortality rate for lung cancer in the United States approaches 90 percent[1] because most of the patients have advanced cancers when first diagnosed or when they come for treatment. The first major attempt in the United States to detect lung cancer by routine screening of the smoker at high risk was carried out by Boucot and Weiss in Philadelphia.[11,12] They reported in 1973 on 6,136 smoking males who were recruited in 1959. They were cigarette smokers and were scheduled to have chest photofluorograms every 6 months for 10 years. One hundred twenty-one lung cancers were found; 33 were removed surgically. Eight percent of the cancer patients survived for 8 years. It was the conclusion of this study that screening chest x-rays for high-risk individuals was deemed not valuable in detecting lung cancer for cure.

Because screening chest x-rays was believed not to be useful, the National Cancer Institute in the early 1970s embarked on a National Lung Program to study the value of sputum cytology in screening individuals at high risk for lung cancer.[13] We had noted[14] that individuals who were expectorating cancer cells in their sputum but who had negative routine chest x-rays did very well in conquering their cancer, provided that the cancers could be found promptly. These so-called occult or T0 lung cancer patients were not common. Prior to the advent of the flexible fiberoptic bronchoscope T0 cancers were not always easily found by routine bronchoscopy. Most of these patients have an epidermoid carcinoma that tends to be in the portions of the tracheobronchial tree now visible with the flexible bronchoscope. If the tumors were promptly found, the patients had a good survival rate after surgical excision. As time passed it became evident that there was a tendency for new tumors to appear. The good results in these patients pointed out the value of sputum cytology.

A prospective study was set up with the cooperation of Johns Hopkins Hospital,[15] the Mayo Clinic,[16] and the Memorial Sloan Kettering Cancer Center/Strang Preventive Medicine Institute.[17] The proposal was that individuals smoking cigarettes and presumed to be at high risk for lung cancer would all be studied by routine chest x-rays. A test group composed of half the group would also be studied by sputum cytology, with the hope that the curability of the patients who developed lung cancer could be enhanced.

In the early 1970s each institution recruited 10,000 men over the age of 45 years who had smoked more than one pack of cigarettes per day for more than 20 years. The Johns Hopkins group was somewhat intermediate in age between the Mayo Clinic and Memorial Hospital groups.

When the experiments were set up, the research plan for Johns Hopkins and Memorial Sloan Kettering was the same. In each project the 10,000 men were divided into 5,000 pairs by statisticians and epidemiologists. All 10,000 in both institutions had an annual posteroanterior and lateral chest x-ray for 10 years. In the 5,000 matched pairs, "control" group A had chest x-rays alone and "experiment" group B had sputum examinations every 4 months cytologically for the 10 years.

The Mayo Clinic project was different. In their control group, each enrollee was to have an annual chest x-ray (which could be either posteroanterior and lateral or stereoscopic chest x-rays) and an annual sputum cytology test. These tests were usually not done at the Mayo Clinic but were recommended to be obtained locally. It was requested that chest x-rays and sputum cytology tests be done every 4 months in the experiment group. These tests and the results were reviewed at the Mayo Clinic.

The results in the first screen of 31,360 males at all three institutions were as follows: 79 lung cancers were found at Johns Hopkins, 91 lung cancers were found at the Mayo Clinic, and 53 lung cancers were found at Memorial Sloan Kettering, for a total of 223 "prevalent" lung cancers. One hundred five of these patients (47 percent) were so-called stage I. The 5-year survival with this group was overall 92 of 233 (41 percent) well at 5 years. This fact seems to have been overlooked by the critics who stated that screening "x-rays" did no good in this study.[18] These critics have also convinced some physicians not to use screening chest x-rays for lung cancer detection. (Suemasu K: personal communication, Tokyo, 1987).

The subsequent "incidence" of lung cancers in the Johns Hopkins study amounted to a total of 396 cancers, about half in group A and half in group B. At Memorial Sloan Kettering 235 patients were found in the incidence group, again about half and half in groups A and B. The Johns Hopkins and Memorial Sloan Kettering studies found that the sputum cytology added little to the detection of early lung cancer, with these individuals who all were getting annual chest x-rays.

Melamed[17] reported that in the Memorial Sloan Kettering study in which 288 lung cancers were detected (Tables 3-1 and 3-2), 40 percent of the cancers were stage I. This group had a 70 percent 5-year survival rate. The T1, N0, M0 with small tumors had an 85 percent survival rate at 8 years (Figs. 3-1 and 3-2). The overall survival rate in all patients with cancers detected in the Memorial

Table 3-1. Cancer by Cell Type (MSKCC Screen, 288 Cancers)

Cell Type	Cases (%)
Small cell	15
Non-small cell	85
Adenoca	48
Squamous	31
Large Cell	6

Abbreviation: MSKCC, Memorial Sloan-Kettering Cancer Center.
(From Melamed et al.,[17] with permission.)

Table 3-2. Lung Cancers by Stage (MSKCC Screen, 288 Cancers)

Stage	Number of Cases	Percentage of Cases
I	117	41
II	18	6
III (and IV)	153	53

Abbreviation: MSKCC, Memorial Sloan-Kettering Cancer Center.
(From Melamed et al.,[17] with permission.)

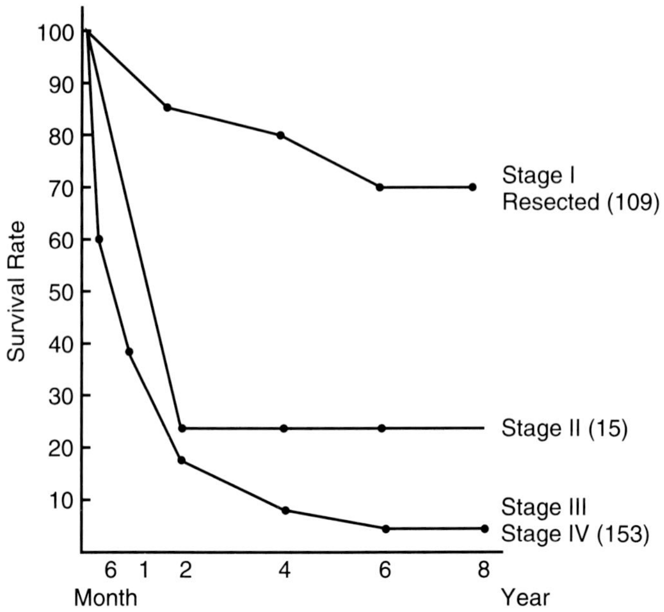

Fig. 3-1. Final results in the Memorial Sloan-Kettering study of 288 lung cancers as reported by Melamed et al. in 1984. (From Melamed et al.,[17] with permission.)

Sloan Kettering study group, was 35 percent compared with 8 percent in the Philadelphia study.[11] Melamed's conclusion was "thus the weight of evidence at this time supports the prudent medical practitioner who recommends regular screening of the asymptomatic person at high-risk of lung cancer."

Much was made of the fact that the Mayo Clinic reported in their frequent (every 4 months) dual-screen experiment with sputum and chest x-rays that there was a 40 percent 5-year survival rate in the patients with lung cancers detected. However, in their yearly dual-control group the 5-year survival rate was only 15 percent. This was interpreted by the epidemiologists and biostatisticians to mean that the frequent screening at Mayo Clinic was finding cancers earlier but not curing them. The critics claimed that the improved Mayo Clinic survival results were due to "lead time bias."[18]

The fact is that, even with its problems, the screening chest x-ray has remained the best means of early detection of lung cancer. The incidence of lung cancer in the 55-year-old smoking group is four times that of the 45-year-old smoking group. In the 65-year-old smoking group, the lung cancer incidence is eight times that in the 45-year-old smoking group. What has not been done is to encourage the smoking males (especially in the 55- and 65-year-old age group) to have an annual chest x-ray, with the individual smoker paying for the chest x-ray. The average cigarette smoker smokes up to two packs per day for 365 days per year. The smoker spends over $1,000 a year on this smoking habit. It would be relatively easy for these smokers not to smoke one pack of cigarettes per week and to put this money in a "save-your-life" account to purchase an annual chest x-ray. A change in a chest x-ray from normal to abnormal is a significant alteration. Unfortunately, the American Cancer Society is not encouraging smokers to seek screening chest x-rays, although all women aged 50 or older are encouraged

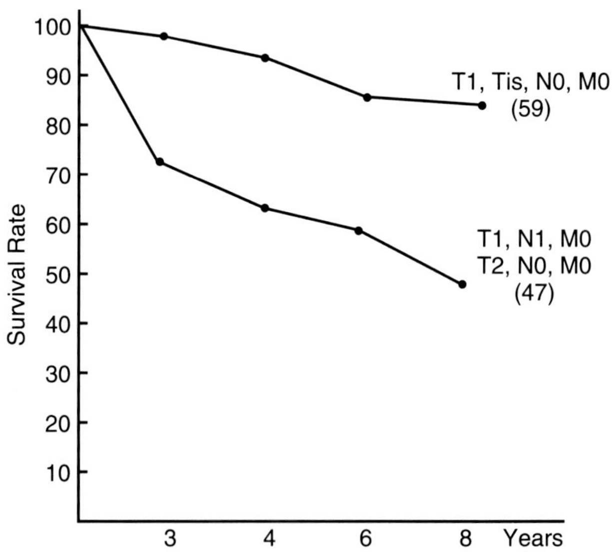

Fig. 3-2. Final results of the Memorial Sloan-Kettering study showing specifics of staging. (From Melamed et al.,[17] with permission.)

to have annual mammograms for life. Yet more American women are now dying annually from lung cancer than from breast cancer. It is interesting that in April 1987 a Japanese committee and the Japanese government fiscally supported annual screening chest x-rays for Japanese smokers over the age of 40 (Suemasu K: personal communication, Tokyo, 1987).

Mulshine et al.,[19] in reviewing the current status of lung cancer screening, have pointed out that "randomized trials that use a mortality endpoint eliminate the need for considering selection, lead time, and length bias in evaluating benefit." Tockman has reported two cancer-associated monoclonal antibodies to stain sputum samples retrospectively in the Johns Hopkins National Lung Project.[15] In 8 years of the Johns Hopkins lung study, 626 individuals showed moderate or greater atypia in their sputum cytology. The sensitivity of the test was 91 percent in those who developed lung cancers, and the specificity was 88 percent among those who remained free of lung cancer. It would seem that newer techniques in studying sputum cytology must be evaluated. The lung cancer study group individuals had a 3 percent per year incidence of new primary lung cancers in the cured stage I patients. These individuals are a good population for the Tockman monoclonal antibody study of sputum.

If individuals do not get annual chest x-rays, there is an advantage to using sputum cytology as a periodic screen. Minna et al., in studies of expectorated cells, found genetic changes predictive of development of small cell lung cancer.[20] This may prove profitable in the future.

There is no question that individuals should not smoke cigarettes. Not smoking is undoubtedly the best way to prevent lung cancer. Unfortunately, even if not one more cigarette were lit in the United States, by the year 2000 we would still have one million lung cancer victims who can be expected to die of their disease.[21]

DIAGNOSIS

THE ASYMPTOMATIC PATIENT

In the asymptomatic patient the most common finding to suggest the diagnosis of lung cancer is an abnormal chest x-ray. A lung cancer can produce almost any variation in the abnormality of a chest x-ray. Any abnormality in the chest x-ray of an older cigarette smoker is particularly suspicious, especially if it represents a change from what was seen on a previous chest x-ray. Our own rule is that an abnormality persisting for 1 month requires accurate diagnosis. Occasionally a sputum check will find cancer cells at a time when the routine chest x-ray is negative. Some of the patients may have an occult lung cancer; probably most have a head and neck cancer. If the bronchial washings contain cancer cells, a thorough systemic bronchoscopic study of the 18 segmental orifices and their subdivisions will usually identify the tumor location. If the tumor is not readily located, the use of photofluorescent compounds to help identify the lesion with the bronchoscope may be helpful. Rarely, tumor markers or metastases elsewhere will suggest an occult lung cancer to be the source.

THE SYMPTOMATIC PATIENT

Most lung cancers detected in the United States are symptomatic and in an advanced stage when found. This explains our current high mortality rate. The most common symptom is a cough or change in a cough, since most cigarette smokers already have a cough. Sputum production also is common, with most smokers producing sputum whether or not they expectorate. Hemoptysis is not the rule, although blood streaking in the sputum may develop. The sight of blood in the sputum usually brings the patient to a physician straight away. Blood in the sputum is indication for examination, chest x-ray, and endoscopy.

Fever, cough, and sputum are common accompaniments of an obstructing cancer. Dyspnea is common if a lung is already emphysematous from smoking. A pleural effusion can greatly handicap breathing. Pain tends to be a serious prognostic sign since it may mean pleural, chest wall, spine, or mediastinal involvement. Hoarseness may mean involvement of the recurrent laryngeal nerves. Since the left nerve descends to the ligamentum arteriosum in the left chest, it is more vulnerable to involvement by lung cancers. The right recurrent nerve only enters the upper thorax and is therefore less vulnerable to involvement by a right-lung cancer. A paralyzed diaphragm suggests involvement of the phrenic nerve and implies direct invasion or metastasis to the mediastinum. Systemic changes, such as pulmonary osteoarthropathy, can occur, as can generalized abnormalities secondary to abnormal hormone production or biochemical changes.

Diagnosis begins with a complete history and physical examination. Examination of eyes, ears, nose and throat, breast, rectum and pelvis must not be neglected. Medical, social, and family histories are important. Routine complete blood counts, differential white blood cell smears, platelet counts, so-called SMAC-20, biochemical studies, urinalysis, electrocardiogram, CT scans of the chest, arterial blood gases, ventilation tests, and split function tests, if there is any chance a pneumonectomy might be done, are all important. If surgery is considered, prothrombin time, partial thromboplastin time, and tumor markers should also be measured.

Any clues to abnormality in any of the major organ systems require careful evaluation of that particular system. Most tumors that metastasize outside the chest will go to the brain, skeleton, or liver. In consequence one must be very careful about the history and examination of potential brain metastases. A history of bone pain or elevation of the alkaline phosphatase level would require a bone scan. Ordinarily the computed tomographic (CT) scan of the chest includes the liver and adrenal glands. Any abnormality in liver function tests requires further evaluation of the liver. However, in the evaluation of a potential stage I lung cancer it is not customary to take CT scans of the head, bone scans, or further liver tests if none of the aforementioned abnormalities exist. However, once a lung cancer has been clearly established and even a so-called stage I lung cancer has been treated, we do obtain these scans so that we have baselines in case of further problems in the follow-up of the patient.

The most important problem in treating lung cancer is to establish accurate diagnosis and an accurate staging of disease.

There are four ways to obtain material for pathologic or cytologic examination for the diagnosis. The first is to collect sputum. If the patient has productive sputum, a sample for bacteriologic study and a sample fixed in 50 percent alcohol for cytologic study should be collected. If there is no obvious sputum the best technique is to collect a pooled A.M. sputum for three mornings. The patient is instructed to raise whatever sputum is possible first thing upon waking and expectorate it directly into alcohol. This sample is checked for sputum cytology. If there is no sputum or no diagnosis is made from the sputum, the second major diagnostic step is a bronchoscopy. Nowadays this is usually performed with the flexible fiberoptic bronchoscope. Some tumors can be seen directly and samples biopsied for diagnosis. Many of the lesions are peripheral and are not in view, but appropriate brushings and washings can be taken from the segmental or subsegmental bronchus to the lesion. At times the fluoroscope is valuable in guiding a brush or needle for biopsy into the region of the lesion. If there is evidence of mediastinal lymphadenopathy a transbronchial needle biopsy may establish the status of N1 or N2 lymph node metastases. The third approach, if these two fail (and particularly if the patient is such a poor surgical risk that thoracotomy would be inadvisable unless one were certain of a tumor), is a percutaneous needle biopsy. If the lesion is visible in the fluoroscope, and especially if it is close to the surface of the lung, our interventional radiologists are skilled at obtaining needle biopsies that, by cytologic examination from a skinny needle, may give us a diagnosis of carcinoma, and perhaps of the cell type. A negative needle biopsy is not of help. Whether a percutaneous needle biopsy should be done is a matter for good judgment. With the skinny-needle biopsy a minority of our patients get significant pneumothoraces. Some 5 percent require chest tube drainage because of the volume of the pneumothorax. We seldom see significant bleeding resulting in either hemothorax or hemoptysis with the use of the skinny needle. Needling lesions around the hilum or near major blood vessels is more likely to cause bleeding. The fourth and final method of establishing a diagnosis is exploratory thoracotomy. At thoracotomy one can either do a wedge excision if the lesion is small or take a biopsy with a so-called true cut or Vim-Silverman needle. This technique can get a biopsy large enough for frozen-section diagnosis. It is wise to be certain about the diagnosis before proceeding with a lobectomy and especially before proceeding with a pneumonectomy.

STAGING OF LUNG CANCER

An important advance in the study of lung cancer was the adoption of the TNM system (Table 3-3), which is presently used by most experts in the care of the lung cancer patient. The patient is first evaluated by history and physical examination, routine laboratory work, and posteroanterior and lateral chest x-rays. This is usually followed by a CT scan of the chest. With this information at hand, the clinical staging of the tumor is carried out. The T denotes the size and extent of the tumor. Any tumor under 3.0 cm in diameter surrounded by lung tissue is a so-called T1; the same tumor over 3.0 cm in diameter is a T2. If the tumor involves the visceral pleura it is T2; if it involves parietal pleura it is T3; if it is within 2.0 cm of the carina it is T3; if it involves the entire lung it is T3; and if it is extensive and thought to be nonresectable it is T4 (Table 3-3).

The N signifies lymph nodes and indicates the status of the lymph nodes in the thorax and base of the neck. If no lymph nodes are enlarged or involved with tumor, the disease can be staged clinically as N0. Tumor involvement of lymph nodes in the lung or on the bronchi is classified as N1. Tumor involvement of lymph nodes in the ipsilateral mediastinum bounded by the plane of the first rib, the diaphragm below, and the mediastinal pleura laterally is classified as N2. If lymph nodes are involved on the contralateral side of the mediastinum, the stage is designated as N3. If the lymph nodes in the base of the neck (prescalene area) are involved, it is also classified as N3.

M refers to metastases, generally outside the thorax. The most common site for metastases in the lung cancer patient is the brain, followed by the skeleton and liver. Other organs as well as the whole body can be involved, but the adrenal glands are notable as potential sites of metastatic involvement. If no metastases can be found, the cancer is

Table 3-3. American Joint Committee on Cancer Staging for Lung Carcinoma

Primary Tumor (T)

TX	Primary tumor cannot be assessed, or tumor proven by the presence of malignant cells in sputum or bronchial washings but not visualized by imaging or bronchoscopy
T0	No evidence of primary tumor
Tis	Carcinoma in situ
T1	Tumor 3 cm or less in greatest dimension, surrounded by lung or visceral pleura, without bronchoscopic evidence of invasion more proximal than the lobar bronchus[a] (i.e., not in the main bronchus)
T2	Tumor with any of the following features of size or extent: More than 3 cm in greatest dimension; Involves main bronchus, 2 cm or more distal to the carina; Invades the visceral pleura; Associated with atelectasis or obstructive pneumonitis that extends to the hilar region but does not involve the entire lung
T3	Tumor of any size that directly invades any of the following: chest wall (including superior sulcus tumors), diaphragm, mediastinal pleura, parietal pericardium; tumor in the main bronchus less than 2 cm distal to the carina[a] but without involvement of the carina; or associated atelectasis or obstructive pneumonitis of the entire lung
T4	Tumor of any size that invades any of the following: mediastinum, heart, great vessels, trachea, esophagus, vertebral body, carina; or tumor with a malignant pleural effusion[b]

Regional Lymph Nodes (N)

NX	Regional lymph nodes cannot be assessed
N0	No regional lymph node metastasis
N1	Metastasis in ipsilateral peribronchial and/or ipsilateral hilar lymph nodes, including direct extension
N2	Metastasis in ipsilateral mediastinal and/or subcarinal lymph node(s)
N3	Metastasis in contralateral mediastinal, contralateral hilar, ipsilateral or contralateral scalene, or supraclavicular lymph node(s)

Distant Metastasis (M)

MX	Presence of distant metastasis cannot be assessed
M0	No distant metastasis
M1	Distant metastasis

Stage Grouping

Occult carcinoma	TX	N0	M0
Stage 0	Tis	N0	M0
Stage I	T1	N0	M0
	T2	N0	M0
Stage II	T1	N1	M0
	T2	N1	M0
Stage IIIA	T1	N2	M0
	T2	N2	M0
	T3	N0, N1, N2	M0
Stage IIIB	Any T	N3	M0
	T4	Any N	M0
Stage IV	Any T	Any N	M1

Abbreviations: T, primary tumor; N, regional lymph nodes; M, distant metastasis.

[a] The uncommon superficial tumor of any size with its invasive component limited to the bronchial wall, which may extend proximal to the main bronchus, is also classified T1.

[b] Most pleural effusions associated with lung cancer are due to tumor. However, there are a few patients in whom multiple cytopathologic examinations of pleural fluid are negative for tumor. In these cases, fluid is non-bloody and is not an exudate. When these elements and clinical judgment dictate that the effusion is not related to the tumor, the effusion should be excluded as a staging element and the patient should be staged T1, T2, or T3.

(Adapted from Beahrs et al.,[120] with permission.)

staged at M0. If metastases outside the chest are found the condition is staged as M1. It is helpful to segregate and classify these patients appropriately and to separate solitary M1 from multiple M1. One should note where the solitary M1 is located. At present, lesions in the opposite lung that are thought to be metastatic from the primary lung cancer (rather than a double primary, which is sometimes difficult to establish) are also classified as M1. Likewise, a metastasis in the lobe or lung on the ipsilateral side is classified as M1, although it seems to the authors that a different nomenclature probably should be used. It is our impression that these M1s do better than M1s that are outside the thorax.

Clinical staging is complete after the patient has had an initial screen and the physicians involved have tentatively assigned a TNM staging designation. For example, if this was thought to be an early stage I lung cancer, the nomenclature would be T1, N0, M0c (the "c" signifies that staging is based on clinical findings). Surgical procedures such as scalene node biopsy, mediastinoscopy, and mediastinotomy can be used as diagnostic aids for clinical staging.

When an operation such as exploratory thoracotomy or thoracotomy with lobectomy or other lung resection is performed, the mediastinal lymph nodes should be sampled or removed, depending on the conditions. After the operation, a surgical TNM staging is assigned. For instance, if there was a small tumor with metastases to lymph nodes confined to the right upper lobe bronchus and no tumor lymph nodes were found in the mediastinum, the condition would be staged as T1, N1, M0s (the "s" signifying that staging is based on surgical findings). If the surgical findings agree with the clinical findings, the designation would be T1, N1, M0c,s. If the final pathology report confirms the clinical and surgical staging, the final staging is expressed as T1, N1, M0c,s,p.

When publishing studies involving the staging of lung cancers, authors should indicate whether TNM staging has been used. If it has, it is important to qualify the staging findings by appropriate letters, namely c, s, and/or p. Without these letters, differing clinical and surgical findings cannot be identified. If all cases have not been surgically staged, they can be compared only clinically. Furthermore, clinically staged series and surgically staged series are not comparable. In using TNM staging nomenclature, authors must be careful not to compare the proverbial "oranges and apples."

The CT scan, as stated above, is a major advance in recognizing abnormal disease in the chest. In the lung cancer patient lymph nodes under 1.0 cm tend to be noncarcinomatous. Lymph nodes over 2.0 cm are usually thought to contain malignant tumors, whereas lymph nodes in the range of 1 to 2.0 cm are borderline. This is a helpful guide, but diagnosis cannot be determined solely on the basis of any chest x-ray. The scientific physician or surgeon caring for the patient must ensure that appropriate microscopic confirmation is carried out. This cannot be stressed too much. All cancer patients, if they are to be treated with hope for cure, deserve appropriate, accurate pathologic diagnosis and correct TNM staging.

TREATMENT OF PRIMARY LUNG CANCER

As we have indicated previously the most important problem in treating lung cancer is to establish accurate diagnosis and an accurate staging of disease.

STAGE I

Under this stage I heading there are three major types: the so-called T0, N0, M0, the T1, N0, M0, and the T2, N0, M0. The T0, N0, M0 patient expectorates cancer cells but has a negative routine chest x-ray. A careful head and neck examination is done to ensure that the cancer is not coming from the head and neck region. Then a bronchoscopy is carried out to be certain that the bronchial washings contain cancer cells. If bronchial washings are localized to one lung, careful inspection of the segments and subsegments usually will show the lesion. If not, washings and brushings from all the subsegments is indicated until the T0 lesion is found. Usually these are small superficial bronchial lesions, and mostly they are squamous or epidermoid carcinoma (non-small cell lung cancers). Once the lesion is found it is not longer T0 but gets the appropriate T designation.

Most of the T1, N0, M0 lesions are coin lesions less than 3.0 cm in diameter surrounded by lung tissue. In 1977 Martini and Beattie[22] reported experiences with 691 consecutive non-small cell lung cancers first seen and treated at the Memorial Sloan-Kettering Cancer Center (Table 3-4). Of this group 198 had thoracotomy; there were no surgical deaths. Ultimately, 124 of 691 (19 percent) were found to have stage I lung cancers (Fig. 3-3), and 115 of these tumors were resected. (One pa-

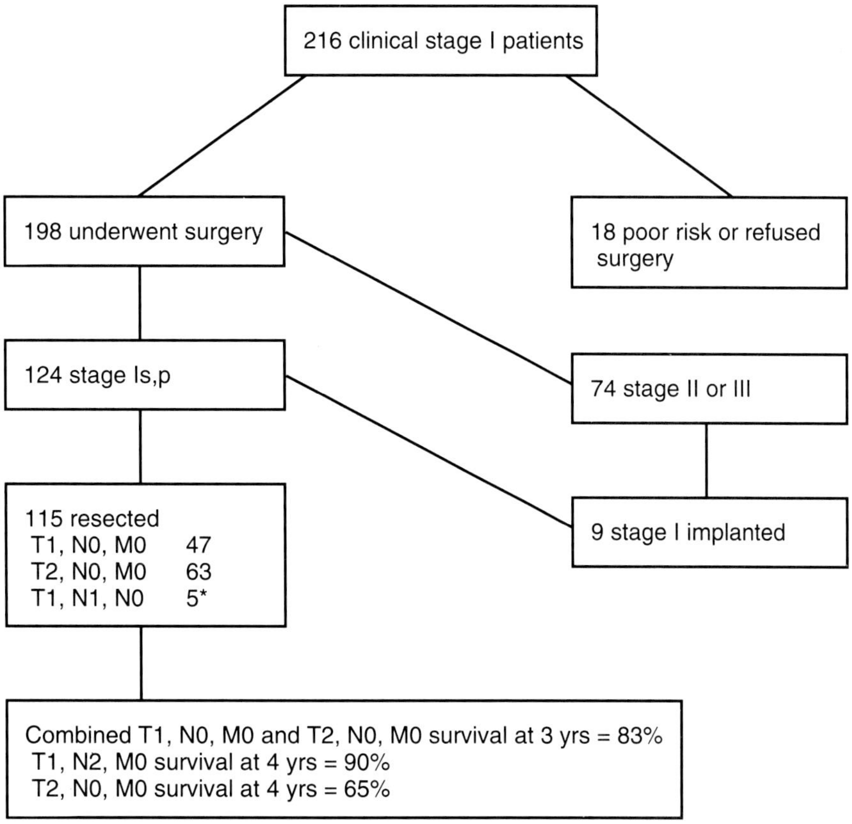

*Now no longer considered stage I.

Fig. 3-3. Treatment course and outcome of 216 clinical stage I patients treated at Memorial Sloan-Kettering between 1973 and 1976. (From Martini and Beattie,[22] with permission.)

tient with presumed T1, N0, M0 lung cancer refused operation; therefore 124 patients were used in these statistics.) Thus 74 (37 percent) of clinical stage I patients were upstaged at thoracotomy. In addition to these 124, 10 patients were T0, N0, M0, showing negative chest x-rays but positive sputum tests. Tumors were small and were located by bronchoscope. Resection was carried out in all 10 patients, with good results. Not to prejudice this series, these T0, N0, M0 cases were eliminated when we reported on the 124 patients. The T1, N0, M0 group ultimately was found to have a 5-year survival rate of 85 percent. Most of the T2, N0, M0 lesions were coin lesions in excess of 3.0 cm in diameter and were surrounded by lung tissue, or else they were lesions smaller than 3.0 cm involving the visceral pleura. Thus they were upstaged to T2, N0, M0.

Table 3-4. Clinically Staged Non-Small Cell Lung Carcinomas

	No. with			
Year	Stage I	Stage II	Stage III	Total
1973	35	3	118	156
1974	44	3	83	132
1975	66	5	120	196
1976	71	7	126	207
Total	216	18	447	691

(From Martini and Beattie,[22] with permission.)

In 1977, when we first reported on these patients, who had undergone surgery between 1973 and 1976, the 3-year survival rate free of disease was 83 percent. Figure 3-4 shows the 4-year survival of T1, N0, M0 patients to be 90 percent, whereas the 4-year survival of T2, N0, M0 patients was below 65 percent. Throughout the period of this study our routine operation in low-risk patients was a lobectomy plus careful staging of the mediastinum. We began to use an anatomic staging map patterned after consultation with our

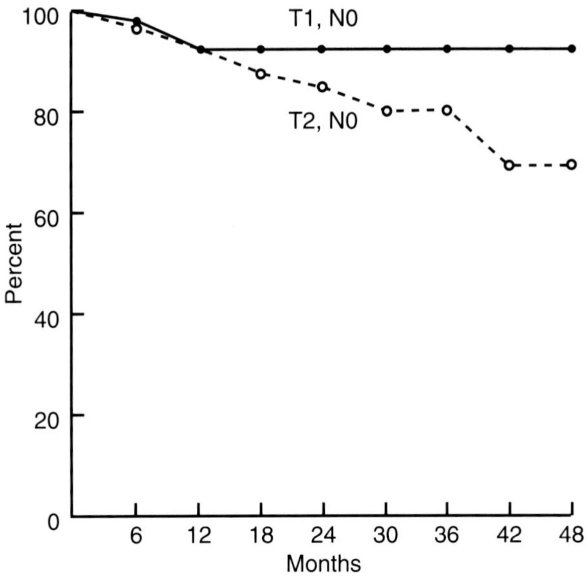

Fig. 3-4. Four-year survival curves in the 47 T1, N0, M0 and 63 T2, N0, M0 tumors resected, as reported by Martini and Beattie in 1977. (From Martini and Beattie,[22] with permission.)

Japanese colleagues at the National Cancer Center Hospital, Tokyo, wherein the lymph nodes in the mediastinum were numbered 1 through 9 from the top to the bottom of the chest (Fig. 3-5). Lymph nodes inside the pleural cavity were designated levels 10 through 13, with 10 being at the mainstem bronchus, 11 at the lobar bronchi, 12 at the segmental level, and 13 at the subsegmental levels. We found that when doing a lobectomy, it was essential to attempt to remove and sample all these nodes to be certain that N0 was truly N0.

It was found ultimately that the 5-year survival rate free of disease with surgical excision alone was approximately 60 percent for T2, N0, M0 lesions. The 5-year survival rate in the entire group of stage I lung cancer is largely dependent on the mixture of T1 and T2 lesions. We later found that the average 5-year survival rate for stage I overall was 70 percent.

Even though T1, N0, M0 patients have an 85 percent 5-year survival rate and T2, N0, M0 patients have a 60 percent 5-year survival rate, better adjuvant therapy would increase these rates. The cancer deaths in this stage were from disease outside the chest since we found no recurrent disease in the chest in 1977. The presumption is that in these cases the tumor has already metastasized outside the chest even though there was no evidence of involvement of the mediastinal or lung

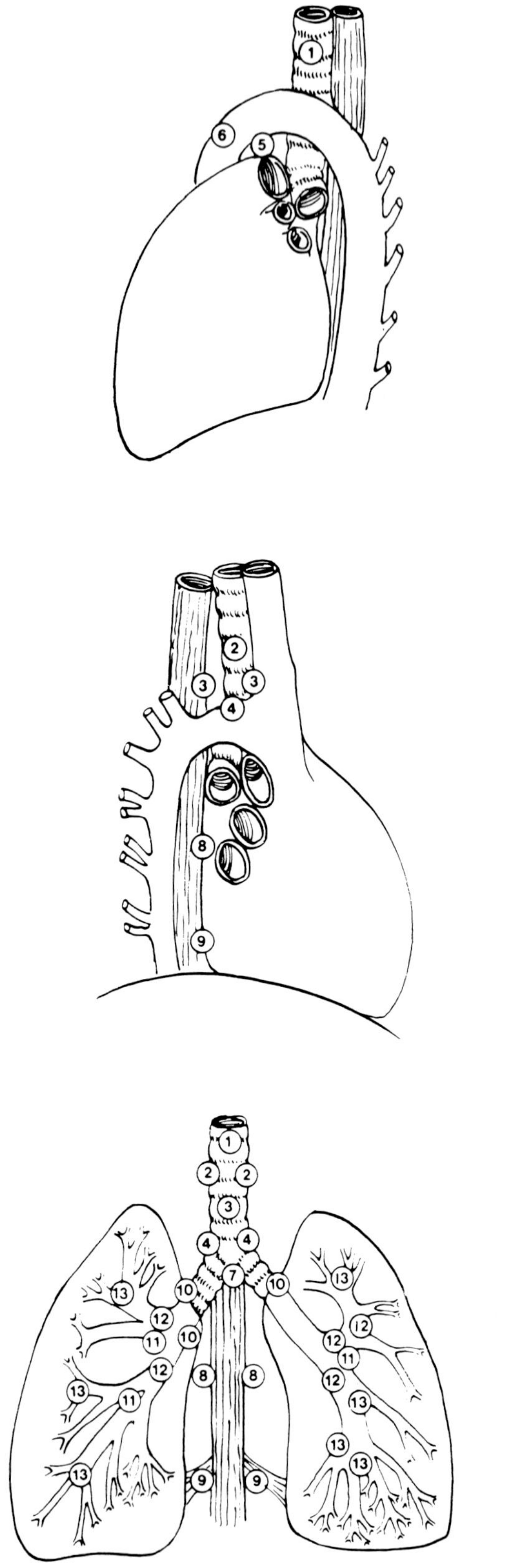

Fig. 3-5. Anatomic staging map with lymph nodes of the mediastinum numbered 1 to 9. (From Beahrs et al.,[120] with permission.)

lymph nodes. These tumors are prone to metastasize to the brain, skeleton, and/or liver. In 1977 brain metastasis was the leading cause of death. A worth research project would be to identify which patients in this stage I group would not be cured by surgery alone and to develop better means of adjuvant therapy to improve the survival rate.

Not all patients can tolerate a lobectomy, especially if they have diminution of respiratory reserve. Another question is whether these patients require a lobectomy, i.e., whether a segmental resection or even a wedge excision would give similar cures. If the tumor was truly localized and was completely removed by either a wedge resection or a segmentectomy, the ultimate 5-year survival rate should be the same. The National Lung Study Group has been conducting a prospective randomized trial comparing lobectomy with segmentectomy; their results so far are not published, but segmentectomies and certainly wedges seem less curative.

In our own experience with wedge resections reported in 1969,[23] 25 wedge excisions done before we were using accurate mediastinal staging resulted in a 5-year survival rate of 25 percent. It is our impression that a segmentectomy, which carries a parenchymal wedge of tissue down to the hilum of the lobe, is superior to wedge excision for treatment of stage I lung cancer. Since patients with stage I lung cancer are usually heavy smokers and may have emphysema, the standard technique of doing a segmentectomy by controlling the hilum and stripping the segment out is complicated by prolonged air leaks. An alternative is to use a stapling device to wedge out the appropriate bronchopulmonary segment after the hilum of the segment has been controlled.

The alternative treatment to wedge excision, segmentectomy, or lobectomy in the seriously compromised respiratory patient with a high degree of emphysema is the use of internal radiotherapy. In this situation one normally implants iodine-125 (I-125) seeds in the tumor at 1.0 cm equidistance from each other for a good dose distribution of radiation effect. As long as the tumor is under 6.0 cm in one dimension, internal implant radiotherapy may be used. The success rate is about 80 percent of that of surgical excision. This means that T1, N0, M0 tumors that normally have an 85 percent success rate with lobectomy would have 80 percent of 85 percent, or approximately 65 percent 5-year survival rate, if implanted with radioactive I-125 seeds. In similar fashion the 60 percent 5-year survival rate of T2, N0, M0 tumors would achieve 80 percent of 60 percent or about 50 percent 5-year survival rate, if implanted.[24]

STAGE II

About 5 percent of NSCLC patients are stage II patients. In this group of patients tumor has spread to the lung or hilar lymph nodes. Therefore the group is classified as N1. To be called stage II, the T component can be either T1 or T2 associated with N1 disease, but without metastases, and therefore M0. In this group of patients our recommendation to date has been a lobectomy with dissection and removal of all the hilar and mediastinal lymph nodes possible. Presumably all the gross disease is removed by this treatment. It has been our policy to recommend postoperative radiation therapy to patients with N1 disease. Martini et al.[25] reported 75 of these relatively uncommon stage II patients. Of these, 47 were men and 28 were women (1.7/1.0) (Table 3-5). Seventeen patients were T2, N1, M0 with 56 percent 5-year survival, and 58 were T2, N1, M0 with 48 percent 5-year survival. The 5-year survival rate overall with surgical excision plus external radiation therapy was 50 percent. More recently we have tried chemotherapy combined with radiation therapy in the hope that the 5-year survival rate will be improved.

We are not certain that the combination of chemotherapy and radiotherapy postoperatively can increase the 5-year survival rate in excess of 50 percent. Other attempts to use this treatment have not resulted in a higher survival rate.

STAGE III

The stage III group of patients makes up a large percentage of the individuals with lung cancer. Since no more than 30 percent of our more recent

Table 3-5. Results of Treating N1 Lung Cancer[a]

Tumor Type	Male	Female	Total Patients
Adenocarcinoma	20	18	38
Epidermoid Carcinoma	26	10	36
Large Cell Cancer	1	0	1
Total Patients	47	28	75

[a] Overall 49 percent five-year survival: 17 T1, N1, M0 (56 percent) and 58 T2, N1, M0 (48 percent).

(From Martini et al.,[25] with permission.)

patients have stage I and 5 percent have stage II cancer, 65 percent are in stages III and IV. If chest x-rays are obtained more frequently, a larger number of these patients will be found in stage III than in stage IV with metastases outside the chest.

Stage III has recently been subdivided into stage IIIa and stage IIIb. The "a" group in general is believed to have a better chance for "cure" and 5-year survival than the "b" group, in which disease is more difficult to control. The main feature of the stage III group is that all patients are M0 with no known metastases outside the chest and no metastases in the contralateral lung. The latter condition is unusual in our experience unless there is a considerable amount of gross disease in the mediastinum. In the group of patients with M0 disease who are classified as stage III there is a T3 group in which either the tumor is less than 2.0 cm from the carina or more than one lobe or the parietal pleura is involved. All of these are potentially removable for cure and are classified as T3. Provided that there are no metastases to mediastinal lymph nodes or only to hilar lymph nodes, the staging T3, N0, M0 or T3, N1, M0 represent a potentially curable stage IIIa tumor. Surgical excision, which might be lobectomy or pneumonectomy with or without chest wall resection, should be done. With surgical excision, chest wall involvement alone with no involvement of lymph nodes is associated with a 5-year survival rate in the 30 to 40 percent range.[26,27] The individual with chest wall involvement who also has hilar or mediastinal lymph nodes involved drops to a much worse classification, with a 5-year survival rate in the range of 5 percent.

There was a time when it was thought that N2 involvement was not surgically curable. Curability depends on the extent of N2 involvement and the facility with which the tumor can be surgically dissected. In 1983 Martini et al.[28] reported a series of 151 patients with N2 disease selected from a consecutive group of 1,598 lung cancer patients of whom 706 had N2 disease; 151 of these cancers could be surgically removed. In this group of patients 90 percent received postoperative radiation therapy. Twenty-seven percent of these 151 patients were alive and well 8 years later despite N2 disease (Fig. 3-6). Although the majority of these patients had disease in the lymph nodes, they did not have gross widening of the mediastinum and did not have extensive mediastinal lymph node metastases. The majority of these 151 patients had adenocarcinomas. Until then, patients with adenocarcinomas in lymph nodes were given a

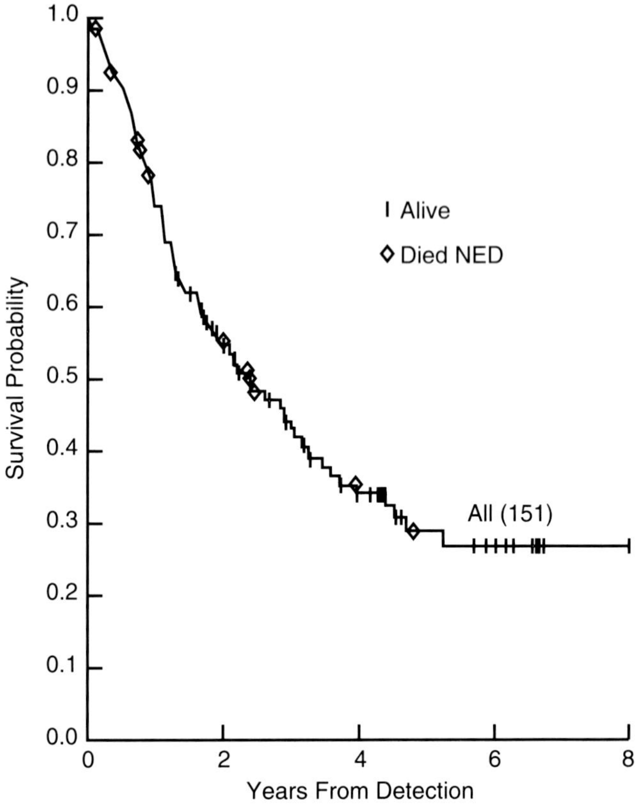

Fig. 3-6. Survival curve in N2 resected lung tumors, as reported by Martini et al. in 1983. NED, no evidence of disease. (From Martini et al.,[25] with permission.)

grave prognosis. We found no significant difference in the survival of these N2 patients by cell type (Fig. 3-7).

The gross involvement of the mediastinal lymph nodes in N2 disease and especially if the lymph node involvement has extended above the clavicle to the prescalene area (N3) or if the lymph node involvement has extended across the midline to the contralateral side of the mediastinum (also N3) places the patient in the stage IIIb category, where the chances of cure after surgical excision become poor. It is in this group of patients particularly that neoadjuvant treatment has come into vogue. Neoadjuvant treatment began with preoperative chemotherapy. More recently it has been augmented to combine chemotherapy with radiotherapy in the chemotherapy-radiotherapy "sandwich" used preoperatively in the neoadjuvant setting. The routine use of a CT scan of the chest for patients with lung cancer has been helpful in identifying enlarged hilar and mediastinal lymph nodes. In stage III patients we wish to have lymph nodes sampled if enlarged nodes are found. If one does

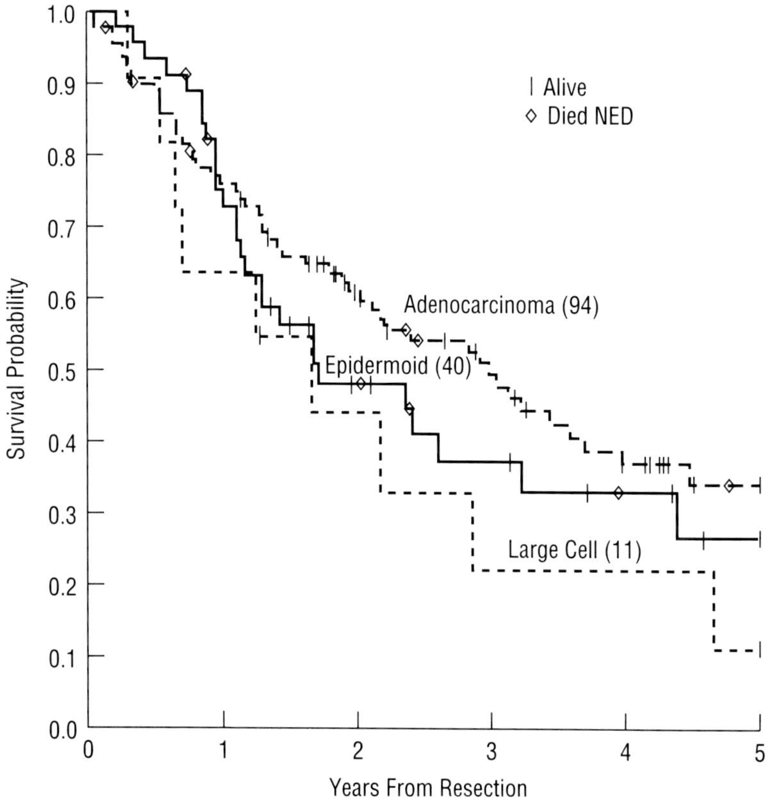

Fig. 3-7. Survival from resection of N2 lung cancer by cell type, as reported by Martini et al. in 1983. NED, no evidence of disease. (From Martini et al.,[25] with permission.)

not know with certainty the status of the mediastinal lymph nodes in advance, it is difficult to evaluate the efficacy and the indications for the use of the neoadjuvant chemotherapy-radiotherapy. We try to do transbronchial needle biopsy before resorting to either a mediastinoscopy or a mediastinotomy. If N2 disease can be demonstrated our current practice is to give the patient two cycles of the chemotherapy-radiotherapy sandwich (see Chemotherapy). After that we reevaluate the patient. It is essential to know the status of the brain CT scan and the bone scan. The CT scan of the chest should include the liver and the region of the adrenal glands. If these seem clear, and especially if there has been a response to treatment by chemotherapy-radiotherapy, these stage III patients are considered eligible for surgical exploration. In our recent experience 60 to 75 percent of non-small cell lung cancer patients will have an improvement in their status with this neoadjuvant treatment. A majority of these are minor (25 percent) or partial (50 percent) responses. With chemotherapy-radiotherapy we have seen complete responses in 25 percent of the patients.[29–32]

If, at the end of two cycles of chemotherapy-radiotherapy, there has been no improvement and the situation still seems formidable, or if the disease has extended outside the thorax, a third cycle of chemotherapy-radiotherapy is given. Another alternative if it is believed that the tumor cannot be completely removed is to use internal radiotherapy with permanent implantation of I-125 seeds and/or the combination of temporary afterloading radiotherapy with the placement of catheters for iridium-192 (Ir-192) therapy.

In 1985 Hilaris et al.[32] reported our preliminary experience in treating 100 stage IIIa and IIIb patients with surgical exploration, surgical resection, and internal radiotherapy supplemented by postoperative external radiotherapy (Fig. 3-8). Approximately half of these patients were stage IIIa and half were stage IIIb. The overall results were that 22 of the 100 patients were alive and well, seemingly free of disease, 4 to 8 years after treatment. The survival rate was 30 percent in the stage IIIa and 12 percent in the stage IIIb groups (Fig. 3-9). In this group of patients chemotherapy was not used. This represented the best efforts of surgery plus combined internal-external radiation therapy. In approximately 75 percent of the patients, regardless of whether they were stage IIIa or IIIb, the thoracic tumor was controlled for the life of the patient. The recurrent disease that caused death was primarily disease outside the chest. It is

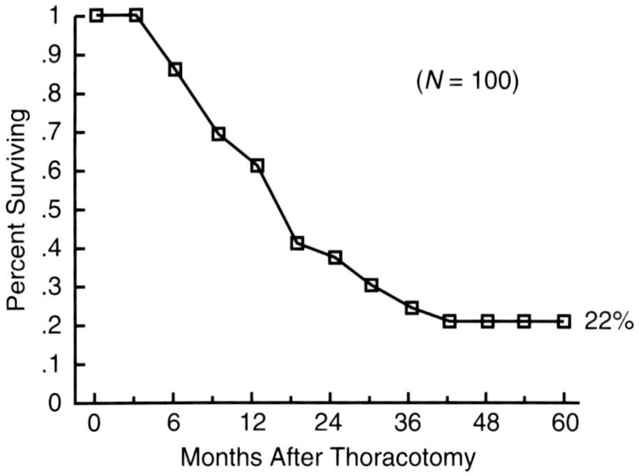

Fig. 3-8. Survival of 100 patients staged IIIa and IIIb whose therapy combined surgery with internal and external radiation. (From Hilaris et al.,[32] with permission.)

not known yet whether the neoadjuvant chemotherapy-radiotherapy in these stage IIIa and IIIb patients will be successful in decreasing the number of deaths from metastases outside the chest (M1 disease).

A worsening of the T factor produces T4 lung cancer. In these situations the extent or location of the tumor is such that it is thought that the tumor cannot be removed successfully for cure or long-term survival. A classic example is the malignant pleural effusion in which the tumor has spread over the parietal and visceral pleura. Fluid is produced, and usually there are more implants on the parietal pleura than on the visceral pleura. This extent of disease makes cure by surgery highly unlikely if not impossible.

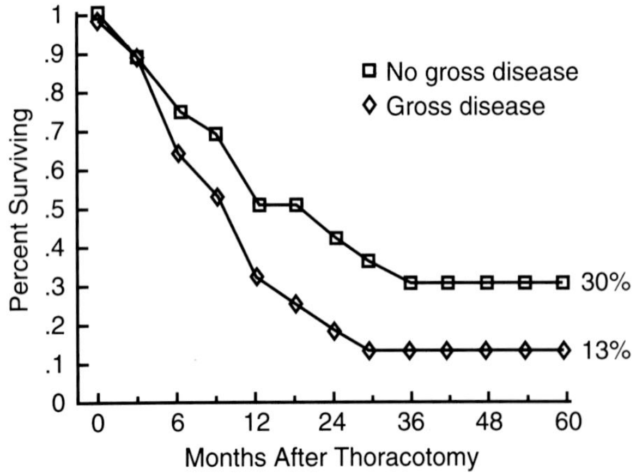

Fig. 3-9. Survival of 100 patients treated with surgery and internal and external radiation and reported by gross disease or as gross disease left after surgical resection. (From Hilaris et al.,[32] with permission.)

There are other examples of T4 disease, such as some tumors in the superior sulcus location. Tumors in this location have a tendency to expand into the neck rather than metastasizing to hilar lymph nodes. Only some 15 percent of superior sulcus carcinomas are associated with hilar lymph node metastases.[33] Involvement of the stellate ganglion with a Horner syndrome and erosion of ribs in the chest wall with resulting pain are frequent. At times the brachial plexus is directly involved with tumor. The tumor may invade the spine itself. It is possible in some circumstances to excise these spinal tumors by performing laminectomies in collaboration with neurosurgeons and removing en bloc the tumor, the costospinal articulation with the pedicles, transverse processes, and bodies of vertebra (Fig. 3-10).[34] Ordinarily it is not considered valuable to resect more than the lowest cord of the brachial plexus since it would result in a flail arm or loss of the extremity. This is an area where preoperative radiation therapy combined with internal radiotherapy in a certain number of cases can be beneficial.[32,35–38] The pain can be controlled, and at times the tumor can be "cured" or controlled for prolonged periods. Some patients with tumors in the superior sulcus location with some brachial plexus involvement and Horner syndrome may do well with external radiation therapy alone. These tumors occupy a small volume, and

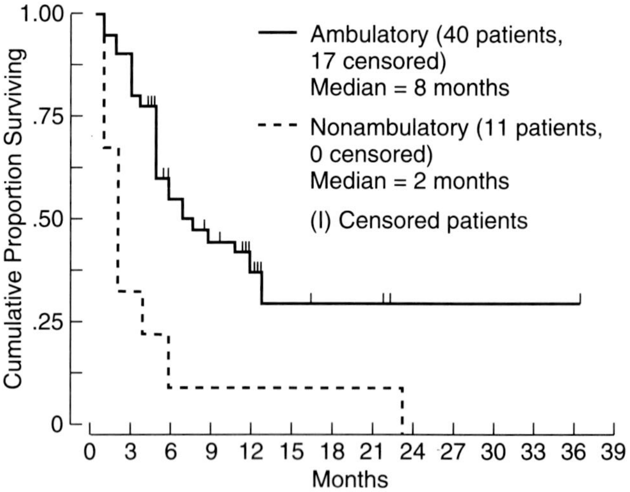

Fig. 3-10. Survival analysis following treatment of lung cancer by spine resection. The difference in survival between patients who were ambulatory following surgery and those who were nonambulatory is statistically significant ($P < 0.01$). (From Sundaresan et al.,[34] with permission.)

radiation can be relatively intense while sparing the spinal cord.

T4 tumors may also grow through the pulmonary veins and grow inside the left atrium. It is possible in some cases to resect part of the left atrium with or without cardiopulmonary bypass. A minority of the patients may benefit and have prolonged periods of control. The intrapericardial pneumonectomy is useful to treat these and other extensive lesions. Tumors that involve the pericardium and the pulmonary veins may be resectable for cure. The T4 classification is usually reserved for involvement of part of the heart that is not readily excised.

At times the tumor may involve the tracheal carina or the trachea itself. This would be considered a T4 lesion. Modern techniques of "sleeve resections" in which one can resect the lung and carina and reapproximate the other lung onto the trachea by a variety of methods can be carried out. A minority of these patients do well.[39,40] One of the most serious complications of lung cancer in the T4 classification is tumor involvement of the superior vena cava. Most attempts to reconstruct the superior vena cava have not been successful. However, smaller pieces can be removed with success. This can be done by partially occluding the cava with a Satinsky clamp, which will permit removal and suturing. Another useful technique if one wishes to resect a piece of the superior vena cava without stenosis is to place a heart bypass venous drainage catheter in the right auricular appendage and pass it into the right innominate vein. The right and left innominate veins and the superior vena cava can be occluded with tapes around this internal shunt. With appropriate holes in the catheter, the cerebral venous drainage passes through this shunt into the right atrium. A sequestered area of the superior vena cava can be approached surgically, and a segment can be resected. If necessary it can be patched or replaced with an autologous vein graft. If there is full-blown superior vena caval syndrome, the disease is most often too extensive for mass resection of the superior vena cava. The survival rate of surgery for this syndrome is such that internal radiotherapy seeds, seed sutures, and afterloading catheters supplemented by external radiotherapy seem to be better palliation.[41]

Tumor invading the esophagus also warrants a T4 classification. In highly selected cases it might be valuable to resect a lung cancer with a portion of the esophagus. In most situations the tumor is so extensive that it is not practical to do so. Such a tumor involving the esophagus may result in a tracheoesophageal or bronchoesophageal fistula. If untreated, these patients have a survival time of about 1 month with aspiration pneumonias. There are certain selected fistula patients in whom a colon bypass can be used to defunctionalize the esophagus by closing the esophagus above the fistulous connection. When the colon interposition is placed connecting the stomach to the cervical esophagus, it is necessary to ligate the cardia to prevent regurgitation of gastric contents into the esophagus from below. The fistulous connection to the airway persists, but the patient can tolerate the small amount of esophageal secretion. External radiation therapy can be used postoperatively for tumor control for a time. These patients, if they survive the procedure, are more comfortable without the constant cough that is caused by a fistula. They can continue to eat and drink normally for the remainder of their lives. In poor-risk patients an internal stent may be placed to block the fistula, with some comfort and palliation.

STAGE IV

In stage IV patients the deciding factor is the presence of metastases outside the chest. The patient is classified as M1. If there are metastases into the opposite lung the classification is M1. If there are metastases from one lobe to the other lobe in the same lung, this is also considered M1. One must be careful in applying the M1 stage to lung lesions, as the occurrence of simultaneous double primaries is not uncommon. The experience of the lung cancer study group and others[42] in stage I patients who had undergone resection for potential cure found an incidence of new second primaries at the rate of 3 percent per year. Thus in a 5-year follow-up period, approximately 15 percent of the patients had new tumors. Our 115 stage I lung cancers[23] had 33 (29 percent) multiple primary cancers. A mistake that is not infrequent in the cancer patient is to call a new cancer metastatic disease. One must be careful not to do this. It is better and safer for the patient involved to assume that subsequent cancer may be a new and separate cancer. The cancer patient is prone to get cancer.

The question is whether metastases from lung cancer can be cured. The most common form of distant metastasis in the lung cancer patient is metastasis to the brain. Most of these metastases are multiple. If there are multiple brain metastases, it is ordinarily impractical to remove these lesions, and these patients are treated with whole-brain radiation therapy. However, long-term survival is possible in lung cancer patients who have solitary brain metastases that are accessible to surgical removal. If a solitary lesion is found in the brain on a CT scan of the head, it should be evaluated by a neurosurgeon to determine whether it can be removed safely. If the tumor is removable, if the patient is a relatively good surgical risk, and if the primary lung cancer is apparently controlled or controllable, it is worthwhile to remove the brain lesion. Since the brain metastasis usually is more of a pressing matter than the primary lung tumor, these patients are usually started on steroid therapy. The neurosurgeon is encouraged to remove the lesion by a craniotomy by careful enucleation of the tumor mass. This is followed by whole-brain radiation therapy, usually on the order of 4,500 rads of radiotherapy with continued steroid protection.[43,44]

The chest lesion can be treated after the brain lesion has been taken care of. Treatment depends upon the stage of disease. Some patients have brain metastases with stage I and stage II disease, although the majority of patients with metastases have stage III disease in the chest. The magnetic resonance imaging (MRI) brain scan is particularly helpful in the early diagnosis of brain metastases, since metastasis is usually detectable in the MRI some time ahead of the CT scan.

In 1985 Sundaresan and Galicich[45] reported on 125 patients with solitary brain metastases who underwent surgery (Table 3-6). Fifty of these had lung cancer primary tumors. In approximately half

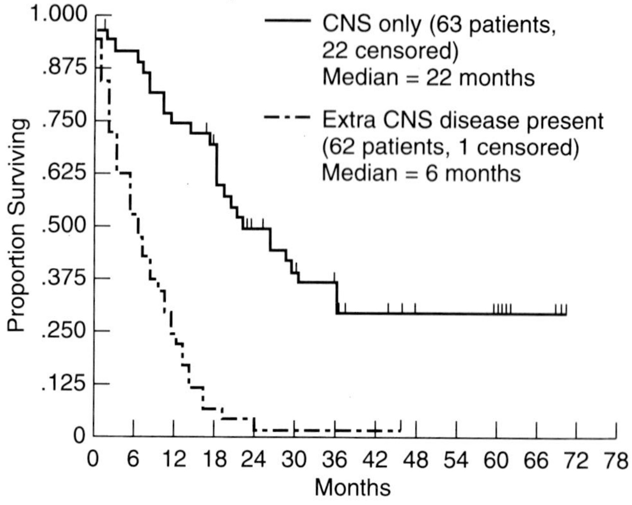

Fig. 3-11. Survival by extent of systemic disease. CNS, central nervous system. (From Sundaresan and Gralicich,[44] with permission.)

of the patients, the primary tumor was controlled. In this group of patients with the brain metastasis removed and the primary tumor controlled, the 6-year survival rate was 27 percent (Fig. 3-11). A series of patients was reported from the Henry Ford Hospital,[46] where lung cancer patients with solitary metastases were treated with appropriate surgery. There was a 22 percent 5-year survival rate after treatment of both lesions. These results are better than the results with whole-brain radiation therapy alone.

Should multiple brain metastases be resected? This would depend on the status and the wishes of

Table 3-6. Clinical Parameters by Primary Site of Tumor in 125 Patients

		Distribution				Neurologic Grade		
Primary Site	Total	Supra-	Infra-	Early Onset	CNS Only	I	II	III
Lung	50 (40%)	47	3	35	30	17	23	10
Skin (melanoma)	14 (11.2%)	13	1	2	5	3	7	4
Kidney	14 (11.2%)	10	4	5	7	4	8	2
Colon	10 (8.0%)	7	3	3	2	1	7	2
Soft-part sarcoma	10 (8.0%)	7	3	2	4	2	4	4
Breast	8 (6.4%)	7	1	3	6	5	3	0
Unknown primary site	6 (4.8%)	4	2	3	3	2	3	1
Miscellaneous	13 (10.4%)	11	2	9	6	3	8	2

Abbreviations: Supra-, supratentorial; Infra-, infratentorial; CNS, central nervous system; CNS only: disease limited to CNS. (From Sundaresan and Galicich,[44] with permission.)

the patient and the accessibility of the lesions. We believe that superior palliation may be achieved but have no 5-year survivors.

Treatment of other systemic metastases has been tried, but with little success. Solitary bone lesions should be diagnosed by a needle biopsy. One would be hesitant to do major excisions of long bones for metastases. Many of these metastases require pinning of the bone so that pathologic fractures do not occur. At that time a combination of cryotherapy to freeze the tumor followed by external radiation therapy can give prolonged benefit. Bone metastatic lesions tend to be multiple rather than solitary.

The adrenal gland is an area where solitary metastases may appear outside the chest. We have resected a few, but unfortunately we have no prolonged survivals because other metastases appeared later. Investigation should continue. Future development of better neoadjuvant therapy could change this picture.

SMALL CELL LUNG CANCER

It is estimated that 20 percent of the lung cancer seen annually in the United States is small cell lung cancer (Table 3-7).

On rare occasions small cell lung cancer presents as a coin lesion shadow in the lung, with no evidence of any enlargement of mediastinal lymph nodes or disease elsewhere. These tumors should be treated as any other coin lesion cancer, by appropriate resection. Lobectomy should be performed in patients with satisfactory risk factors, and the mediastinal lymph nodes should be removed for staging purposes. If there is no apparent involvement of the lymph nodes by small cell lung cancer it is still generally recommended that these patients receive postoperative chemotherapy for a significant length of time. These rare lesions have 5-year survival rates greater than 50 percent.[47]

Unfortunately, most small cell lung cancer is considerably more advanced when diagnosed. The next stage of small cell lung cancer is that which is advanced in the chest but with no evidence of disease outside the chest is staged as limited disease (LD). In this group of patients chemotherapy is the first line of attack. There is still some controversy about the potential role of surgery in treating this condition. In good-risk patients in whom the primary lesion is localized to a lobe and it seems that a lobectomy would be well tolerated, we have favored carrying out a lobectomy after the chemotherapy has produced a satisfactory response. Then, since the primary tumor has been excised, the follow-up of external radiation therapy to the mediastinum can be given without the need for radiation of the primary part in the lung. The alternative is not to remove the primary lesion in the lung but, after an appropriate course of chemotherapy, to use radiation therapy to the mediastinum and to the appropriate lung in a pattern that will cover all of the known disease.

At any rate, this aggressive approach of chemotherapy-external radiotherapy or chemotherapy, surgery, and external radiotherapy in a small number of limited-disease small cell lung cancer

Table 3-7. Primary Lung Cancer

Parameter	NSCLC	SCLC	Bronchial Carcinoids	Adenoidcystic Carcinoids	Mucoepidermoid Carcinoma
Incidence	80% of lung cancer (120,000/yr)	20% of lung cancer (30,000/yr)	1–2% of lung cancer	Rare	Rare
Sex	M : F = 2 : 1	M : F = 2 : 1	M = F	M = F	M = F
Age (yr)	60s	60s	Childhood to 50s	30–65	40–50s
Location	Adenocarcinoma: peripheral Epidermoid: central	Mostly central	Central	Central	Central
Growth	Variable, 40% slow	Usually rapid	Slow	Slow	Slow
Curability	Good for stage I, poor for advanced	Usually advanced and poor	Usually good	Moderate	Moderate

Abbreviations: NSCLC, non-small cell lung carcinoma; SCLC, small cell lung carcinoma; M, male; F, female.

will produce 5-year survival rates of about 20 to 30 percent.[48] There is a significant mortality rate from the aggressive chemotherapy-radiotherapy. Again, the major fear is that these patients will develop brain metastases at some point. It is thought that in this group of small cell lung cancer patients with limited disease who are treated for potential cure and who are doing well, one should use prophylactic whole-brain irradiation to forestall any subsequent injury or death from the brain metastases.[49] As these modalities improve, it is hoped that more and more of the limited-disease small cell lung cancer patients will be saved.

Unfortunately a significant number of small cell lung cancer patients have extensive disease when first seen. In these circumstances the disease frequently involves the bone marrow and the brain. Here the treatment again is aggressive chemotherapy with appropriate radiation therapy to the brain and mediastinum or any other symptomatic area that has not been controlled or palliated with the chemotherapy. In general the survival rate in this disease is poor.

Johnson et al.[50] at the National Cancer Institute studied 252 patients with small cell lung cancer. Thirteen percent survived free of cancer for 2 years or more, 5 percent survived for 10 years free of cancer, and 10 patients were alive and free of cancer more than 10 years after the original treatment. These patients were treated with combination chemotherapy with or without radiation from 1973 to 1978.

BRONCHIAL CARCINOID

In 1972 Turnbull et al. reported a group of bronchial carcinoids in patients at the Memorial Sloan-Kettering Cancer Center.[51] They listed 44 patients with bronchial carcinoids, 5 patients with adenoid cystic carcinoma, and 12 patients with mucoepidermoid carcinoma (Tables 3-8 and 3-9). In this particular series 59 percent of the patients with bronchial carcinoid, 60 percent of the patients with adenoid cystic carcinoma, and none of the patients with mucoepidermoid carcinoma survived for 5 years. This strongly indicated that these tumors, especially in the stage when we saw them, had a serious prognosis. Clearly they should be called by their appropriate proper names and the inclusive former term of bronchial adenoma be abandoned.

PULMONARY METASTASES

Surgery for pulmonary metastases for cure was first reported in the United States by Barney and Churchill in 1939.[52] Churchill had performed a right middle lobe lobectomy for what was thought to be a primary lung tumor. The pathology report indicated that the tumor in the right middle lobe was metastatic from the kidney. A nephrectomy was subsequently done, and the patient lived for 23 years. Thoracic surgeons then began to treat individuals with solitary pulmonary metastases if the primary tumor was controlled or controllable. Relatively large series[53] were reported, and the long-term survival rate was in the range of 35 percent for both metastatic carcinoma and metastatic sarcoma.

Our own interest in the treatment of pulmonary metastases came to focus on multiple pulmonary metastases in the lungs of children with osteosarcoma. Marcove et al.[54] had reported 145 osteosarcomas that had occurred in the extremities of patients under 21 years of age who were treated by amputation with hope for cure. Only 17 percent of these patients were alive and well 5 years postoperatively. The others developed pulmonary metastases, which were untreated in those days, and soon died. Of those individuals not cured by amputation, 95 percent were dead within 3 years of the amputation.

In 1965, at Marcove's suggestion, we began an aggressive surgical approach to these patients with pulmonary metastases. In 1971, Martini et al.[55] reported our experience in 28 patients. In 22 it was possible to remove all the pulmonary metastases. After 3 years, instead of a 5 percent survival rate in the untreated pulmonary metastases group, we found a 45 percent 3-year survival rate if the pulmonary metastases had been removed, even if multiple bilateral thoracotomies were required. Of the 22 patients reported at that time, only 6 had a solitary metastasis. At the time of our report in 1971, these 22 patients had had 58 thoracotomies ranging from one to six thoracotomies per patient.

In a 20-year follow-up report by Beattie et al.[56] one patient had no evidence of disease and was lost to follow-up after 10 years. One patient had died of the consequences of a new osteosarcoma in the opposite knee, 16 years after the first primary knee tumor. A third patient was well at 22 years; a fourth patient was well at more than 23 years and was also well after a new histiocytic lymphoma of

Table 3-8. Clinical Findings in 59 Patients at Hospital Admission for Bronchial Adenoma, Memorial Sloan-Kettering Cancer Center, 1926–1969

	Type of Neoplasm		
Clinical Finding	Carcinoid (44 patients)	Adenoid Cystic (5 patients)	Mucoepidermoid (12 patients)
Hepatomegaly	3	—	4
Pneumonia	7	1	—
Bone metastases	—	—	4
Hemiparesis	—	—	2
Aphasia	—	—	1
Visual field defect	—	—	1
Digital clubbing	—	1	2
Superior vena cava obstruction	—	—	1
Vocal cord paralysis	1	—	2
Diaphragm paralysis	—	—	1
Horner's syndrome	—	—	1
Empyema	1	—	—
Bronchiectasis	1	—	—
Lymphadenopathy	2	—	—
Cutaneous metastases	—	1	—
Pleural effusion	1	—	—

(From Turnbull et al.,[51] with permission.)

the mediastinum that had been found 9 years previously. A fifth patient was free of osteosarcoma 24 years after amputation only to succumb to a breast carcinoma 2.5 years after diagnosis. The final patient had survived hemipelvectomy and six thoracotomies with 33 metastases resected and then had 10 months of chemotherapy. She was well from 3 until 17 years postamputation. She then developed recurrent osteosarcoma in the right upper lobe 14 years after her chemotherapy. She had a repeat excision of the metastatic disease but ultimately died of disease almost 20 years posthemipelvectomy. The 10-year survival of our patients with bilateral pulmonary metastases from osteosarcoma was 27 percent, and the 15-year survival was probably also 27 percent. However, at 20 years one patient had died of a new osteosarcoma and another of recurrent osteosarcoma. One patient

Table 3-9. Age and Sex Distribution of 61 Patients with Bronchial Adenoma, Memorial Sloan-Kettering Cancer Center, 1926–1969

Type of Neoplasm	Average Age and Range (yr)	Sex
Carcinoid	49 (22–73)	22 M/22 F
Adenoid cystic carcinoma	47 (40–53)	4 M/1 F
Mucoepidermoid carcinoma	59 (49–69)	9 M/3 F

Abbreviations: M, male; F, female.
(From Turnbull et al.,[51] with permission.)

had died of breast carcinoma and another had survived a second malignant tumor, histiocytic lymphoma. The fifth patient was well and the sixth patient, lost to follow-up.[57]

This experience demonstrates the inadequacy of the 5-year follow-up and shows why tumor registries and follow-up of patients with cancer should be continued for life. This appears to be especially true in pediatric patients, who normally would have a long life span. These patients appear to be at increased risk. Cancer centers should monitor their pediatric cancer patients indefinitely.

We found from these patients that the sarcoma metastases to the lung did not metastasize to mediastinal lymph nodes. Instead, they grew locally and, if not removed, could metastasize outside the chest via the systemic circulation. Additionally, they tend to be located on the surface of the segment involved. It is therefore important to treat the tumors before they have grown through the visceral pleura, where they can develop pleural effusions (frequently bloody), which makes cure more unlikely. These tumors invade blood vessels and it is important to remember that they may grow through the pulmonary veins inside the heart. We have seen two such patients, both of whom died of this complication.

The carcinoma metastases to the lung, conversely, can metastasize to hilar and mediastinal lymph nodes. It is important, therefore, that these lesions, especially if they are multiple, be removed promptly. Otherwise, if multiple lymph nodes are involved bilaterally, cure from local resection becomes highly doubtful.

When operating on a patient with a presumed solitary carcinoma metastasis, one should do a cancer operation. That is, one should do a segmentectomy or lobectomy and the hilar lymph nodes and mediastinal lymph nodes should be removed for staging and for treatment. One has to be careful at the time of surgery to remove a solitary pulmonary metastasis for carcinoma not to be misled by a frozen section report that the carcinoma is metastatic. The pathology report may be changed, and the final report may identify a new lung carcinoma that could have been inadequately treated by wedge excision.

DIAGNOSIS

If a patient has had a malignant tumor and then is found by chest x-ray to have multiple lesions, the supposition that this represents pulmonary metastases is reasonable. However, metastases must be confirmed by tissue diagnosis. A "solitary metastasis" is more difficult to prove, and it is better to presume that there are two separate diseases until proven otherwise. Either way, it is important that physicians as well as thoracic surgeons know that patients with multiple or solitary metastases can be cured if the metastases can all be removed. The criteria for surgical treatment of metastases have been constant for decades.

The overwhelming majority of metastases are asymptomatic when found. Symptomatic metastases tend to be of a late stage and not curable. Routine chest x-rays should be used to screen for metastases; waiting for symptoms to appear is not recommended.

The use of routine posteroanterior and lateral chest x-rays taken frequently, i.e., every 2 to 3 months has been the standard way of detecting pulmonary metastases after treatment of a primary tumor or of pulmonary metastases themselves. One should remember that a lesion must be almost 1.0 cm in diameter to be seen in a routine posteroanterior and lateral chest x-ray. Once a lung lesion or lesions have been seen, it is customary to get a CT scan of the chest. Lesions as small as 3 mm can be detected by CT scan, but approximately half the time the lesions found are not tumors. Additionally, tumor seedings of 1 to 2 mm in size that can readily be felt by the surgeon at thoracotomy are not seen even in the CT scan. The tomogram that we formerly used is now seldom employed. It is able to detect lesions of a size intermediate between those seen on the CT scan, which is more sensitive, and those seen on a standard chest x-ray, which is less so.[57–59]

After all of the metastatic tumors have been surgically removed, it is valuable to have a new baseline CT scan of the chest taken 1 to 2 months postoperatively.

Ordinarily the primary tumor is found and treated before the metastases occur. This is particularly true if the metastases are multiple. Occasionally the metastasis or metastases are found before the primary source.[52] However, if the metastases are multiple, the primary source should be sought.

The chief difficulty occurs when there is a solitary lung lesion synchronous with a primary tumor elsewhere. Here there may be two separate primary tumors instead of one primary tumor with one lung metastasis. If this occurs, the more serious lesion is treated first. One example would be the patient who has a new primary tumor in the lung and also seemingly has a new primary colorectal tumor. Another example would be the patient who is discovered to have a probable brain metastasis associated with a coin lesion or some other symptomatic lesion in the chest that is presumably consistent with a primary lung cancer.

FACTORS AFFECTING SURVIVAL

The most important factor affecting survival is the complete removal of all metastases.

The tumor-free interval (TFI) has been calculated.[60] Theoretically, the longer the time until the development of metastases the better, but we (with Mountain) have not found this somewhat controversial question to be a very significant factor. Also, statistics mean less in one patient.

The tumor doubling time (TDT)[61] is an attempt to estimate whether the metastases double every 20, 20 to 40, or more than 40 days. According to Joseph et al.,[61] if tumors double in under 20 days surgical cure is unlikely, but if they double in more than 40 days surgical cure is much more likely. Generally, rapidly growing tumors are more serious, but we have seen numerous individual exceptions and believe that it is not a rule to be universally applied.

As adjuvant therapy, ordinarily chemotherapy is effective. When successful chemotherapy is available, pulmonary metastases may be prevented, or they become more curable with or without surgery. In treating multiple pulmonary metastases, conventional external radiotherapy has little role. However, if one or two metastases are not too large (well under 6 cm) but so located that removal would be too destructive, internal radiotherapy can be used with some hope for prolonged survival.[38]

SURGICAL APPROACH

In our original bilateral thoracotomies, we used left and right lateral approaches. An advance has been the use of the median sternotomy,[62–64] which permits metastases to be removed from both lungs during one operation. We concur with the opinion that if the lesions are not too numerous, there is an advantage for the patient in approaching these lesions by median sternotomy. Clearly a persistent attack on the tumors is worthwhile. Our present indication for operating on pulmonary metastases is the meeting of these four criteria:

1. The patient must be able to withstand the surgery planned.
2. It must be possible to remove all of the metastases at operation.
3. The primary tumor must be controlled or controllable.
4. There is no other treatment available that offers a chance for cure.

With these criteria, we have seen over the years a changing picture in the treatment of pulmonary metastases. Metastatic germ cell tumors from the testes have responded to chemotherapy for cure.[65] The same is true for metastases from choriocarcinoma of the uterus.[66] Osteosarcoma has responded to chemotherapy.[67] It is to be hoped that more advances such as this will make surgical removal of more pulmonary metastases unnecessary.

However, with chemotherapeutic successes a new problem arises if there is a persistent shadow in the lung. After control of a metastatic testicular tumor, it may be necessary to remove the shadow for diagnostic purposes. Metastatic germ cell tumors can differentiate back into benign teratomas. They still continue to grow, and they require surgical removal.[66]

There has been great improvement in the control of osteosarcomas. As chemotherapy improved, the approach changed to tumor biopsy, followed by neoadjuvant chemotherapy. After establishing the sensitivity of the tumor to chemotherapy, the primary tumor in the extremity was resected, hopefully avoiding limb amputation. Any metastases that are apparent or become visible in the lung by chest x-ray or CT scan are removed surgically. The chemotherapy is continued or modified. If the lung lesions have persisted or grown in spite of the chemotherapy this is a warning to the medical oncologist to try to strengthen the chemotherapy protocol. However, since osteosarcomas can contain bone, one cannot tell by x-ray whether there is active tumor or "tombstones" present. Operation is required to inform the medical oncologist of whether it is safe to stop the chemotherapy. Marcove, a bone tumor surgeon, and Rosen, a pediatric oncologist, played a key role in developing this program that took childhood osteosarcoma from a 17 percent cure with amputation to an 80 percent "cure" usually with limb preservation.[67]

At operation for sarcoma a wedge excision with clear margins suffices for treatment. The surgeon must be as sparing as possible in preserving lung parenchyma when multiple pulmonary metastases are present. This can be done with a stapling device or by hand suturing (see Atlas section for details). At times we have used the electrocautery when lesions were small and numerous.[57]

Metastases tend to exist at the periphery of the pulmonary segment involved. If they are near the visceral pleura, they are simple to treat. If they are deep in the lung parenchyma, treatment is more complicated. At times one can open the intersegmental plane to excise deeply situated lesions. Otherwise a cone excision may have to be done with the electrocautery or laser.

McCormack and Martini have followed the pulmonary metastases resected at Memorial Sloan Kettering Cancer Center.[66] In 1979 they listed the sites of primary tumors in 448 patients (Table 3-10). They reported the thoracotomies per patient (Table 3-11). There were more thoracotomies per patient in the sarcomas. The number of thoracotomies varied from 1 to 10 per patient. In two of my personal patients there were 12. The case study of one of these patients, B.J.B., is presented in Chapter 10. He survived a total of 23 years. Table 3-12 lists McCormack's reported 5-year survival in patients with carcinomas. The rate varied from colon carcinoma at 14 percent to testis carcinoma at 51 percent. Since surgery for testis pulmonary metastases has been markedly decreased by successful chemotherapy, head and neck cancers at 47 percent now head the list for success. The 5-year survival for sarcoma metastases (Table 3-13) was just under 30 percent, except for neurosarcomas (18 percent).

McCormack et al. have continued to update the Memorial Sloan Kettering series of pulmonary metastases.[57,58] In 1989 they reported 208 sarcomas metastatic to the lungs treated from 1960 to 1983[57] (Table 3-14). This excludes the osteosarcomas, which have been collected separately. The 5-year survival rate was 29 percent for synovial sarcomas, 27 percent for leiomyosarcomas, 21 percent for fibrosarcomas, and 20 percent for the remainder. The operative mortality rate remained at 2 percent.

In 1991 McCormack and Martini reported 397 carcinomas metastatic to the lung[58] seen from 1960 to 1984 (Table 3-15). In this time interval colon and rectum cancer had become a more common source of the pulmonary metastases in the series treated. The survival rate in the colorectal metastases group is affected by the Duke classification in which the primary tumor is better for A and least good for C. The present 5-year survival rate for the colorectal metastases to the lung treated in the McCormack series is now approximately 30 percent (P. McCormack: personal communication, 1992).

We conclude that it is reasonable that in rela-

Table 3-10. Presentation of Pulmonary Metastases in 448 Patients

Type of Metastasis	Carcinoma	Sarcoma
Unilateral solitary	138	66
Bilateral solitary	3	5
Unilateral multiple	73	77
Bilateral multiple	32	54
Total	246	202

(From McCormack and Martini,[66] with permission.)

Table 3-11. Number of Thoracotomies per Patient[a]

Thoracotomies/patient	Carcinoma	Sarcoma	Total
1	200	107	307
2	39	63	204
3	4	17	63
4	2	11	52
5	—	1	5
6	—	2	12
10	1	2	20

[a] 663 Thoracotomies in 448 patients; 298 in 246 carcinoma patients (1.2/patient); 355 in 202 sarcoma patients (1.75/patient).

(From McCormack and Martini,[66] with permission.)

Table 3-12. Five-Year Survival Rate by Site of Disease in Patients with Carcinoma

Site of Disease	5-Year Survival Rate (%)
Testis	51
Head and neck	47
Breast	30
Renal	28
Melanoma	19
Colon	14

(From McCormack and Martini,[66] with permission.)

Table 3-13. Five-Year Survival Rate by Cell Type in Patients with Sarcoma

Cell Type	5-Year Survival Rate (%)
Synovial sarcoma	29
Fibrosarcoma	21
Neurofibrosarcoma	18
Osteosarcoma	25
Leiomyosarcoma	27

(From McCormack and Martini,[66] with permission.)

Table 3-14. Resection of Metastatic Soft Tissue Sarcoma in Lung, Memorial Sloan-Kettering Cancer Center, 1960–1983

Soft Tissue Sarcoma	Number of Patients
Synovial sarcoma	38
Leiomyosarcoma	38
Malignant fibrous histiocytoma	21
Fibrosarcoma	19
Rhabdomyosarcoma	17
Malignant peripheral nerve tumor	15
Liposarcoma	14
Spindle cell sarcoma	12
Alveolar soft part sarcoma	11
Miscellaneous	23
Total	208

(From McCormack et al.,[57] with permission.)

tively healthy patients in whom the primary tumor is controlled or controllable and no other treatment is available, a very aggressive approach should be taken in removing both solitary and multiple metastases to the lung even if multiple surgical procedures are required.

RISK AND COMPLICATIONS OF SURGERY

The risk of surgery depends in large measure on the status of the patient, the stage of the tumor, and the extent of the procedure planned. It is important that the surgical team attempt to measure these factors in advance so that a risk/benefit ratio can be estimated.[68–70] It is this estimate that forms the basis of so-called good surgical judgment. Most otherwise healthy patients with a diagnosis of a growing lung cancer can be expected to die of their disease if untreated.[1] The survival time of the untreated patient is stage dependent. Generally the median survival of patients in stage III and stage IV is 6 months. Treated patients in these classifications tend to live longer than untreated patients. Surprisingly, some patients will be alive 5 years later.[25,29]

Table 3-15. Origin of Primary Carcinomas, 1960–1984

Site	Total
Colon and rectum	78
Testis	75
Melanoma	59
Breast	52
Head and neck	47
Kidney	41
Bladder	13
Uterus	10
Cervix	9
Lung	3
Ependymoma	1
Duodenum	2
Esophagus	1
Sweat gland	1
Ovary	4
Adrenal	1
Total	397

(From McCormack and Martini,[58] with permission.)

Patients who have major organ damage are at greater risk than "healthy" patients. Coronary artery disease, cardiac failure, and arrhythmias must be well evaluated and controlled prior to lung surgery. Liver disease such as cirrhosis may be a major contraindication. Renal failure may be hazardous. Lung impairment in particular must be evaluated, and the lung should be well prepared for an elective operation.

We usually quote our surgical risk of death from operation as the "30-day surgical mortality." This figure is largely a function of the condition of the patient and the severity of the surgical procedure. Most of our patients who are elderly and have smoked cigarettes for years are not good surgical risks. Pneumonectomies and esophagectomies are serious operations. Over the years and on the average, our mortality rate for thoracic surgery has been approximately 2 percent overall. This rate increases to 3 to 4 percent if patients are over the age of 70. A right pneumonectomy that removes 55 percent of the vascular bed and breathing capacity is worse than a left pneumonectomy. The mortality rate of a right pneumonectomy may be as high as 5 to 10 percent.[69–72]

PERIOPERATIVE PRECAUTIONS

Cigarette smoking should be stopped for a minimum of 1 week prior to surgery. Bronchial spasm and/or any lung infection must be controlled. Since patients tend to be terrified by the diagnosis of lung cancer, great attention must be paid to gaining the confidence of the patient and family. This requires compassionate, gentle honesty without conflicting statements that can only upset the patient more. The recommended treatment, the alternative treatment if any, the reasonable risks, and the course of events to expect are important issues to discuss with the patient. Frank presentation of this information tends to make the patient less tense and more cooperative.

It is important that the anesthetist evaluate the patient for problems with intubation. Intubation must be done with the patient awake if doing otherwise would be considered hazardous. Rarely a tracheostomy is needed. An available bronchoscope of the correct size is a necessary accessory for intubation of single-lumen tubes in difficult situations, and/or in the positioning of a double-lumen tube into the left main bronchus.[73,74]

We favor giving 24 hours of prophylactic antibiotics just before operation in most patients having pulmonary resections. Care must be taken to ascertain any past history of allergic reactions.

A true surgical adage is that there is no substitute for the correct operation done at the right time. Assuming that this has been done, we find a simple mnemonic valuable for the team to recite as the chest closure is begun. It is "A, B, C, D, E."

"A" is for air leak. Air leaks are looked for by filling the thorax with sterile water along with inflating the lung by the anesthetist. Any repairable air leak must be fixed.

"B" is for bleeding. In similar fashion, bleeding is looked for when the thorax is filled with clear water. The lung, pleura, intercostal vessels, mediastinal vessels, and rib ends all must be scrutinized. Bleeding must be controlled. In this day of human immunodeficiency virus (HIV) risk, transfusions are to be avoided. Blood loss should have been measured in the suction bottles and the weight gained from the use of dry sponges. If necessary, undue blood loss should be replaced. Autologous blood transfusion, up to 2 units, can be prepared in nonanemic patients having elective thoracotomies.

"C" is for collapse. The residual lung must be fully inflated, with no areas of atelectasis.

"D" is for drainage. Ordinarily two chest tubes are placed. They must be zigzagged in so that there will not be an open hole into the chest when the tubes are removed. The tip of one tube should be in the apex to drain air. One tube should have its bottom opening in the bottom of the chest to drain fluid. They should be sewn in with two sutures each.

E is for empty. There must be no sponges left in the chest, or tucked away anywhere under the chest wall or the incision. The sponge count must be done and must be correct. If not, a portable chest x-ray must immediately be taken while the chest is still open. After chest closure the chest tubes must be securely attached to the waterseal drainage.

Postoperatively one must first ensure that there is no bleeding and that respiration is adequate. Monitoring vital signs, watching chest tube drainage on an hourly basis, checking the hemoglobin, checking oximeters, and/or measuring the arterial blood levels, as well as getting a postoperative chest x-ray to be certain the lung is expanded without pneumothorax, hemothorax, or gastric dilatation, are all essential.

POSTOPERATIVE COMPLICATIONS: PREVENTION AND TREATMENT

PAIN AND ATELECTASIS

The first two important problems postoperatively are the control of pain and prevention of atelectasis. All thoracotomies hurt, and the two intercostal catheters aggravate the pain. If the pain is not relieved, the patient is uncomfortable, uncooperative, and unforgiving and is unable to cough or to move freely. Ten milligrams of morphine sulfate given every 4 hours intramuscularly is the standard for pain relief. It is the surgical team's responsibility to see that the pain is relieved. Analgesic dosage can be adjusted for size and condition or changed to smaller doses more frequently given such as 2.5 mg of morphine sulfate every hour (or given in an intravenous drip) until a safe comfort level is established. Patients tolerant to analgesics need higher doses. If pain is not relieved, higher doses are in order. If pain is relieved but relief is of short duration, more frequent medication is needed.

Analgesic agents administered through epidural catheters can help if done well and personally monitored by the anesthetist. However, epidermal catheters ordinarily are used only in intensive care locations. Nerve blocks or intrapleural installations of anesthetic agents can be used, but the pain must be relieved. Surgeons must be familiar with injected versus oral effectiveness of analgesic agents. Methadone is unique in that it is almost equally effective by injection or by mouth. Morphine is 10 times more effective by injection. Meperidine (Demerol) is very ineffective by mouth. Demerol, 50 mg, by mouth has the same analgesic effectiveness of aspirin, 600 mg, by mouth.

If the pain is not relieved, atelectasis is almost certain to ensue. Atelectasis is best prevented by a good cough, which is best taught preoperatively. If atelectasis occurs and is not shortly corrected, infection will supervene. Hospitals are reservoirs of pathologic bacteria, and minor complications may thereby become major complications. Aseptic nasotracheal aspirations or sterile bronchoscopies may be needed. Appropriate cultures must be taken.

SEPSIS

Sepsis such as wound infection, empyema, and pneumonia is a third major problem. Preoperative bronchoscopy cultures are valuable in knowing the bacteriology of the patient. It is important to treat significant pathologic bacteria before and during surgery. It is also important to be as aseptic as possible in handling the patient with bronchoscopes, suction catheters, and airways.

RESPIRATORY INSUFFICIENCY

Respiratory insufficiency is a complication to be feared. That is why preoperative assessment is essential and caution must be used in removing excessive lung parenchyma. This risk of respiratory insufficiency in the impaired patient is why we favor the use of internal radiotherapy that can treat the patient for cure without excising lung parenchyma. Our aim is to have a patient removed from the respirator as soon as possible postoperatively. At times, respiratory support of a complicating pneumonia may be lifesaving.

Best results are obtained when the predicted postoperative FEV_{10} is greater than 40 percent of predicted normal; a postoperative FEV_{10} less than 30 percent of predicted normal generally precludes resection of lung parenchyma.[70] Implant and internal radiotherapy are valuable in patients who are not candidates for resection.[62]

BRONCHOPLEURAL FISTULAS

Bronchopleural fistulas are serious complications in pneumonectomies.[75] They occur in as many as 5 percent of pneumonectomies. If a fistula occurs early, reoperation may be successful, especially if there is a bronchial stump remaining. The use of the omentum may be helpful in prevention or treatment. Otherwise these patients are treated by immediate closed drainage followed by chronic open drainage when the mediastinum is stable. Some small leaks may be sealed with so-called transbronchoscopy "glue."[76]

CARDIAC ARRHYTHMIAS

Cardiac arrhythmias are not uncommon; consequently we favor preoperative digitalization in the age group over 50 years.[77] Low-dose heparin, 5,000 U subcutaneously every 12 hours, is started on hospital admission the night before operation. This is continued until discharge of the patient. Pulsating compressive devices are used on the lower extremities, both legs and thighs, during operation and continued in the immediate postoperative period.[78] We have not recognized any major pulmonary emboli while using this regimen.

RADIOTHERAPY

Recent developments in computer technology and the introduction of high-energy linear accelerators have created the tools for precise definition of tumor target volume and calculations of high doses of radiation.[79]

Ionizing radiation can be electromagnetic or particulate. Electromagnetic radiation is divided into two types: Roentgen rays and γ rays. The difference between the two types is the way in which they are produced. γ rays are the effect of changes in the nucleus, while Roentgen rays are produced by electrons interacting on the outer structures of the atoms. Radioactive isotopes like I-125, Ir-192, and cesium-137 (Cs-137) are γ-ray emitters by way of decay.[80,81]

The effects of radiation on cells are random. The random effects are assumed to occur at the DNA level, compromising the reproductive integrity of tumor cells. Other important effects of radiation are due to changes on the cell membrane or in the cytoplasm. Cells that lose their reproductive integrity may divide once or more before all the progeny are rendered reproductively sterile. This means that an irradiated cell does not appear damaged until it faces at least the first division. This damage may be repaired or modified by repair, as in osteosarcoma, in which cancer cells have a great capacity to reverse the effects of radiation. Elkind and colleagues plotted a survival curve for different mammalian cells to determine the dose per fraction and total dose assumed to be sufficient to counteract these repairs (see Hall[82]). The dose needed shows variation for different cell types and different volume of cancer. Five thousand cGy is sufficient to eradicate subclinical disease; tumors over 5 cm theoretically should receive doses of 10,000 cGy to achieve 70 to 80 percent control.[81] This then exposes the patient to high incidence of radiation-induced side effects. The precision of the technique, the route of delivery, and the combination of different energies and modalities such as intraoperative, endobronchial, and external irradiation are the protagonists in minimizing these side effects.

DEFINITIVE IRRADIATION

Patients referred for radiation therapy usually have conditions that are nonresectable because of the extent of the tumor or the medical condition of the patient. Candidates for curative irradiation are as carefully selected as they are for surgery. Patients whose disease is confined to the chest are considered for curative treatment. Evaluation for radiation therapy includes physical examination, blood test, chest x-ray, and CT of the chest including the liver and adrenal glands. Lung function is carefully evaluated, along with the patient's performance status. Histologic confirmation of malignant tumor by means of biopsy or cytology is required. Liver-spleen scan, bone scan, and CT of the head are not routinely indicated because, in the absence of signs or symptoms, the investigation is mostly unrewarding.[83]

Patients with severe obstructive lung disease, congestive heart failure, or recent myocardial infarction need a very careful design of radiation treatment because of the high risk of acute and late complications, but they can also be treated with curative intent.[79] In designing treatment portals, diagnostic or planning CT scans are used for the precise delineation of tumor volume. Custom-made blocks are created for each patient to exclude as much normal tissue as possible from the high-dose radiation field. To ensure a homogeneous dose distribution, computer-generated isodose curves are used to prescribe the daily and total doses. The spinal cord dose is calculated by using lateral x-ray films. The dose to the cord is kept under 4,500 cGy by using special wedges or tissue-equivalent compensators. Treatment is started with anteroposterior and posteroanterior fields. These fields cover the primary tumor and the relevant lymph node bearing areas such as the ipsilateral hilum, mediastinum, and paratracheal lymph nodes. If the tumor is located in the upper lobes, the supraclavicular areas are included in the treatment field. In selected cases the contralateral hilum also is included in the treatment field. Approximately 3,600 cGy is given with 180- to 200-cGy daily fractions to the anteroposterior and posteroanterior portals, and then the beam direction is changed to avoid the spinal cord. This arrangement also includes less lung tissue within the zone of high dose radiation. Five thousand cGy is usually prescribed to the mediastinum but the primary tumor receives 6,400–6,600 cGy. With this dose complete responses of 35 percent for stage I, II, and IIIa patients and a 7 percent 5-year recurrence free survival has been reported[79,84,85] (Fig. 3-12).

INTRAOPERATIVE IRRADIATION

To improve local control in unresectable or incompletely resected tumors, intraoperative radiotherapy with artificial isotopes as radioactive sources was pioneered by Henschke at Memorial Hospital in New York. He postulated that a much higher dose can be delivered to the tumor with less damage to normal tissues with implantation than with external irradiation alone.[80] A combination of surgery, brachytherapy, and external irradiation was promoted and further refined by Hilaris et al.[36] I-125, with a superior radiation safety factor, a convenient half-life, and easy application, was introduced.[87] Removable implants involving Ir-192 seeds to treat the superior mediastinum were used in selected cases. Locoregional control was observed in 76 percent of the patients. The median survival was 26 months, with an impressive 2-year actuarial survival of 50 percent.[36–38]

A similar approach has been used since 1985 for unresectable lung cancer patients at Beth Israel Medical Center. Eighteen patients received an intraoperative I-125 implant followed by external irradiation in 1985 and 1986. Of these patients, 33 percent were alive and well at 3 years after treatment (Tables 3-16 and 3-17). This is a modest but

Table 3-16. Stage of Disease and Treatment

Treatment	Unresectable	Lobectomy	Total
S + I + E	9	6	15
S + I	3	0	3
Total	12	6	18

Abbreviations: S, surgery; I, internal radiation therapy; E, external radiation therapy.

Table 3-17. Patterns of Failure

Treatment	NED	L + D	L	D
S + I + E	6	5	2	2
S + I	0	2	1	0
Total	6	7	3	2

Abbreviations: S, surgery; I, internal radiation therapy; E, external radiation therapy; NED, no evidence of disease; L, local; D, distant.

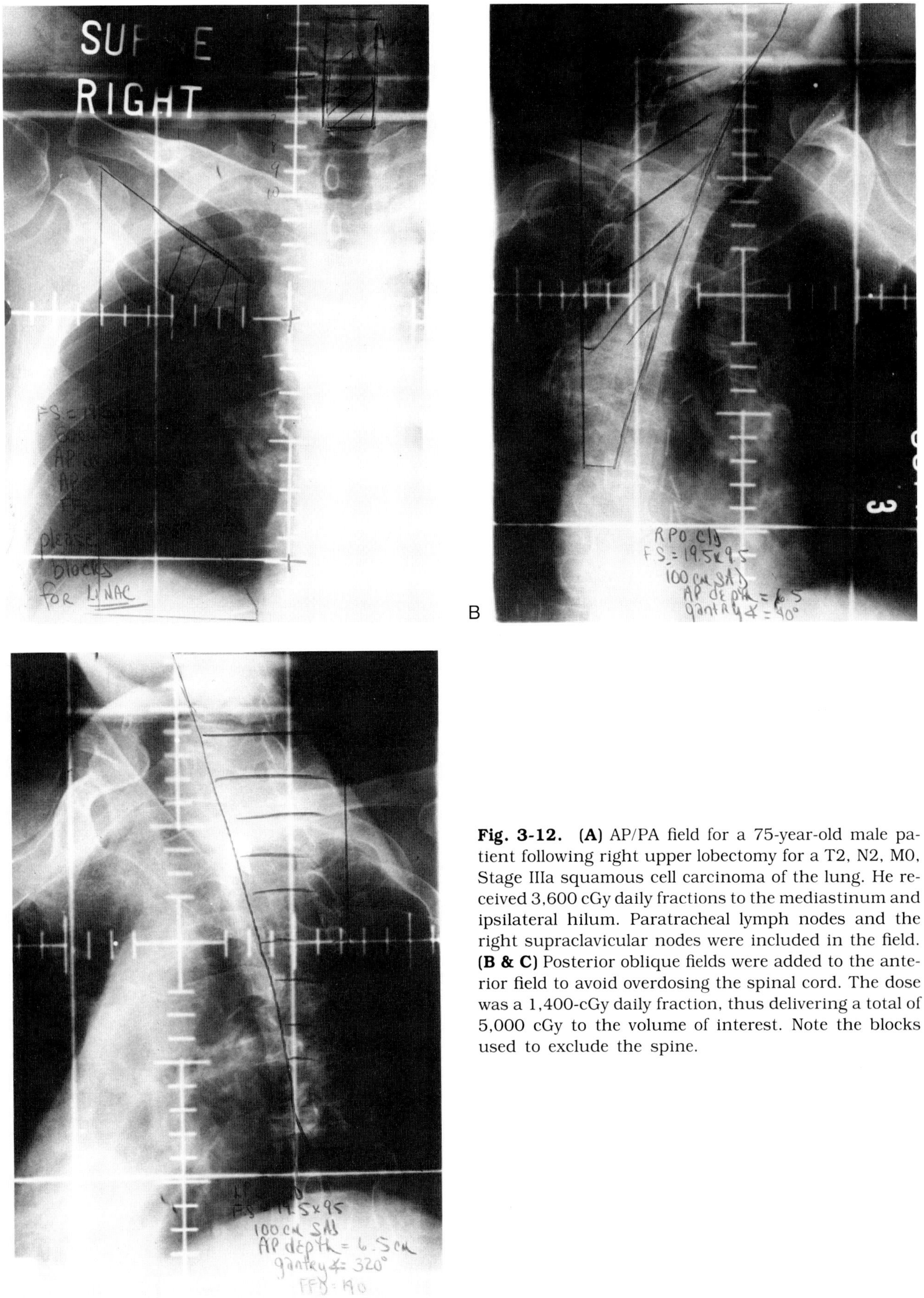

A B C

Fig. 3-12. **(A)** AP/PA field for a 75-year-old male patient following right upper lobectomy for a T2, N2, M0, Stage IIIa squamous cell carcinoma of the lung. He received 3,600 cGy daily fractions to the mediastinum and ipsilateral hilum. Paratracheal lymph nodes and the right supraclavicular nodes were included in the field. **(B & C)** Posterior oblique fields were added to the anterior field to avoid overdosing the spinal cord. The dose was a 1,400-cGy daily fraction, thus delivering a total of 5,000 cGy to the volume of interest. Note the blocks used to exclude the spine.

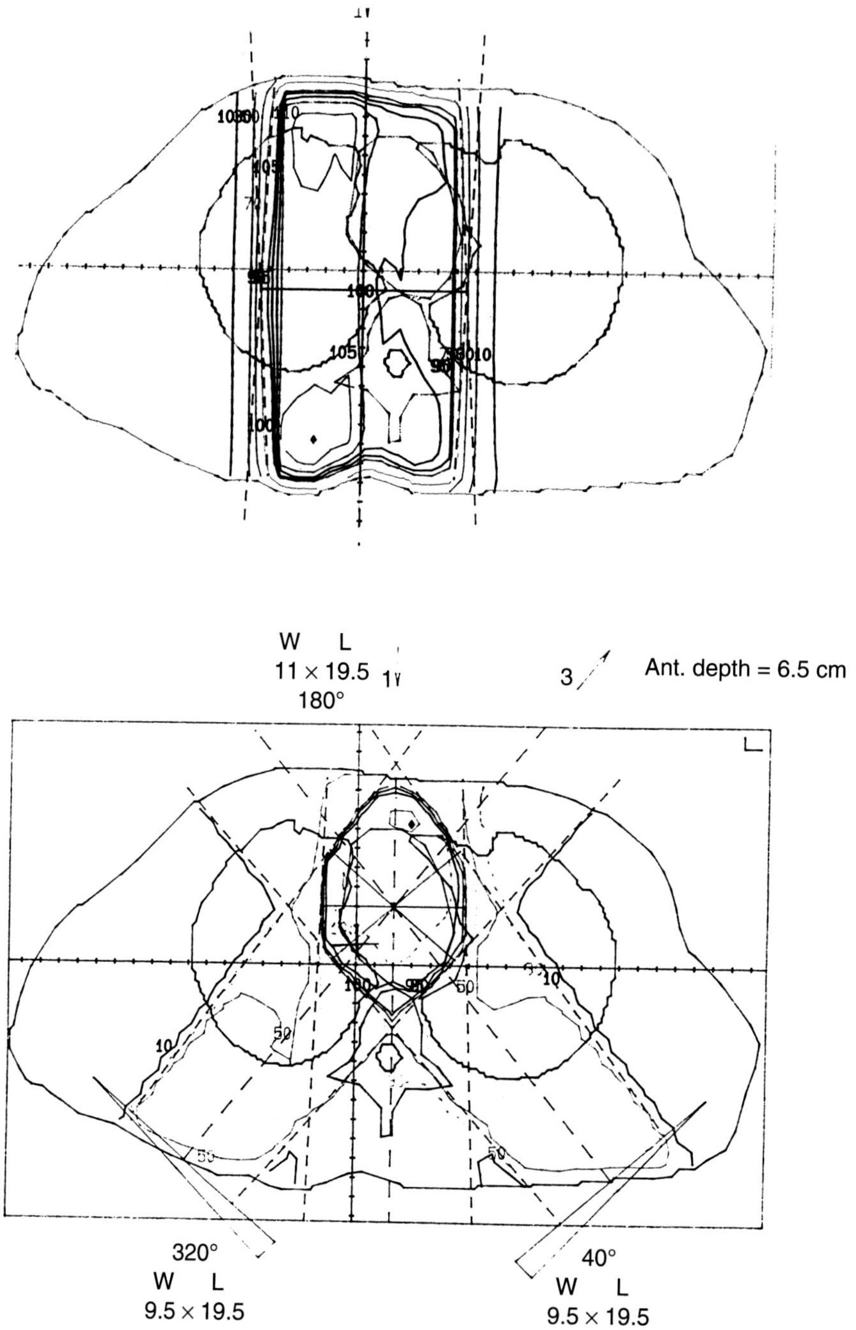

Fig. 3-12 (*Continued*). **(D)** Isodose curves for the same patient showing the area of interest in the 95 percent isodose curve and showing that the spinal cord is in the high-dose area. **(E)** Composite isodose curves, including the dose delivered with AP and PA fields plus the dose from the oblique fields. The target volume received over 5,000 cGy, whereas the spinal cord dose was under 4,200 cGy.

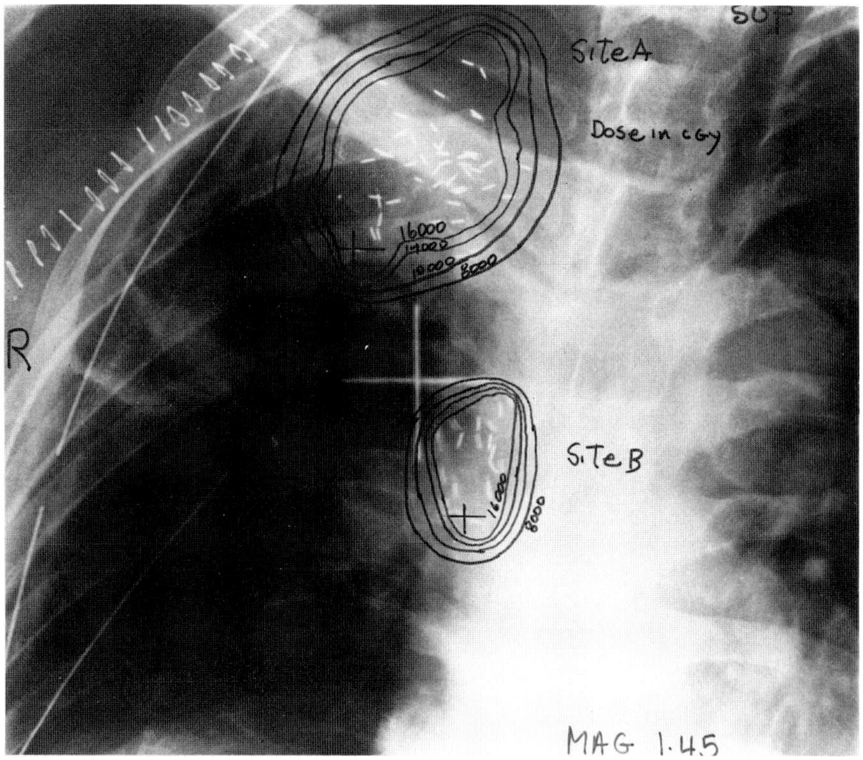

Fig. 3-13. PA view of 50-year-old man with a nonresectable T4, N2, M0 adenocarcinoma of the right upper lobe. Sixty I-125 seeds were implanted into the tumor, and 20 in the node positioned in the right hilum. The dose is equal to 6,000 cGy in 30 fractions. External irradiation was added to the mediastinum 4 weeks posttreatment.

solid improvement for unresectable disease over external irradiation alone[79] (Fig. 3-13).

POSTOPERATIVE IRRADIATION

The role of posteroperative irradiation in the management of lung cancer has been evaluated extensively. The incidence of involvement of hilar and mediastinal lymph nodes by metastatic disease has been in the range of 30 to 60 percent in surgical series, even after thorough staging work-up was done, including mediastinoscopy.[88,89] Autopsy studies have shown that the incidence of residual or recurrent carcinoma in the lymph nodes of the mediastinum varied from 25 to 55 percent depending on the length of survival after surgery.

Patients with positive regional lymph nodes or incomplete resection have a very poor 5-year survival rate of nearly 0 percent. It is well demonstrated that high doses of radiation therapy are capable of sterilizing lung cancer at the primary site or in the regional lymph nodes. A carefully planned radiation therapy with moderately high doses is able to control residual microscopic disease, but does not effect survival in node-negative patients with the exception of T-3 lesions. The overall actuarial survival for this group of patients is 33 percent at 5 years.[89] Retrospective studies also showed significant improvement in survival in node-positive patients after radiation therapy.[89]

The Lung Cancer Study Group conducted a randomized prospective study for stage II and III epidermoid cancer of the lung. A total of 230 patients were entered, all of whom underwent very careful intraoperative staging. The resection margins were microscopically free of tumor, with the addition that the node proximal or distal to the highest tumor bearing node had to be biopsied and found to be free of tumor. The investigators could not demonstrate that radiation prolonged the overall disease-free survival time or altered the pattern of overall recurrence rate, but there was a statistically significant difference in local recurrence rate, defined as the first recurrence in the ipsilateral lung or mediastinum for stage II patients, and the overall recurrence rate was significantly reduced among patients with N2 disease.[90] The above studies suggest that postoperative irradiation should be considered for patients with T3, N0 and for patients with N1, N2, or N3 disease regardless of the T stage.

IRRADIATION COMBINED WITH CHEMOTHERAPY

The prognosis of patients with advanced lung cancer is determined by failure of local and systemic therapies. With irradiation alone the 2-year survival for clinically staged patients is 13 percent while a somewhat higher survival (15 to 27 percent) is achieved for surgically staged patients.[85] Innovative ways of combining irradiation with chemotherapy had been explored by RTOG, ESTRO, SWOG and the Cancer and Leukemia Group B.[85,91] Choi, Eagan et al., and Weiden were able to show complete responses of 81 to 89 percent in stage III disease,[92,93] and Taylor had a much lower complete response rate in his group of patients.[94] There was a difference between the studies insofar as in Taylor's study once-a-day irradiation with simultaneous cisplatin and 5-fluorouracil (5-FU) infusion was used whereas Choi, Eagan et al., and Weiden employed twice-a-day radiation. These efforts showed a fairly high response rate but a relatively short median survival. They demonstrated that patients with a histologically complete response at resection had a lower local recurrence rate and a somewhat improved 2-year survival. To further improve local control and possibly survival, accelerated, interrupted high-dose irradiation was started at Beth Israel Medical Center. This program was very well tolerated in head and neck cancer patients with an excellent local control rate and survival in one of the studies conducted at the same institution.[95] This served as a basis for the treatment design of lung cancer patients for whom three cycles of treatment were prescribed with the understanding that each patient is evaluated for surgery after the second cycle is completed. A clinically complete response of 38 percent was achieved with moderate acute toxicity. The predicted actuarial survival at 2 years is 56 percent. The results show that this approach is worthy of further exploration with randomized prospective trials and should be offered to patients with advanced unresectable disease.

RADIATION TREATMENT COMPLICATED BY AIRWAY OBSTRUCTION

Airway obstruction due to primary or recurrent endobronchial tumor is a frequent presentation in patients with lung cancer. The effects of airway obstruction are distressing and often morbid. An especially complicated problem is presented by patients who have already received definitive external irradiation to that area. Re-treatment with radiation can be widely used with different time-dose and fractionation schedules. Green and Melbye reported that 74 percent of their patients had a variable objective response on re-treatment with external irradiation.[96] This response was observed for all cell types. The symptom-free interval ranged from 1 to 23 months with a median survival of 8 months for patients with good response.

An alternative form of management of recurrent tumor with an endobronchial component or extrabronchial compression is endoluminal brachytherapy by using a high-dose rate remote afterloading device (HDR-microSelectron). Patients presenting with cough, hemoptysis, and postobstructive pneumonia are good candidates for this modality. The endobronchial extent of the tumor can be determined by bronchoscopic examination or by limited high-resolution CT scan examining the area in question. The procedure is carried out with a large-channel bronchoscope, guiding the afterloading catheter to the appropriate position. The dose and depth of prescription depend on the location and extent of tumor as well as on the previous treatment. As a rule a depth of 1 cm is chosen in the trachea and mainstem bronchus while 0.5 cm is preferable in the lobar bronchus. The dose most often prescribed is 500 or 1,000 cGy. Higher doses are not advocated because of potential complications. This treatment is then repeated at 1- or 2-week intervals once or twice based on the clinical judgement of the radiation oncologist.

Intraluminal high-dose rate brachytherapy is also used in patients with primary lung cancer presenting with symptoms of bronchial obstruction or bleeding. Patients with bulky tumor and a high grade of obstruction can receive YAG laser resection to control the acute symptoms and facilitate placement of the afterloading catheter. Multiple catheters can be placed if more than one bronchus is at risk. This treatment then should be followed by external irradiation or surgery, whichever is feasible. Macha reported that 75 percent of his patients had endoscopy-proven tumor regression resulting in clinical improvement. Pulmonary function test, blood gas analyses and perfusion showed highly significant improvement.[97] Seagren found that cough and hemoptysis were more responsive than dyspnea and pneumonia. At least 50 percent tumor regression was seen in all of their patients on rebronchoscopy.[98] Complications from this procedure are generally low. Seagren et al. report no radiation-induced tracheitis, bronchitis, pneumonitis, or esophagitis. Only one patient developed clinical evidence of transient pericarditis 3 weeks posttreatment (Fig. 3-14).

The advantages are the short treatment time (5 to 15 minutes), nil radiation to personnel, elimi-

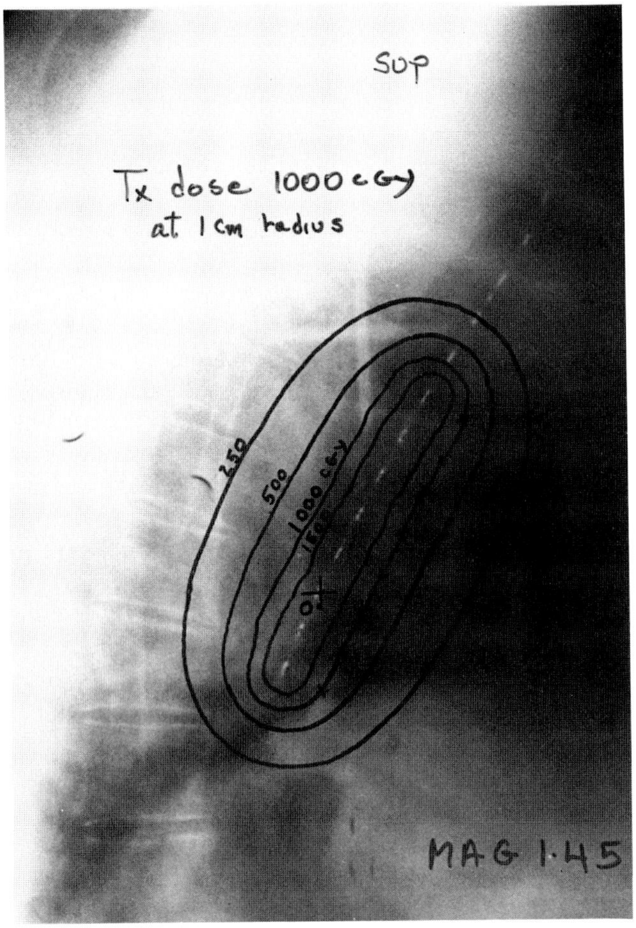

Fig. 3-14. Lateral view of a 55-year-old man with T3, N2, M0 squamous cell carcinoma, who presented with obstructive symptoms. He underwent bronchoscopy to aid afterloading catheter placement. He received 1,000 cGy to a 1.0-cm depth with the HDR microSelectron device. This view shows computer-aided isodose calculation to different depths from the source (isotope is Ir-192 with 15- to 20-Ci activity). This treatment was followed by external irradiation.

nation of operating room and hospital admission, and the ability to treat multiple areas simultaneously.

ACUTE AND LATE TOXICITY FROM IRRADIATION

Acute side effects of radiation therapy include esophagitis, bronchitis, and erythema of the skin. Bronchitis secondary to irradiation or infection may require antibiotics and cough medication. Dysphagia is well controlled with aspirin, Tylenol, or xylocain viscous 2 percent.[99]

Subacute and chronic complications include pneumonitis. The incidence and degree of pneumonitis vary in accordance with the patient's cardiorespiratory status and the technique used for treatment.[82] Symptoms of radiation-induced pneumonitis include low-grade fever, cough, and shortness of breath. On chest x-ray interstitial infiltration might be seen. Auscultation is usually normal, but pulmonary function tests show restrictive ventilatory defect. In the chronic phase there is a well-outlined area of fibrosis corresponding to the field of radiation. Bed rest, oxygen administration, and corticosteroids are helpful in controlling acute symptoms. Antibiotics are indicated when infection is strongly suspected. Corticosteroid treatment should be tapered carefully to avoid rebound reaction. Careful selection of patients for irradiation may ensure that the gain in local control and survival is not offset by serious pulmonary complications.

CHEMOTHERAPY

NON-SMALL CELL LUNG CARCINOMA

The discovery of Cvitkovic et al. that by tripling urinary output, triple the dose of cisplatin could be administered without risk[100] opened a new era in combination chemotherapy for non-small cell lung cancer. Successful protocols in the last decade have generally been cisplatin based. In 1983 Itri et al.[101] reported using CVB (cisplatin, vindesine and bleomycin) on 54 patients with advanced non-small cell lung cancer. Twenty patients (38 percent) had complete or partial remission, with a median duration of survival of 8 months. Also in 1983 Gralla[102] reported that five doses of 2 mg of metoclopramide per kg given over 9 hours beginning 30 minutes before administration of cisplatin, 120 mg/m^2, could control the emesis related to chemotherapy. Thus began a series of responses in non-small cell lung cancer patients with chemotherapy protocols containing cisplatin especially in regimens made more tolerable with control of the emesis.

In 1986 Kris et al.[103] reported data on 90 patients with stage III non-small cell lung cancer treated with cisplatin (120 mg/m^2), vindesine (3 mg/m^2), and mitomycin C (8 mg/m^2). They found major responses in 80 percent of the patients.

In 1988 Gralla and Kris[104] summarized the major response rates that had been found with newer combination chemotherapy regimens in non-small cell lung cancer (Table 3-18). It can be seen that major response rates in these numerous com-

Table 3-18. Major Response Rates with Newer Combination Chemotherapy Regimens in Non-Small Cell Lung Cancer

Regimen	Number of Patients	Major Response Rate (%)	Reference
Mitomycin C + vindesine + cisplatin (120 mg/m^2)	52	54	Gralla et al.[105]
Mitomycin C + vinblastine + cisplatin (100 mg/m^2)	45	77	Folman et al.[106]
Mitomycin C + vindesine + cisplatin (60 mg/m^2)	79	35	Joss et al.[107]
Mitomycin C + vinblastine + cisplatin (40 mg/m^2)	121	31	Ruckdeschel et al.[108]
5-Fluorouracil + cisplatin (100 mg/m^2)	21	66	Wheeler et al.[109]
5-Fluorouracil + cisplatin (60 mg/m^2)	24	33	Yanagihara et al.[110]

(From Gralla and Kris,[104] with permission.)

binations varied from 33 percent to as high as 77 percent.[105,110]

In 1988 chemotherapy combinations began to be used as neoadjuvant regimens delivered prior to definitive surgical resection. A study from Memorial Sloan Kettering Cancer Center[111] investigated 41 patients, later increased to 73 stage III non-small cell lung cancer patients treated with preoperative chemotherapy. There were 49 patients who showed a partial response (67 percent) and 7 patients who showed a complete response (10 percent), a response rate of 77 percent overall. Subsequently 58 percent of the patients were explored and 44 patients were reported to have a complete surgical resection. This figure represented 60 percent of the total patients or 70 percent of the responding patients. The median survival rate for these patients was subsequently found to be 19 months. There was a 26 percent survival rate at 3 years. Individuals who had a complete surgical resection had a 44 percent survival rate at 3 years compared with those with incomplete resections, none of whom survived 3 years.

More recently there have been an increasing number of reports of chemotherapy combinations used in the neoadjuvant setting. Table 3-19 is a summary by Gralla and Kris concerning recent preoperative chemotherapy trials in non-small cell lung cancer patients.[112–118] In the first three of these cited series, the median survival varied from 9 to 19 months. In the last three series cited the resection rate varied from 45 to 60 percent.

From 1983 to 1985 a study was reported by Sridhar et al. at the University of Miami.[29–31] In these series 25 patients with stage IIIb or marginally resectable stage IIIa tumors were reported. The preoperative chemotherapy protocol included cisplatin, VP-16 (etoposide) and 5-FU. Patients received either two or three cycles of chemotherapy prior to surgical exploration. Of 25 patients, 17

Table 3-19. Recent Preoperative Chemotherapy Trials in Non-Small Cell Lung Cancer

Regimen	Number of Patients	Findings	Reference
Vinca alkaloid + etoposide + cisplatin	20	Median survival, 9 mo[a]	Bitran et al.[112]
Various	44	Median survival, 18 mo[a]	Takita et al.[113]
Mitomycin C + vinca alkaloid + cisplatin	25	Median survival, 19 mo[a]	Spain et al.[114,115]
5-Fluorouracil + cisplatin + radiation therapy	55	Resection rate, 49%	Trybula et al.[116]
Vinca alkaloid + cisplatin + radiation therapy	20	Resection rate, 60%	Strauss et al.[117]
Mitomycin C + vinca alkaloid + cisplatin	20	Resection rate, 45%	Kris et al.[118]

[a] Radiation therapy instead of surgery after chemotherapy in many patients.
(From Gralla and Kris,[104] with permission.)

were partially responsive to preoperative chemotherapy. Of the 25 patients, 23 were surgically explored. Nineteen patients were rendered disease free after surgery. Patients who had responded to chemotherapy generally did not need brachytherapy. Brachytherapy was used for any situation in which there was believed to be incomplete surgical removal. Fourteen patients received postoperative radiation therapy; 15 patients received postoperative chemotherapy. Eleven patients are alive and disease free, including five patients with a minimum follow-up of 4 years. Of the first 10 patients with stage III disease treated in this fashion, 5 are alive with a minimum follow-up of within 5 years. The projected 5-year survival rate of the entire group is approximately 35 percent. Four patients died tumor free, including one who died of pulmonary embolism 30 days postsurgery. Sridhar's chemotherapy protocol regimen is outlined in Table 3-20.

In our recent years at Beth Israel Medical Center, the response rate of stage III non-small cell lung cancer to chemotherapy has been approximately 60 percent. For the past 2 years a preoperative neoadjuvant chemotherapy protocol combined with accelerated radiation therapy has been used (Fig. 3-15). The patient is admitted to the hospital and receives 5 days of chemotherapy together with two radiation therapy treatments a day for 5 days, totaling 200 cGy/week. After a 2-week rest this cycle is repeated, and the patient is reevaluated at 6 weeks. Patients with 50 percent or greater reduction undergo exploration and either complete surgical resection or resection plus internal brachytherapy. Patients with less than 50 percent reduction in tumor mass after two cycles receive a third cycle of chemotherapy-radiotherapy sandwich. After the third cycle patients are reassessed and a decision is made regarding surgery or other alternatives.

At the time of surgery, if it is not possible to carry out complete resection, brachytherapy is used. This consists either of I-125 implantation in residual tumor in the lung or mediastinum or of I-125 seed sutures placed around areas whence tumor has been removed, and/or the use of temporary afterloading catheters for Ir-192 across the mediastinum where there is residual tumor or margins had been suboptimal. Whether or not postoperative external radiotherapy can be used depends on the total dose of radiation therapy already received. If there had been a response to chemotherapy, three or four additional cycles of chemotherapy are recommended postoperatively, so that these patients receive a total of six cycles. Approximately 75 percent of patients will have a partial or complete radiologic response to this chemotherapy-radiotherapy "sandwich". Approximately 25 percent of patients given this protocol will have no tumor found in the specimen at the time of surgery, but 5-year follow-up has not yet been reached.

Table 3-20. Chemotherapy Non-Small Cell Lung Cancer

Day	Drug[a]
1	Cisplatin 50 mg/m^2 (raise to 75 and 100 mg/m^2)
2, 3, 4	5-Fluorouracil, 40 mg/m^2/hr × 72 hours
2, 3, 4	VP-16 (etoposide), 80 mg/m^2/day × 3 days
	Repeat every 21 days

[a] Tumor response rate, 56 percent.
(From Sridhar et al.,[29] with permission.)

SMALL CELL LUNG CARCINOMA

Small cell lung cancer has three recognizable stages. Rarely it presents as a so-called coin lesion, with no evidence of any spread to lymph nodes in the mediastinum or systemically. At this stage surgical excision and postoperative chemotherapy achieve a relatively good 5-year survival rate (approximately 65 percent).[47] More commonly the tumor is advanced in the chest alone, designated limited disease. Here a combination of chemotherapy and external radiotherapy has produced 3-year survival rates as high as 40 to 50 percent. There is still controversy about whether surgery plays a role in limited disease small cell lung cancer. It has been found that after induction chemotherapy, the primary lesion in the lung can frequently be resected, preferably by lobectomy.[48] Resection obviates the need for radiation. External radiotherapy can then be used to the mediastinum alone with continued systemic chemotherapy.

The majority of patients with small cell lung cancer have extensive disease, with metastases to brain, bone, liver, or bone marrow. In these instances, although the tumor usually responds to chemotherapy, the chance for long-term survival free of disease remains poor. Chemotherapy and radiotherapy used in this situation are often designed for palliation while investigation with more intense dose schedules incorporating bone marrow transplant or the newly available colony-stimulating factors continue to attract interest.[50]

The role of prophylactic brain irradiation (PBI)

Cycle 1

	5-FU					
	VP-16	VP-16	VP-16	—	—	Rest period of 14 days
	X	X	X	X	X	
	X	X	X	X	X	
Days	1	2	3	4	5	6 to 19

Cycle 2

	5-FU					
	VP-16	VP-16	VP-16	—	—	6-week reevaluation
	X	X	X	X	X	
	X	X	X	X	X	
Days	20	21	22	23	24	

Note: X = radiation therapy treatment (RT)(2 doses each day)

Stage IIIA	Postoperative
IIIB	Neoadjuvant, preoperative, and postoperative
Chemo/RT	Regimen
5-FU	900 mg/m^2, constant infusion, qd days 1–4
VP-16	80 mg/m^2, IVPB, qd x 3, days 1–3
Cisplatin	30 mg/m^2, qd x 3, days 1–3
RT	200 cGy bid x 5, days 1–5
	Repeat cycles q21 or q28d, dependent on recovery of WBC to 2,000 and of platelets to 100,000.

Stage IIIA	Three full cycles postoperative (two with radiation to mediastinum, if total resection)
Stage IIIB	Assessment of response after two cycles: >50% reduction: proceed to surgery, and follow with last cycle of combined chemo/RT and three cycles of chemotherapy <50% reduction: deliver third cycle, and reassess response; thoracotomy possible for either definitive local resection and/or brachytherapy

---

Stage IV

Chemo/RT	Regimen
5-FU	1,000 mg/m^2, constant infusion, days 1–4
VP-16	80 mg/m^2, IVPB, days 1–3
CDDP (Cisplatin)	100 mg/m^2, day 1
	Repeat cycles q21–28d

Fig. 3-15. Chemotherapy protocol used on non-small cell carcinoma.

used to prevent brain metastases from small cell lung cancer remains controversial. State-of-the-art therapy includes PBI early in the management of patients with limited disease, assuming that the majority will be controlled in the thorax with the currently used combinations of chemotherapy and radiotherapy with or without surgery. The use of PBI in patients with extensive disease, however, has not clearly demonstrated an impact on survival or quality of life.[49] Patients who exhibit marked tumor responsiveness to systemic therapy might be considered on an individual basis regarding the value of PBI. It has been found that prophylactic whole-brain radiation therapy will prevent death from symptomatic brain metastases even if it does not cure the patient. Any time brain metastases are found, whole-brain radiation therapy is indicated.

Shank et al.[119] reported 34 patients at Memorial Sloan-Kettering Cancer Center with limited-disease small cell lung cancer. They were treated with cyclophosphamide, doxorubicin, and vincristine alternating with VP-16 and cisplatin. PBI or chest radiotherapy was also used. Twenty-two of 34 patients (65 percent) were complete responders. Nine of 34 patients (26 percent) had local failure. The 3-year survival rate in this group was 33 percent.

REFERENCES

1. Silverberg E, Boring CC, Squires TS: Cancer statistics, 1990. CA 40:9, 1990
2. Doll R, Peto R: The causes of cancer. J Natl Cancer Inst 66:1191, 1981
3. Wynder EL, Hoffman D: Tobacco and health. J Med 300:894, 1979
4. Doll R, Hill AB: A study of the aetiology of carcinoma of the lung. Br Med J 2:1271, 1952
5. Wynder EL, Graham EA: Tobacco smoking as a possible etiologic factor in bronchogenic carcinoma: a study of six hundred and eighty four proved cases. JAMA 143:329, 1950
6. Wynder EL: Smoking and lung cancer. Offentliche Gesundheitwesen 51:733, 1989
7. Hammond EL, Selikoff IJ, Seidman H et al: Asbestos exposure, cigarette smoking and death rates. Ann NY Acad Sci 330:473, 1979
8. Hirayama T: Epidemiology of lung cancer with special reference to cigarette smoking. Kokyu Junkan 38:3, 1990
9. Janerich DT, Thompason WO, Varela LR et al: Lung cancer and exposure to tobacco smoke in the household. N Engl J Med 323:632, 1990
10. Augustus A, Harris RE, Wynder EL: Compensation as a risk factor for lung cancer in patients who switch from non-filter to filter cigarettes. Am J Public Health 79:188, 1989
11. Boucot KR, Weiss W: Is curable lung cancer detected by semi-annual screening? JAMA 224:1361, 1973
12. Weiss W, Boucot KE, Cooper DA: The Philadelphia pulmonary neoplasm research project. Survival factors in bronchogenic carcinoma. JAMA 216:2119, 1973
13. Berlin NI, Buncher CR, Fontana RS et al: The National Cancer Institute cooperative early lung cancer detection program. Results of the initial screen (prevalence). Am Rev Respir Dis 130:545, 1984
14. Beattie EJ: So-called Stage "0" lung cancer. J Jpn Assoc Thorac Surg 20:22, 1972
15. Tockman MS: Survival and mortality from lung cancer in a screened population. The Johns Hopkins study. Chest 89(suppl.):324S, 1986
16. Sanderson DR: Lung cancer screening. The Mayo Study. Chest 89(suppl.):324S, 1986
17. Melamed MR, Flehinger BJ, Zaman MD et al: Screening for early lung cancer. Results of the Memorial-Sloan-Kettering study in New York. Chest 86:44, 1984
18. Eddy DM: Screening for lung cancer. Ann Intern Med 111:232, 1989
19. Mulshine JL, Tockman MS, Smart CR: Commentaries—considerations in the development of lung cancer screening tools. JNCI 81:900, 1990
20. Minna JD, Battey JF, Brooks BJ et al: Molecular genetic analysis reveals chromosomal deletion, gene amplification, and autoimmune growth factor production in the pathogenesis of human lung cancer. Cold Spring Harbor Symp. Quant Biol 51:843, 1986
21. Beattie EJ, Harvey JC: Screening for lung cancer. J Surg Oncol 46:1, 1991
22. Martini N, Beattie EJ: Results of surgical treatment in stage I lung cancer. J Thorac Cardiovasc Surg 74:499, 1977
23. Ramsey HE, Cahan WG, Beattie EJ et al: The importance of radical lobectomy in lung cancer. J Thorac Cardiovasc Surg 98:591, 1969
24. Hilaris BS, Martini N, Batata M et al: Interstitial irradiation for unresectable carcinoma of the lung. Ann Thorac Surg 20:491, 1975
25. Martini N, Flehinger BJ, Nagasaki F et al: Prognostic significance of N_1 disease in carcinoma of the lung. J Thorac Cardiovasc Surg 86:646, 1983
26. McCaughan BC, Martini N, Bains MS et al: Chest wall invasion in carcinoma of the lung. J Thorac Cardiovasc Surg 89:836, 1985
27. McCormack P, Bains MS, Beattie EJ et al: New trends in skeletal reconstruction after resection of chest wall tumors. Ann Thorac Surg 31:45, 1981
28. Martini N, Flehinger BJ, Zaman MD et al: Results of resection in non-oat cell carcinoma of the lung

with mediastinal lymph node metastases. Ann Surg 198:386, 1983
29. Sridhar KS, Thurer R, Raskin N et al: Neoadjuvant chemotherapy (CT) with cisplatin, etoposide, and 5-FU infusion (FED), surgery and radiation therapy in non-small cell lung cancer (abstract). Proc Ann Meet Am Assoc Cancer Res 28:216, 1987
30. Sridhar KS, Varki J, Donnelly E et al: Toxicity of FED chemotherapy in non-small cell lung cancer. Am J Clin Oncol 10:499, 1987
31. Sridhar KS, Thurer R, Beattie EJ et al: Multimodality treatment of non-small cell lung cancer: response to cisplatin, VP-16, and 5-FU chemotherapy and to surgery and radiation therapy. J Surg Oncol 38:193, 1988
32. Hilaris BS, Gomez J, Now D et al: Combined surgery, intraoperative brachytherapy and postoperative external radiation in Stage III non-small cell lung cancer. Cancer 55:1226, 1985
33. Raskin N, Beattie EJ: Superior sulcus tumor. p. 185. In Wanebo HJ (ed): Common Problems in Cancer Surgery. Year Book Medical Publishers, New York, 1990
34. Sundaresan N, Galicich JH, Bains MS et al: Vertebral body resection in the treatment of cancer involving the spine. Cancer 53:1393, 1984
35. Hilaris BS, Martini N, Nori D et al: The place of radiotherapy in the treatment of lung cancer. World J Surg 5:675, 1981
36. Hilaris BS, Nori D, Beattie EJ et al: Value of perioperative brachytherapy in the management of non-oat cell carcinoma of the lung. Int J Radiol Oncol Biol Phys 9:1611, 1983
37. Beattie EJ, Raskin N: Progress in lung cancer: non-oat cell (non-small cell lung cancer). Jpn J Surg 17:5, 1987
38. Hilaris BS, Martini N: The current state of intraoperative interstitial brachytherapy in lung cancer. Int J Radiol Oncol Biol Phys 15:6, 1988
39. Watanabe Y, Shimizu J, Oda M et al: Results in 104 patients undergoing bronchoplastic procedures for bronchial lesions. Ann Thorac Surg 50:607, 1990
40. Tsuchiya R, Goya T, Naruke T et al: Resection of bronchial carcinoma for lung cancer. J Thorac Cardiovasc Surg 99:779, 1990
41. Hilaris BS, Martini N, Batata M et al: Interstitial irradiation for unresectable carcinoma of the lung. Ann Thorac Surg 20:491, 1975
42. van Bodegom PC, Wagenaar SJSC, Corrin B et al: Second primary lung cancer: importance of long term follow up. Thorax 44:788, 1989
43. Sundaresan N, Galicich JH, Beattie EJ: Surgical treatment of brain metastases from lung cancer. J Neurosurg 58:666, 1983
44. Sundaresan N, Galicich JH: Surgical treatment of brain metastases. Cancer 55:1382, 1985
45. Sundaresan N, Galicich JH: Surgical treatment of single brain metastasis from non-small cell lung cancer. Cancer Invest 3:207, 1985
46. Magilligan DJ Jr, Rogers JS, Knight RS et al: Surgical approach to lung cancer with solitary cerebral metastasis: twenty-five years experience. Ann Thorac Surg 42:360, 1986
47. Massen W, Greschychna D, Martinez I: The role of surgery in the treatment of small cell carcinoma of the lung. Recent results. Cancer Res 97:107, 1985
48. Shepherd PA, Ginsberg RJ, Feld R et al: Surgical treatment for limited small cell cancer. The University of Toronto Lung Oncology Group experience. J Thorac Cardiovasc Surg 101:385, 1991
49. Rosen ST, Makuch RW, Lichter AS et al: Role of prophylactic cranial irradiation in prevention of central nervous system metastases in small cell lung cancer. Potential benefits restricted to patients with complete response. Am J Med 74:615, 1983
50. Johnson BE, Grayson J, Makuch RW et al: Ten-year survival of patients with small-cell lung cancer treated with combination chemotherapy with or without irradiation. J Clin Oncol 8:396, 1990
51. Turnbull AD, Huvos AG, Goodner JT et al: The malignant potential of bronchial adenoma. Ann Thorac Surg 14:453, 1972
52. Barney JD, Churchill ED: Adenocarcinoma of the kidney with metastasis to the lungs treated by pulmonary resection. J Urol 42:269, 1939
53. Thomford NR, Woolner LB, Clagett OT: The surgical treatment of metastatic tumors in the lungs. J Thorac Cardiovasc Surg 49:357, 1965
54. Marcove RC, Mike V, Hajek JV et al: Osteogenic sarcoma under the age of 21. A review of 145 operative cases. J Bone Jt Surg 52:411, 1970
55. Martini N, Huvos AG, Mike V et al: Multiple pulmonary resections in the treatment of osteogenic sarcoma. Ann Thorac Surg 12:271, 1971
56. Beattie EJ, Harvey JC, Marcove R et al: Results of multiple pulmonary resections for metastatic osteogenic sarcoma after two decades. J Surg Oncol 46:154, 1991
57. McCormack P, Bains MS, Martini N: Surgical management of pulmonary metastases. p. 263. In Shiu MH, Brennan MF (eds): Surgical Management of Soft Tissue Sarcomas. Lea & Febiger, Philadelphia, 1989
58. McCormack PM, Martini N: A current view of surgical management of pulmonary metastases. p. 246. In Economou S (ed): Adjuncts to Cancer Surgery. Lea & Febiger, Philadelphia, 1991
59. Beattie EJ: Surgical treatment of pulmonary metastases. Cancer 54:2729, 1984
60. Mountain CF, McMurtrey MJ, Hermes KE: Surgery for pulmonary metastasis: a 20-year experience. Ann Thorac Surg 38:323, 1984
61. Joseph WL, Morton DL, Adkin PC: Prognostic significance of tumor doubling time in evaluating operability in pulmonary metastatic disease. J Thorac Cardiovasc Surg 61:23, 1971
62. Johnston MR: Median sternotomy for resection of

pulmonary metastases. J Thorac Cardiovasc Surg 85:516, 1983
63. Regal AM, Antkowiak JG, Hart T et al: Median sternotomy for metastatic lung lesions: 100 cases. p. 128. In: 37th Symp Soc. Surg. Oncol Soc. Head Neck Surg. New York, 1984
64. Roth JA, Pass HI, Wesley MN et al: Comparison of median sternotomy and thoracotomy for resection of pulmonary metastases in patients with adult soft-tissue sarcomas. Ann Thorac Surg 42:134, 1986
65. Einhorn LH, Williams SD, Mandelbaum I et al: Surgical resection in disseminated testicular cancer following chemotherapeutic cytoreduction. Cancer 48:904, 1981
66. McCormack P, Martini N: The changing role of surgery for pulmonary metastases. Ann Thorac Surg 28:139, 1979
67. Rosen G, Capparos B, Huvos AG et al: Preoperative chemotherapy for osteogenic sarcoma: selection of postoperative adjuvant chemotherapy based on the response of the primary tumor to preoperative chemotherapy. Cancer 49:1221, 1982
68. Mitchell C, Garrahy P, Blake P: Postoperative respiratory morbidity: identification and risk factors. Aust NZ J Surg 52:203, 1982
69. Nagasaki F, Flehinger BJ, Martini N: Complications of surgery in the treatment of carcinoma of the lung. Chest 82:25, 1982
70. Markos J, Mullan BP, Hillman DR et al: Peroperative assessment as a predictor of mortality and morbidity after lung resection. Am Rev Respir Dis 139:902, 1989
71. Peters RM: Special problems in preoperative and postoperative management. p. 67. In Delarue NC, Eschapasse H (eds): International Trends in General Thoracic Surgery. Vol I. Lung Cancer. WB Saunders, Philadephia, 1985
72. Ginsberg RJ, Hill LD, Eagan RT et al: Modern thirty-day operative mortality for surgical resections in lung cancer. J Thorac Cardiovasc Surg 86:654, 1983
73. Egbert LD: The value of the preoperative visit by an anesthetist. JAMA 185:553, 1963
74. Ovassapian A, Schrader S: Fiberoptic aided bronchial intubation. Semin Anesth 6:133, 1987
75. Ginsberg RJ, Pearson FG, Cooper JO et al: Closure of chronic post-pneumonectomy bronchopleural fistula using transternal transpericardial approach. Ann Thorac Surg 47:231, 1989
76. York EL, Lewall DB, Hirji M et al: Endoscopic diagnosis and treatment of postoperative bronchopleural fistula. Chest 97:1391, 1990
77. Kirsh MM, Rotman H, Behrendt DM: Complications of pulmonary resections. Ann Thorac Surg 20:215, 1975
78. Hull RD, Raskob GE, Hirsh J: Prophylaxis of venous thromboembolism: an overview. Chest 89:374S, 1986
79. Choi NC: Curative radiation therapy for unresectable non-small cell carcioma of the lung: indications, techniques, results, p. 163. In Choi NC, Grillo H (eds): Thoracic Oncology. Raven Press, New York, 1983
80. Walter J, Miller H, Bomford CK: The production of X and gamma ray beams. p. 17. In Walter J, Miller H: A Short Textbook of Radiotherapy, 4th Ed. Churchill-Livingstone, Edinburgh, 1979
81. Delclos L: Afterloading methods for interstitial gamma ray therapy. p 84. In Fletcher GA (ed): Textbook of Radiotherapy. 3rd Ed. Lea & Febiger, Philadelphia, 1980
82. Hall EJ: Classification of radiation damage. In: Radiobiology for the Radiologist. 2nd Ed. Harper & Row, Hagerstown, Md, 1978
83. Emami B, Perez CA: Carcinoma of the lung. p. 655. In Perez CA, Brady LW (ed): Principles and Practice of Radiation Oncology, JB Lippincott, Philadelphia, 1987
84. Montravadi VP, Gates JO, Crawford JN et al: Unresectable non-oat cell carcinoma of the lung: definitive radiation therapy. Radiology 172:851, 1989
85. Guttman J: Radiation therapy for patients selected at thoracotomy. p. 12. In Choi NC (ed): Lung Carcinoma: Recent Progress and Current Controversies. Refresher course 308, American Society for Therapeutic Radiation Oncology, San Francisco, 1989
86. Henscke UK: Interstitial implantation in the treatment of primary bronchogenic carcinoma. Am J Roengenol Radium Ther Nucl Med 79:6, 1958
87. Marchese MT, Hall EJ, Hilaris BS: Clinical, physical and radiobiological aspects of encapsulated I-125 in radiation oncology. Endocr Hyperthermia Oncol 1:67, 1985
88. Choi NC: Role of postoperative radiation therapy in lung cancer with either metastases to regional lymph nodes (N1 or unforeseen N2) or director invasion beyond visceral pleura (T3). p. 129. In Choi NC, Grillo HC (eds): Thoracic Oncology. Raven Press, New York, 1983
89. Green N: Postresection irradiation for primary lung cancer. Radiology 116:405, 1975
90. The Lung Cancer Study Group: Effects of postoperative mediastinal radiation on completely resected Stage II and Stage III epidermoid cancer of the lung. N Engl J Med 315:1377, 1986
91. Holmes E: Combined modality therapy for non-small cell lung cancer. Adv Oncol 4:4, 1989
92. Eagan RT, Ruud C, Lee RE et al: Pilot study of induction therapy with cyclophosphamide, doxorubicin and cisplatin and chest irradiation prior to thoracotomy in initially inoperable Stage III M_0 non small cell lung cancer. Cancer Treat Rep 71:895, 1987
93. Weiden P: Preoperative chemo-radiotherapy in Stage III non-small cell lung cancer (NSCLC): a phase III study of the lung cancer study group (abstract). Proc Am Soc Clin Oncol 6:185, 1987

94. Taylor SG, Trybula M, Bonomi PD et al: Simultaneous cisplatin-fluorouracil infusion and radiation followed by surgical resection in regionally localized Stage III non-small lung cancer. Ann Thorac Surg 43:1, 1987
95. Vikram B, Malamud S, Gold J et al: Chemotherapy rapidly alternating with accelerated radiation therapy for locally advanced carcinomas of the hypopharynx and upper esophagus. Head Neck 5:415, 1991
96. Green N, Melbye RW: Lung cancer: retreatment of local recurrence after definitive irradiation. Cancer 49:865, 1982
97. Macha HN, Stadler M, Koch K et al: Neue wege der strahlentherapie des bronchialkarcinoms. Dtsche Med Wochenschr 18:111, 1986
98. Seagren S, Harrell JH, Horn RA: High dose rate intraluminal irradiation in recurrent endobronchial carcinoma. Chest 88:810, 1985
99. Coggle JE, Lambert BE, Moores SR: Radiation effects in the lung. Environ Health Perspect 70:261, 1986
100. Cvitkovic E, Spaulding J, Bethune V et al: Improvement of cis-dichlorodiammineplatinum (NSC 119875): therapeutic index in an animal model. Cancer 39:1357, 1977
101. Itri LM, Gralla RJ, Kelsen DP et al: Cisplatin, vindesine and bleomycin (CVB) combination chemotherapy of advanced non-small cell lung cancer. Cancer 51:1050, 1988
102. Gralla RJ: Metoclopramide: a review of antiemetic trials. Drugs 25(suppl. 1):63, 1983
103. Kris MG, Gralla RJ, Wertheim MS et al: Trial of the combination of mitomycin, vindesine, and cisplatin in patients with advanced non-small cell lung cancer. Cancer Treat Rep 70:1091, 1986
104. Gralla RJ, Kris MG: Chemotherapy in non-small cell lung cancer: results of recent trials. Semin Oncol 15(suppl. 4):2, 1988
105. Gralla RJ, Kris MG, Burke MT et al: The influence of the addition of mitomycin to vindesine plus cisplatin in a random assignment trial in 120 patients with non-small cell lung cancer (abstract). Proc Am Soc Clin Oncol 5:182, 1986
106. Folman R, Rosman M, Auerbach S: Mitomycin-C, vinblastine, and cisplatinum in the combined modality treatment of non-small cell lung cancer (abstract). Proc Am Soc Clin Oncol 3:232, 1984
107. Joss RA, Ludwig CH, Alberto P: Combination chemotherapy of non-small cell lung cancer with mitomycin, vindesine, and cisplatin (abstract). Proc IV World Conf Lung Cancer 4:133, 1986
108. Ruckdeschel JC, Finkelstein DM, Ettinger DS et al: A randomized trial of the four most active regimens for metastatic non-small cell lung cancer. J Clin Oncol 4:14, 1986
109. Wheeler C, Ervin T, Come S et al: Platinum, 5-FU and methotrexate: an active regimen in non-small cell lung cancer (abstract). Proc Am Soc Clin Oncol 5:181, 1986
110. Yanagihara R, Rivera R, Kummet T: 5-Fluorouracil, cisplatin, etoposide, and vincristine chemotherapy in non-small cell lung cancer (abstract). Proc Am Soc Clin Oncol 5:173, 1986
111. Martini N, Kris MG, Gralla RJ et al: The effects of preoperative chemotherapy on the resectability of non-small cell lung carcinoma with mediastinal lymph node metastases (N_1M_0). Ann Thorac Surg 45:370, 1988
112. Bitran JD, Golomb HM, Hoffman PC et al: Protochemotherapy in non-small cell lung carcinoma. An attempt to increase surgical resectability and survival: a preliminary report. Cancer 57:44, 1986
113. Takita H, Regal AM, Antkowiak JG et al: Chemotherapy followed by lung resection in inoperable non-small cell lung carcinomas due to locally far-advanced disease. Cancer 57:630, 1986
114. Spain R, Anderson P, Speer J et al: Improved survival with mitomycin-C, cisplatinum and continuous vinblastine infusion plus radiation therapy or surgery over TF alone for Stage III limited, initially inoperable, non-small cell lung cancer (abstract). Proc IV World Conf Lung Cancer 4:33, 1985
115. Spain R, Anderson P, Speer J et al: Improved survival and symptom palliation with mitomycin-C, cisplatinum, and continuous vinblastine infusion plus radiation therapy or surgery over RT alone for Stage III limited, initially inoperable non-small cell lung cancer (abstract). Proc Am Soc Clin Oncol 4:180, 1985
116. Trybula M, Taylor SG, Bonomi P et al: Preoperative simultaneous cisplatin/5-fluorouracil and radiotherapy in clinical Stage III, non-small cell bronchogenic carcinoma (abstract). Proc Am Soc Clin Oncol 4:182, 1985
117. Strauss G, Sherman D, Schwartz J et al: Combined modality therapy for regionally advanced Stage III non-small cell carcinoma of the lung employing neoadjuvant chemotherapy, radiotherapy, and surgery (abstract). Proc Am Soc Clin Oncol 5:172, 1986
118. Kris MG, Gralla RJ, Martini N et al: Trial of preoperative cisplatin plus vinca alkaloid chemotherapy in non-small cell lung cancer patients with clinically apparent, ipsilateral, mediastinal lymph node metastases (abstract). Proc Am Soc Clin Oncol 6:177, 1987
119. Shank B, Saher H, Hilaris BS et al: Increased survival with high-dose multifield radiotherapy and intensive chemotherapy in limited small cell carcinoma of the lung. Cancer 56:2771, 1985
120. Beahrs OH, Henson DE, Hutter RVP, Myers MH (American Joint Committee on Cancer) (eds): Manual for Staging of Cancer. 3rd Ed. JP Lippincott, Philadelphia, 1988

ATLAS OF THORACIC SURGERY

RIGHT HEMITHORAX

The right lung has been removed to show the important anatomic landmarks. The diaphragm makes up the floor of the chest. The spine comes rather more anteriorly into the chest than is generally realized. It can be seen that the intercostal veins join the azygos vein, which, just above the right lung hilum, turns anteriorly and drains into the superior vena cava. The superior vena cava can be seen more anteriorly coming down from the apex of the chest and entering the heart and right atrium. The phrenic nerve runs along the side of the superior vena cava. It passes immediately in front of the right lung hilum and then inserts medially into the junction of the pericardium and diaphragm, where the fibers tend to sweep around the diaphragm anterolaterally. More posteriorly the vagus nerve can be seen entering the chest in the mid-mediastinum. The recurrent nerve branch is given off high in the chest; it passes posteriorly and medially under the subclavian artery. The vagus nerve then continues downward, joins the esophagus, and runs along the lateral side of the esophagus to the abdomen.

Anterior to the superior vena cava is seen the remaining anterior mediastinum, which is larger in its superior aspect. It is bordered laterally by the mediastinal pleura (which is continuous with the costal pleura and diaphragmatic pleura), covers the mediastinum, and forms the mediastinal compartment. Fat, some lymph nodes, and the thymus gland are located in this anterior area. In the mid-mediastinum the trachea descends posterior to the superior vena cava, and below the azygos vein it bifurcates into the right and left mainstem bronchi. The esophagus runs posterior to the trachea and anterior to the vertebral bodies of the spine and runs in this location in the mid-mediastinum. It deviates more to the right chest in its midportion and then more to the left chest in its inferior portion.

The hilum of the lung shows it to be invested with mediastinal pleura. This mediastinal pleura and its two leaves extend down toward the diaphragm and form the inferior pulmonary ligament. In the posterior superior portion of this hilum is seen the right mainstem bronchus, and immediately caudad to that is the inferior pulmonary vein. In the anterior portion of the hilum and slightly cephalad to the mainstem bronchus can be seen two branches of the pulmonary artery, which in turn has come out of the mediastinum posterior to the superior vena cava. In approximately the same plane as the main pulmonary artery and immediately caudal to it is the superior pulmonary vein, shown here with two branches. This vein therefore lies cephalad and anterior to the inferior pulmonary vein. Both of these veins pierce the pericardium, on the back of the heart, and enter the left atrium, which is in fact the posterior atrium.

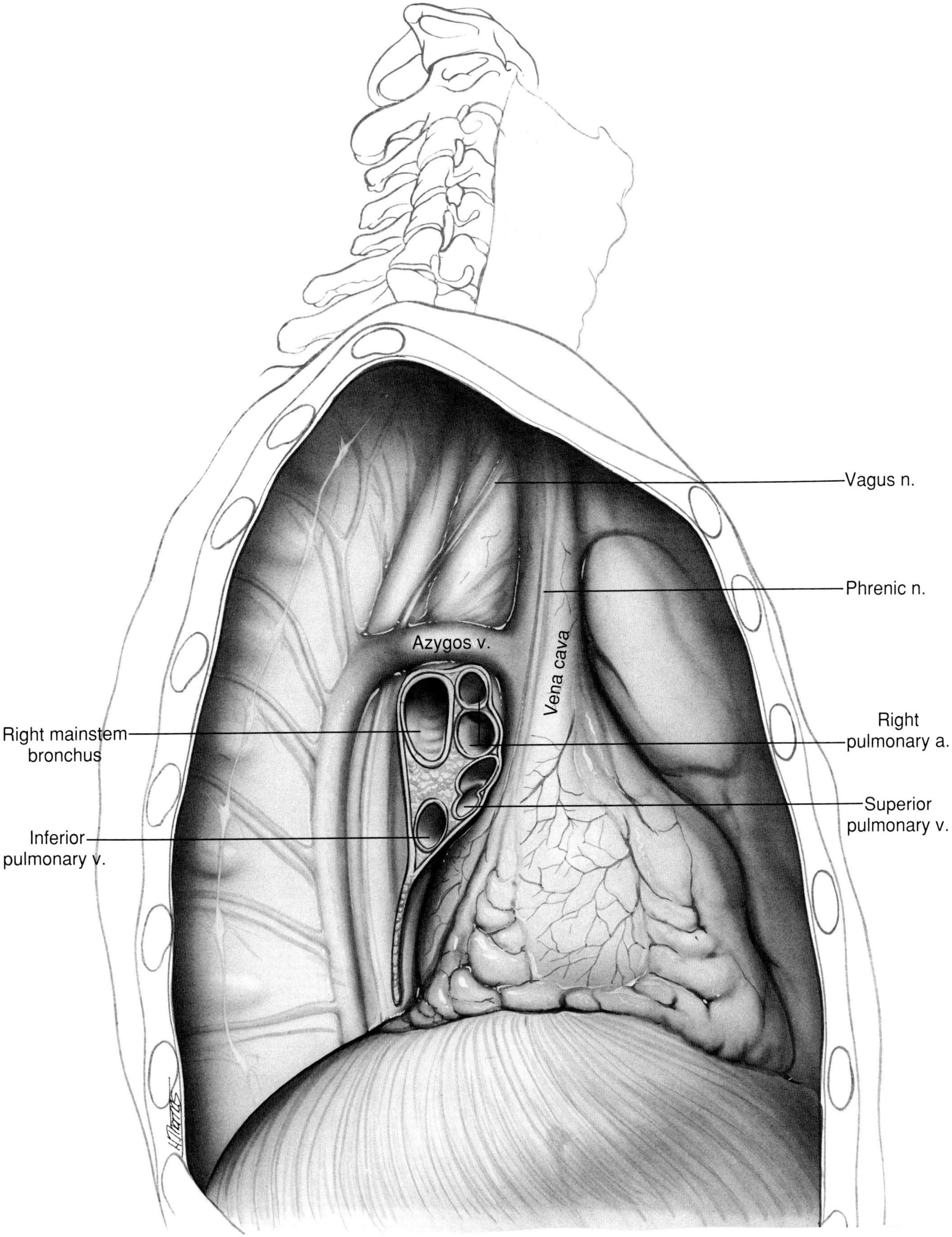
Vagus n.
Phrenic n.
Azygos v.
Vena cava
Right mainstem bronchus
Right pulmonary a.
Superior pulmonary v.
Inferior pulmonary v.

RIGHT LUNG, ANTERIOR OBLIQUE VIEW

We can see the bronchus to the right upper lobe with its trifurcation and its arterial blood supply. The posterior arterial branch to the posterior segment of the right upper lobe can be seen as it comes from the pulmonary artery caudad to the right upper lobe takeoff, rather near the longitudinal fissure. It moves posteriorly and cephalad to supply the posterior segment. This artery branch has to be looked for. It is sometimes hard to dissect and can be a source of trouble to the surgeon. The superior pulmonary vein is well seen anteriorly. The spatial configuration of the bronchi and arteries are shown, whereas the inferior pulmonary vein is seen as a main channel only.

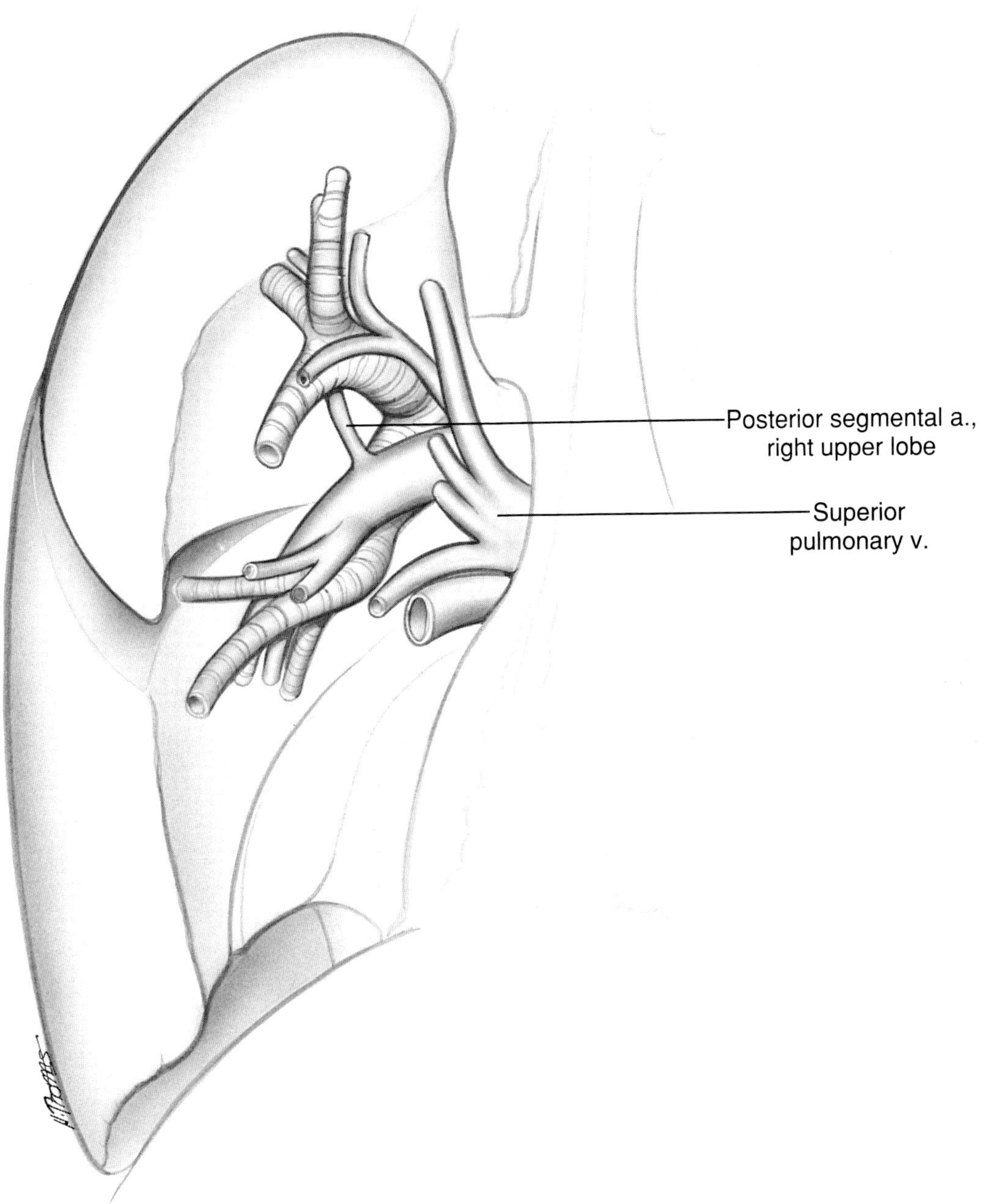

RIGHT LUNG, LATERAL VIEW

The longitudinal fissure follows the course of the sixth rib. The transverse fissue takes origin at the midaxillary line location of the longitudinal fissure and runs horizontally to the sternum. It ends at the fourth interspace.

It is important for the thoracic surgeon to develop a mind's-eye picture of the three-dimensional spatial relationship of the bronchi, arteries, and veins supplying the lung, the lung lobes, and the lung segments. The bronchi and their branches are the key to the location of the various subdivisions of the lung. These subdivisions or segments have certain anatomic variations, but the standard location is that after the right upper lobe bronchus has taken origin shortly below the tracheal carina, the right upper lobe bronchus trifurcates into an anterior branch, posterior branch, and apical branch. They are clearly defined here. The bronchus intermedius then continues caudad and bifurcates into right lower lobe and right middle lobe bronchi. An important point is that the superior segmental bronchus of the right lower lobe comes off posteriorly almost even with or frequently only slightly more caudad than the right middle lobe bronchus. This relationship can be well seen here. The right lower lobe bronchus continues downward and, on the right side, ordinarily branches into four basal segments with the anterior, lateral, and posterior basal bronchi traveling more laterally and the fourth branch, the medial-basal segmental bronchus, traveling more medially toward the heart.

The pulmonary artery is anterior for the most part and slightly cephalad to these bronchi, so that if the various bronchial segments are identified, one or more arterial branches accompany the segment. The veins, however, form and collect in the intersegmental planes and pass from the intersegmental planes to the collecting veins, which lead to the superior and inferior pulmonary veins. The superior pulmonary vein drains primarily the right upper lobe but usually also has a branch drainage from the right middle lobe. In similar fashion, the inferior pulmonary vein drains primarily the lower lobe, but it often has a venous drainage tributary from the right middle lobe. The veins as depicted here tend to be anterior but more medial to their bronchial spatial relationship.

Although this is the standard anatomy, there are numerous variations, and the careful thoracic surgeon must be aware of the anatomy present rather than the textbook pictures of the anatomy. The lung, like the liver, has two blood supplies. As demonstrated here the major blood supply for the function of the lung is the pulmonary artery system and the pulmonary venous system. However, the nutrient vessels to the lung parenchyma, especially the bronchi, are the bronchial arteries, which are branches of the aorta or intercostal arteries. The bronchial veins drain along the bronchi and are systemic veins that tend to drain into the azygos and hemiazygos systems. These two systems, one of which is a low-pressure "blue" blood system, namely the pulmonary artery system, contrasts with the bronchial vascular sytem, which is a systemic pressure system with arterialized blood. At the bronchiole levels there are collateral connections between the bronchial arterial system and the pulmonary arterial system. This is a protective mechanism so that the lung will not become necrotic with the ligation of either vascular system. If, however, the pulmonary artery is obstructed or ligated on a permanent basis, there is a very great enlargement of the bronchial arterial system, which can function like a peripheral arterial venous fistula.

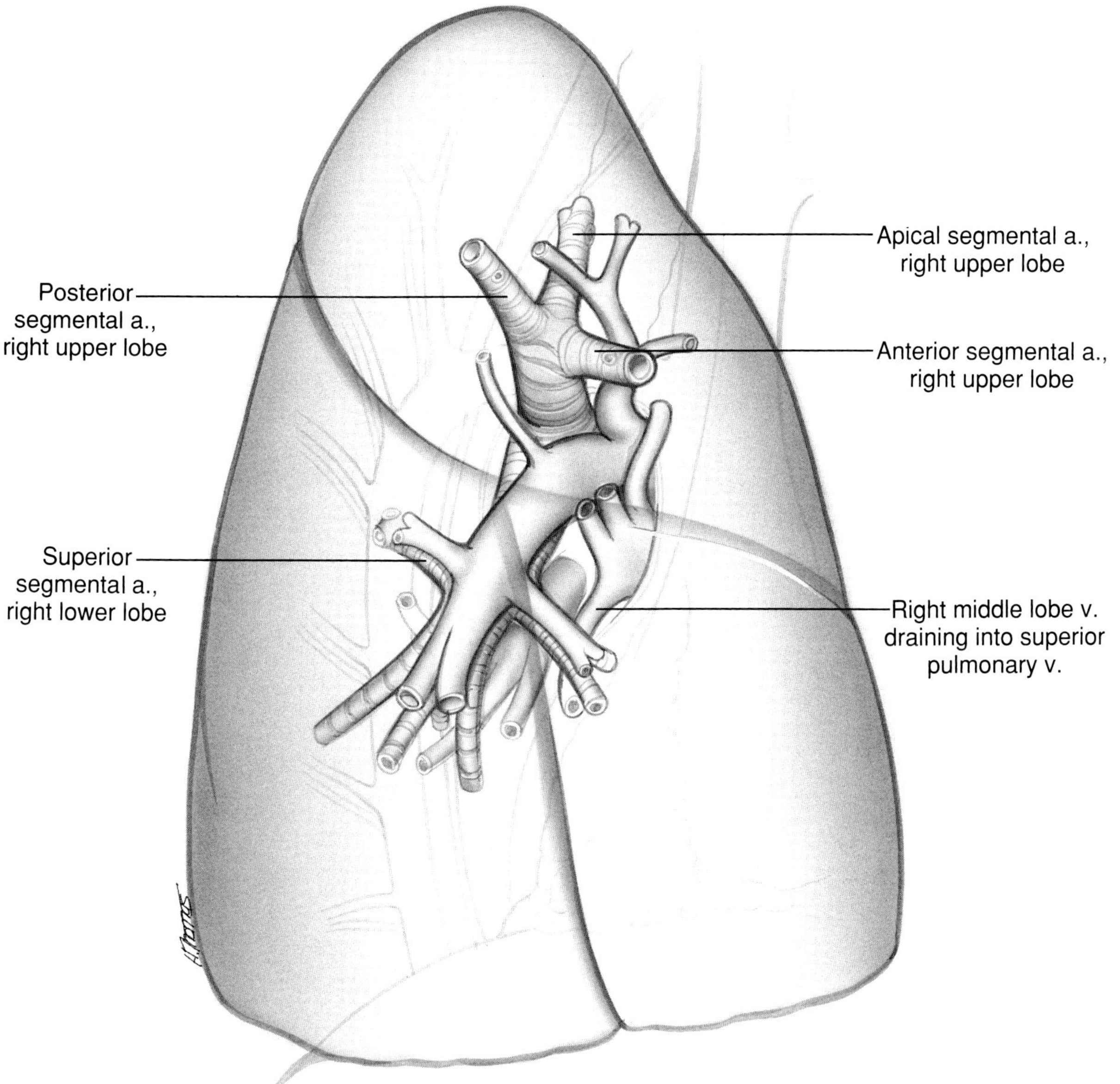
Apical segmental a.,
right upper lobe
Posterior
segmental a.,
right upper lobe
Anterior segmental a.,
right upper lobe
Superior
segmental a.,
right lower lobe
Right middle lobe v.
draining into superior
pulmonary v.

RIGHT LUNG, POSTERIOR VIEW

The fissure outlining the superior segment of the right lower lobe comes up quite high since this is a rather voluminous segment. The anatomy of the bronchus is seen. The cartilaginous horseshoes all face forward with their open hoops posteriorly connected by the membranous portion. This means that one has always to exercise more care in dissecting the thin posterior membranous portion of the tracheobronchial tree than the tougher anterior-cartilagenous portion of the tracheobronchial tree. It is relatively clearly shown how one can approach from posteriorly the right upper lobe bronchus since the arterial and venous supplies to the right upper lobe are primarily anterior to this lobe. It can also be seen that the main pulmonary artery runs lateral and anterior to the bronchus down the lung. The inferior pulmonary vein is primarily caudad to the bronchus intermedius. As already mentioned, these veins drain from the intersegmental planes and tend to be caudal to the bronchi in this location.

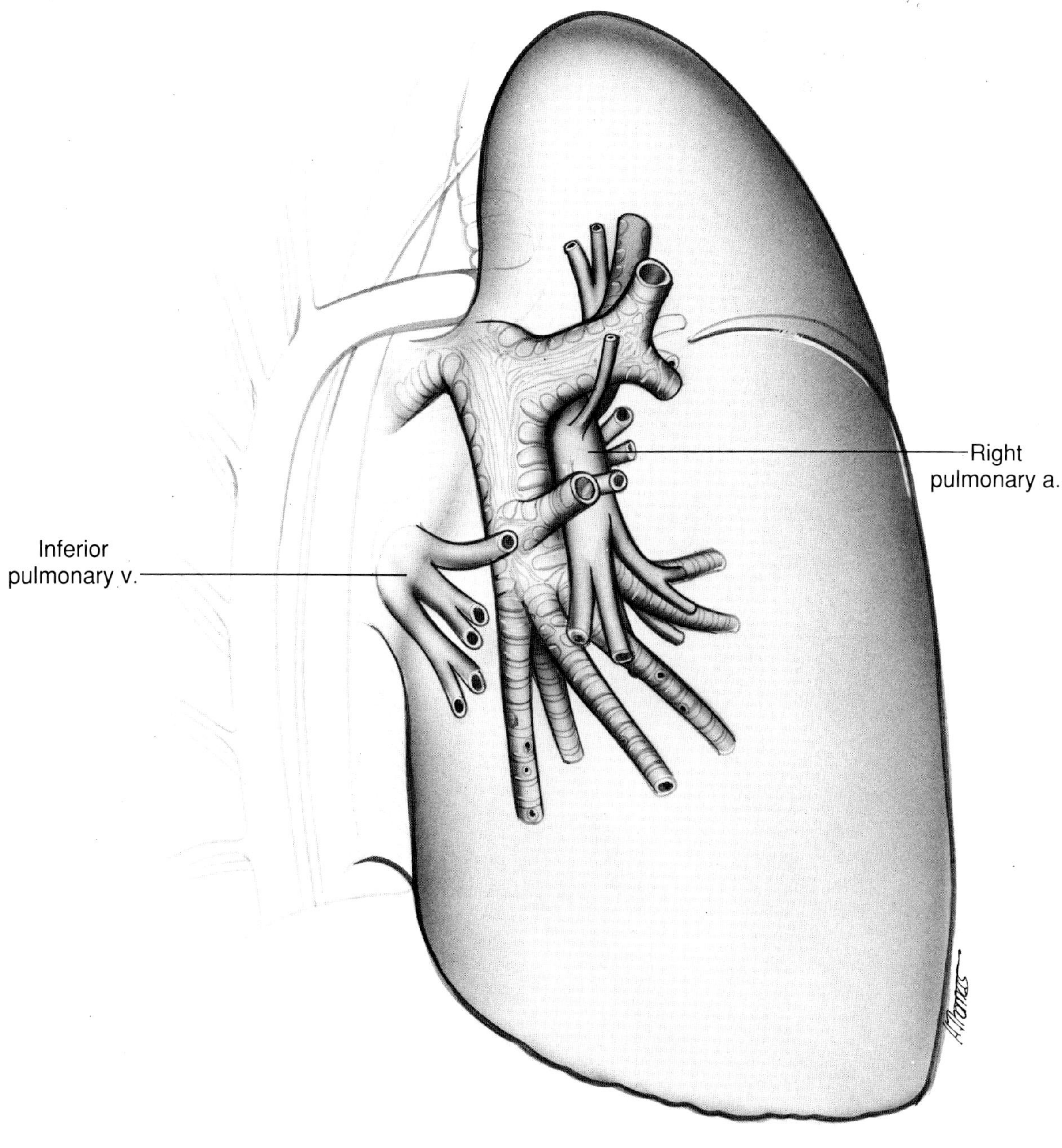

LEFT HEMITHORAX

Here we are looking into the empty left chest, the left lung having been removed. The mediastinum is lined by mediastinal pleura, which again is continuous with the costal pleura and the diaphragmatic pleura to make the thoracic cavity.

The left chest is the arterial chest, whereas the right chest is the venous chest. One can see the ascending aorta arising from the heart, sweeping around posteriorly, and running caudad immediately adjacent to the anterior bodies of the spine. Running upward on the spine and collecting the intercostal venous drainage is the hemiazygos system, analogous to the azygos sytem on the right side. Here this system drains into the left innominate vein, which can be seen anterior to the carotid artery, which is the first branch of the aortic arch. Immediately posterior to this is the subclavian artery, which arches out of the apex of the chest and crosses the first rib posterior to the scalene tubercule, which is on the midportion of the concave side of the first rib. The internal mammary artery is the first branch from this subclavian artery and runs down the anterior chest less than 1 cm lateral to the border of the sternum. The phrenic nerve can be seen entering the chest lateral to the innominate vein, which is the landmark for it. One must be very careful with surgery in the anterior superior mediastinum not to injure these two structures, the left and right phrenic nerves. These nerves swing posteriorly as they enter the chest and run directly anterior to the lung hila. Therefore, to avoid injury, the phrenic nerve can be found anterior to the hilum of the lung and traced cephalad or caudad so that its course is known.

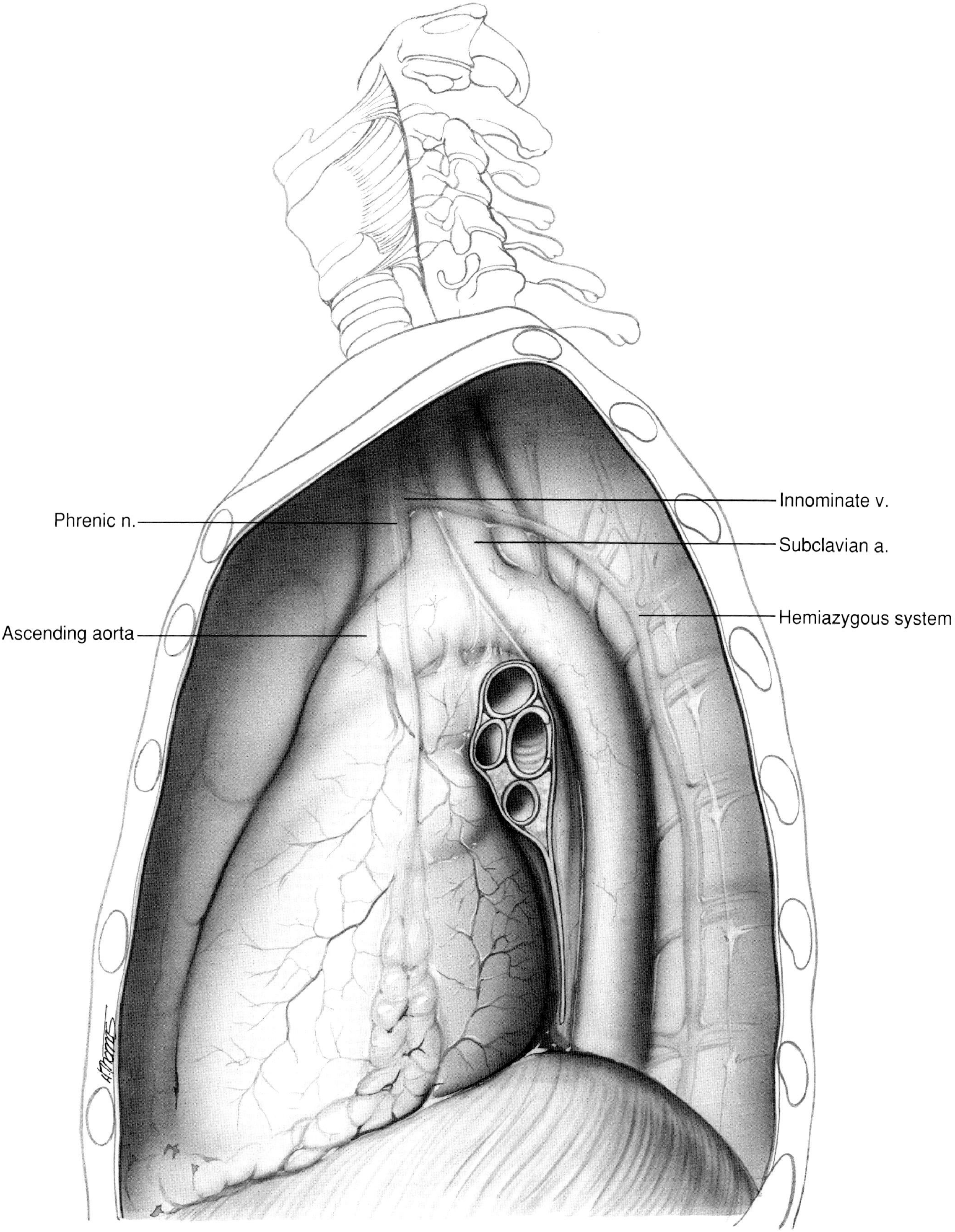

Innominate v.
Phrenic n.
Subclavian a.
Hemiazygous system
Ascending aorta

LEFT LUNG, ANTERIOR VIEW

In the cephalic part of the hilum is the main pulmonary artery, which comes out and swings around to descend in the longitudinal fissure between the upper and lower lobes. Its first branch is usually the apical branch. The artery gives off several branches to the left upper lobe before continuing down in the fissure to supply the lower lobe. The structure that is immediately caudad but slightly anterior to the plane of this pulmonary artery is the superior pulmonary vein. Here we see three main branches that enter and make up the superior pulmonary vein. The highest venous drainage branch can be seen to cross up over the first branch of the pulmonary artery. This can be troublesome in exposing the first arterial branch if tumor lymph nodes are close. It is often necessary to divide this branch to expose safely the first arterial branch. The other branches of the superior pulmonary vein continue their course and drain from the lingula upwards. Posterior to the superior pulmonary vein and caudal to the pulmonary artery is the left mainstem bronchus, which branches into the left upper and lower lobes. The left upper lobe bronchus soon branches into the superior and inferior divisions. The inferior division makes up the superior and inferior segments of the lingula, whereas the superior division bifurcates and gives off the anterior branch and the apical-posterior branches. The left lower lobe bronchial branch runs in the fissure but medial to and hidden by the main pulmonary artery. Its first branch, not well shown here, is the superior segmental branch. It continues downward to give three basal segmental bronchi, one of which is the anteromedial bronchus. The inferior pulmonary vein is in the caudal part of the hilum next to the main bronchus, and below that is the inferior pulmonary ligament.

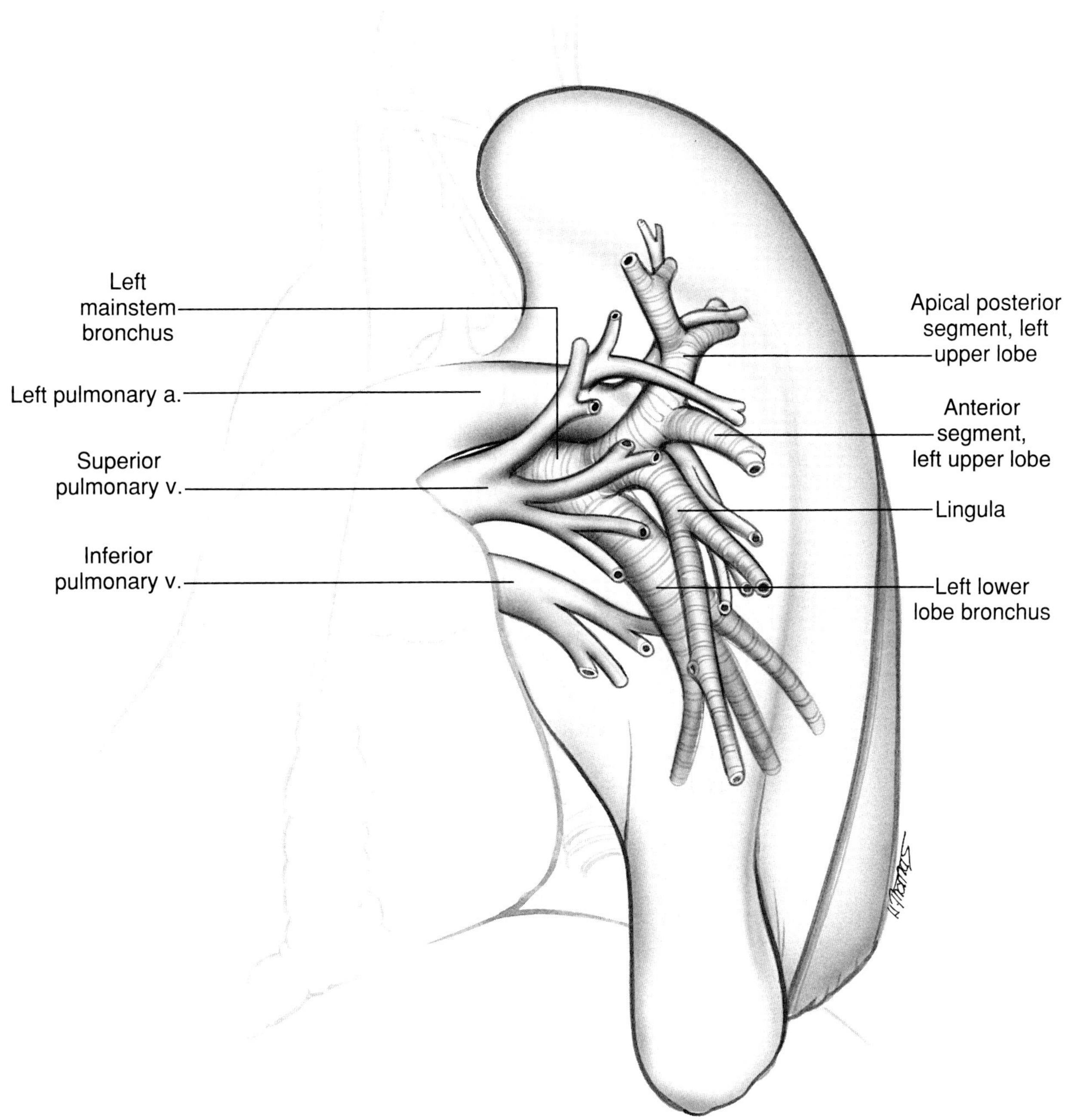

Left mainstem bronchus
Left pulmonary a.
Superior pulmonary v.
Inferior pulmonary v.
Apical posterior segment, left upper lobe
Anterior segment, left upper lobe
Lingula
Left lower lobe bronchus

LEFT LUNG, LATERAL VIEW

This is the lateral view of the left lung. The artist has drawn in the standard anatomy which the surgeon should be familiar with and look for. As one opens the longitudinal fissure, the structure seen first is the main pulmonary artery. Here one can see the lingular artery branch, which runs anteriorly in the lowest portion of the left upper lobe. There is a more proximal arterial branch going up to the anterior segment and a branch to the posterior segment. As mentioned already, these branches are variable. The superior segmental branch can be seen running to the superior segment of the left lower lobe. The bronchus is very hard to expose in this area until the necessary branches of the pulmonary artery are divided so that the bronchus can be uncovered. The left upper lobe bronchus with its inferior division lingula and superior division containing the rest of the upper lobe segments is clearly seen. The superior segmental bronchus and then the continuation into the left lower lobe basal segmental bronchus are also seen. The inferior pulmonary vein is hidden and is not readily visible in this approach, although one can see some of it slightly anterior and caudal to the bronchus.

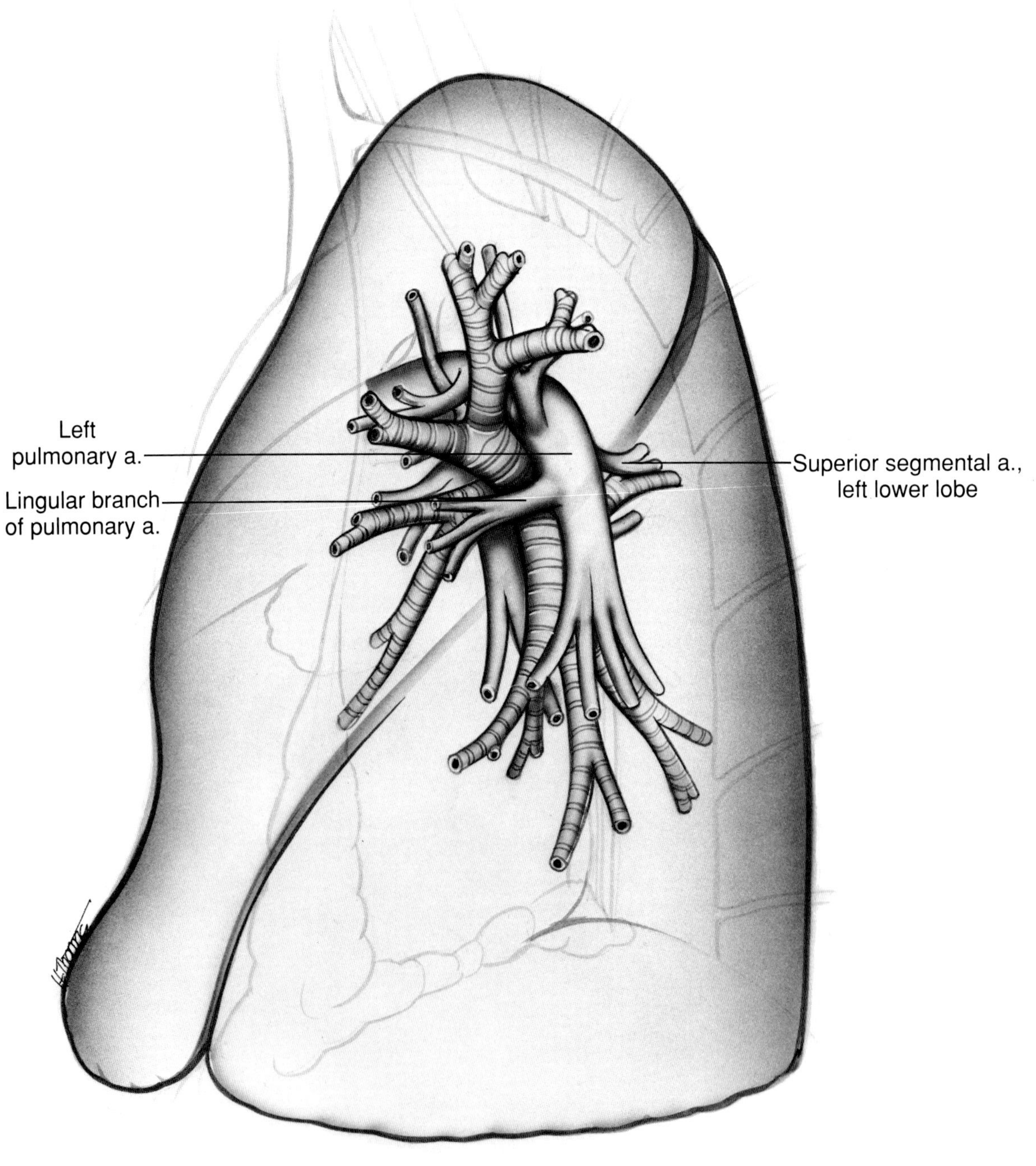

LEFT LUNG, POSTEROLATERAL VIEW

In this view we see the hilar anatomy from the rear. Here the pulmonary artery is seen to be the highest portion of the hilum. Caudal to that in roughly the same plane is the left mainstem bronchus. The tracheal carina is rather high near the aortic arch in this approach. The inferior pulmonary vein can be well seen here since it is in the same plane as the bronchus and caudal to it. The various branches of the upper lobe and lower lobe bronchi are well depicted. The surgeon should be very familiar with the standard anatomy in any approach to the lung but should be alert for anatomic variations, which are all too common.

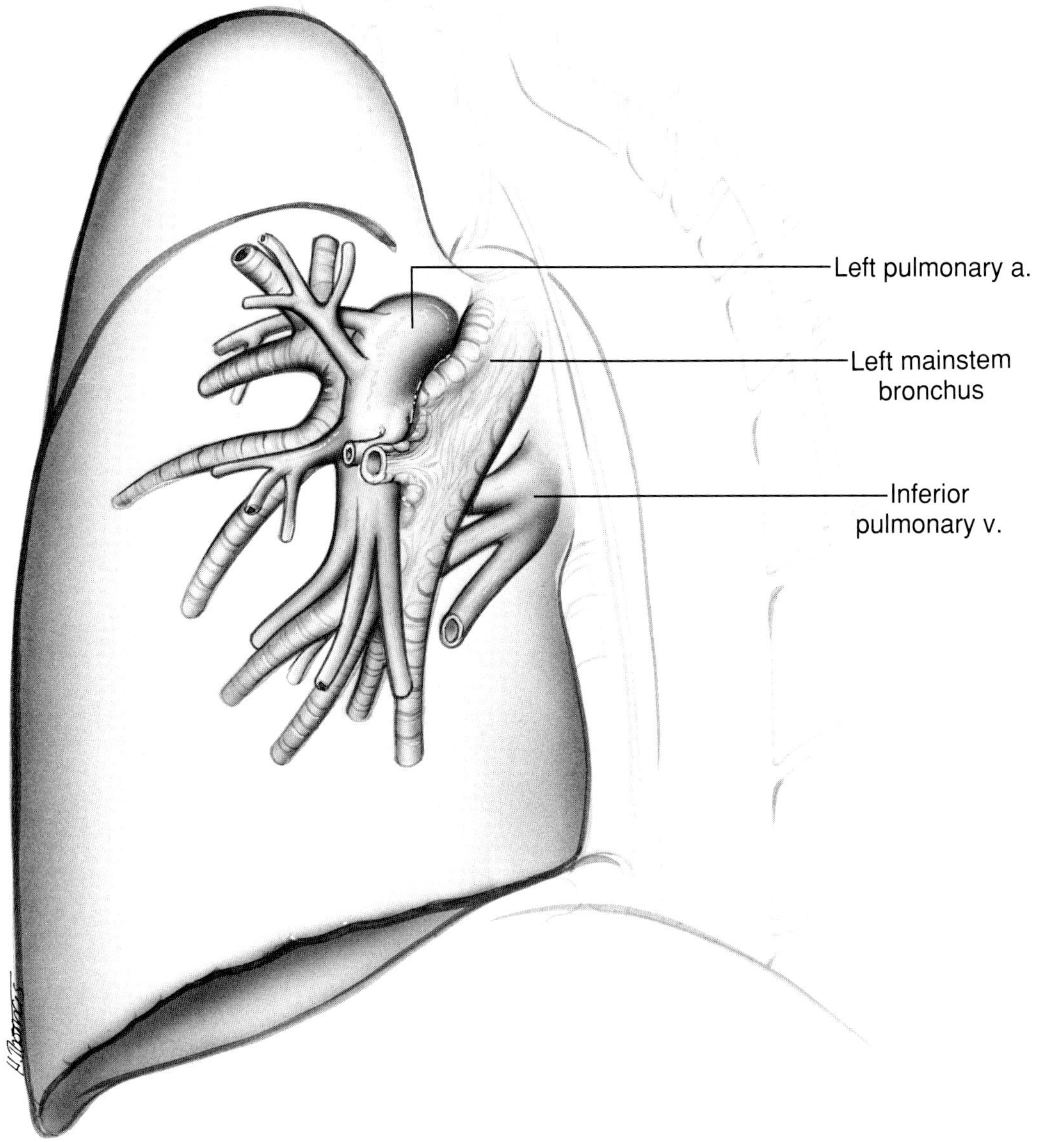

LEFT LUNG, WITH FISSURE SPREAD

Here we are approaching the left lung laterally, and the fissure has been spread. The artist has ghosted in the anatomy in the proper relationship. Note that the key feature is the pulmonary artery running down the fissure. The first posterior branch of the pulmonary artery is the superior segmental branch, which is matched by the superior segmental bronchus immediately medial to it. It can be seen that the bronchi are somewhat medial to the artery as depicted here and that the venous drainage that comes from the intersegmental planes goes to the caudal and medial portions of the bronchial drainage. In similar fashion, it can be seen that in the left upper lobe the artery branches are posterior to the bronchi. The bronchi are midway between the arteries posteriorly and the venous drainage anteriorly.

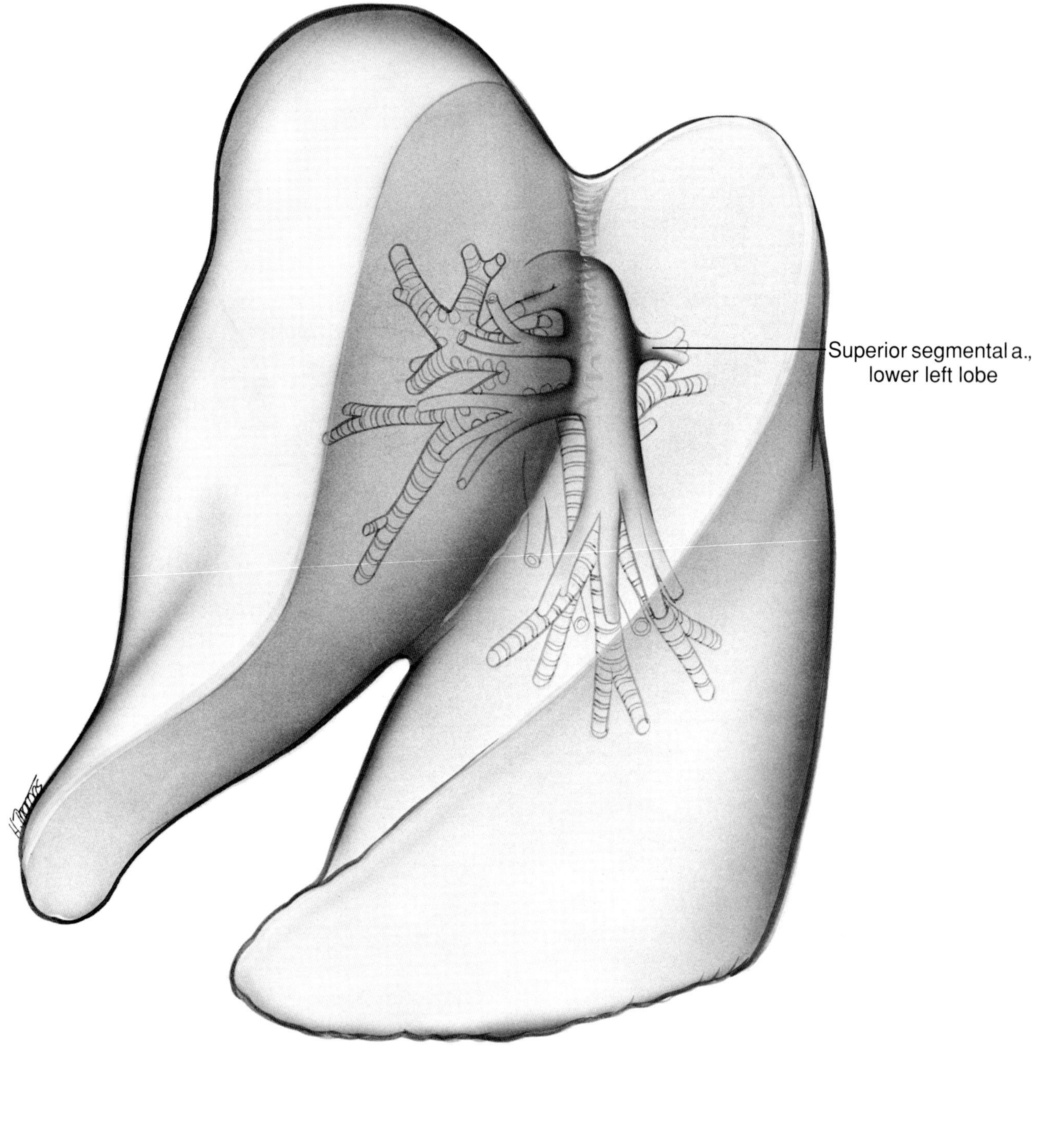

LEFT LUNG, ARTERIAL BRANCHES EXPOSED

Here the fissue has been opened and the sheath over the pulmonary artery has been cut so that one can see the arterial branches to the left upper lobe. The inferior portion of the longitudinal fissure and the lung parenchyma between the left lower lobe and right lower lobe in the inferior portion of the hilum is still intact. The circle around this shows what has to be opened, but it can be seen that great care must be taken not to injure the lingular arterial branch and to watch out for the branches draining into the superior pulmonary vein and inferior pulmonary vein, since there may be vessels that cross this fissure. Once this plane has been identified anteriorly and the surgeon has seen all the pertinent and chief anatomic features, a stapler can readily and safely open up this fissure to give a further view of whichever of these lobes or segments the surgeon wishes to approach surgically.

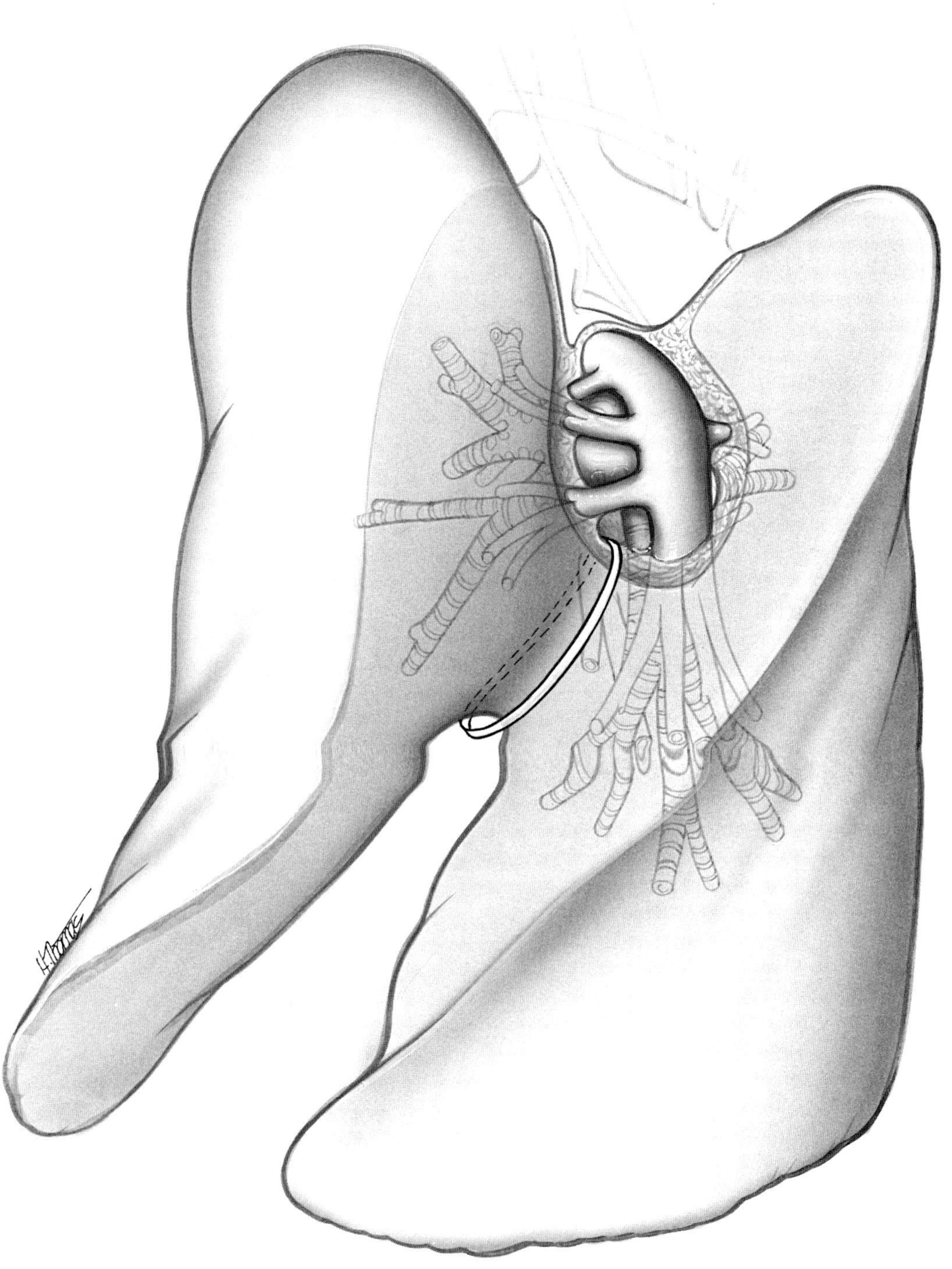

LOCATION OF LYMPH NODES IN THE LUNGS AND MEDIASTINUM

In this drawing the upper diagram shows the general location of the lymph nodes. The lower left drawing shows the lateral view in the right chest. The lower right drawing shows the view within the left chest. The operating thoracic surgeon must be aware of this system. He is responsible for sampling or removing all the nodes possible and ensuring that they are appropriately labeled. The pathologist should know which location these nodes came from. A good technique used in Japan is for the scrub nurse to have on the operating table a compartmentalized box where lymph nodes of various numbers can be placed. Further information is obtained when the pathologist reports the status of these lymph nodes and reports whether the tumor is within the lymph node, notes the size of the lymph node, and ascertains whether the tumor has broken the capsule of the lymph node.

Mediastinal lymph nodes are numbered 1 through 9; double-digit numbers indicate lymph nodes in the lungs. Double-digit nodes must be identified by location, specifying which lobes, segments, and/or subsegments are involved.

Mediastinal Lymph Nodes

1, superior or highest
2, paratracheal to right / left
3, pretrachael / posterior tracheal
4, tracheobronchial, at right azygos vein
5, aortic window, on the left
6, para-aortic on ascending aorta on left
7, subcarinal
8, paraesophageal, left or right, below carina
9, inferior pulmonary ligament, left or right

Thoracic Lymph Nodes

10, hilar, left / right mainstem bronchus
11, interlobar area
12, lobar, located on upper lobe, middle lobe, and lower lobe
13, segmental, 10 on right, 8 on left
14, subsegmental, peripheral nodes where segments bifurcate

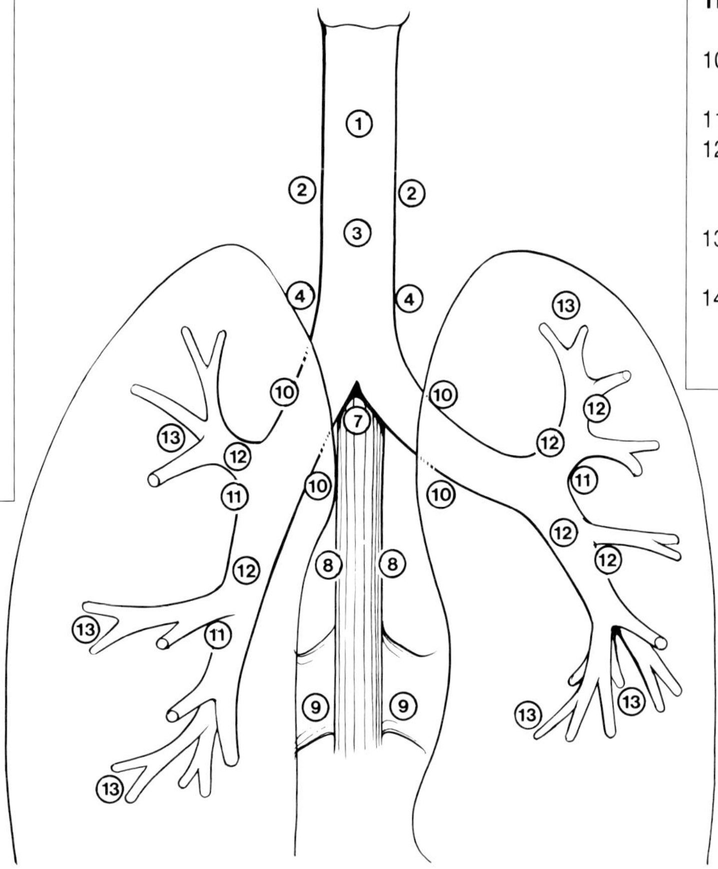

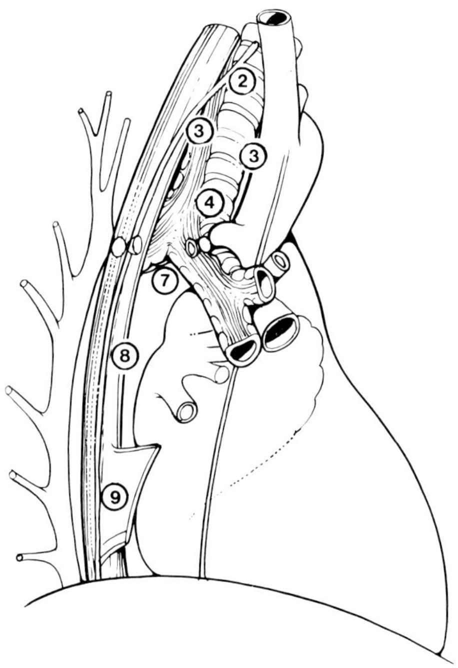

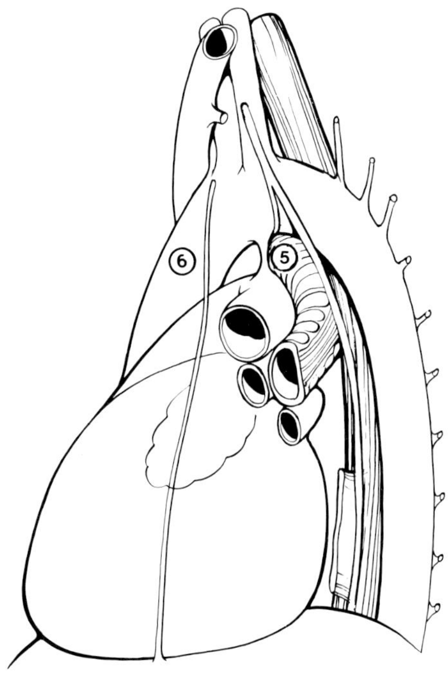

BRONCHOPULMONARY ANATOMY

Learning about bronchopulmonary segments was an important contribution to thoracic surgery. It was especially important when operations to remove bronchiectasis and pulmonary tuberculosis were common. In surgical oncology, lung tissue often must be conserved, and bronchopulmonary segment resection of tumor may be the best way to do so. This is true if there is significant emphysema or when multiple pulmonary metastases are present.

There are three segments in the right upper lobe, two segments in the right middle lobe, and five segments in the right lower lobe. There are four segments in the left upper lobe and four in the left lower lobe. To find these segments the surgeon dissects the hilum of the lobe to identify the bronchus to the segment in question. When the bronchus has been dissected free, the anesthetist can then aspirate the lung. The surgeon then can use a noncrushing clamp to occlude the segmental bronchus in question. The anesthetist reinflates the lobe and lung. By watching which surface portion of the lobe inflates, the surgeon can identify the proper bronchus and segment. When the segment is identified, one can divide the arteries accompanying the bronchus and either strip the segment out or wedge it out with stapling devices.

An alternative but less satisfactory approach is to keep the lung inflated and, by the knowledge of the surface anatomy of the segments, open up the fissures with stapling devices. The segment is isolated to the hilum, which is taken last.

BRONCHOPULMONARY ANATOMY

TRACHEOBRONCHIAL TREE, ANTEROPOSTERIOR VIEW

This drawing demonstrates the 10 segmental bronchi on the right and the 8 segmental bronchi on the left. There is considerable variation in these bronchi, but this drawing shows the most usual situation. Each of these bronchi promptly bifurcates or trifurcates. It can be seen by comparing this drawing with the highlight box that the nomenclature for the segments is correlated to the "B" numbers. We would refer the reader to a textbook of bronchology for further analysis of this nomenclature. The subdivisions of the "B" numbers are B1a, B1b, B1c, etc.

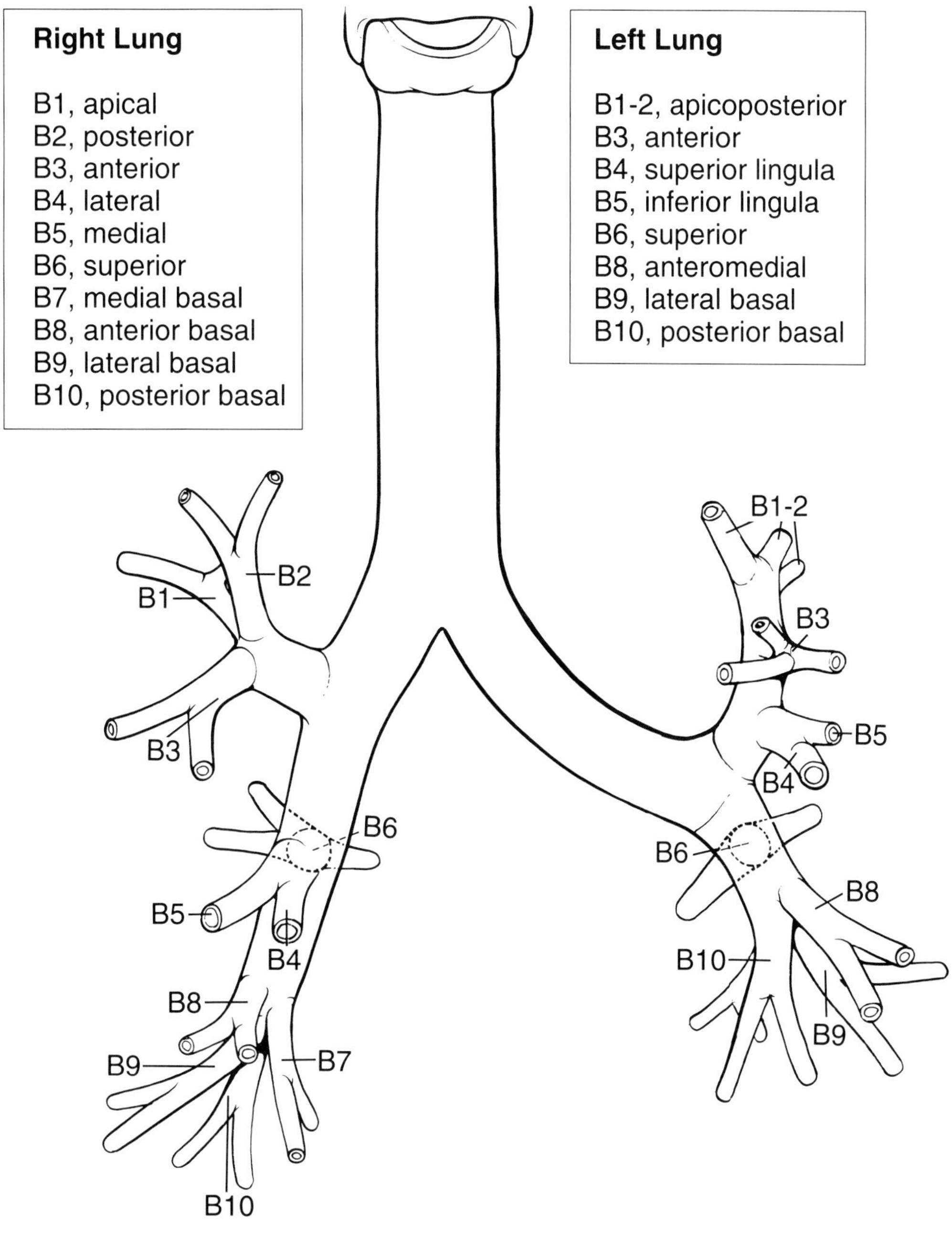
Right Lung
B1, apical
B2, posterior
B3, anterior
B4, lateral
B5, medial
B6, superior
B7, medial basal
B8, anterior basal
B9, lateral basal
B10, posterior basal
Left Lung
B1-2, apicoposterior
B3, anterior
B4, superior lingula
B5, inferior lingula
B6, superior
B8, anteromedial
B9, lateral basal
B10, posterior basal
B2
B1
B3
B6
B5
B4
B8
B9
B7
B10
B1-2
B3
B5
B4
B6
B8
B10
B9

BRONCHOPULMONARY ANATOMY

BRONCHIAL SEGMENTS, LATERAL VIEW

This drawing shows the bronchial segments marked with their appropriate "B" numbers. In this case we have added the subsegment terminology "a" and "b." If there is a trifurcation it ordinarily would be a "c" number.

Lateral projections of the right and left lungs are drawn to show the surface representation of the bronchopulmonary segments. In the right lung are seen the apical segment B1, the posterior segment B2, and the anterior segment B3, of the right upper lobe. In the right middle lobe the medial segment is B5 and the lateral segment is B4. In the right lower lobe the largest segment is the superior segment B6. The anterior basal segment B8, the lateral basal segment B9, and the posterior segment B10 are seen. Not seen is the medial basal segment B7, which goes medially toward the mediastinum. Each of these basal segments has representation on the diaphragmatic surface as well.

The left lung is a smaller lung since the heart is in the left chest. In the left upper lobe the bronchus branches into the superior division containing the anterior segment B3 and the combined apicoposterior segment, which is B1-2. The inferior portion of the left upper lobe is the lingula, with the superior lingula B4 and the inferior lingula B5. The large superior segment of the left lower lobe is B6. There is no separate medial basal segment since the heart occupies space in the left chest. B8 is the anterior (or anterior medial) basal segment with B9 and B10 the lateral basal and the posterior basal segments, respectively. It is important that the thoracic surgeon operating on lungs be familiar with the segmental anatomy, the anatomy of the bronchi, and the correct terminology.

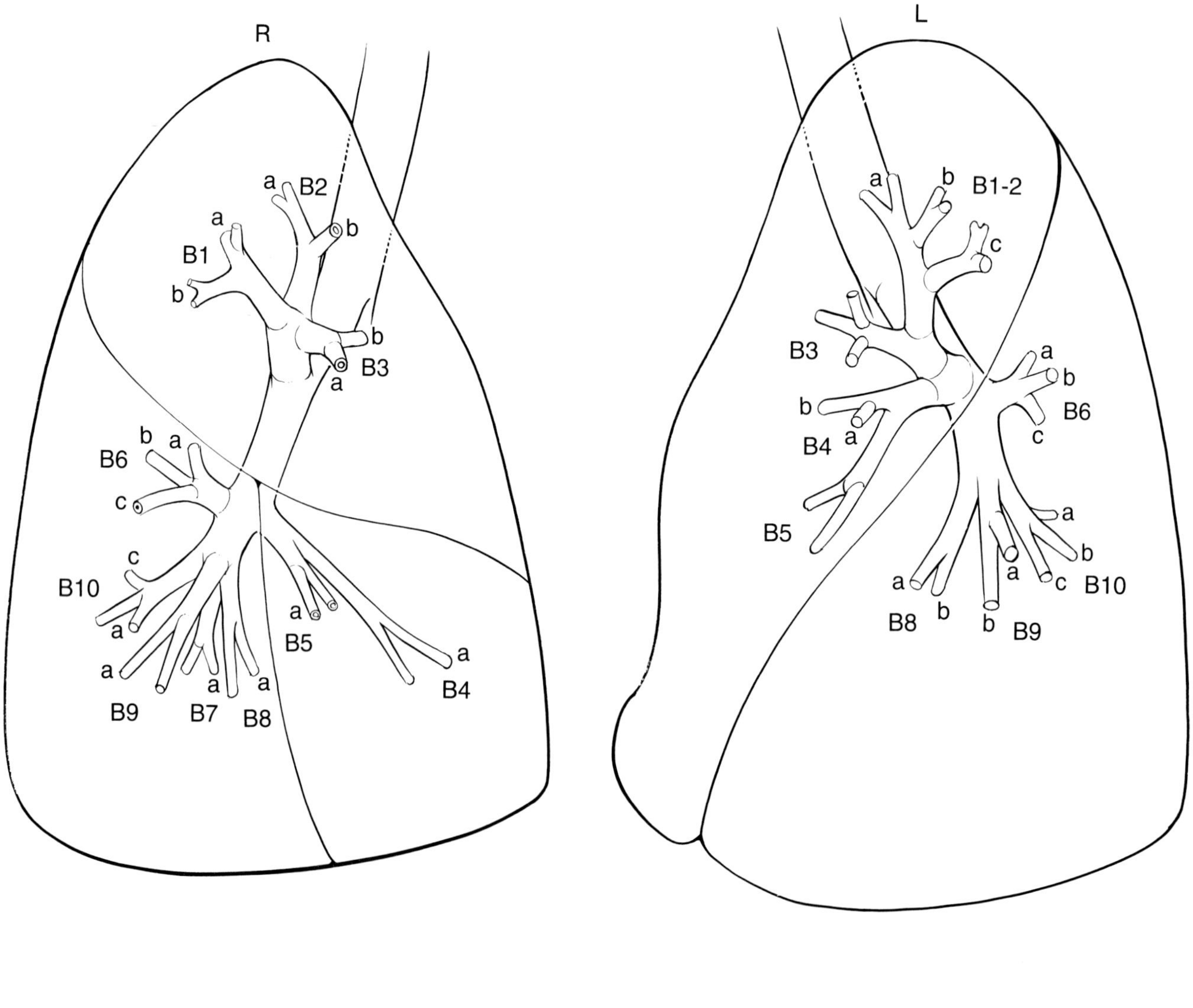

BRONCHOPULMONARY ANATOMY

BRONCHOPULMONARY SEGMENTS, LATERAL VIEW

On the left of this drawing is a lateral view of the right lung showing the bronchopulmonary segments. Areas marked 1, 2, and 3 are, respectively, the apical, posterior, and anterior segments of the upper lobe; 4 and 5 are the lateral and medial segments; 6, 8, 9, and 10 are the superior, anterior basal, lateral basal, and posterior basal segments of the lower lobe; and 7, the medial basal segment of the lower lobe, is not visible. On the right is the view of the left lung, showing its eight bronchopulmonary segments; 1-2, 3, 4, and 5 represent respectively the apicoposterior, anterior, superior lingula, and inferior lingula segments of the upper lobe; 6, 8, 9, and 10 are the superior, anteromedial, lateral basal, and posterior basal segments of the lower lobe.

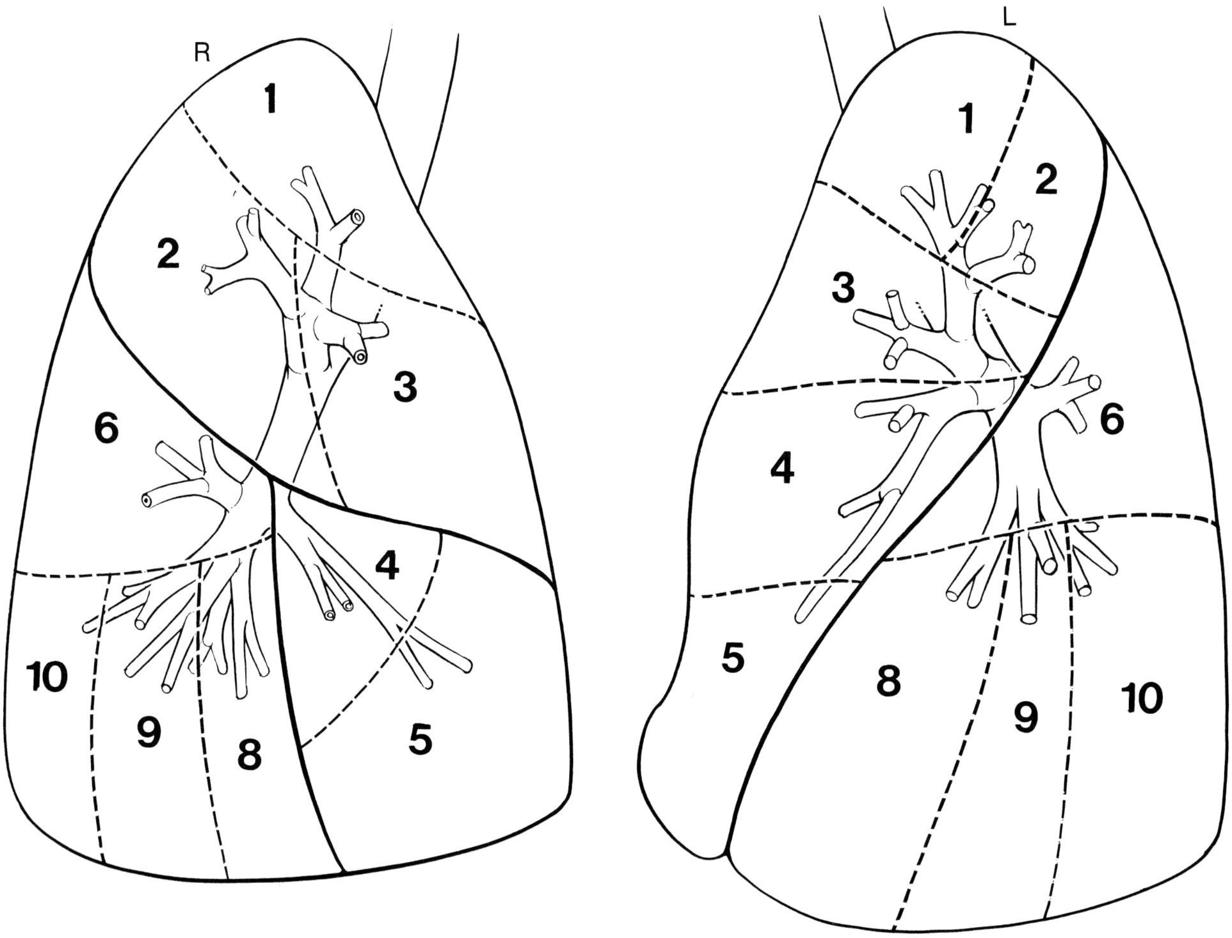

VIEWS SEEN ON BRONCHOSCOPY

The first view in the right main bronchus is of the right upper lobe, where the apical (B1) bronchus is at about 3 o'clock with the anterior (B3) bronchus toward 11 o'clock and the posterior (B2) bronchus toward 7 o'clock.

The next view down the bronchus intermedius is of the right middle lobe anteriorly and the right lower lobe posteriorly. The carina between should be sharp. The right middle lobe branches into the medial (B5) and the lateral (B4) segments.

In the right lower lobe bronchus the superior segment (B6) moves immediately posterior (6 o'clock). The basal segments are arranged medially to laterally as medial basal (B7), posterior basal (B10), lateral basal (B9) and anterior basal (B8).

When the bronchoscope enters the left main bronchus, the left upper lobe and left lower lobe are seen straight ahead with their carina running from 2 o'clock to 8 o'clock.

The left upper lobe is seen to the left and anteriorly. It promptly divides into the superior and inferior division (lingula), about 9 o'clock and 3 o'clock, respectively. These in turn divide left to right into segments apicoposterior (B1-2), anterior (B3), and then superior lingula (B4) and inferior lingula (B-5).

Similar to the right side, the superior segment (B6) of the left lower lobe goes directly posteriorly (6 o'clock). The other three basal segments are also arranged left to right as anterior (B8), lateral (B9), and posterior (B10).

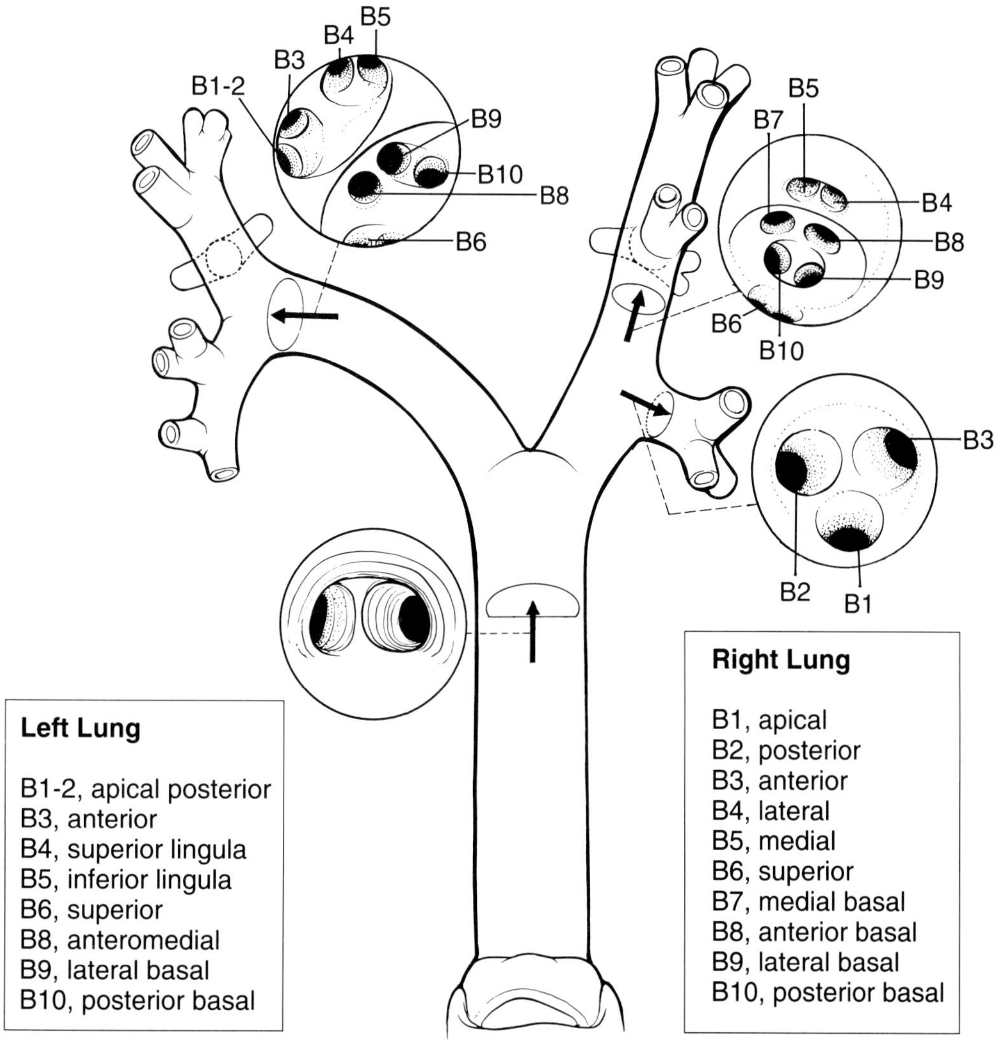

THORACOTOMY

THE POSTEROLATERAL INCISION

In this drawing the patient is lying in the left lateral position and the right chest is diagrammed. The incision is just below the angle of the scapula, and the anterior portion of the incision curves anteriorly toward the nipple. In the male the nipple is in the fourth interspace. The posterior portion of the incision curves cephalad but stays midway between the spinous processes and the medial portion of the spine for whatever distance is believed to be necessary.

The muscles being cut are seen posteriorly. The first is the trapezius, and deep to the trapezius are found the rhomboids. More anterior to the trapezius are the latissimus and the serratus, which is well depicted here. This is usually carried out by a scalpel incision of skin followed by electrocautery cutting and coagulation of the muscle groups down to the thoracic wall.

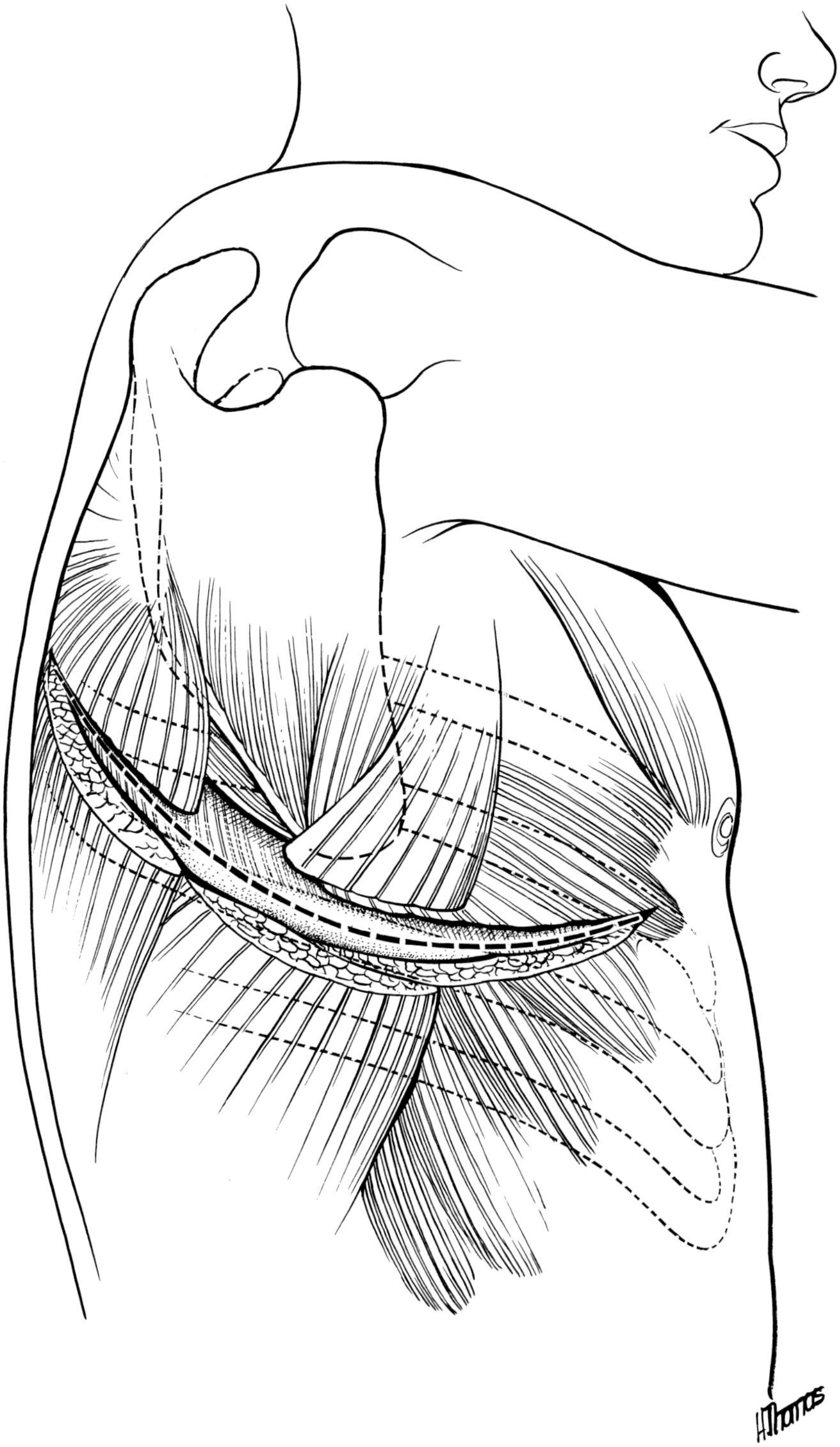

THORACOTOMY

DIGITAL PROBE BETWEEN PLEURAL LAYERS

In this view the chest wall muscles have been cut. The scapula is retracted cephalad, usually by a scapula retractor. The surgeon has felt under the scapula up to the second or first rib to find the exact interspace that he wishes to enter.

In this drawing the intercostal muscles have been divided in the interspace along the cephalic edge of the lower rib so as to avoid the intercostal bundle, which runs under the caudal border of each rib. The parietal pleura has been exposed and an incision has been made in the parietal pleura. The index finger is being inserted to ascertain the presence or absence of adhesions between the visceral and parietal pleura.

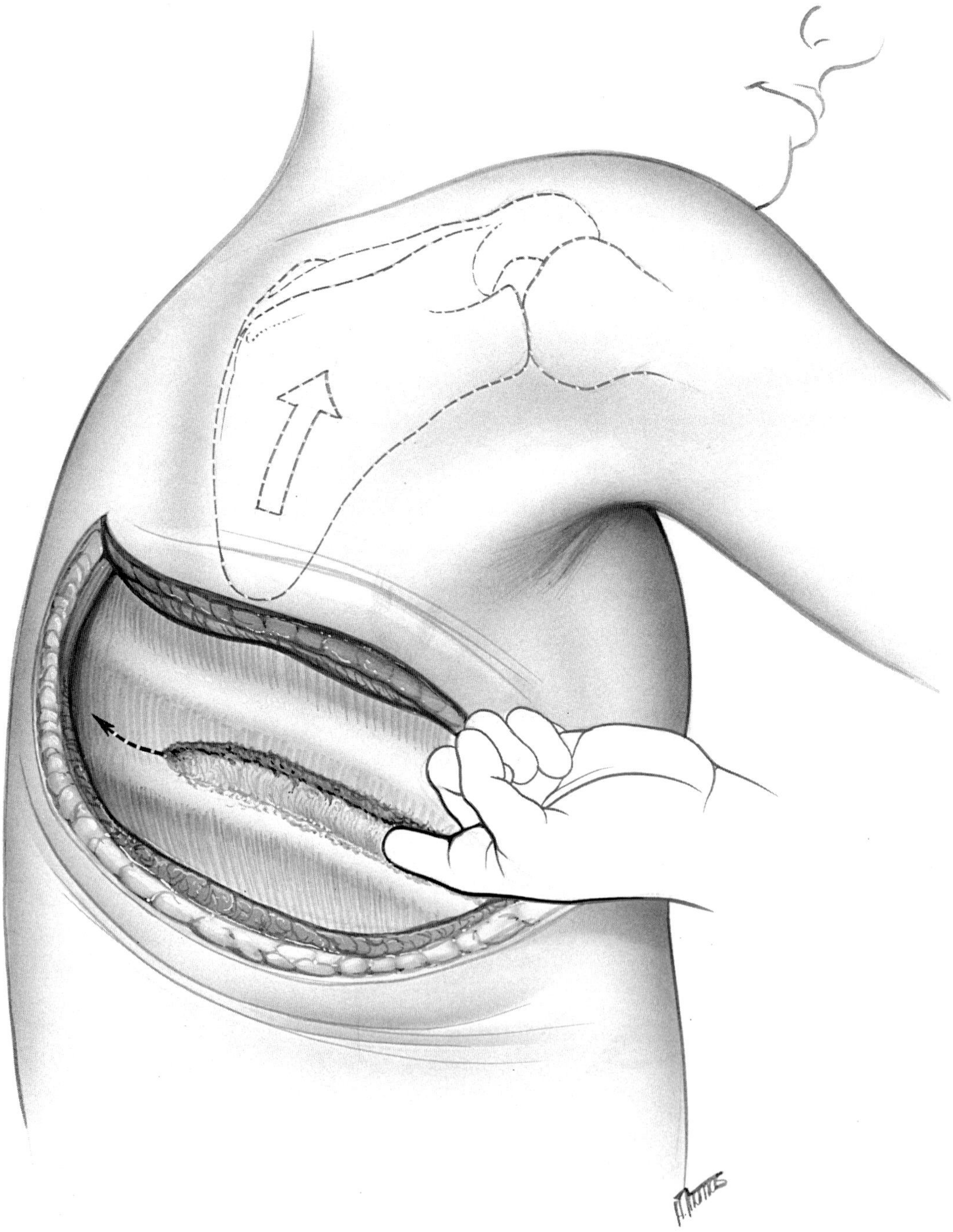

THORACOTOMY

PROBE, CROSS-SECTIONAL VIEW

This illustration could well be combined with the previous one. The upper drawing shows the anatomy of the chest wall. Medically and caudally under each rib runs the intercostal bundle, which consists of the vein most cephalic followed, as one moves caudad, by the artery and nerve. The view shows the external and internal intercostal muscles and the parietal pleura. The black space is the potential space between the visceral pleura of the lung and the parietal pleura of the chest wall.

In the lower drawing the index finger is inserted into the pleural space. The intercostal muscles have been cut from the cephalic side of the lower rib. The finger is exploring and finding that there are no adhesions between the parietal and visceral pleura, so that the incision and opening up of the parietal pleura can continue.

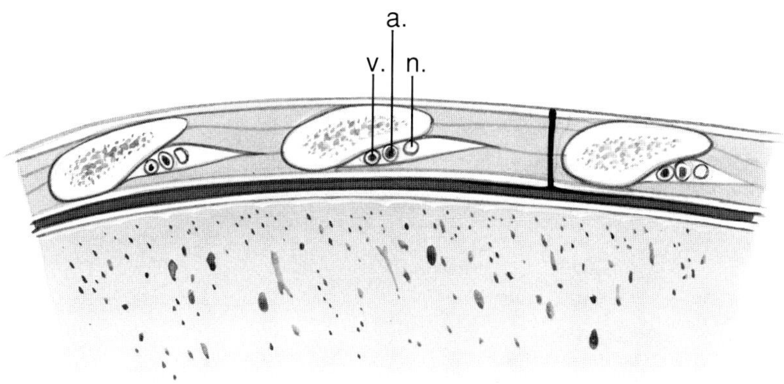

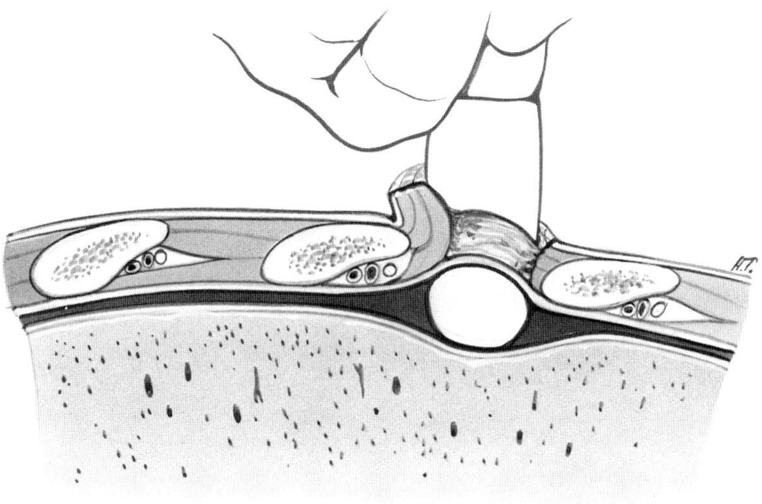

THORACOTOMY

INSERTION OF THE RIB SPREADER

Since the chest wall cephalad includes the scapula, it is usually thicker than the chest wall caudad. If the patient is large, it is an advantage to have a rib spreader with interchangeable blades so that the large blade can be used cephalad and a smaller blade caudad. After its placement, the rib spreader is opened slowly and gently in an effort not to break any ribs. If there is resistance to the ribs being spread and more space is needed, it is better to "shingle" the upper or lower rib posteriorly to gain relaxation. It is somewhat better to cut the caudal rib to preserve the intercostal bundle; ordinarily if one cuts the cephalalic rib it is usually necessary to ligate the intercostal bundle. This ligature may cause increased pain unless the intercostal nerve is free of the ligature. The drawing shows the chest open over the region of the longitudinal fissure with the transverse fissure running anteriorly from it.

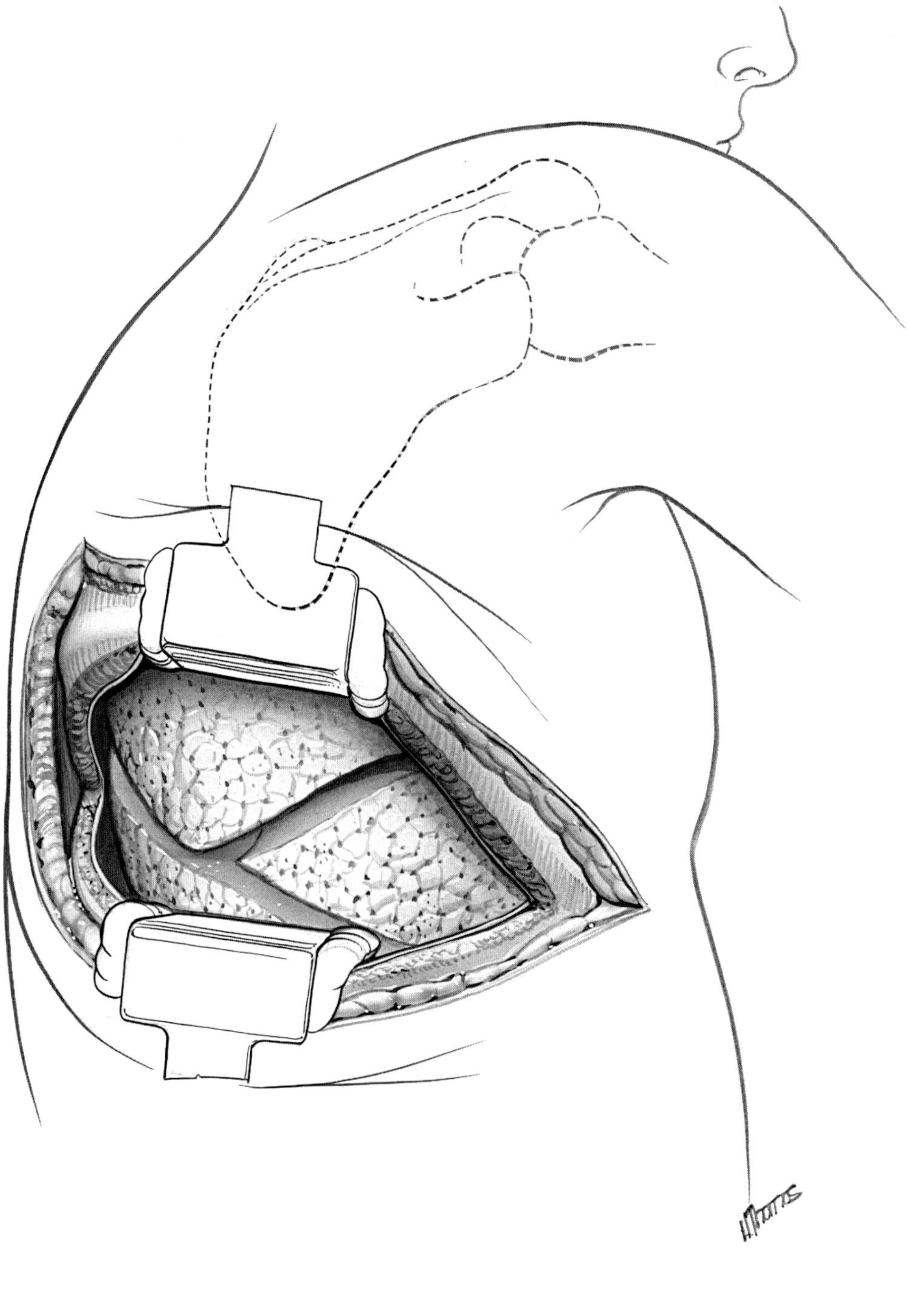

THORACOTOMY

RETRACTION OF THE LUNG

In this drawing, which is quite similar to the previous one, we have retracted the lung anteriorly to show the anatomy of the mediastinum. The view shows the mediastinum with the azygos vein coursing caudad to cephalad. It is being joined by the intercostal veins. It will turn anteriorly and lie directly cephalad to the right lung hilum. It will join the superior vena cava anteriorly to the right lung hilum. The mediastinal pleura, which is not opened in this view, covers the esophagus, which runs down the chest and is anterior to the spine.

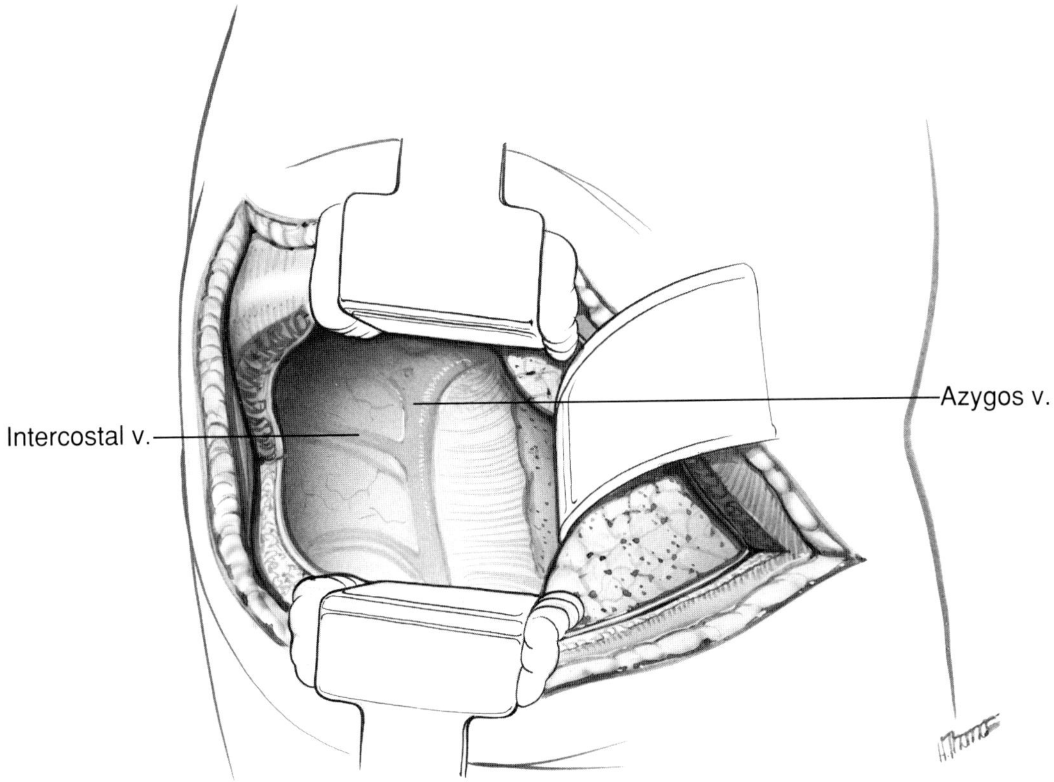

WEDGE EXCISION: STAPLING TECHNIQUE

It is essential that the diagnosis be known before any major resection of lung tissue is carried out. Many times the diagnosis has been proven prior to thoracotomy by finding cancer cells in the sputum, by getting a positive biopsy through a bronchoscope, by obtaining bronchial washings that contain cancer cells, or by performing a percutaneous needle biopsy confirming the presence of cancer. There are times when diagnostic attempts have failed and the surgeon must explore the chest to make a diagnosis. If the lesion is peripheral or accessible, it is a simple matter to carry out a so-called wedge excision.

There are two ways to make a wedge excision: one is with a stapling device, the other is by a hand-sewing technique. In the first method the stapler, after it has been applied to the lung, fires two rows of staples along one side of the intended wedge excision. A blade is then passed to divide the lung tissue between these two rows. Generally two passes of the stapler must be made to permit a wedge excision of the lesion to be examined. One should be careful not to cut across a tumor with the stapling device but to have a free margin. The specimen can then be sent to pathology for frozen-section diagnosis. If there is a possibility that the lesion is benign, it is wise to send it as a sterile specimen so that the pathologist can make a bacteriologic examination.

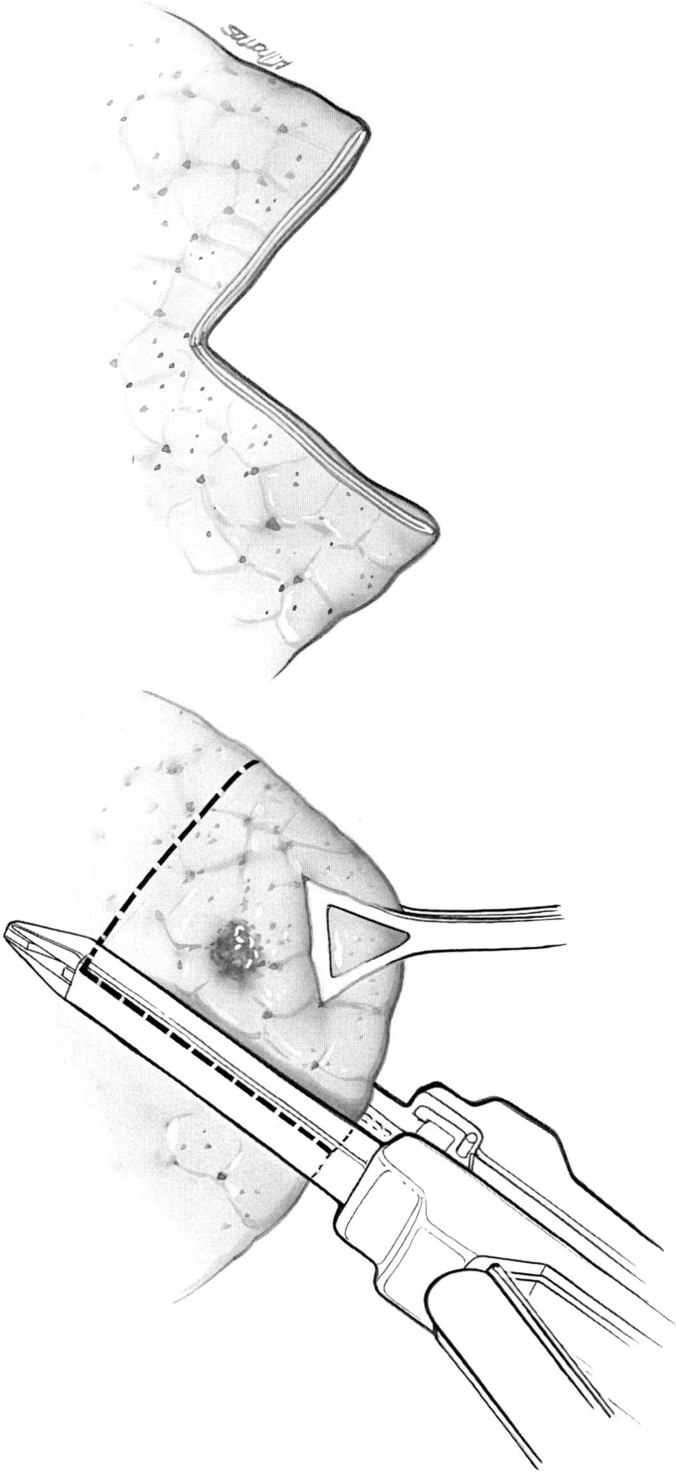

WEDGE EXCISION: HAND-SEWING TECHNIQUE

Here we see the alternative, hand-sewing technique for a wedge excision. **(A)** A small peripheral lesion is seen in the inferior portion of the right lower lobe. **(B)** The lung is drawn gently upward with a Duvall clamp, and two large Rochester peon clamps have been placed to make a V-wedge excision. It is wise to run a continuous suture deep to the clamp. This can be done by starting at the free edge of the lung deep to the clamp and tying the suture at the edge. Then a basting suture is placed to and fro deep to the clamp as the suture is carried to the tip of the clamp. When the tip of the clamp is reached, the surgeon, using a scalpel, can divide the lung tissue relatively flush with the clamp. The incision is carried to the toe of the clamp, and the clamp is removed. The basting suture can be run back over and over the cut lung and tied to the suture where it started. Using a basting stitch, the surgeon places a suture under the other clamp and carries it to the toe. When the lung is again cut and the clamp removed, the over-and-over suture runs back and is tied to the same continuous suture. In drawing B the basting stitch has been placed on the right-hand clamp. **(C)** The basting stitch has been placed deep to the right-hand clamp, and the lung parenchyma is being divided. That stitch will be run back and tied to the original stitch. In this particular drawing the basting stitch also has been placed deep to the left-hand clamp. Here the basting stitch began at the toe of the clamp and was then placed. The lung has been divided, the clamp has been removed, and an over-and-over suture is running back to be tied to the original suture end. One can also tie both continuous sutures together at the toes of the clamp to ensure continuity. **(D)** The specimen has been removed. There is a two-row continuous suture on the right that is based peripherally and a two-row suture on the left that is based medially.

We do not ordinarily wish to do a lobectomy for an unknown lesion that might not be a tumor. At times the lesion is deep and not accessible to wedge excision. The alternative is a needle biopsy. A disposable plastic needle, such as the Vim-Silverman, is used. A core biopsy a few millimeters in diameter and about 2 cm long is obtained. This can be checked by frozen section before the surgeon decides on the extent of operation.

If no diagnosis can be made prior to resection, a surgeon must exercise clinical judgment. However, no diagnostic step must be skipped, and generally a pneumonectomy should be avoided.

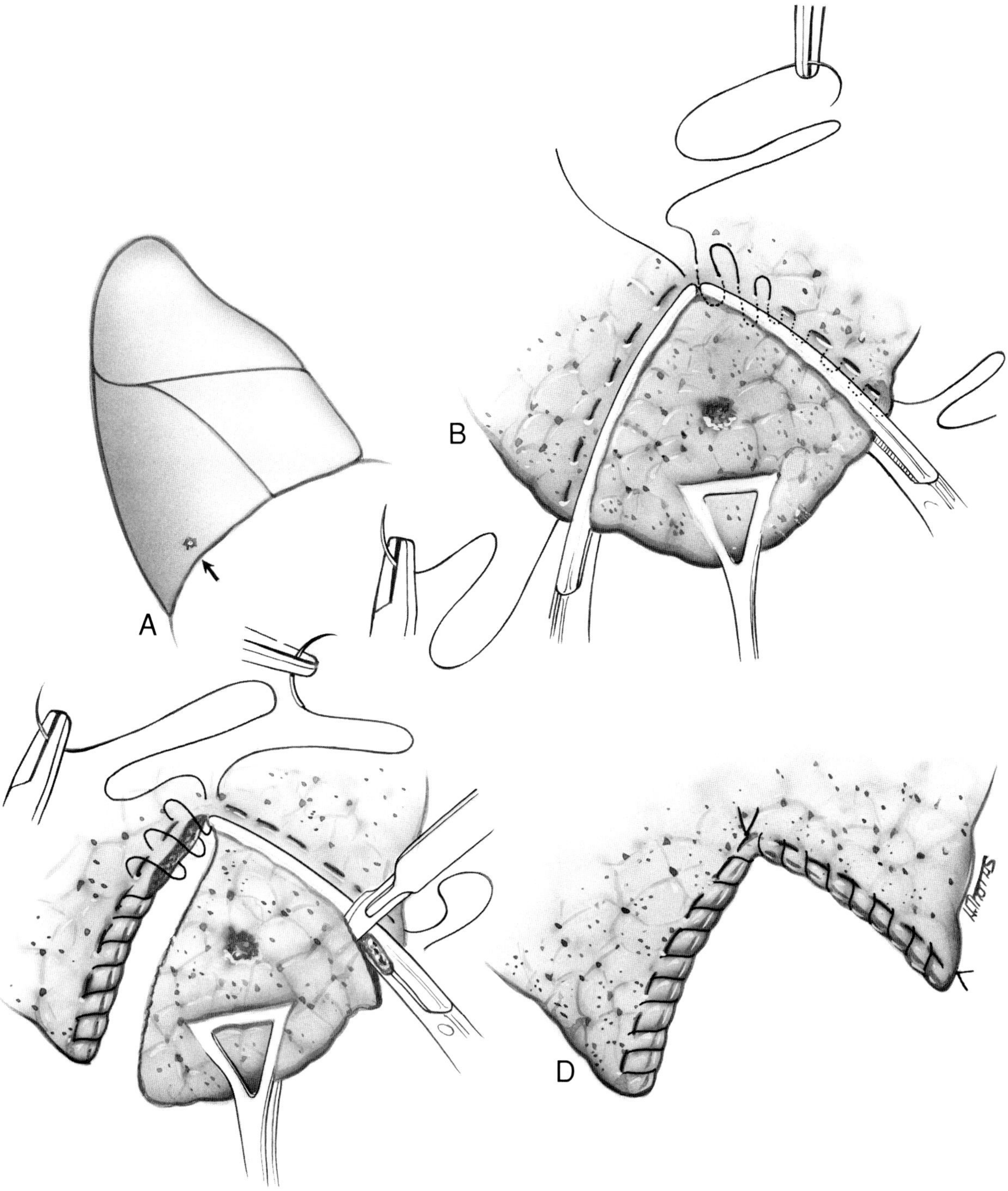
A
B
C
D

METHODS OF LIGATING VESSELS

SUTURE VERSUS STAPLED LIGATURE

This drawing shows some preferred ways of handling blood vessels to or from the lung. In the upper drawings **(A & B)** we have a proximal tie on a major vessel. If this were the superior pulmonary vein, the most proximal tie ordinarily would be one silk. It is wise to tie two overhand knots, i.e., a granny knot, to be certain that the knot is secure. A square knot is placed on top of that, with a total of three or four throws. The branches have been dissected free, and they are tied close to the lung to prevent backbleeding. A suture ligature usually of 3-0 silk has been placed distal to the proximal tie but proximal to the trifurcation. After the suture has been placed through the middle of the vessel, two overhand knots secure half the vessel and then the tie is placed around the entire vessel and ligated. The vessel shown in drawing B is divided distal to the trifurcation but proximal to the ties to prevent backbleeding. In this situation it is difficult for the proximal ties to slip over the enlarged trifurcation. The suture ligature, being fixed, is not likely to slip.

In the lower drawings **(C & D)** the vessel has been stapled. Ordinarily the stapler is left in place after it has been closed. The distal ties for backbleeding are placed on the branches. After the stapler is fired, the vessel is cut relatively close to the stapler. While there should be a remnant of intact vessel distal to the two staple lines placed by the stapler, it should not be unduly long, as this will delay healing. When the stapler is opened and removed, the surgeon and team must be ready with vascular clamp, thumb forceps, and sucker to grasp this vessel in the unlikely event of a significant leak. For a large vessel where there is adequate exposure, it is our preference to use the stapler. The surgeon, however, must be prepared to use any appropriate technique.

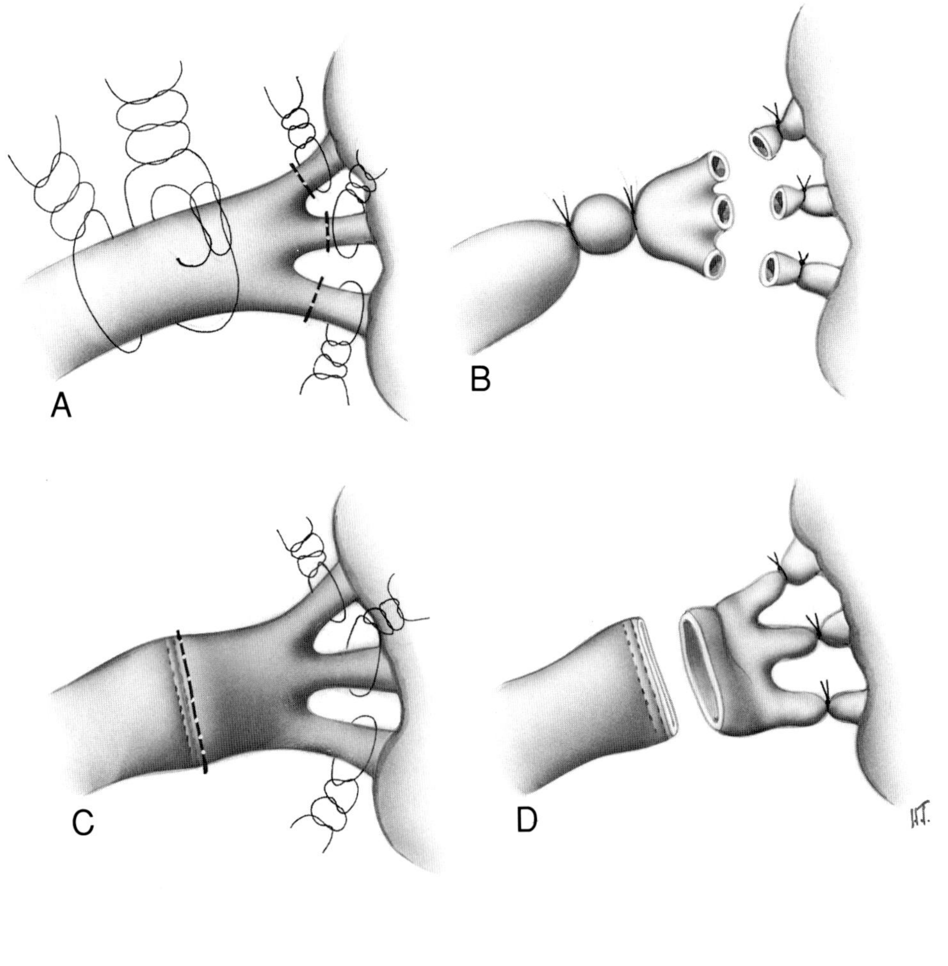

METHODS OF LIGATING VESSELS

SUTURE-LIGATURE WITHOUT VESSEL BIFURCATION

In this drawing a tumor obstructs a branch vessel at a point near where it joins a main vessel. In attempting to dissect the branch vessel, the surgeon runs the risk of spilling tumor cells into the main vessel. However, in this case, the vessel between the tumor and the bifurcation is long enough to allow use of our usual suture-ligature technique. Here a 2-0 silk ligature has been placed proximally. Distal to this ligature is placed a suture ligature, usually 3-0 suture. Ordinarily a ligature will be placed distally to prevent back-bleeding; however, this is not shown in this drawing. The vessel is cut, either with scissors or with a scalpel, leaving a proximal length sufficient to prevent the suture ligature slipping over the cut end of the vessel.

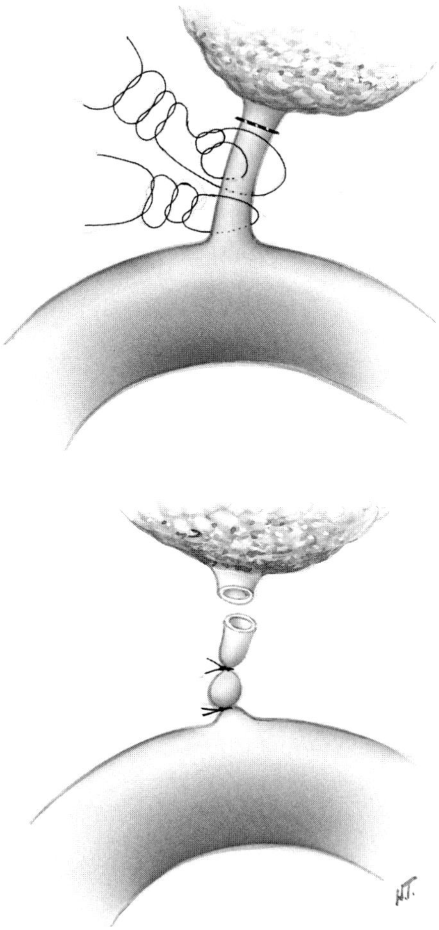

METHODS OF LIGATING VESSELS

SUTURE-LIGATURE OF MAIN VESSEL

This drawing shows an alternative technique for closing the main pulmonary artery if a stapler cannot be used and if a standard technique of ligature plus suture proximal to the branches would not suffice. The alternative is to oversew the arterial stump. **(A)** A vein retractor gently draws the superior vena cava toward the mediastinum to expose the right main pulmonary atery, which enters the right chest posterior to this vessel. An appropriate vascular clamp has been placed on the pulmonary artery; the surgeon is going to carry out a suture ligation of this vessel. One must be certain that this vascular clamp will not slip. A ductus clamp or coarctation clamp is ideal. **(B)** Providing there is adequate room to place the suture safely, the clamp is placed and the vessel is cut. Usually a 5-0 vascular suture is used. The first bit is close to the corner of the vessel and is tied around the side with a number of knots appropriate for the suture material. **(C)** A continuous over-and-over suture is run to the other side of the vessel, and care is taken that one of the sutures goes around the other side. **(D)** The same suture is run back to the first corner. The second-row bits are usually taken between the previous bites and again to a reasonable depth. One must not put these bites too close together, as this may weaken the tissue. After the suture is returned to the first corner, it is tied to the original suture. At this point, with good exposure, the vascular clamp is gently removed. If there is some small bleeding from the vascular stump, it is best to compress the vessel gently with a sponge. This lets the continuous suture equalize its pressure as the vessel stump distends. A short wait permits clotting to occur in the needle holes. Usually after a few minutes of gentle pressure, all bleeding has stopped. If bleeding is significant, the bleeding point or points are noted and the vascular clamp replaced. An appropriate mattress suture(s) can be placed to control the bleeding point.

One of the danger points in carrying out lung surgery is the inadvertent tearing or breaking of a pulmonary vessel, whether an artery or vein. Since these are low-pressure vessels, they tend to be rather fragile; in elderly patients, may be very fragile. This is especially true if chemotherapy and/or radiotherapy has been given preoperatively. In the event that an unexpected catastrophe occurs and a vessel is torn or lacerated, the surgeon must be quick to respond. The best practice is to grasp the bleeding vessel with thumb and index finger and gain control. The team must be organized to provide adequate exposure to obtain proximal control cautiously. Then, depending on circumstances, the surgeon proceeds with the resection or repairs the laceration with 5-0 vascular suture. The important point is to remain calm. A good deal of blood can be lost quickly with rents in these vessels. As a precautionary measure, blood for transfusion must be available. If the patient sustains an unexpected blood loss, blood transfusion should be started and the patient's condition stabilized before proceeding with the repair. Crushing clamps that must remain in the patient should not be placed on vessels injudiciously. In cases of backbleeding, however, it is perfectly proper to clamp. Generally ligatures or suture ligatures can be placed to control any sort of backbleeding.

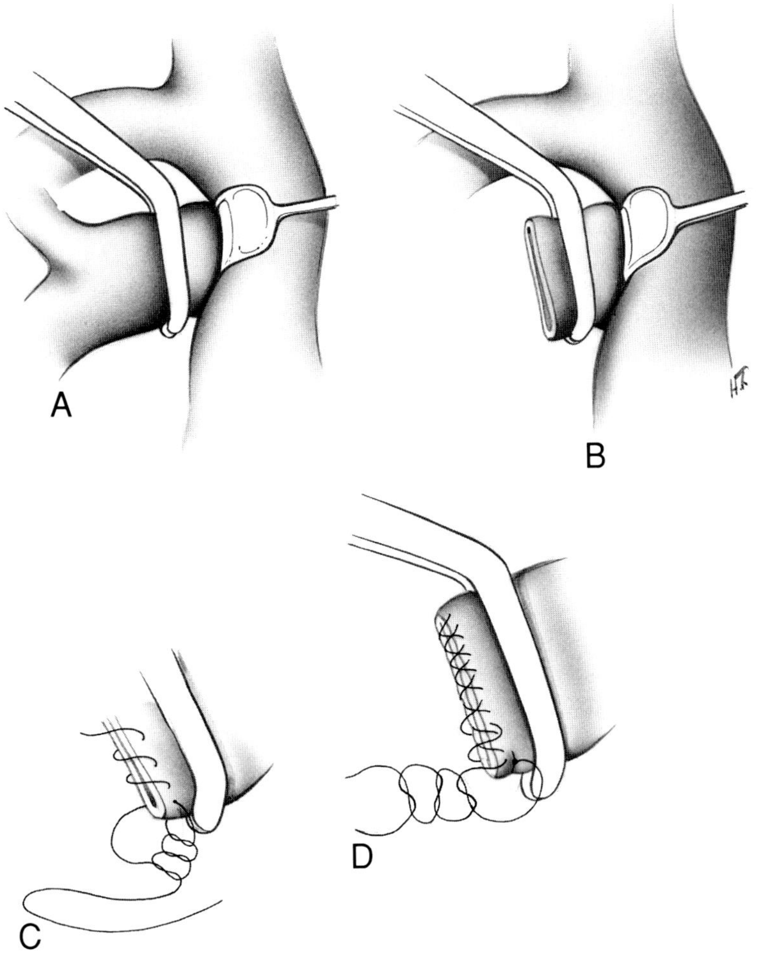
A
B
C
D

METHODS OF LIGATING VESSELS

SUTURE-LIGATURE OF SHORT VASCULAR BRANCH

In this situation a branch of a major vessel cannot be removed. The branch is short and wide and cannot be dissected with sufficient length to be safely tied off, as in the previous drawings. Also, it may be that the tumor is close to the takeoff of this particular vessel.

A partially occluding clamp, such as a Satinsky, is valuable. **(A)** Here the main vessel is continuing to perfuse. This is particularly important if the patient has impaired lungs, and the blood flow through the main pulmonary artery cannot be shut off. **(B)** After the vascular clamp is placed, the vessel is cut free, leaving enough proximal vessel to be sutured and to handle backbleeding. If a distal ligature cannot be placed, one can place a suture ligature after the vessel has been cut. **(C)** A suture is started at one end and tied. It is run as a continuous suture to the opposite end and side. **(D)** It is then run back with bites between these sutures, and ligated with the original end. After the vessel is sutured, the vascular clamp is removed. Gentle pressure with a dry sponge is used until the suture is equalized and there is no bleeding from the suture line. Should there be persistent bleeding from one spot, the clamp can be replaced. A suitable 5-0 mattress suture will usually control the bleeding spot.

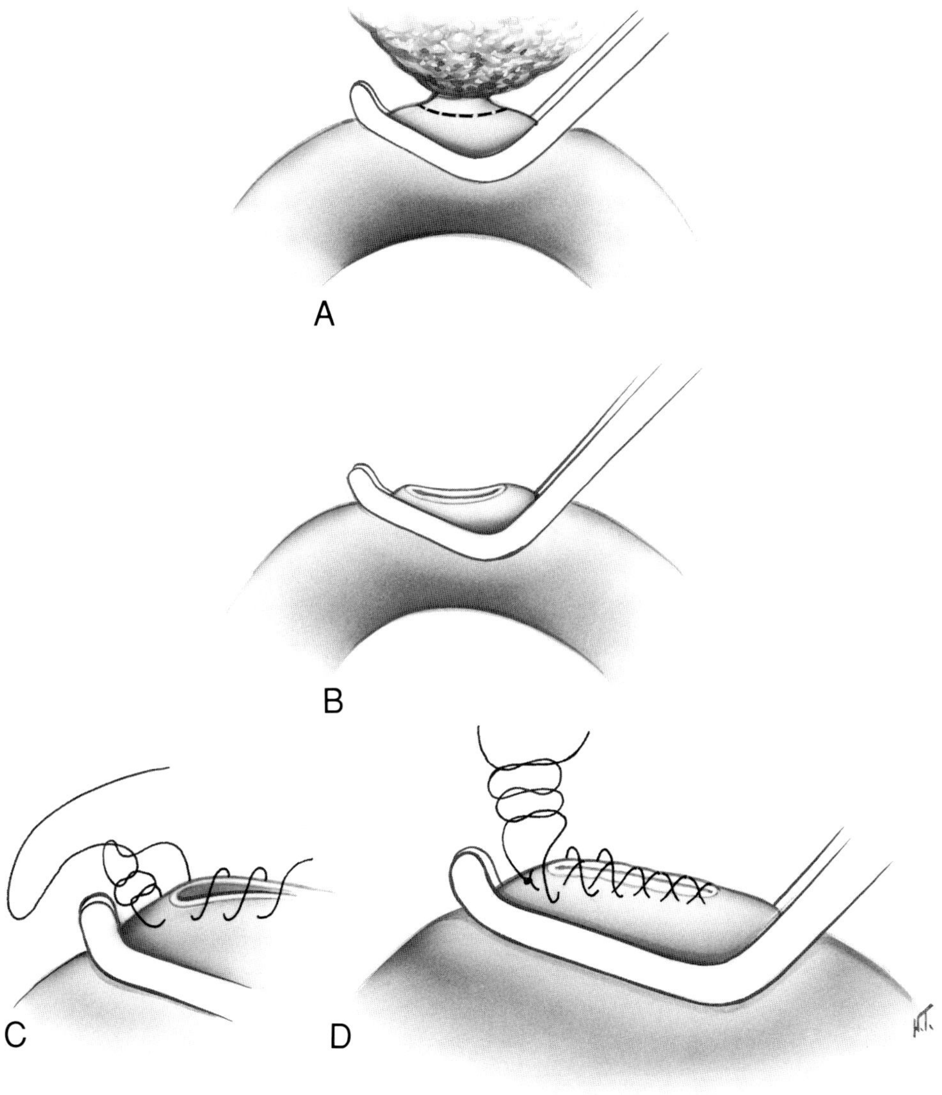

METHODS OF LIGATING VESSELS

SUTURE-LIGATURE OF MAIN VESSEL WHEN BRANCH CANNOT BE LIGATED

In this situation it is not feasible to ligate the branch vessel coming off the main artery. In addition, there may not be room to place a partially occluding clamp and let flow continue through the vessel. In the surgeon's judgment, it is satisfactory for the patient if flow through this vessel is temporarily occluded. We have dissected the vessel proximally and distally. **(A)** Vascular tapes (umbilical tape) with RUML tourniquets have been placed. **(B)** The short rubber tubing has been placed over the two ends of the tape and is gently slid down the tape until the vessel is occluded both proximally and distally. Once this is done, the appropriate amount of the vessel side proximal to the tumor is cut free. **(C & D)** A continuous suture of 5-0 vascular material in two layers over and over is placed and tied. The distal tourniquet is released and checked for bleeding from the back pressure. If it seems dry, the proximal tourniquet is gently released. Any persistent bleeding can be handled by a mattress suture, but ordinarily the vessel should be reclosed when this is being done.

We prefer this tape tourniquet technique since it is less injurious to vessels. Awkward clamps in the field are thus avoided, and there is less danger of tearing vessels. Good exposure and gentleness are required at all times. It is much better to avoid trouble than to repair trouble.

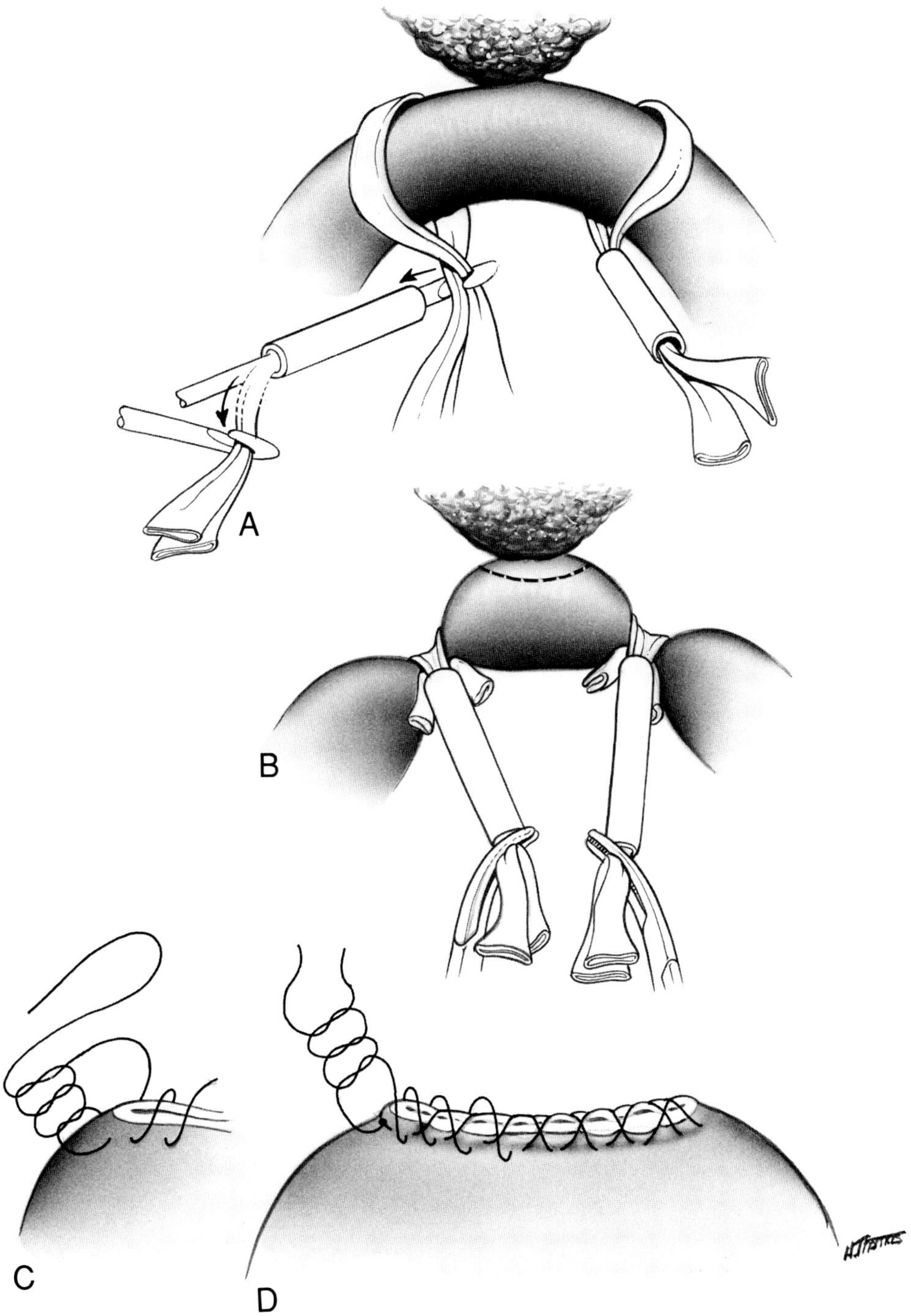
A
B
C
D

STAPLE CLOSURE OF THE BRONCHUS

This drawing shows the use of the bronchial stapler. **(A)** The right upper lobe has been prepared for the stapler. Note that all of the bronchial vessels leading to the right upper lobe have been ligated and divided. One should be careful not to use clips or metallic devices around the bronchus that is to be stapled, as these might interfere with the use of the stapler. It is essential to have adequate room. In addition the tracheobronchial tree must not be devitalized by excessive removal of bronchial vessels. Ordinarily the bronchial stapler is placed so that the bronchus is in the midportion of the stapling device. One compresses the bronchus in what seems to be a comfortable direction. Usually the bronchus is flatter if closed in the anteroposterior direction, as shown in part A. The stapler is applied. For a lobar bronchus or smaller, the stapler setting should be 3.2-mm staple lengths as compared with 4-mm staple lengths or more needed for the pneumonectomy bronchus. The staple is closed but not fired. The anesthetist is asked to aspirate and inflate the lung to be certain that there is no impingement of or interference with aeration in the remaining lobes. When this has been established, the stapler is fired. **(B)** With a scalpel the bronchus is amputated as close to the stapling device as possible. The stapler is removed. It is imperative that the bronchial stump be tested under water, with strong positive pressure being exerted by the anesthetist to be certain that there are no air leaks. It should be noted carefully that there is no bleeding and that there are no untied bronchial vessels that might bleed later if they are temporarily crushed by the stapling device.

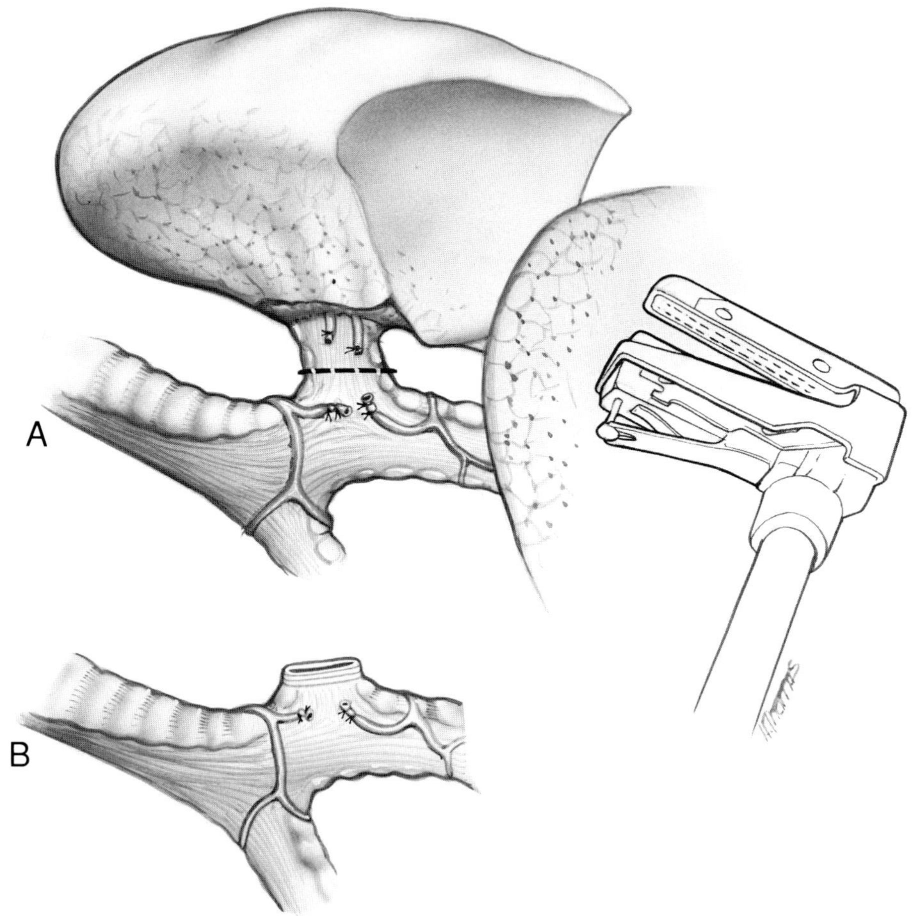

SLEEVE RESECTION, RIGHT UPPER LOBE

DIVISION AND SUTURING

This set of drawings illustrates the sleeve resection of a carcinoma in the right upper lobe orifice. If a standard right upper lobe lobectomy were performed, tumor would be left in the orifice. Consequently, a sleeve resection is an important variation. All other steps of the lobectomy are completed prior to this procedure. It is important that either a double-lumen endotracheal tube be in place so that the left lung will be ventilated through the left channel or a single lumen endotracheal tube be advanced by the anesthetist, with the surgeon's guidance, into the left mainstem bronchus. The tube can be held in place and kept airtight by a balloon in the left main bronchus, or an umbilical tape can be used as a tie around the tube and bronchus in the most proximal part of the left mainstem bronchus. A jet ventilator could also be used here with the jet directed down the left mainstem bronchus. This allows the surgeon to work with an open bronchus during the anastomosis.

In this instance the mainstem bronchus is amputated just distal to the tracheal carina. The necessary bronchial vessels at this point should be ligated. They should not be removed any further up the tracheobronchial tree. The division of the bronchus intermedius distal to the tumor should be done so as to leave an ostium of the bronchus intermedius that approximately matches the size of the proximal right main bronchial opening. Then a series of interrupted bronchial sutures are placed that are usually of 2-0 or 3-0 of an absorbable, long-lasting material. It is usually a good idea to place the two angle sutures in the appropriate ends of the horseshoe cartilagenous rings, laterally and medially. After these angle sutures have been placed, but not tied, and each individually secured with a hemostat, a series of interrupted sutures is begun. They are placed anterior to the bronchus, beginning next to the medial angle. These sutures should be firm bites. They can be either through a major portion of the cartilage or around the cartilage. They are individually placed, although not tied, secured with a hemostat, and as shown in this drawing, looped over an instrument in proper order to make it easy to find and tie each when ready. After all of the sutures have been placed in the cartilagenous horseshoes, the right middle and right lower lobes are manually moved higher in the chest so that the cut bronchi are in close approximation without tension. Next the medial and lateral angle sutures are tied. Then successively the individual sutures, from lateral to medial in reverse order of their placement, are tied. At the conclusion of this step, the sutures in the cartilagenous rings are ligated. Next, the membranous portion, which is relatively fragile and easily torn, is approximated. There must be absolutely no tension on this membranous portion, and the sutures are carefully placed and tied.

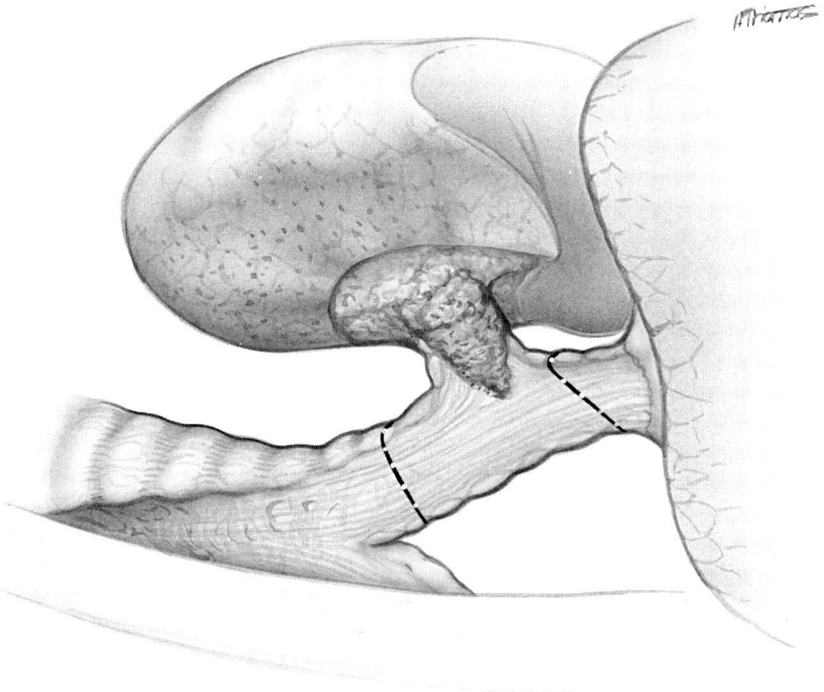

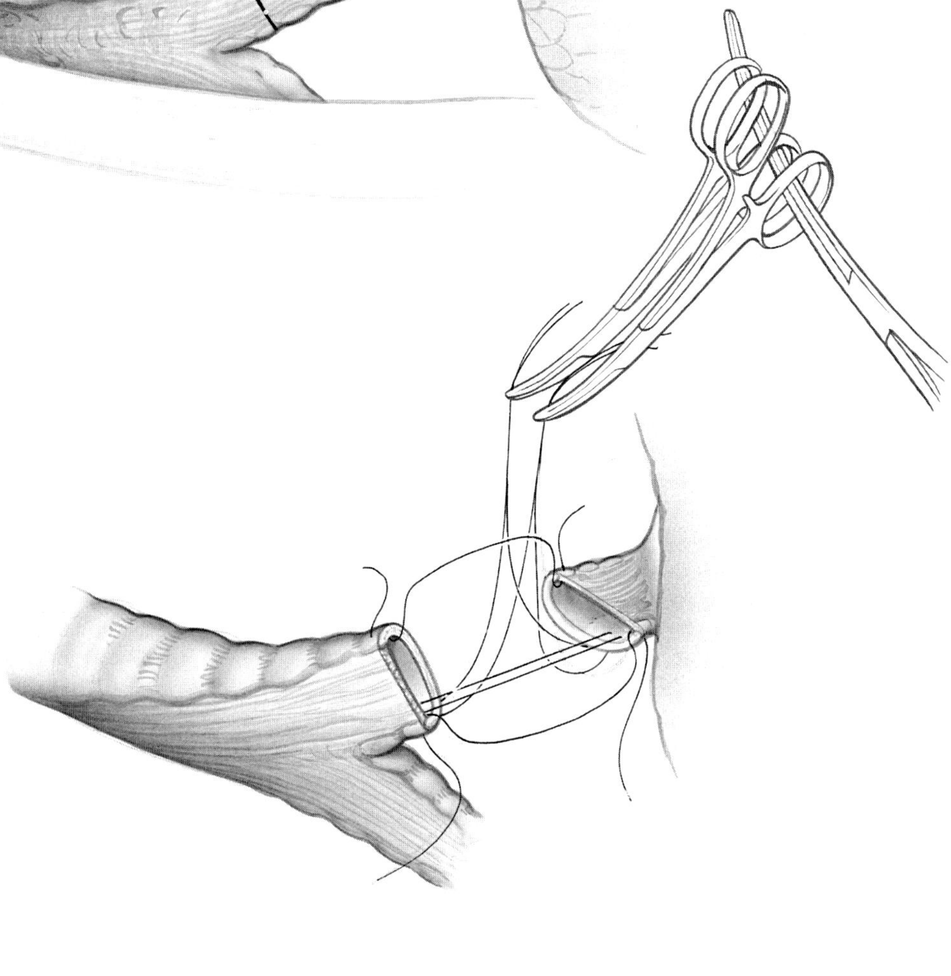

SLEEVE RESECTION, RIGHT UPPER LOBE

DETAIL OF SUTURING

(A & B) These drawings show all of the sutures placed in the cartilagenous area and ligated with the membranous portion not yet sutured. The final drawing **(C)** shows the completed anastomsis. Ordinarily we leave the tied sutures present. The next important maneuver is to test that the anastomosis is airtight. This is done by reinflating the right lung through a double-lumen tube. If there is a single-lumen endotracheal tube, the tube is drawn back into the trachea and the balloon is inflated. The right lung then is reinflated. The anesthetist tests the anastomosis under water with regular expansion and ventilation. Should there be any significant leak, it can be identified between the sutures and fixed with placement of an additional suture.

In the studies that have been reported for lung transplantation, there have been considerable difficulties with the bronchial anastomosis because of the severance of the bronchial blood supply. An advance in this procedure has been the use of the omental pedicle graft brought up from the abdomen and wrapped around the anastomosis. A new blood supply is incorporated into the bronchial anastomosis after a few days. Another technique is to use a viable pedicle graft, such as from the intercostal bundle or from the pericardium. More recently a technique in lung transplant bronchial anastomosis has been developed whereby the donated bronchus is placed for one cartilagenous ring inside the recipient bronchus. The anastomosis is done over two thicknesses of bronchial rings. This has resulted in the anastomosis being more airtight, less stricture prone, and less disruptive. This could be done as a modification of the operation we have described here. The takeoff of the right mainstem bronchus is larger and the bronchus intermedius smaller.

The major secret of tracheobronchial anastomoses is to maintain blood supply, decrease the tension on the anastomosis, and place sutures carefully. Anastomosis can be enhanced by mobilizing the lungs, freeing up the carina to whatever extent possible. If need be, an incision in the neck can release the hyoid bone so that the larynx will drop lower to make more trachea available. If there is significant tension on the tracheal anastomosis, the patient's neck should be kept flexed by whatever device. Sutures from chin to chest for a period can help. If one has later difficulties with stenoses, indwelling silastic stents or Montgomery tubes are extremely valuable in maintaining airways while the strictures are healed or prevented.

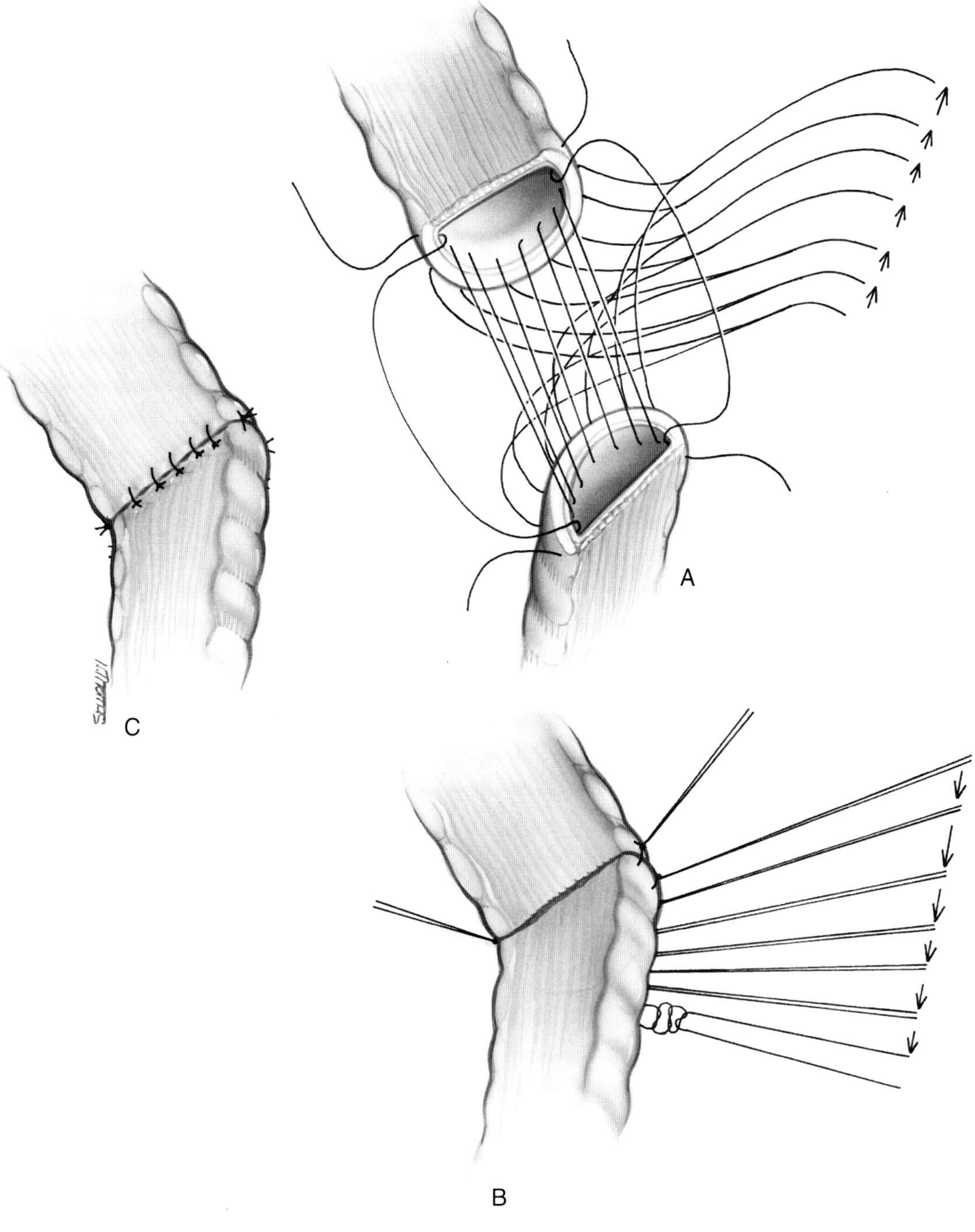
A
B
C

ALTERNATIVE METHOD FOR TRACHEOBRONCHIAL ANASTOMOSIS

This drawing shows an alternative method of performing a tracheobronchial or bronchial reanastomosis. The tumor, for which we plan to carry out a "sleeve resection," is seen in the right upper lobe orifice. The bronchus has been mobilized above and below the right upper lobe bronchus. To ventilate the left lung, either a double-lumen tube is passed into the tracheobronchial tree or a single-lumen endotracheal tube is passed into the left mainstem bronchus.

After the lesion is excised, instead of carrying out an end-to-end anastomosis of the right mainstem bronchus to the distal bronchus intermedius, the smaller bronchus intermedius is telescoped inside the proximal mainstem bronchus. The surgeon uses 3-0 slowly absorbable suture material and places sutures around the outer cartilage and around the bronchus intermedius cartilage. The sutures at the ends of the cartilage horseshoes are placed first. All sutures are placed before any are tied. The cartilage sutures should be tied first, and the sutures in the membranous portions are tied last. It is important that all secretions be aspirated from the bronchus before tying the last sutures. The anesthetist can gently aspirate the lung with the surgeon guiding the suction catheter. The lung is reinflated and examined for air leaks. The chest is partially filled with tepid distilled water. While the anesthetist applies up to 30 to 40 cm of airway pressure into the partially submerged lung, the surgeon looks for air leaks. If a leak is located between the tied but uncut sutures, another suture can be placed.

This technique has evolved from clinical research with lung transplants. In the lung transplant operation the donor lung has no bronchial blood supply. This anastomosis has been found to have fewer air leaks and less tendency to stricture formation.

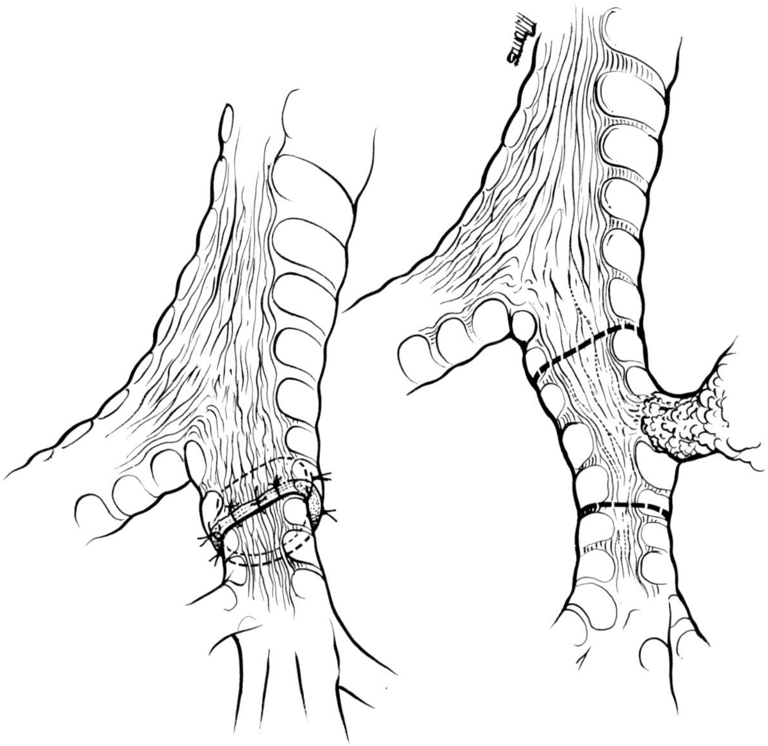

EXCISION TECHNIQUE FOR MULTIPLE METASTASES

Normally if a surgeon finds a peripheral mass in the lung, a wedge excision is indicated for diagnosis. The lesion is removed by a stapling technique or by a clamping and suture method, as depicted in Special Procedures #6 and #7. **(A)** At times a surgeon is faced with the situation in which there are multiple superficial metastases where lung parenchyma must be conserved at all costs. Alternatively, one may find a small, very superficial lesion. In either situation Special Procedure #17 is an alternative means of removing the tumor. **(B)** The electrocautery has made a circular or elliptical incision in the lung around the lesion. **(C)** The lesion is removed and the cutting and cauterization continue under the lesion to include a small uninvolved portion of lung. Usually there are no significant bronchi to produce air leaks at this peripheral location. Blood vessels that bleed in spite of the cautery can be clipped or ligated. If the defect is bloodless and does not leak air, it can be left. **(D)** Alternatively, 3-0 sutures in absorbable plastic or silk can be placed to catch the deep part of the defect to eliminate dead space. A laser knife may be used in place of the electrocautery.

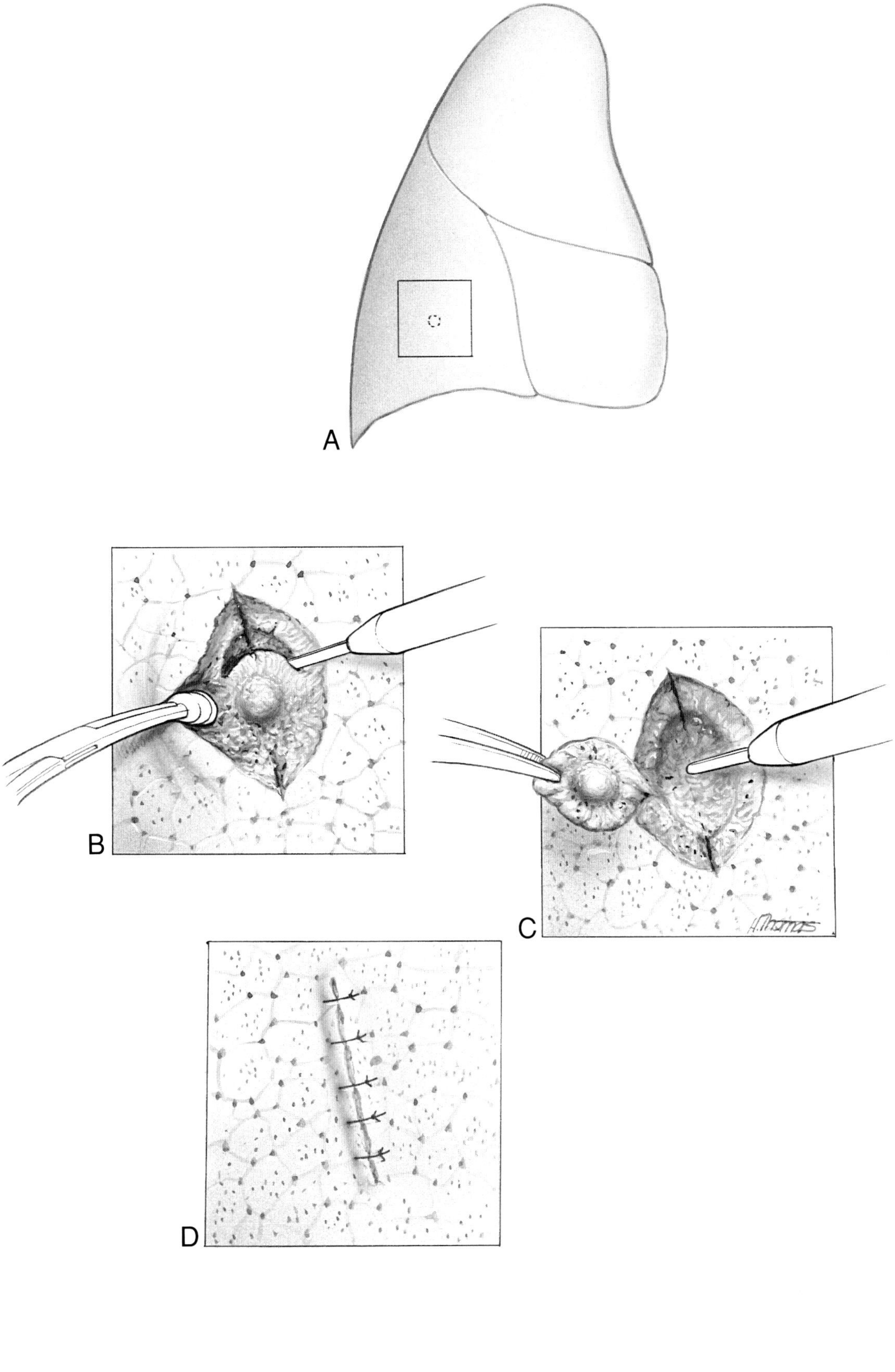
A
B
C
D

RIGHT UPPER LOBECTOMY

ANATOMIC ORIENTATION

This is a lateral-view diagram which shows the right upper lobe, right middle lobe, and right lower lobe exploded so that the anatomy of the three lobes is shown in detail. It is apparent that in the longitudinal fissure the main structure that one encounters first in opening the visceral pleura is the pulmonary artery, which can be seen giving its first and highest right upper lobe branch, anterior and cephalad to the right upper lobe bronchus. The next branch of the pulmonary artery is the posterior artery branch of the right upper lobe. The pulmonary artery continues down the fissure and gives off anteriorly the right middle lobe branch and posteriorly the superior segmental branch of the right lower lobe. The artery continues on and ultimately makes four branches to the four basal segments, in this case by two bifurcations. The bronchus, which is medial to the artery, shows the right upper lobe bronchus with its trifurcation and three segments. The bronchus intermedius comes down caudad and gives off the right middle lobe branch anteriorly with the medial and lateral right middle lobe segments. Opposite posteriorly is the superior segmental bronchus and, continuing caudad, the four anterior, lateral, posterior, and medial basal segments. Also faintly ghosted in by the artist is the superior pulmonary vein visible anteriorly in the transverse fissure between the right upper lobe and right middle lobe. The artist has shown these portions of the transverse fissure, the posterior longitudinal fissure, and the anterior longitudinal fissure that will have to be opened up to expose the hilar anatomy of the right lower lobe.

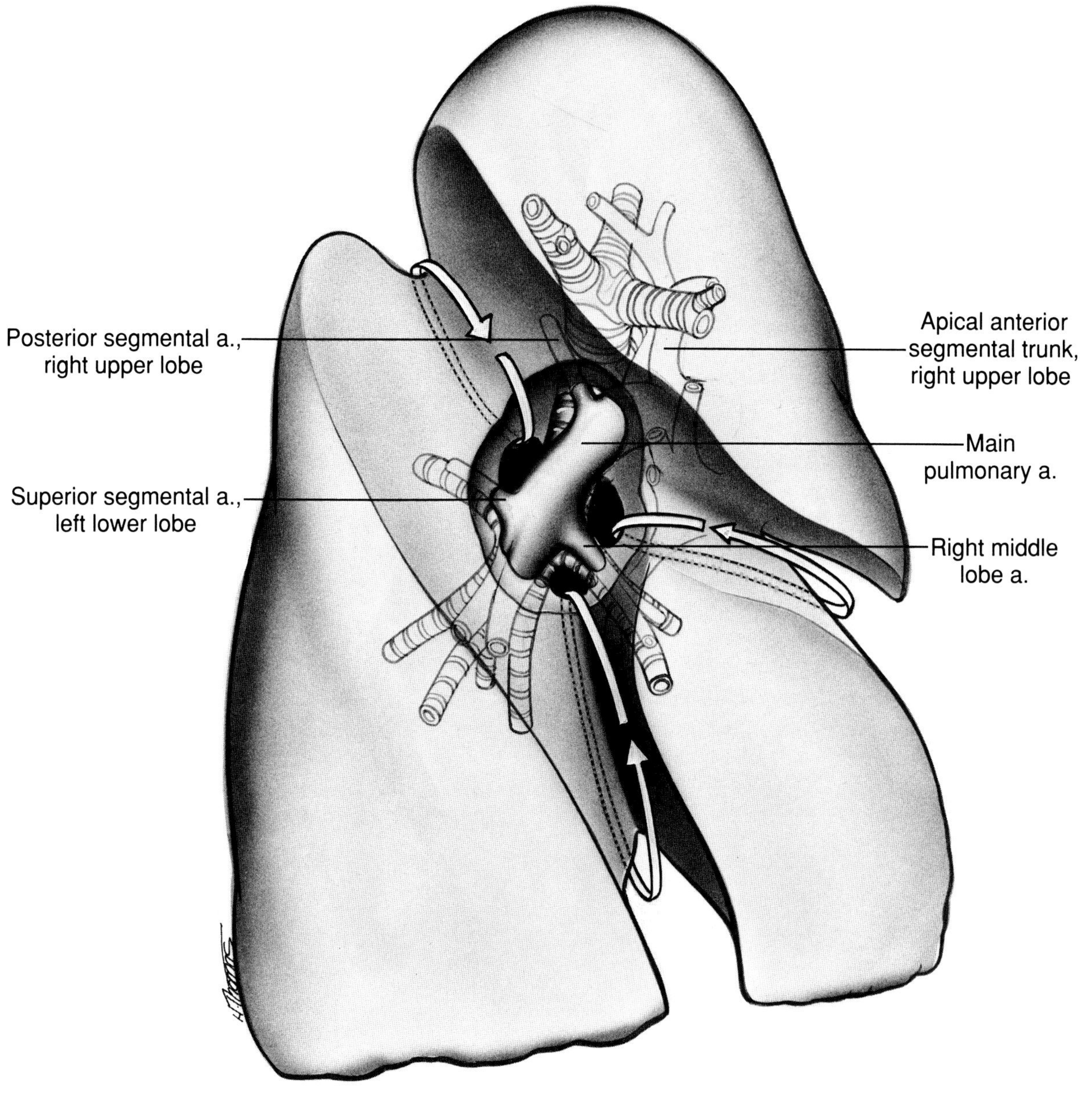
Posterior segmental a., right upper lobe
Superior segmental a., left lower lobe
Apical anterior segmental trunk, right upper lobe
Main pulmonary a.
Right middle lobe a.

RIGHT UPPER LOBECTOMY

OPENING OF THE VISCERAL PLEURA

In this view the chest has been opened. We are looking at the anterior hilum of the right lung with the right lung displaced posteriorly. The phrenic nerve running along the superior vena cava and pericardium anterior to the hilum is visible. The scissors are cutting the visceral pleura over the hilum reflected from the mediastinal pleura onto the lung.

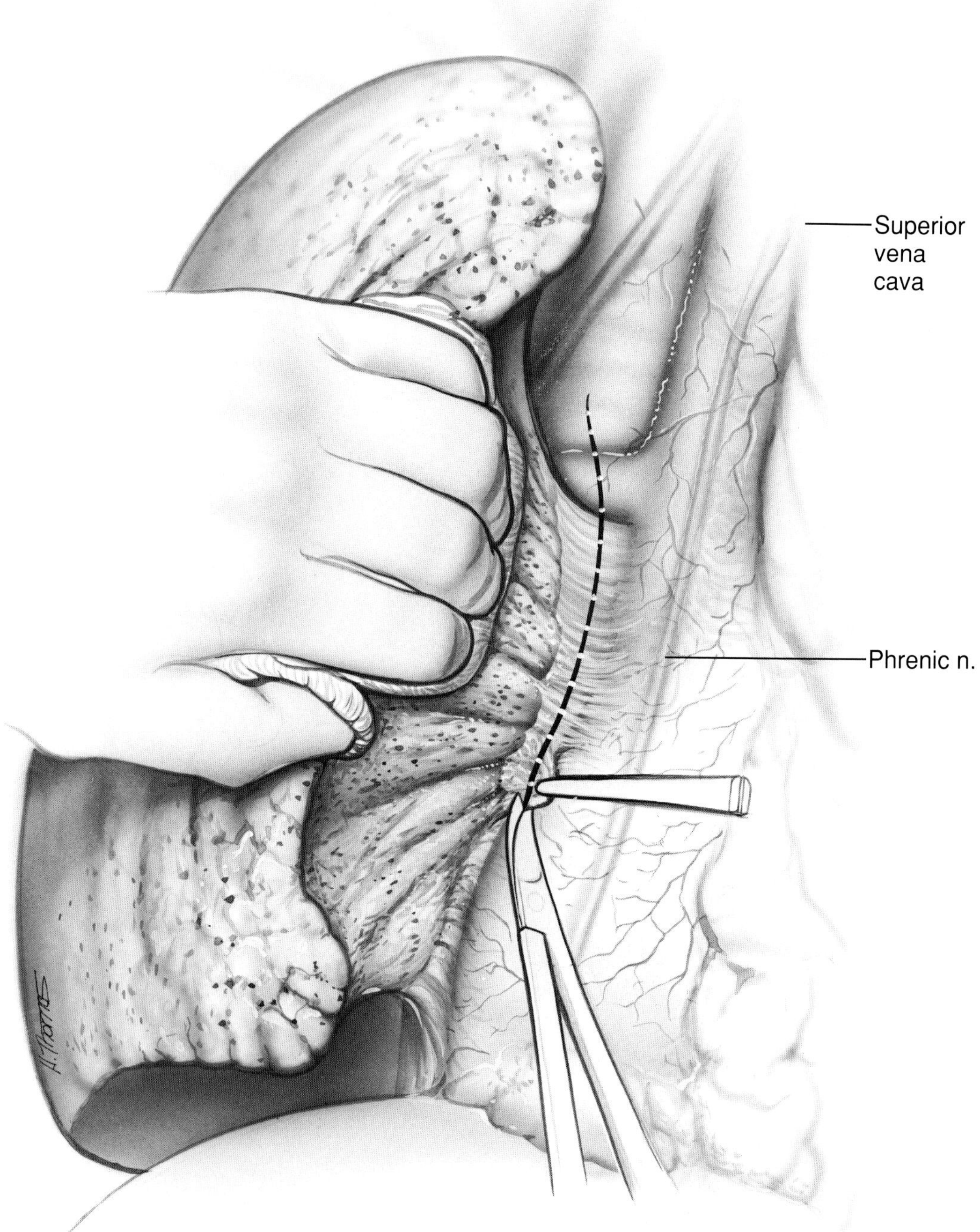

RIGHT UPPER LOBECTOMY

EXPOSURE OF PULMONARY ARTERY AND VEIN

We are still looking at the anterior portion of the hilum. The pleura has been opened so that the most cephalic structure is the azygos vein running from posterior to anterior to insert into and join the superior vena cava. The pulmonary artery can be seen and the superior pulmonary vein as the dissecting sponge delineates the inferior branch of the superior pulmonary vein. It can be seen that the highest branch of the superior pulmonary vein drains across and partially obscures the view of the right upper lobe bronchus.

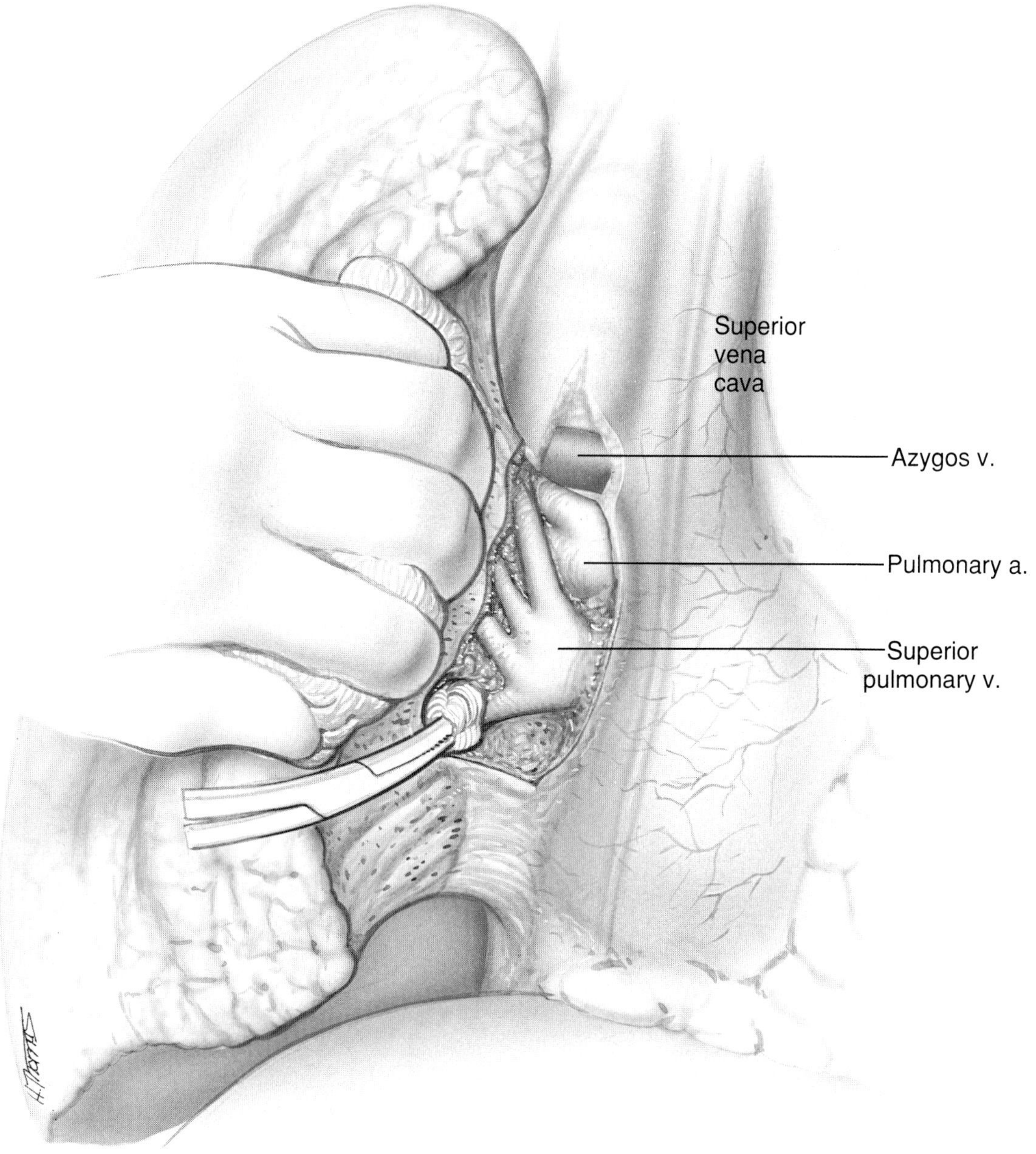

RIGHT UPPER LOBECTOMY

OPENING THE PLEURA POSTERIORLY, EXPOSING THE BRONCHUS

We are now laterally approaching the fissure between the right upper lobe and the right lower lobe. With the scissors we are incising the visceral pleura over the main pulmonary artery. One must be careful that this is free, and usually it is picked up with a pair of thumb forceps while it is being cut.

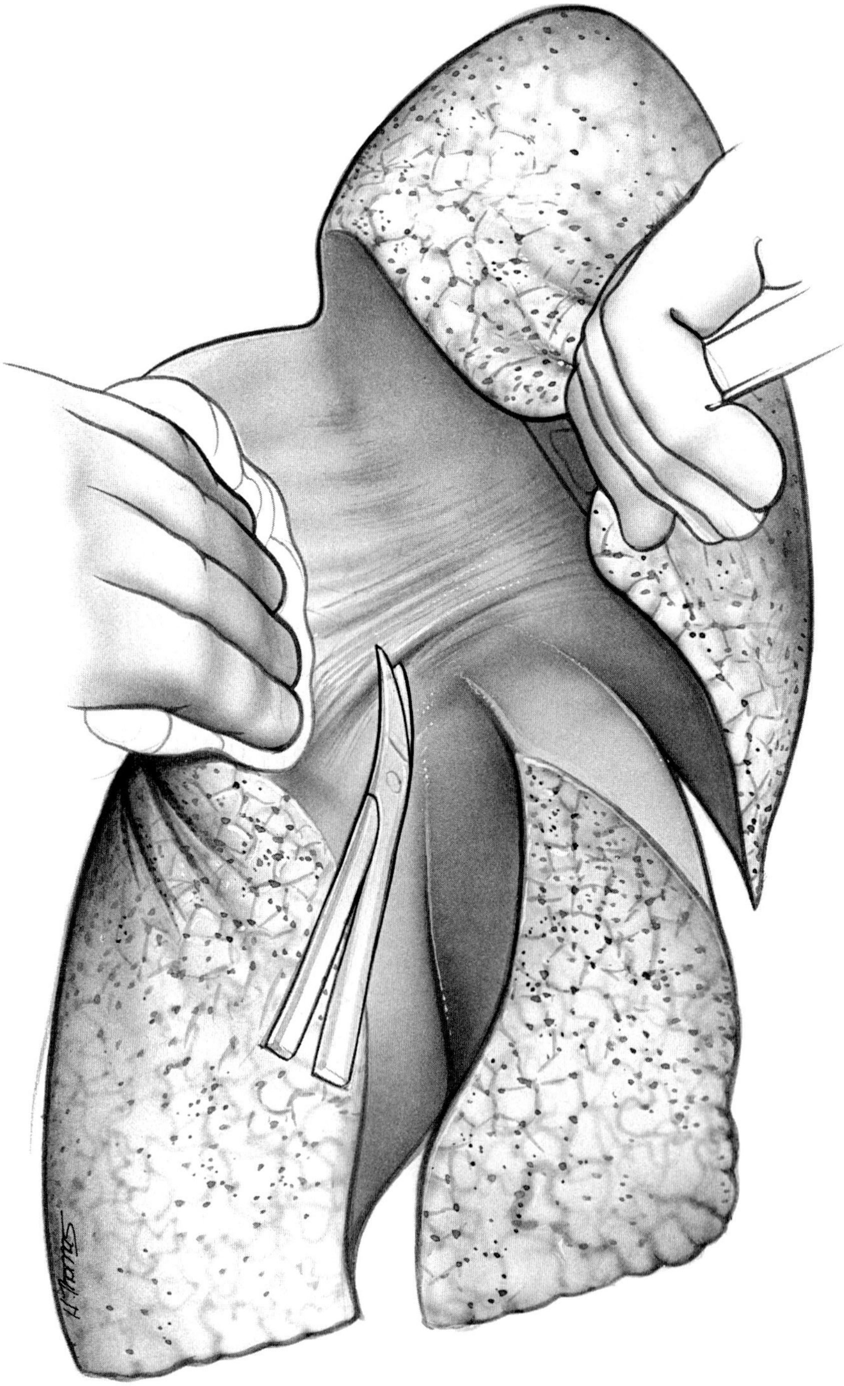

RIGHT UPPER LOBECTOMY

EXPOSURE OF THE AZYGOS VEIN

In this view we have retracted the lung forward. We have opened the mediastinal pleura over the azygos vein above and extending down just in front of the esophagus so that we can see the back of the carina and the right upper lobe bronchus and bronchus intermedius. The esophagus and vagus nerve can be seen coursing posteriorly. The vagus nerve branches that normally run across the mediastinum to the right upper lobe bronchus have been divided. Also in this view we have ligated any bronchial vessels accompanying the right upper lobe bronchus, which can be rather sizeable. The subcarinal space and the inferior pulmonary vein have not yet been dissected.

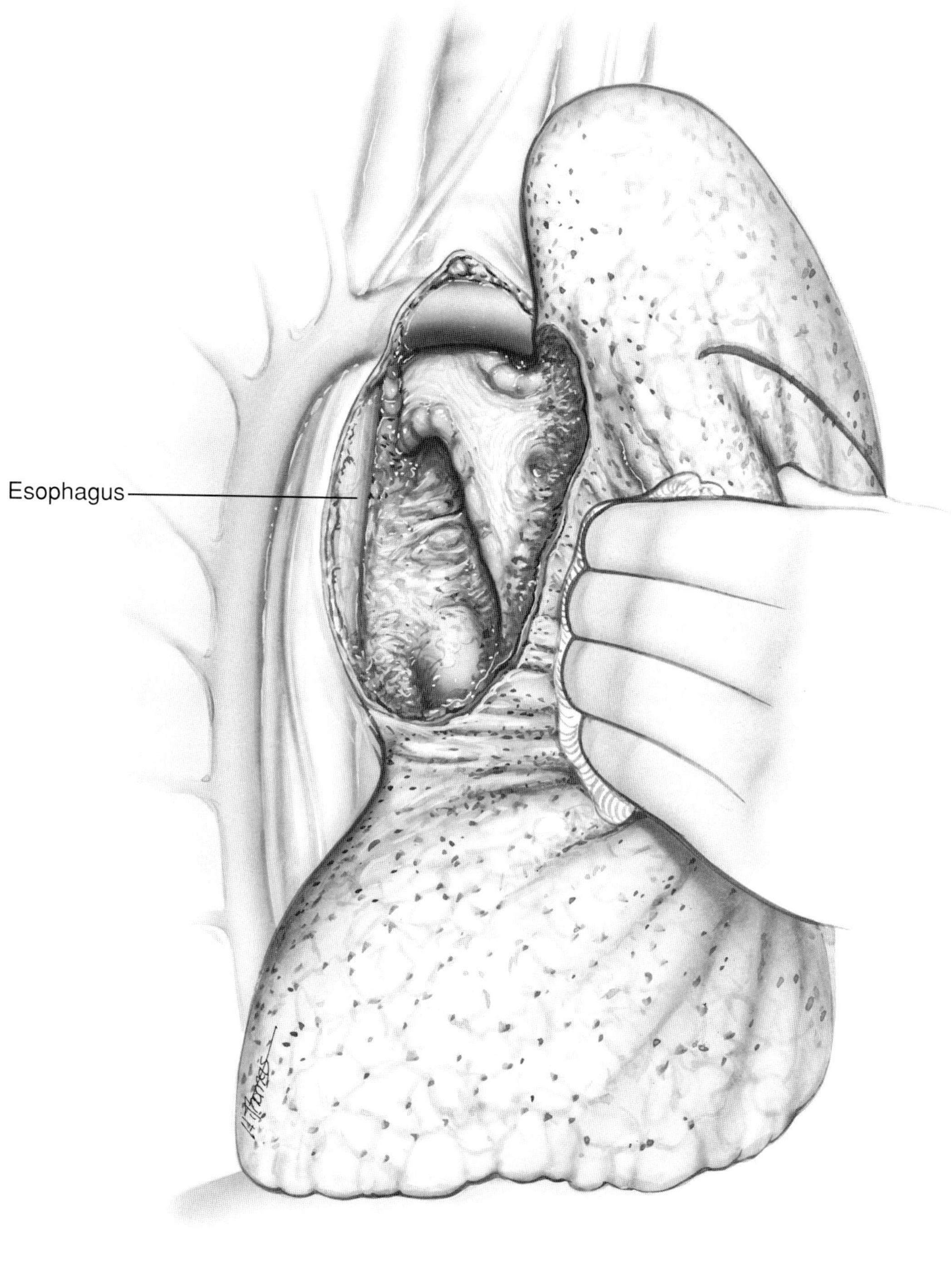

RIGHT UPPER LOBECTOMY

FREEING THE UPPER LOBE BRONCHUS

In this view, with our dissecting sponge we are freeing up the caudal side of the right upper lobe bronchus and preparing to go around anteriorly in front of the right upper lobe bronchus. Care must be taken not to injure the posterior segmental artery branch, which comes off usually as about the second or third branch of the pulmonary artery and runs cephalad and anteriorly in this location anterior to our dissecting sponge to supply the posterior segment of the right upper lobe. The main structure anterior to the bronchus at this point is the first branch of the pulmonary artery going to the apex and anterior segments of the right upper lobe. There may be two branches here. One must ensure that there are not also tumor lymph nodes in this location.

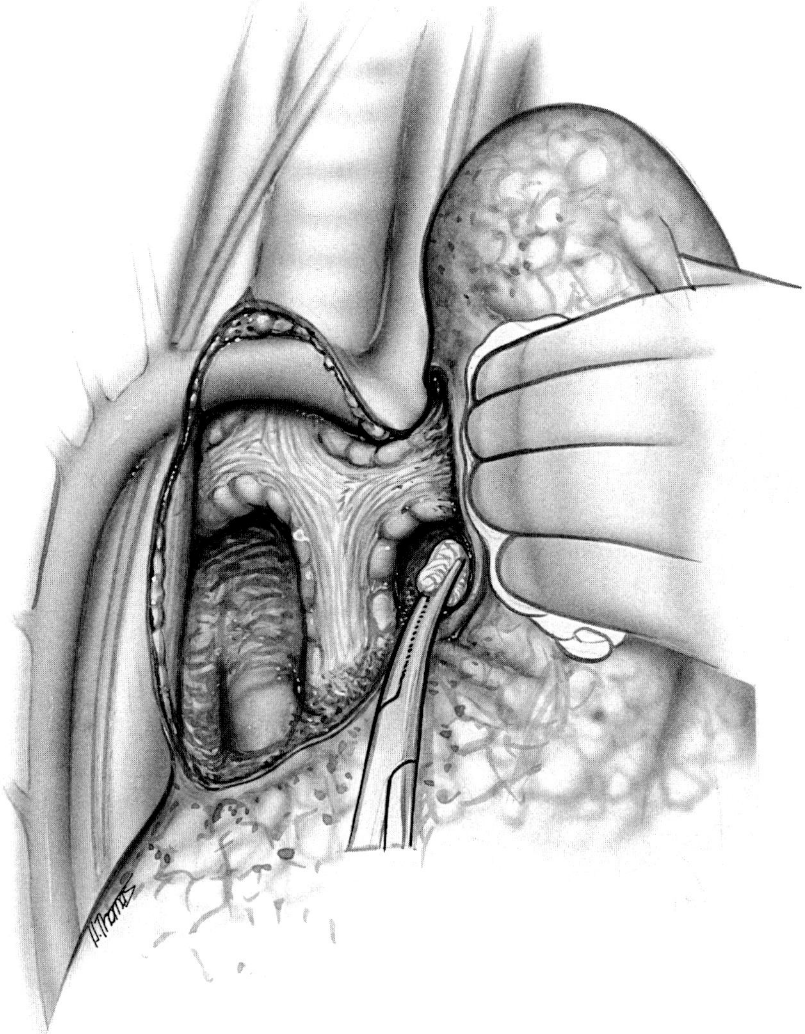

RIGHT UPPER LOBECTOMY

FREEING THE FIRST BRANCH OF THE PULMONARY ARTERY

Here we are looking at the cephalic aspects of the right hilum. The mediastinal pleura which had been opened in front in the fissure and posteriorly has been continued around. We can see the azygos vein cephalad. The superior vena cava and phrenic nerve is anterior. The dissecting sponge is freeing up the first branch of the pulmonary artery. Care must be taken to identify the main pulmonary artery. If there is any question, the dissection should focus on the distal portion of this first arterial branch, since if any tears or blood vessel leaks should occur, it is much better to have them distal than proximal.

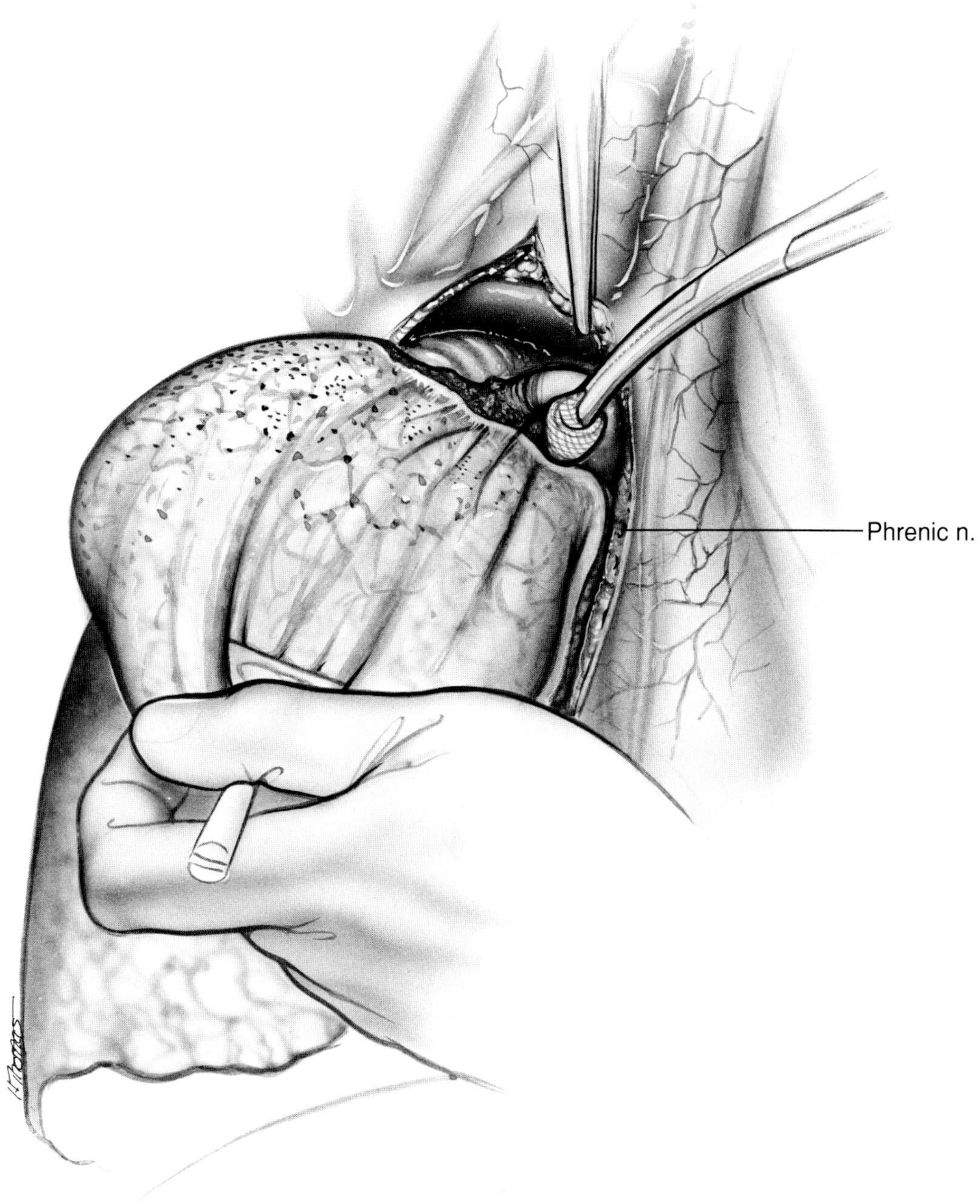

RIGHT UPPER LOBECTOMY

PLACEMENT OF SUTURE LIGATURES

In this view the first branch of the main pulmonary artery, which is coursing down and will be the main structure in the longitudinal fissure, has been proximally ligated. Here the artist has put suture ligatures distal to the bifurcation into two branches with additional ligatures distally to prevent backbleeding. Ordinarily, if there is room it is best to place these suture ligatures proximal to the bifurcation, just distal to the first proximal branch, and to divide the vessels distal to the bifurcation of the artery.

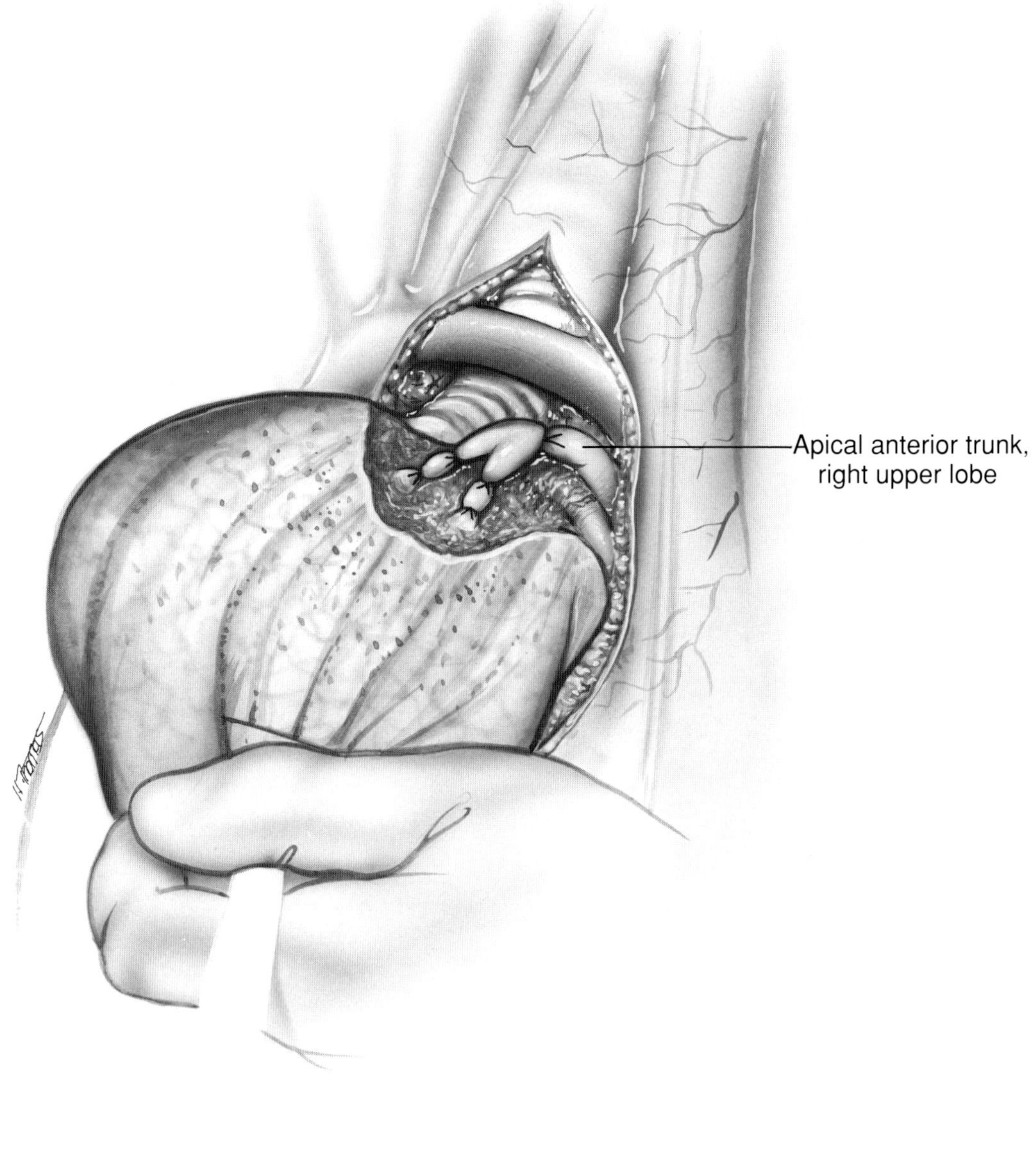

RIGHT UPPER LOBECTOMY

LOCATING THE MAIN PULMONARY ARTERY

In this view we are now again in the longitudinal fissure, making certain that we have located accurately the main pulmonary artery. The artist has ghosted in the course of the artery from the mediastinum to this point and has also shown the approximate location of the posterior segmental arterial branch going to the posterior segment of the right upper lobe. The right middle lobe branch just slightly proximal to but almost opposite the superior segmental artery branch can be seen, as well as the depiction of the continuation of the main pulmonary artery. This dissection is usually straightforward once the sheath has been opened so that this vessel can be seen.

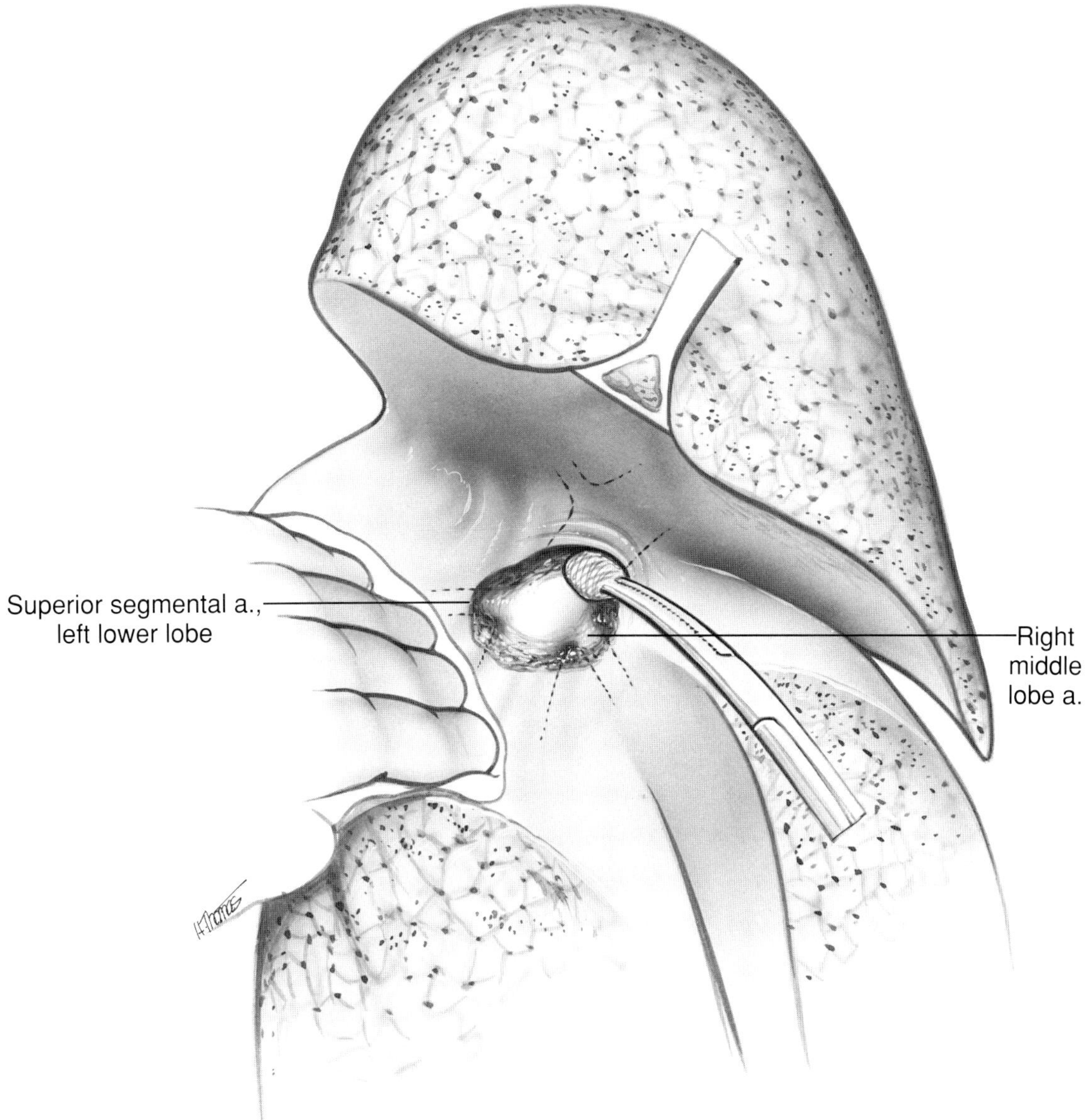

RIGHT UPPER LOBECTOMY

EXPOSURE OF THE MAIN PULMONARY ARTERY

In this view, after having identified the artery and the position of the right upper lobe bronchus, we have stapled open the incomplete fissure with a stapler. We have a proximal ligature, which normally we would have slightly more flush with the main pulmonary artery reinforced with a suture ligature with a distal tie since there did not appear to be any branches here. This will be cut close to the distal tie as the next maneuver.

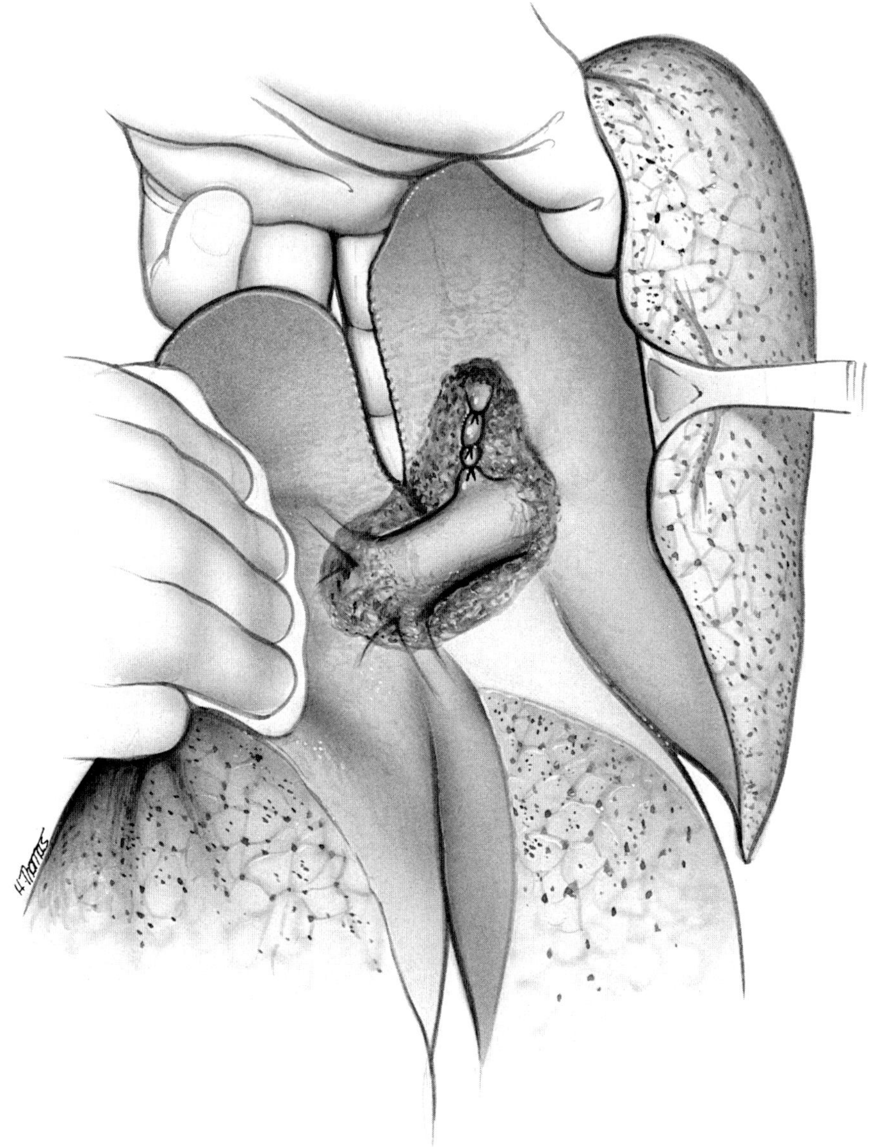

RIGHT UPPER LOBECTOMY

FREEING THE PARENCHYMA AROUND THE HILUM

Here the posterior segmental artery has been divided. The areolar tissue and lung parenchyma around the hilum of the right upper lobe have been dissected free or divided. The transverse fissure has been opened. The hilum of the right upper lobe, which consists of the superior pulmonary vein and bronchus, are gradually being cleared.

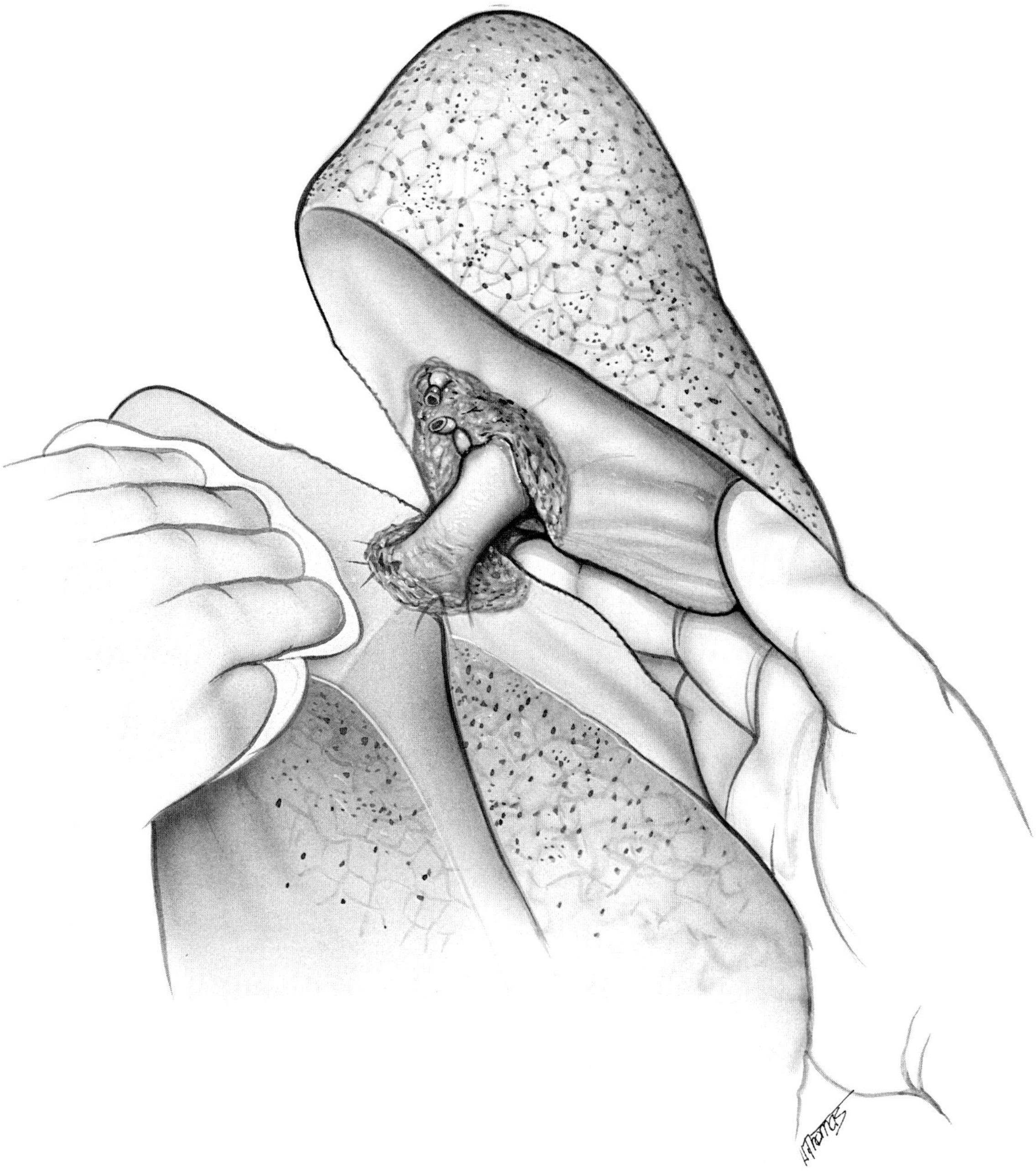

RIGHT UPPER LOBECTOMY

CLOSING THE UPPER LOBE BRONCHUS

In this view we have gone back and stapled the right upper lobe bronchus at its takeoff from the bronchus intermedius. The stapler was applied and closed but not fired. The anesthetist aspirated and reinflated the right lung, demonstrating good inflation of the middle and lower lobes with no inflation of the right upper lobe. The stapler was fired and cut distal to the staple line. Here we can see the open bronchus; we can also see the highest pulmonary artery branch, which has been ligated and the distal ties. The right upper lobe is still being held in place by the superior pulmonary vein, which here is shown to have three branches. Faintly depicted is a right middle lobe venous tributary draining into the base of the superior pulmonary vein, which has been protected and saved.

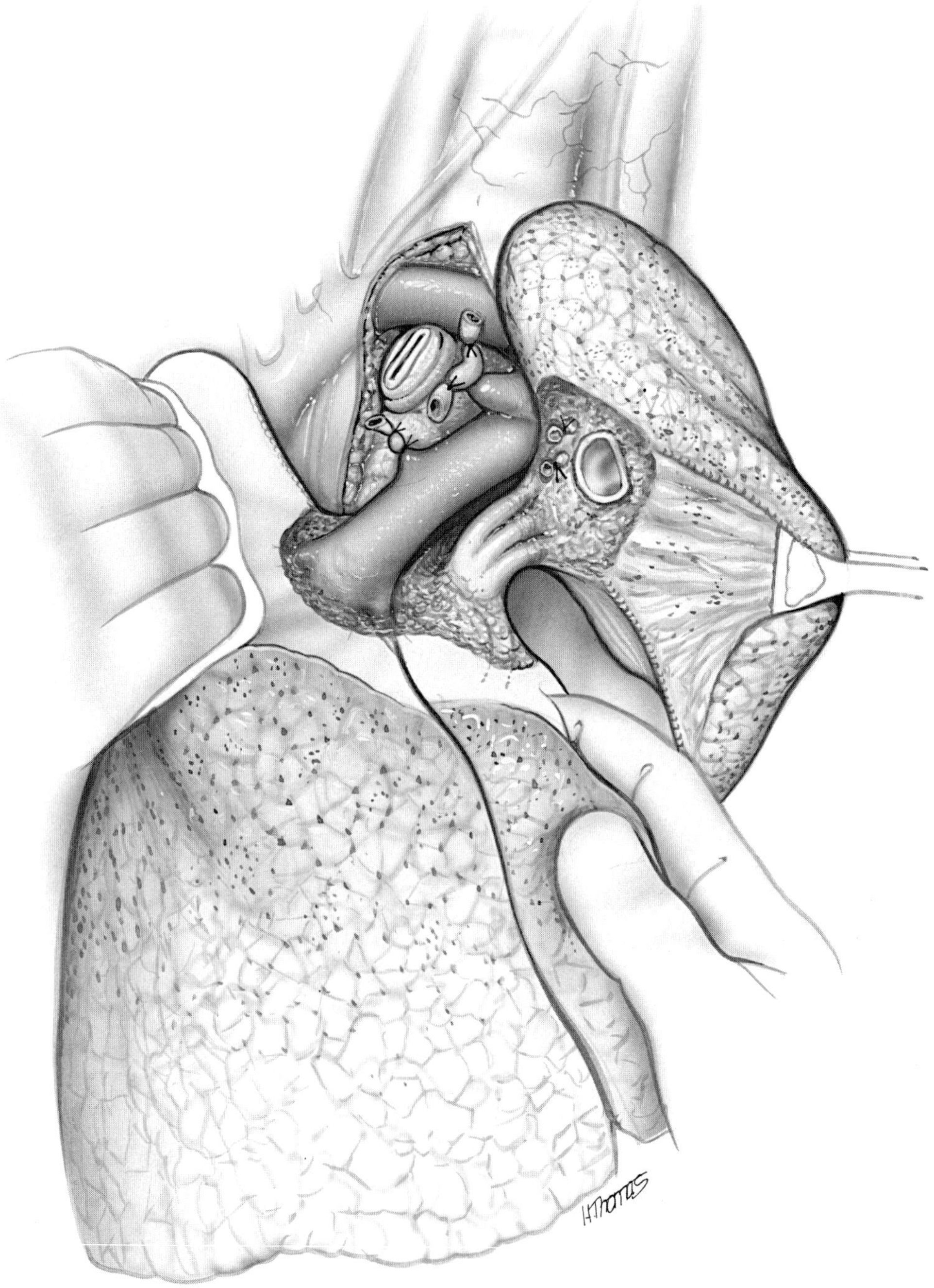

RIGHT UPPER LOBECTOMY

VEIN DISSECTION

Here the lung has been moved posteriorly, and we are once more looking at the anterior hilum of the lung. The three veins draining the right upper lobe are seen, and the finger is aiding in the dissection of this vein, which has still some areolar tissue attached to it posteriorly.

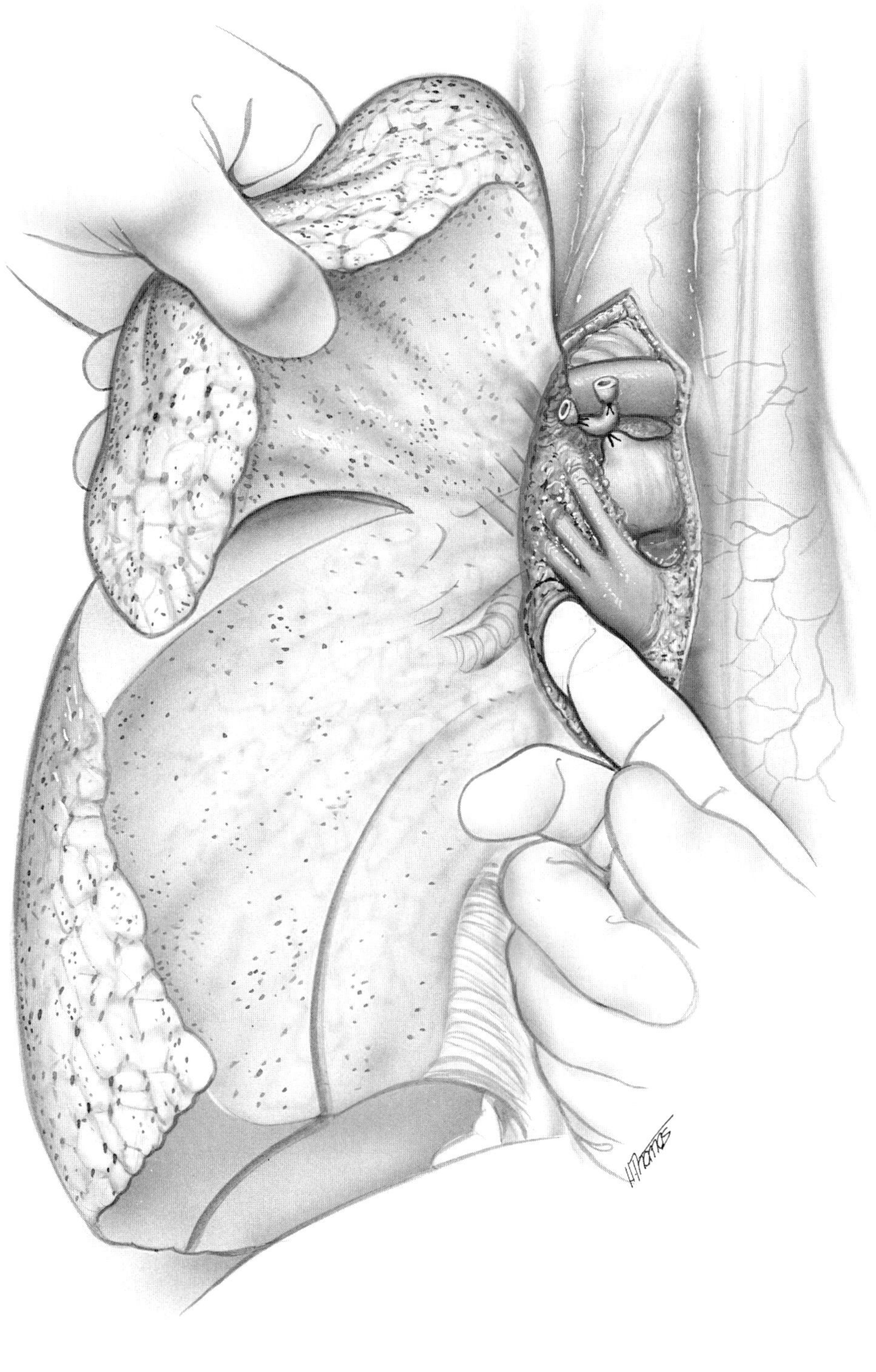

RIGHT UPPER LOBECTOMY

REMOVAL OF THE SPECIMEN

We are still looking at the anterior portion of the hilum. The three tributaries draining into the superior pulmonary vein have a proximal ligature and a proximal suture ligature. The vessels have been cut. The specimen has been removed. We can see the pulmonary artery coursing down to the remaining right middle and right lower lobe. We can see the bronchus continuing down as well; we can also see the venous drainage from the right middle lobe, which is still safely draining into the superior pulmonary vein. The next step is ensure that the inferior pulmonary ligament is divided so that the residual lobes may rise safely into the chest. If the right middle lobe is "floppy" at times, we place two mattress sutures to reclose the anterior longitudinal fissure to prevent any torsion of the right middle lobe. The space will be irrigated to ensure that there are no blood or air leaks that should be fixed before closing the chest.

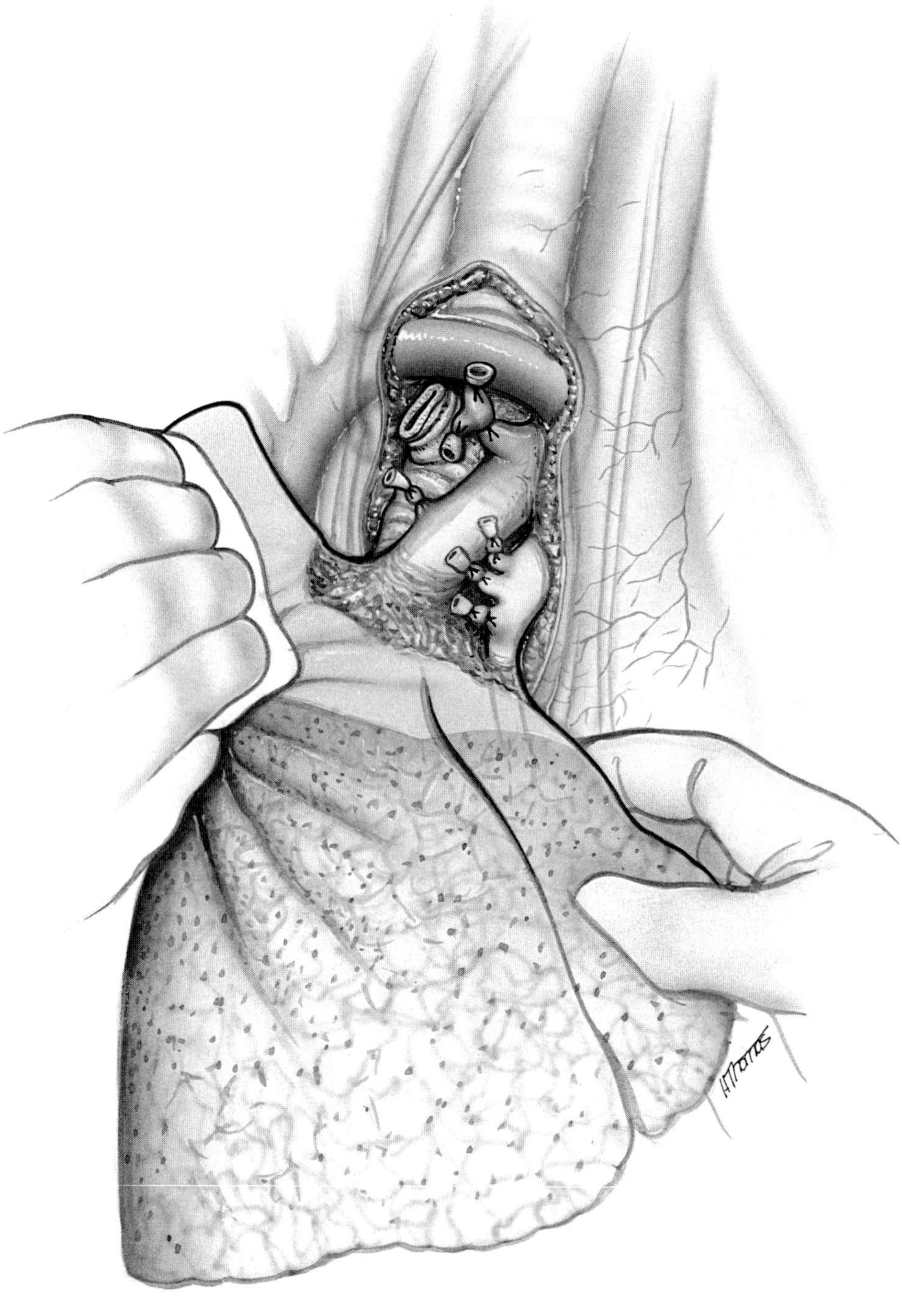

RIGHT MIDDLE LOBECTOMY

ANATOMIC ORIENTATION

In this view we are approaching the anterior portion of the right lung. The azygos vein joining the superior vena cava, which is coursing down to the heart along with the phrenic nerve, is seen to the top and right in the drawing. The left hand is elevating the right upper lobe. The right index finger is demonstrating the anatomy in the hilum of the right middle lobe. The fissure and the visceral pleura have been opened. The superior pulmonary vein is visible with one branch adjacent to the right index finger draining the upper right middle lobe. A branch of the pulmonary artery coursing down the fissure can be seen diagramatically coming to the right middle lobe, and between the two vessels deeper is the right middle lobe bronchus.

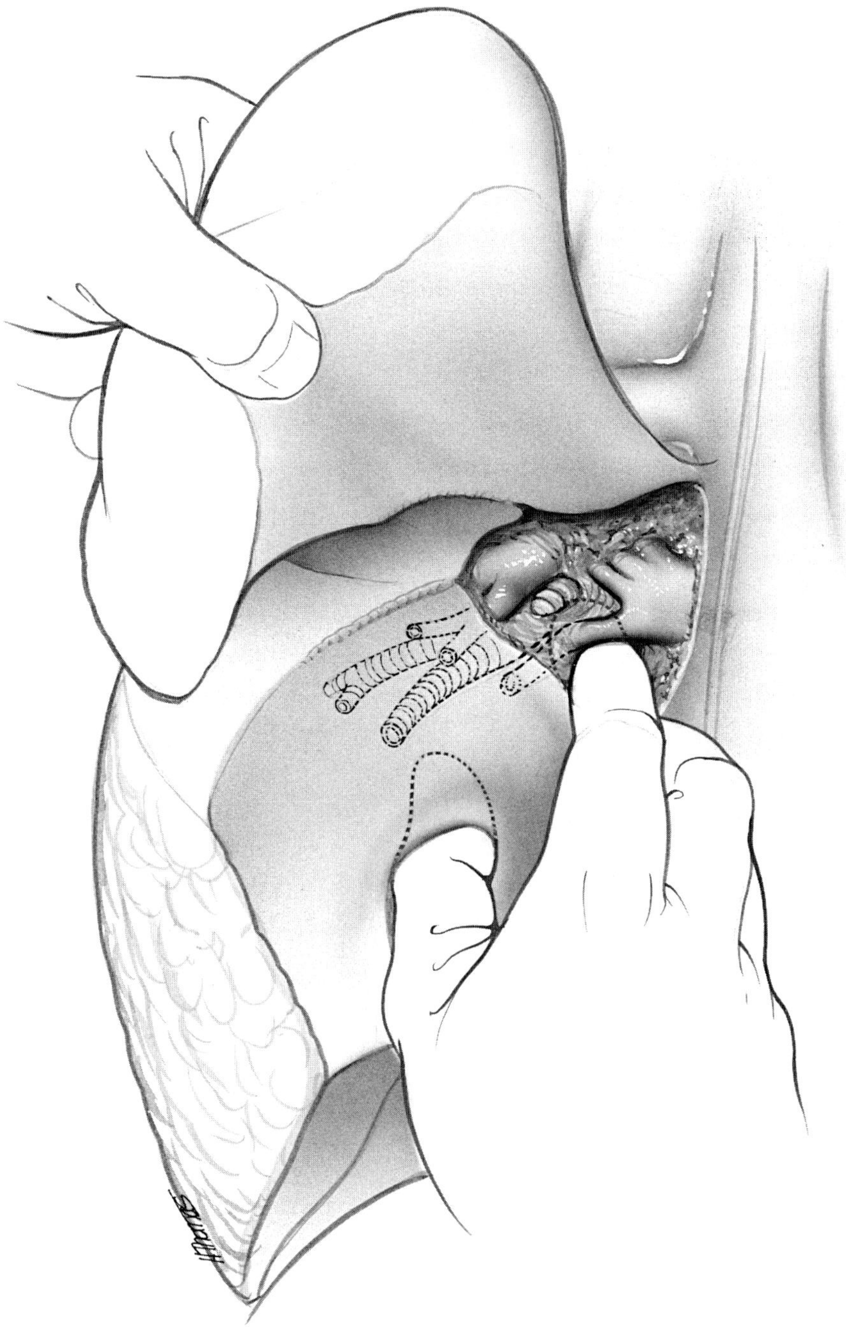

RIGHT MIDDLE LOBECTOMY

LIGATION AND SUTURING OF THE ARTERIAL BRANCH

We are looking at the lateral view of the right lung. The Duval lung clamp is lifting the right upper lobe out of the way. We are viewing the fissure between the right middle lobe and the right lower lobe. The finger demonstrates the arterial branch to the right middle lobe. It has been tied close to the main pulmonary artery. Suture ligature distal to that and another distal ligature have been performed so that we are ready to divide the right middle lobe artery. The venous drainage into the right superior pulmonary vein is hidden behind the right middle lobe in this illustration.

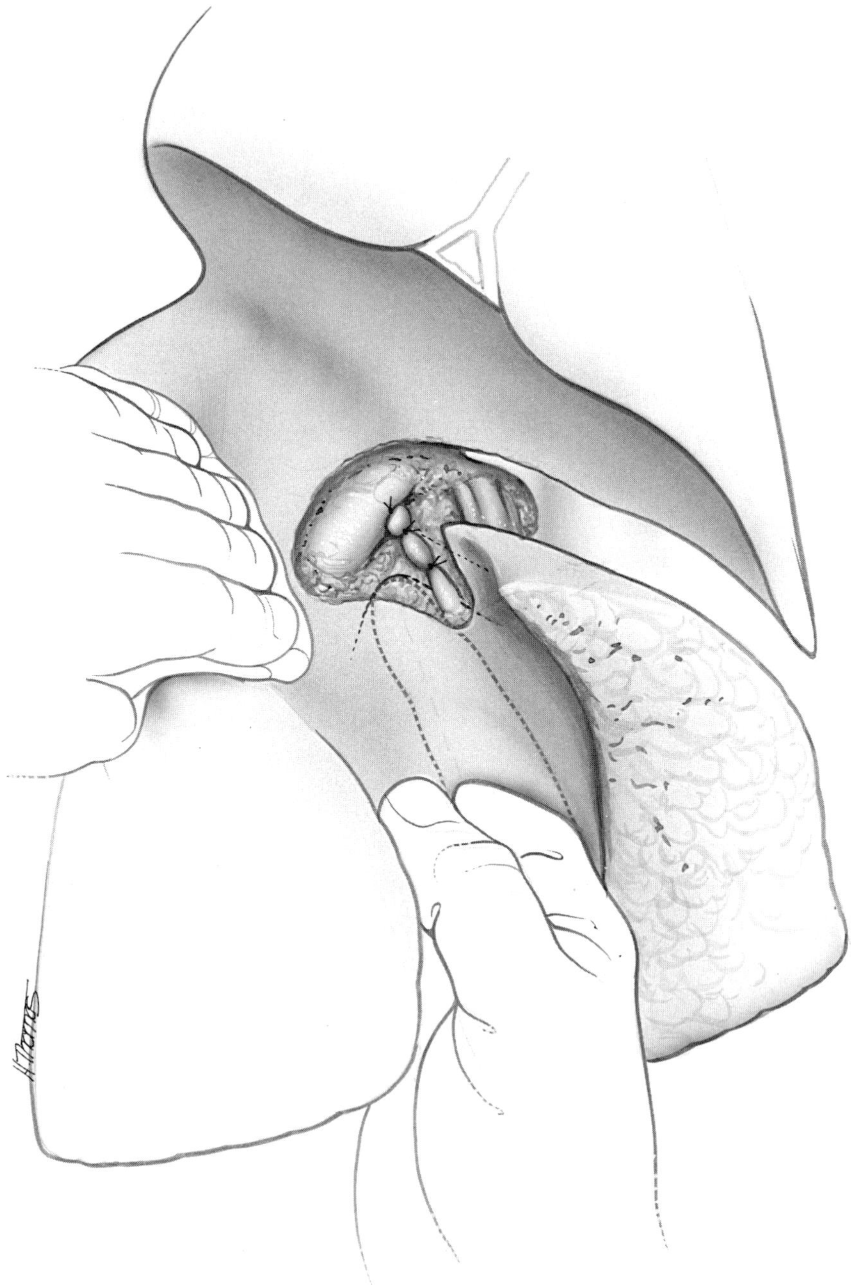

RIGHT MIDDLE LOBECTOMY

PREPARING TO DIVIDE THE MIDDLE LOBE BRONCHUS

In this view the right middle lobe remains attached via the right middle lobe bronchus. The right middle lobe artery stump is seen. The residual venous drainage from the right upper lobe is visible. The right middle lobe is under traction.

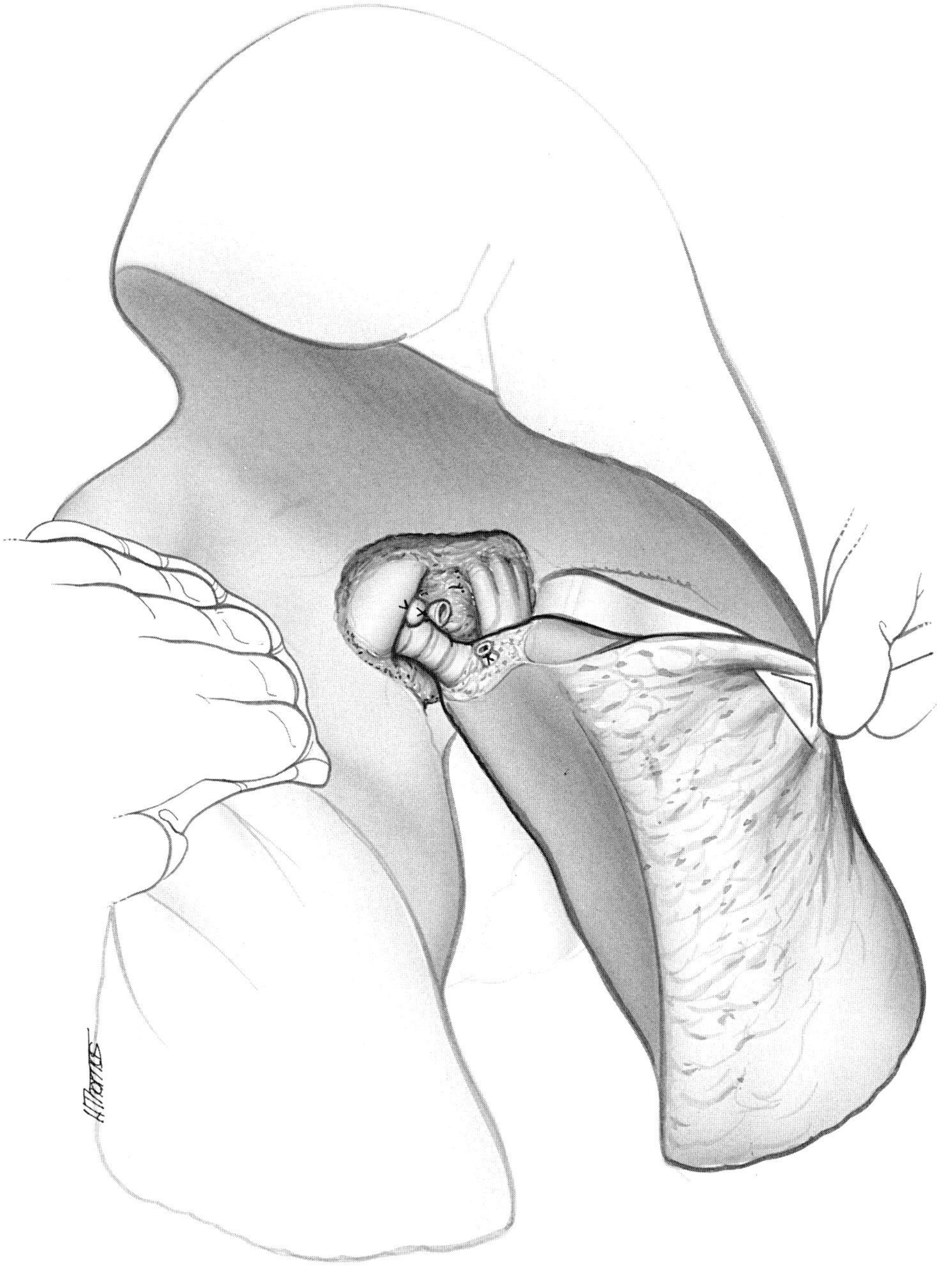

RIGHT MIDDLE LOBECTOMY

REMOVAL OF THE MIDDLE LOBE

The bronchus to the right middle lobe has been divided and sutured over its end. The specimen is free except for the attachment of the right middle lobe vein draining into the superior pulmonary vein. One must also look for venous drainage into the right inferior pulmonary vein. If such exists, it, too, must be divided. All available lymph nodes should be removed and numbered.

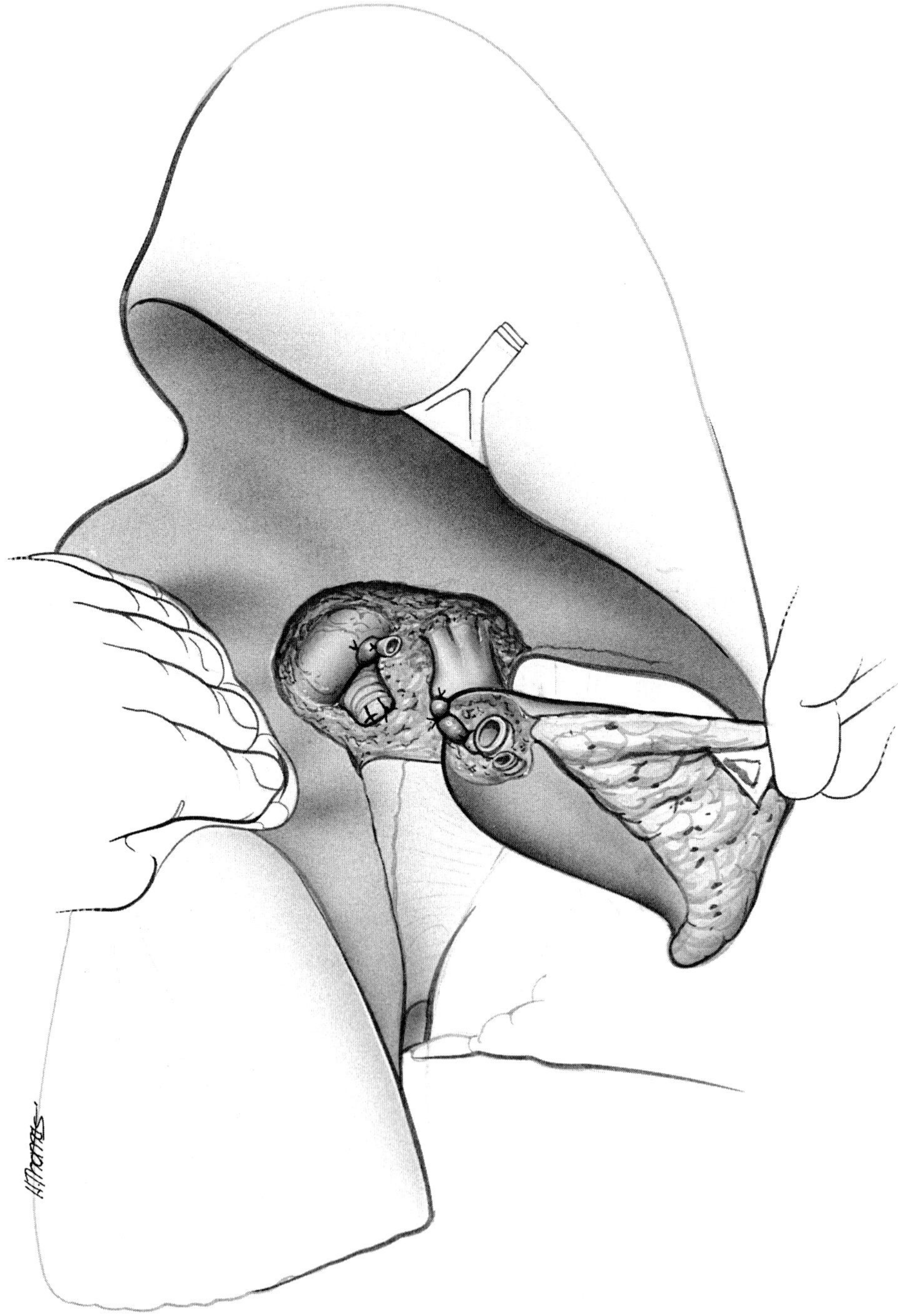

RIGHT MIDDLE LOBECTOMY

ASSESSMENT FOR LEAKAGE

The right lung is retracted posteriorly. The right middle lobe artery stump, bronchial stump, and venous stumps are all seen. It is not ordinarily necessary to cover lobar bronchial stumps, because the inflation of the remaining lung will suffice. All stumps are checked under water for leakage. The size of the bronchial stump dictates the number of sutures needed. Two or three suffice for small bronchi. Four or five usually suffice for a bronchial stump.

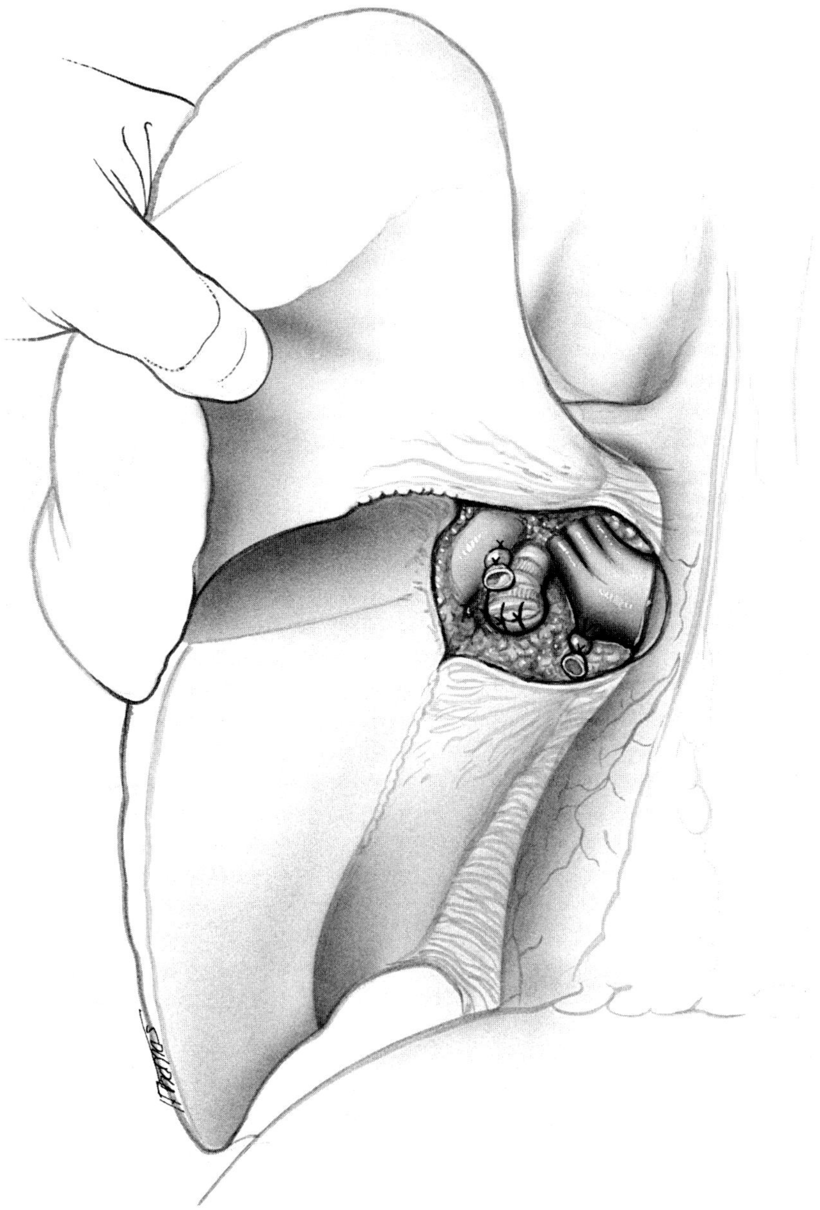

RIGHT LOWER LOBECTOMY

EXPOSURE OF THE MAIN PULMONARY ARTERY

In this view we are approaching the right lung laterally. The right lower lobe is to the left; the right upper lobe and right middle lobe are to the right. The longitudinal fissure is almost completely open, and in the fissure we see the main pulmonary artery running from right to left, cephalad to caudad. The sheath of the vessel has been opened. We have dissected out the superior segmental branch artery to the superior segment. There is a proximal ligature, proximal suture ligature, and distal tie. The surgeon is about to divide this vessel.

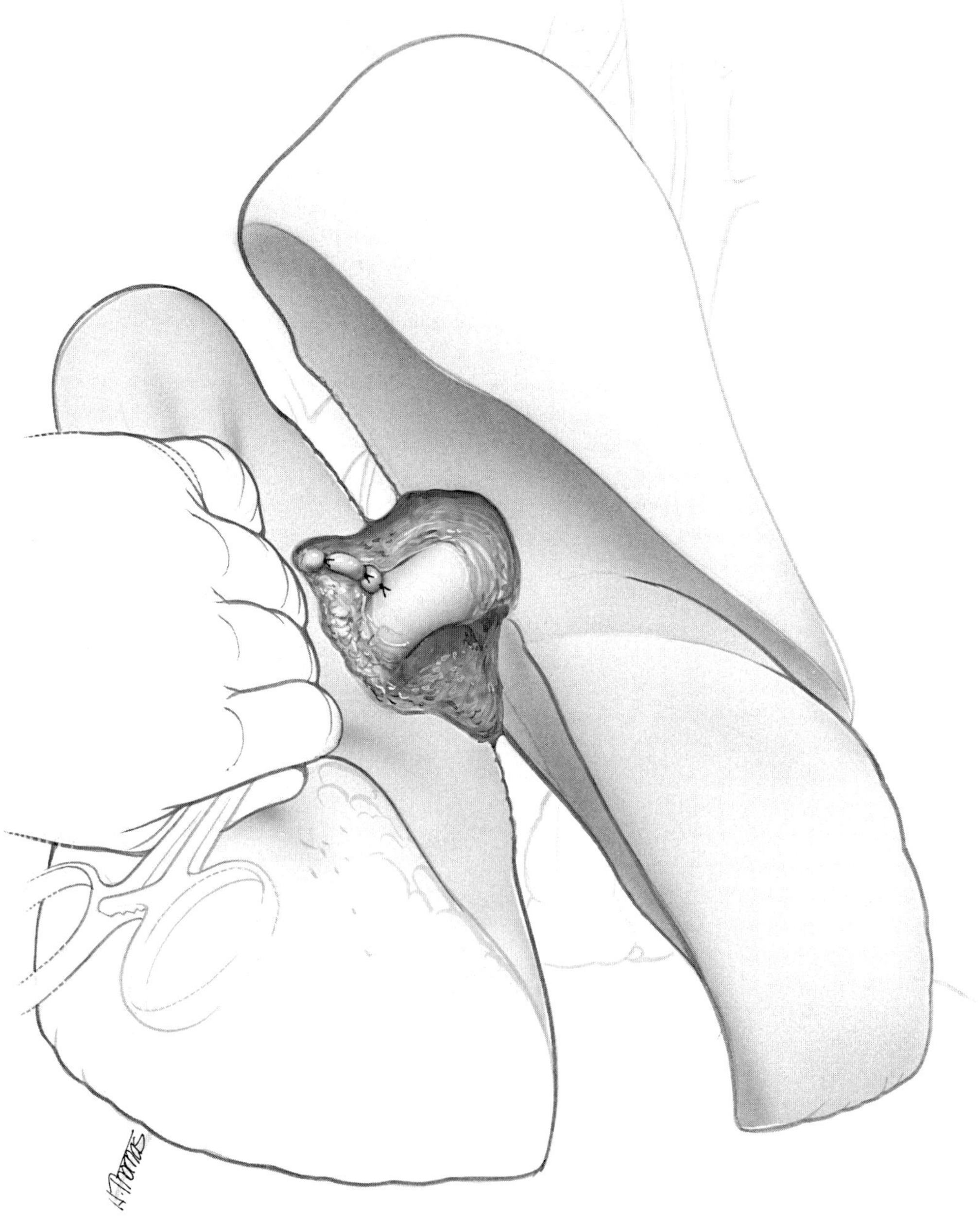

RIGHT LOWER LOBECTOMY

DIVISION OF THE SUPERIOR SEGMENTAL BRONCHUS

In this situation, after having divided the superior segmental bronchus the surgeon has identified the branches of the pulmonary artery to the remaining right lower lobe, in this case two to the basal segments. They have been suture ligated proximally and divided distally. With very gentle displacement of this stump, one can see the right bronchus intermedius running to the right lower lobe. A branch to the superior segment is seen, and a major branch is running to the basal segments. The right middle lobe bronchus ordinarily comes off the bronchus intermedius opposite and slightly proximal to the superior segmental branch. Its location determines whether the lower lobe bronchus can be handled with one placement of the stapler.

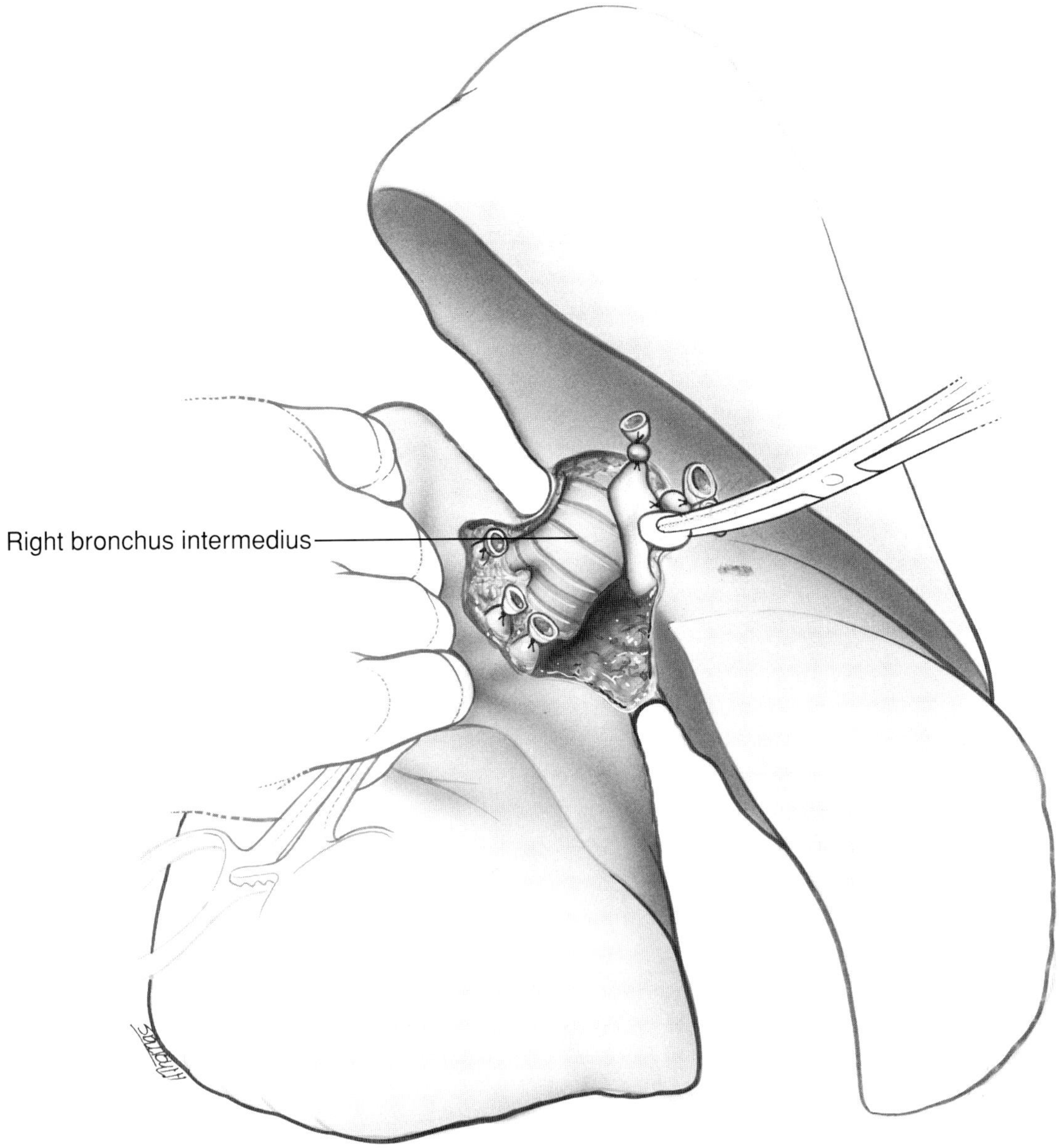

RIGHT LOWER LOBECTOMY

DIVISION OF THE LOWER LOBE BRONCHUS

In this view the approach and exposure are the same as in the previous drawing. We have stapled the right lower lobe bronchus inasmuch as the right middle lobe bronchus is safely more proximal and the stapler will not occlude the airway to the right middle lobe or the posterior portion of the right upper lobe. If there is difficulty in doing this, the right lower lobe bronchus may have to be divided at the superior and basal segmental levels if the tumor surgery permits. At times it may be necessary to remove the middle lobe along with the lower lobe if there is tumor encroachment at this level. In this situation the bronchus intermedius can be divided close to the upper lobe branches and the stump length can be increased significantly by resecting the middle and lower lobes together. Also in this view one can see the right middle lobe artery branch, which has been preserved. Although the dissecting sponge shows displacement of the vessel to make the anatomy clear, one must exercise due caution in handling these pulmonary arteries, which are more the consistency of veins.

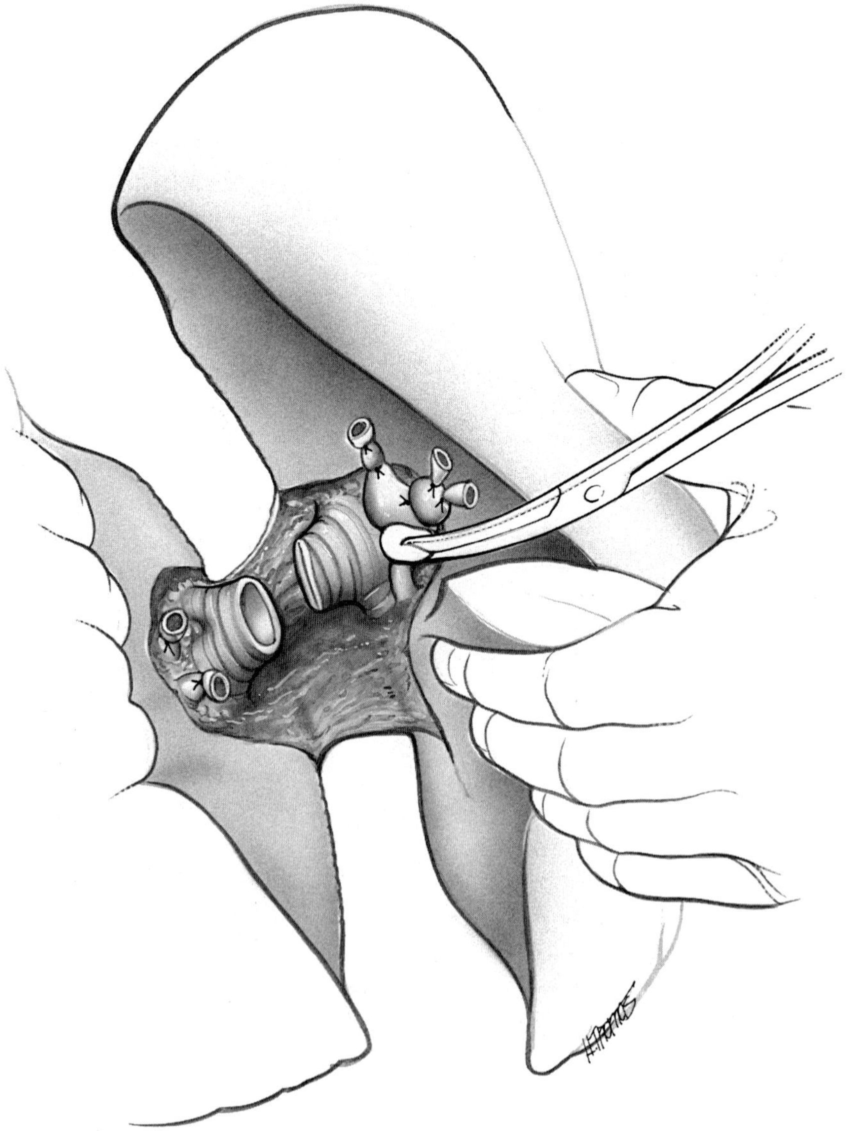

RIGHT LOWER LOBECTOMY

OPENING OF THE INFERIOR PULMONARY LIGAMENT

In this view the right lower lobe has been reflected anteriorly and is being lifted cephalad. The inferior pulmonary ligament has been opened, and we can see the inferior pulmonary vein. We should have looked for any venous drainage from the right middle lobe into this vein at the time we were exposing this area in the previous drawing. As shown, there is no middle lobe venous drainage into this vein.

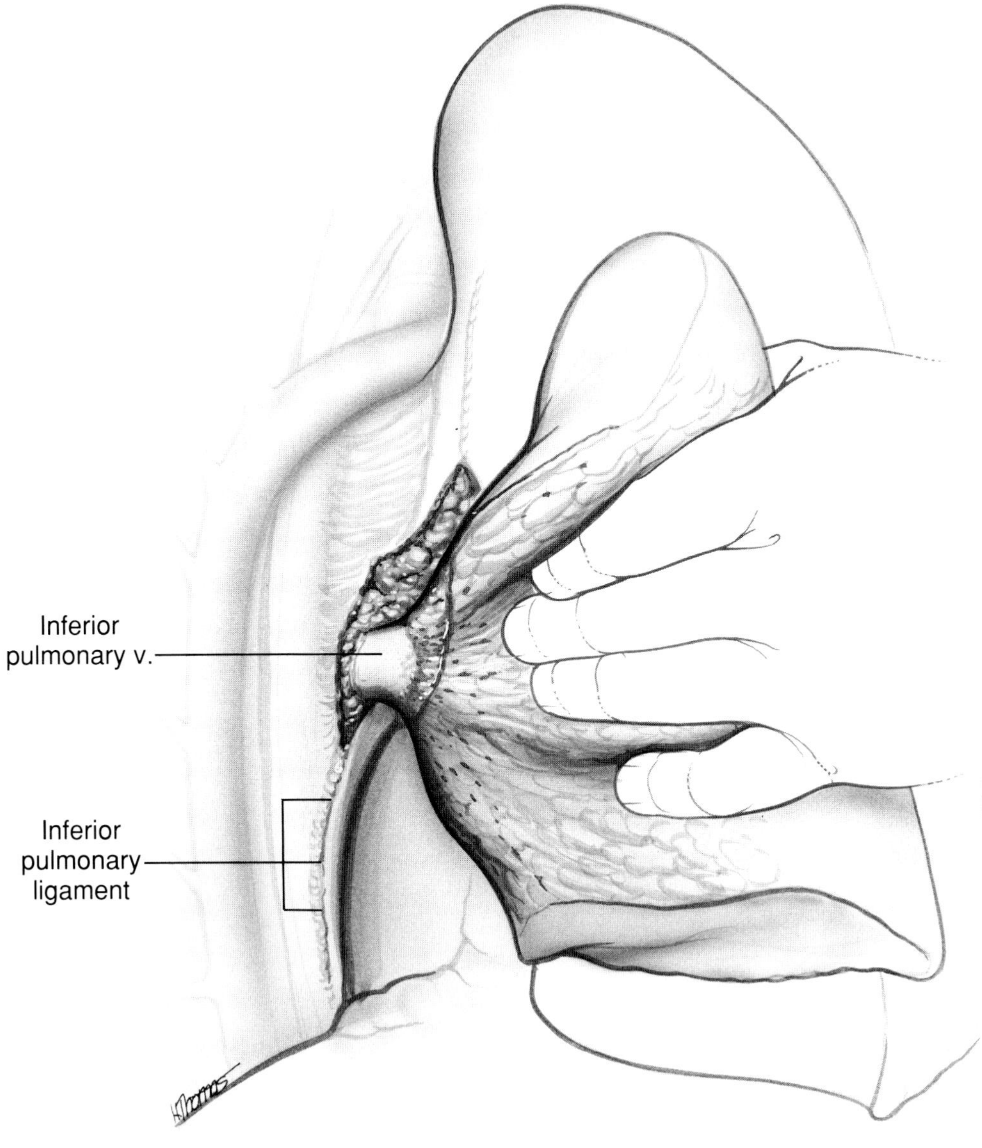

RIGHT LOWER LOBECTOMY

DIVISION OF THE INFERIOR PULMONARY VEIN

This view depicts the right middle lobe being displaced anteriorly and upward. The right upper lobe is in the upper portion of the drawing. The right lower lobe has been removed. We are looking at the hilum of the right lower lobe, and in the posterior inferior portion we see the ligated inferior pulmonary vein. In this instance there must be a heavy ligature proximal, a suture ligature more distal, and either quite an adequate venous stump or the division of the inferior vein at the level of the branches. To a certain extent this is controlled by the location of the tumor, and if the tumor were close to the vein one might very well not be able to preserve the branching still attached to the inferior vein. If there is every any question and a stapler cannot be used, an alternative approach is to place a vascular clamp on the inferior pulmonary vein close to the pericardium and left atrium and then ligate the vein distally. When the vein is divided between the vascular clamp and the distal tie, it is oversewn with 5-0 vascular suture in a two-row continuous mattress fashion to ensure safe control of this vessel.

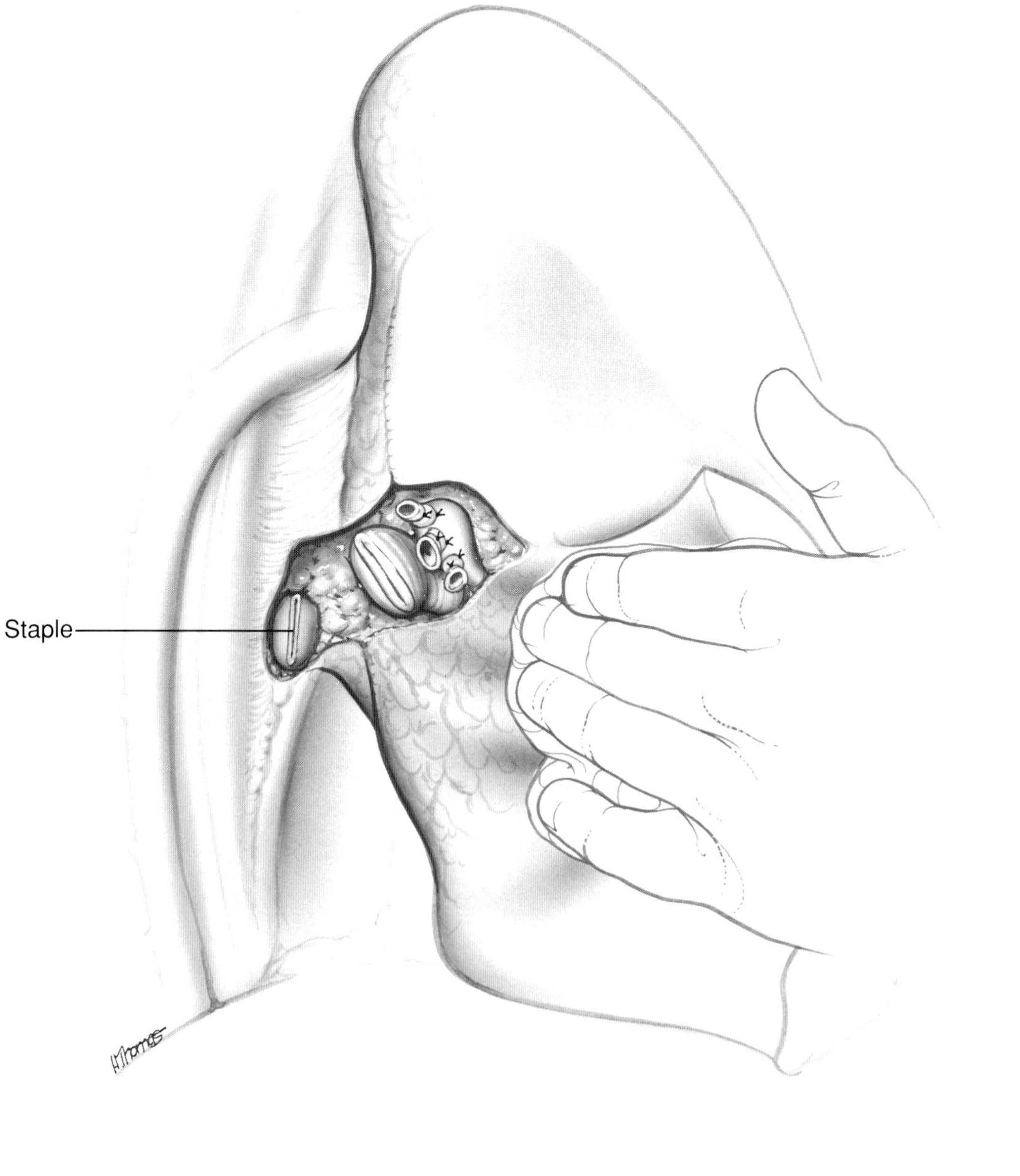

RIGHT PNEUMONECTOMY

EXPOSURE OF THE MAIN BRONCHUS

In this view the patient is in the left lateral position. The thorax has been entered through the right fifth interspace. The lung has been moved anteriorly, and the mediastinal pleura has been opened posteriorly. Visible in the cephalic portion of the incision is the azygos vein traveling from the spine posteriorly to the superior vena cava anteriorly. The right mainstem bronchus has been exposed posteriorly, and we are close to the tracheal carina. The membranous portion of the tracheobronchial tree is posterior in this position. This must be dissected with some care since it is a relatively thin layer. In doing a pneumonectomy the bronchial blood supply should be ligated proximally with 3-0 or 2-0 silk ligatures. We are using the small dissecting sponges to demonstrate the inferior pulmonary vein which lies immediately caudad to the plane of the right main bronchus. More posteriorly is the esophagus, and the vagus nerve can be seen coursing down the esophagus. On this side the recurrent nerve has taken off at the top of the chest and gone posteriorly around the subclavian artery. The vagus nerve also gives branches to the lung hilum, which have to be divided. Small vessels may accompany these branches. In a pneumonectomy, the mediastinal lymph nodes should be removed in continuity or for staging. This is shown in separate drawings.

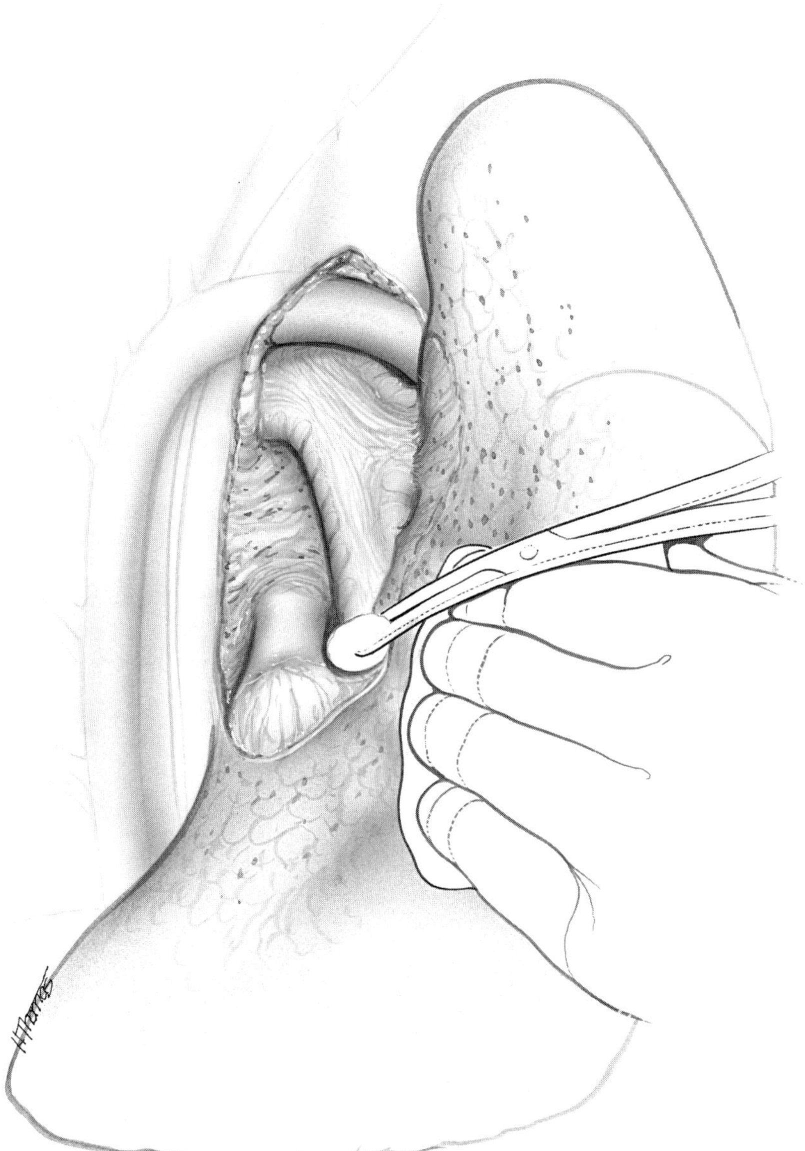

RIGHT PNEUMONECTOMY

EXPOSURE OF THE PULMONARY ARTERY

In this view the lung has been moved posteriorly and we are dissecting the anterior part of the hilum. Again in the cephalic part of the dissection the azygos vein can be seen joining the superior vena cava. On the superior vena cava is the cephalic phrenic nerve. It runs rather close to the anterior lung hilum, and in tumors in this region it may easily become involved with tumor. The heart is caudal to the superior vena cava.

In the hilum immediately caudal to the azygos vein and running anteroposteriorly from under the superior vena cava is the main pulmonary artery. In this situation one can see two ligatures on the first branch of the pulmonary artery to the right upper lobe. Immediately cephalad to the pulmonary artery is the superior pulmonary vein, which drains the right upper lobe and usually part of the right middle lobe directly into the left atrium. The highest branch of the superior pulmonary vein has been suture ligated and divided with an adequate stump. The distal vein is ligated to prevent backbleeding. This vein frequently must be divided to get satisfactory exposure of the arterial supply to the upper lobe.

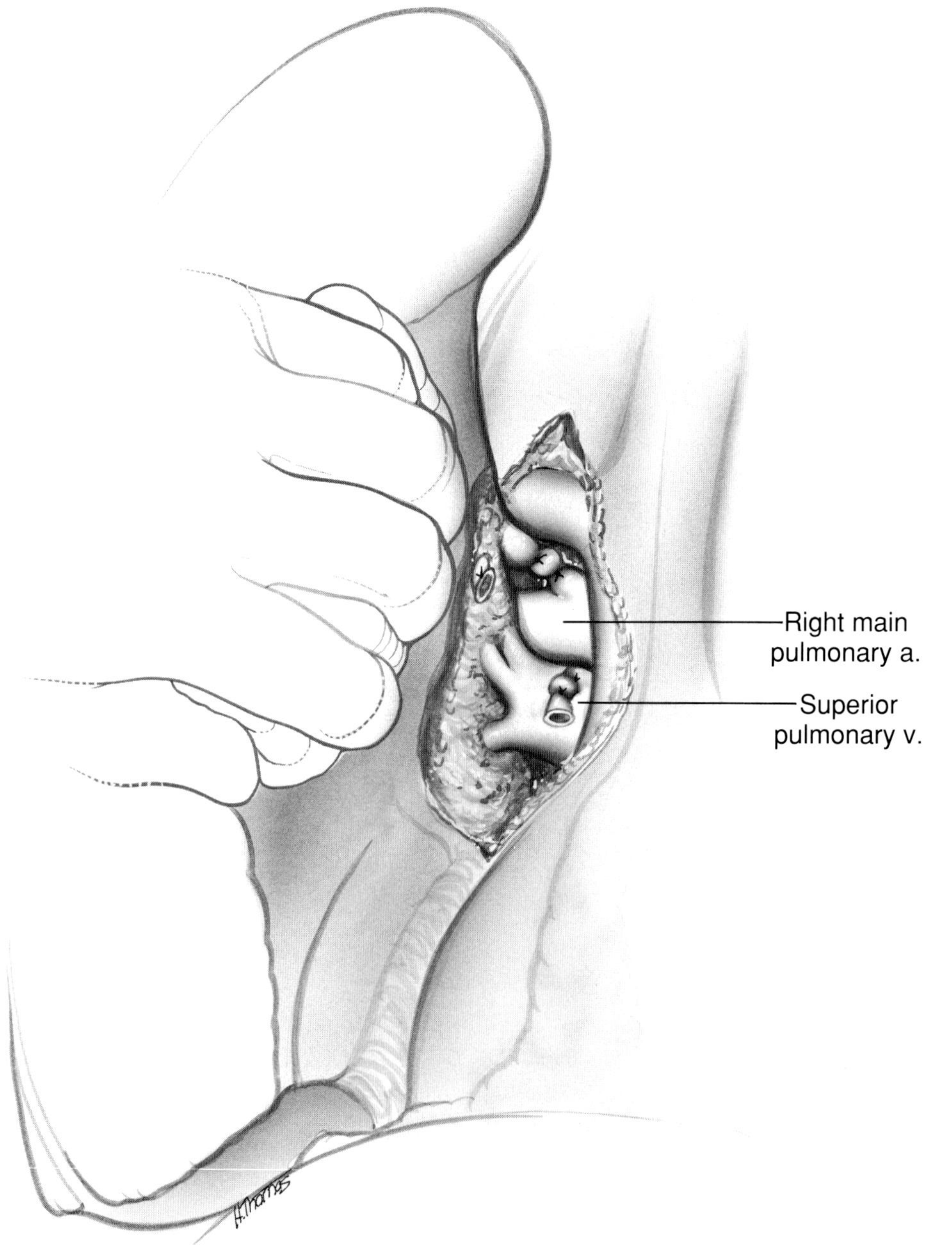

RIGHT PNEUMONECTOMY

DIVISION OF THE MAIN PULMONARY ARTERY

In this view we are still working on the anterior hilum. The main pulmonary artery has been dissected free and has been stapled proximally. The distal pulmonary artery stump has been ligated to prevent backbleeding. The pulmonary artery has been divided. In similar fashion the superior pulmonary vein has been dissected free. It has been ligated closer to the lung, and the stapler has been used proximally. Following this the vein has been divided. It is easier and less blood is lost if the arterial supply to the lung is occluded prior to occluding or dividing the venous drainage. On theoretical grounds in cancer surgery it is wise to close off the venous drainage as soon as feasible to minimize chances for tumor embolization via the venous system. Good judgment must be used when applying this concept since obstructing the venous drainage to an organ as large as the lung prior to control of the arterial input will result in distention of the lung with blood, and a considerable amount of blood will be sequestered and lost to the circulation with this maneuver. Therefore the arterial supply is usually occluded first. However, in dissecting lung cancers the surgeon should avoid undue trauma and pressure to the tumor while it is being removed.

The still intact bronchus can be seen. In freeing the pulmonary artery and the superior pulmonary vein, the major cleavage plane of dissection is the separation of these structures from the bronchus.

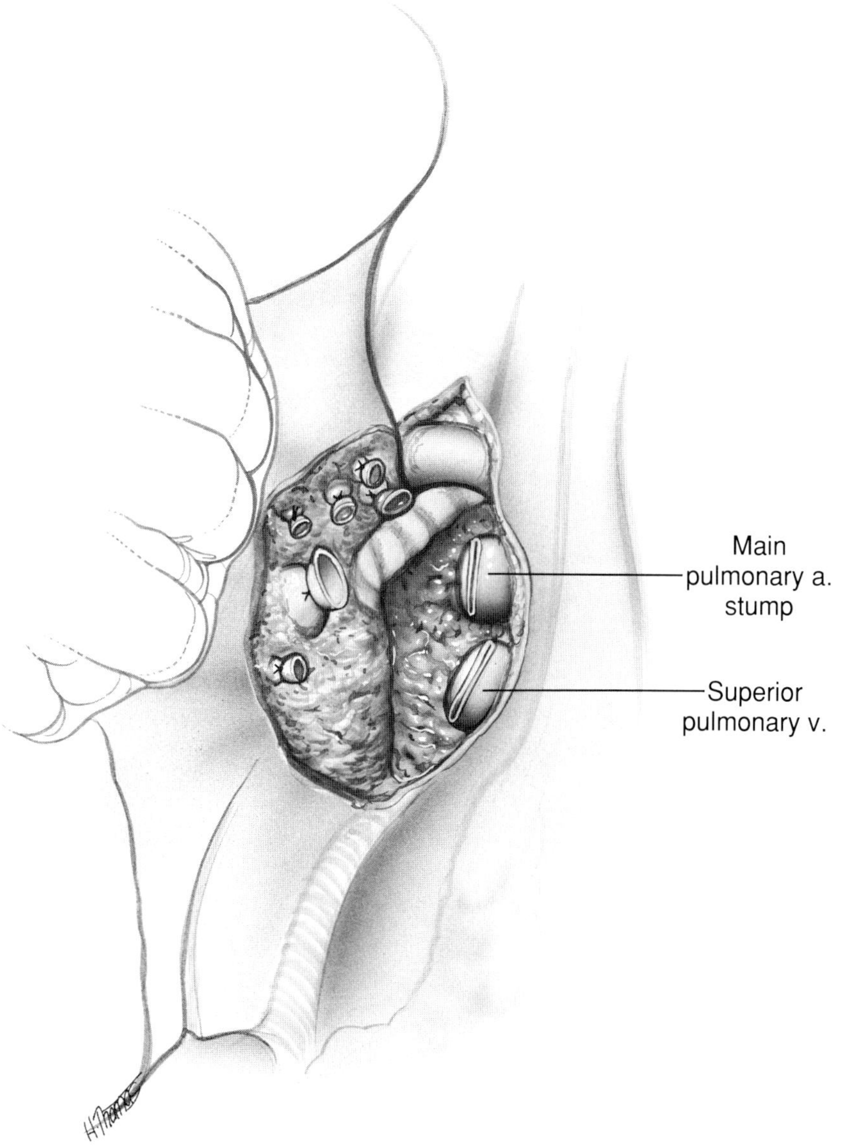

RIGHT PNEUMONECTOMY

PREPARING TO DIVIDE THE MAIN BRONCHUS

Again we are approaching the hilum from posteriorly. The inferior pulmonary ligament, which is a thin structure with reflections of anterior and posterior mediastinal pleura, has been divided. This ligament contains a small bleeder or bleeders which must be ligated, clipped, or coagulated. Lymph nodes in this ligament are position 9. Lymph nodes in the region of the inferior pulmonary vein are position 8, and in the subcarinal space they are position 7. Pictured here the inferior pulmonary vein has been stapled proximally and two branches distally have been ligated to prevent backbleeding. The right mainstem bronchus has been dissected free. We can see the carina and several rings of the left mainstem bronchus disappearing out of sight in the mediastinum to the other side. The azygos vein can be seen coming up from the diaphragm along the spine. Between the azygos vein, spine, and inferior pulmonary ligament runs the esophagus with the accompanying vagal nerve. The areolar tissue that is still seen in the hilum is directly on the pericardium posterior to its piercing by the two pulmonary veins.

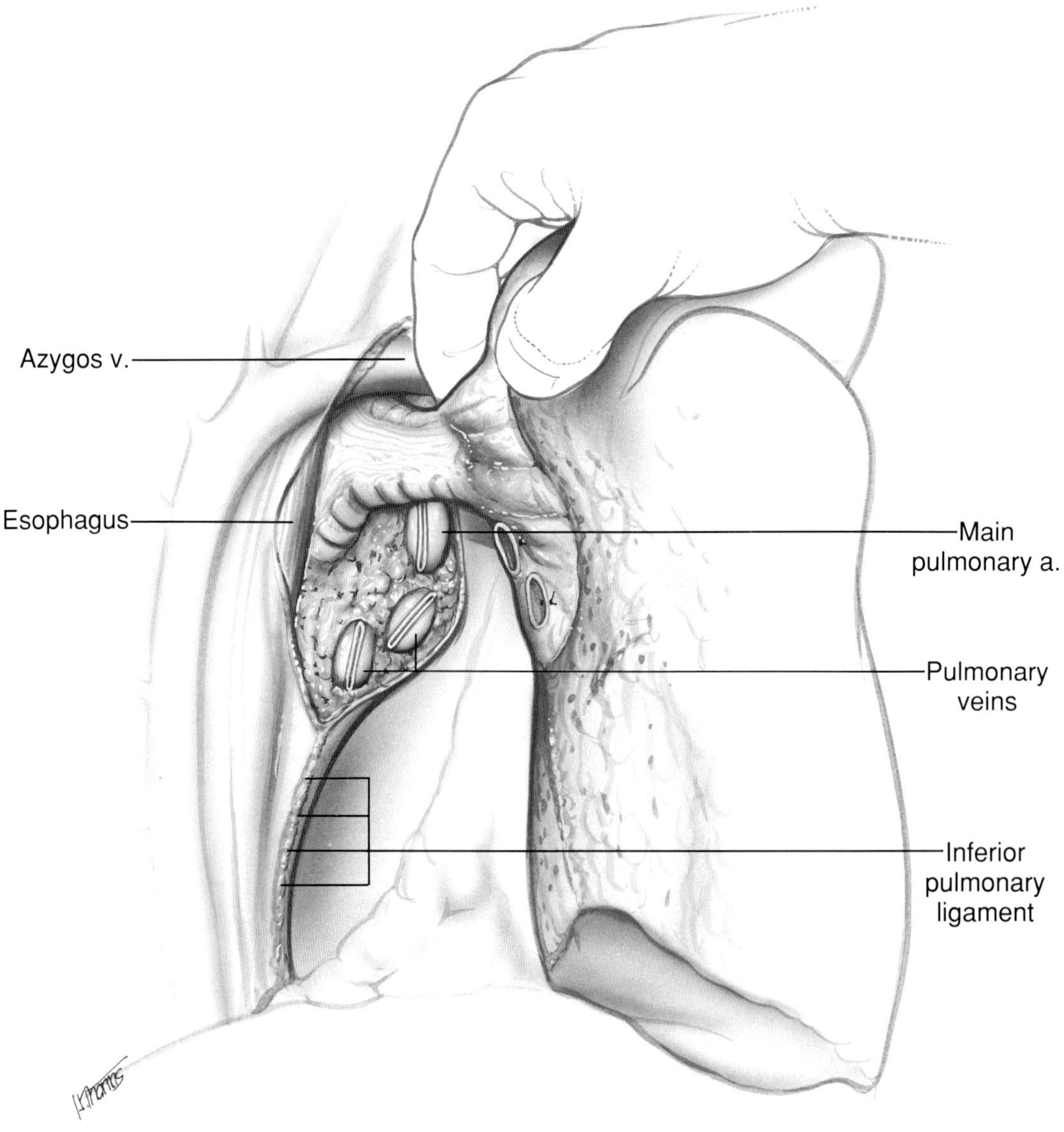

RIGHT PNEUMONECTOMY

CLOSURE OF THE MAIN BRONCHUS

In this view the pneumonectomy has been completed. The right main bronchial stump has been stapled closed. The drawing insert shows the approximate position of the stapler on the right main bronchus. This indicates that the staple has been relatively flush and close to the tracheobronchial junction. It is believed to be important not to leave significant bronchial stumps. One must be very careful not to stenose the tracheobronchial junction to the left lung, especially in small individuals. Again the dissection of the mediastinal lymph nodes is shown in a separate illustration, but is an important part of the operation. If there is available pleura we usually cover the bronchial stump. If the stump healing is doubtful, the mobilized omental pedicle graft brought up from the abdomen is the best buttress.

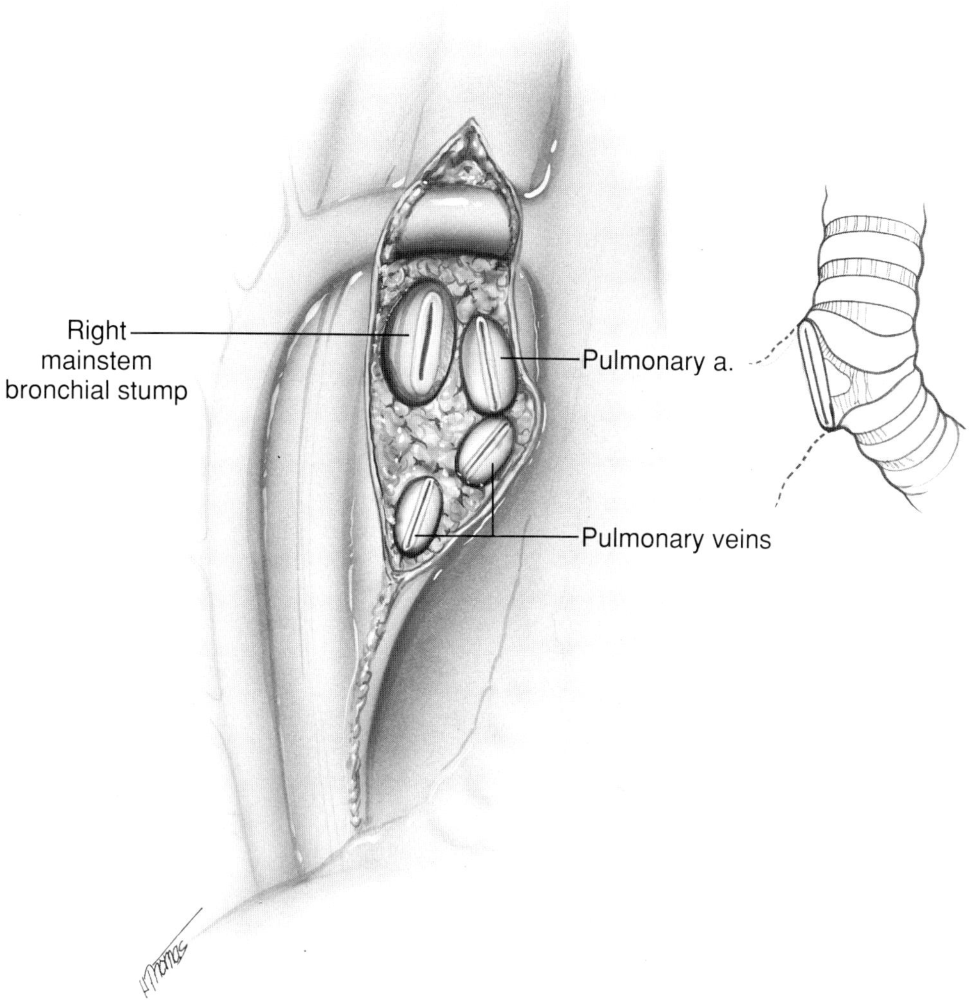

RIGHT PNEUMONECTOMY, VARIATION

In the first drawing, the tumor in the right lung involves the hilum close to the pericardium so that a pneumonectomy is needed. Again it is not possible to dissect the pulmonary artery and the pulmonary veins with safe surgical margins outside the pericardium. Here the pericardium has been opened wide in front of the hilum. The phrenic nerve runs close to the front of the right hilum on its way caudad. The surgeon must make a decision whether the incision should be anterior or posterior to the phrenic nerve. If the phrenic nerve is involved with tumor and the patient can tolerate a right pneumonectomy, it is reasonable to remove the phrenic nerve en bloc with the lung and the necessary subjacent pericardium. If the phrenic nerve can be preserved without interfering with the cancer cure, the phrenic nerve can be spared by moving it gently forward or opening the mediastinal pleura and pericardium posterior to the phrenic nerve. With this approach the pulmonary artery can be dissected free in the upper portion of the incision. The azygos vein should be divided to give better access to the mid-mediastinal area. The pulmonary artery is found coming out posterior to the distal superior vena cava. The surgeon will usually have to dissect around the left atrium to obtain a free margin to secure the pulmonary veins. It is important to remember that the pericardium is free anterior and posterior to the veins to the lung. However, at the cephalic and caudal margins there are reflections, which the surgeon must be careful to dissect free without injuring the vessels. With this approach the surgeon can staple the pulmonary artery and/or the left atrium. If necessary (if the stapler will not fit), a vascular clamp can be placed and a two-layer running 5-0 vascular suture placed distal to the clamp for the closure of the appropriate structure.

In the second drawing of this approach, we have a situation in which the pulmonary artery is obscured lateral to the superior vena cava with the tumor close to the superior vena cava. If the superior vena cava is gently dissected and retracted laterally, one can see that the right pulmonary artery lies posteriorly with the aorta medially and the vena cava laterally. Here the pulmonary artery can be encircled with an occluding tape or can be ligated. Staplers must be used with care in this region since there may not be enough room. One can ligate the pulmonary artery here if there is an emergency situation with improper control of the artery laterally. After this ligation and proximal control, one could mobilize the superior vena cava medially to expose the pulmonary artery distal to the already ligated pulmonary artery. A suture oversewing with two rows of 5-0 suture material could be done to ensure the safe division of the main pulmonary artery.

If there is inadvertent laceration of a major vascular structure, one should try to control the situation locally by grasping the vessel with the fingers or using some form of pressure, if a vascular clamp cannot be placed. After this local control, more proximal control must be obtained, possibly intrapericardially as exemplified in these two drawings.

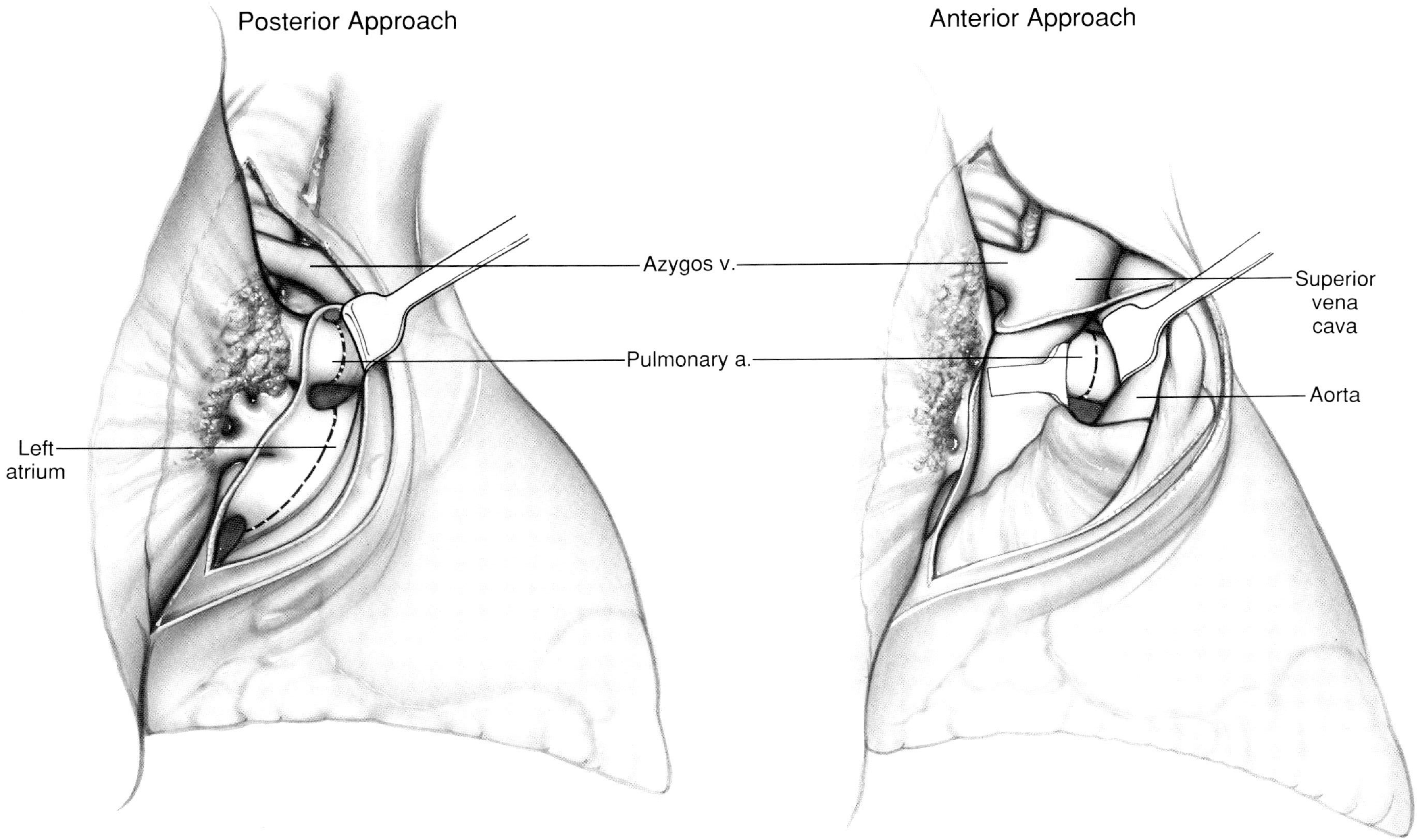
Posterior Approach
Anterior Approach
Azygos v.
Pulmonary a.
Left atrium
Superior vena cava
Aorta

LEFT UPPER LOBECTOMY

APPROACH TO THE HILUM

The left chest is opened. We are approaching the hilum of the lung cephalad to the lung, with the left lung shown largely deflated. The mediastinal pleura over the main pulmonary artery is being grasped with the forceps and incised with the scissors. The left upper lobe is to the operator's left and the left lower lobe to the right. The aortic arch can be seen cephalad with the phrenic nerve crossing anteriorly and the vagus nerve with the recurrent nerve crossing posteriorly toward the posterior position of the hilum.

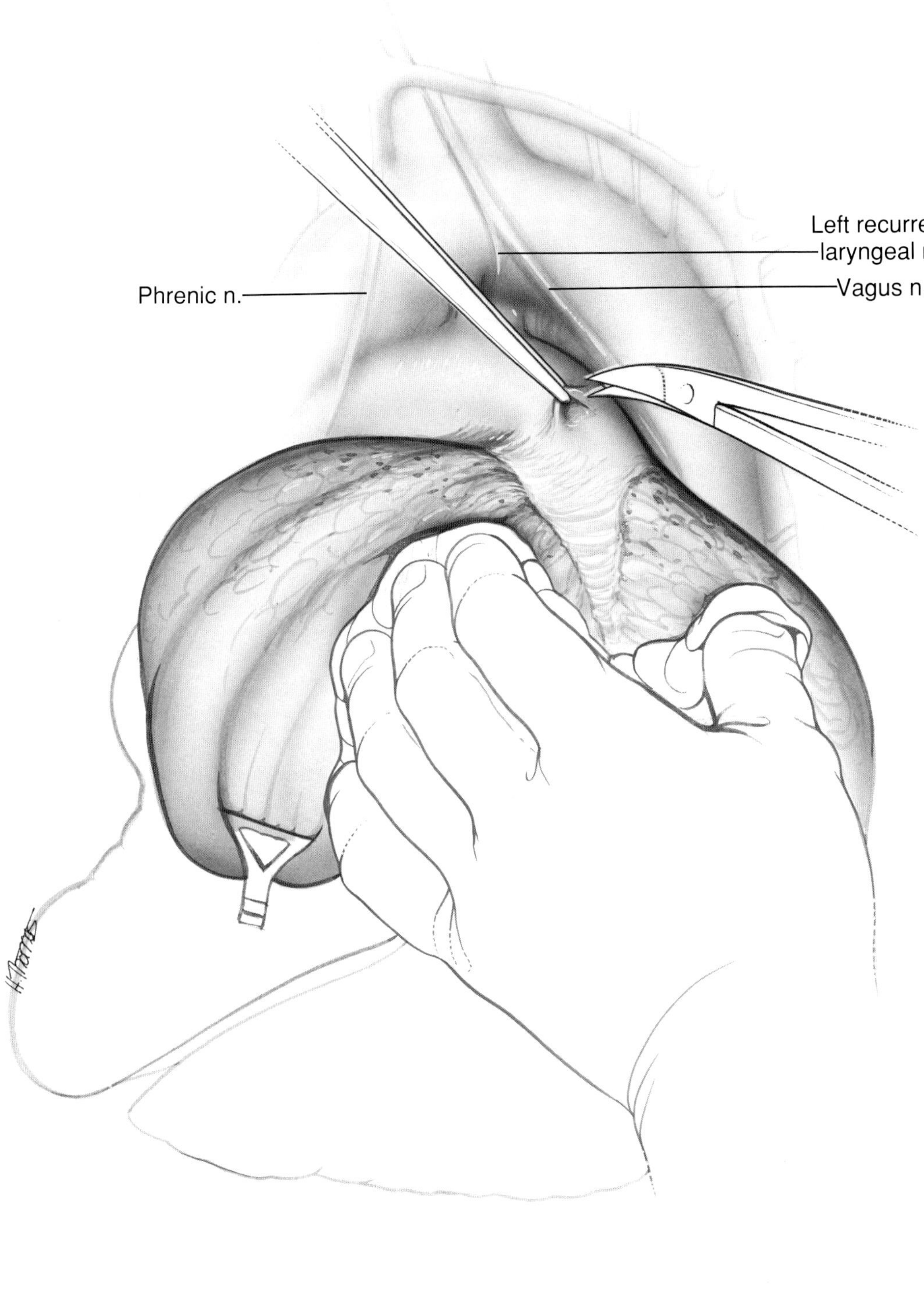

LEFT UPPER LOBECTOMY

EXPOSURE OF THE PULMONARY ARTERY

In this view the position and exposure are the same as in the previous drawing. The pleura and sheath over the pulmonary artery have been opened. The Mixter clamp is a good way to elevate the pleura and sheath in the longitudinal fissure so that the tissue can be divided without injuring the subjacent main pulmonary artery trunk. In situations in which the patient has had preoperative chemotherapy or radiotherapy or both, this plane may be difficult and sometimes even dangerous to achieve. It is very important, therefore, that the operator establish this plane before cutting the tissue in this step. This is best done by grasping the tissue with thumb forceps and, with gentle blunt dissection with a dissecting sponge, attempting to separate and depress the pulmonary artery from this area. If it is potentially hazardous, one may by necessity have to control the blood flow by passing a Rummel tourniquet around the pulmonary artery in a safe proximal location so that this can be done in a rather bloodless field.

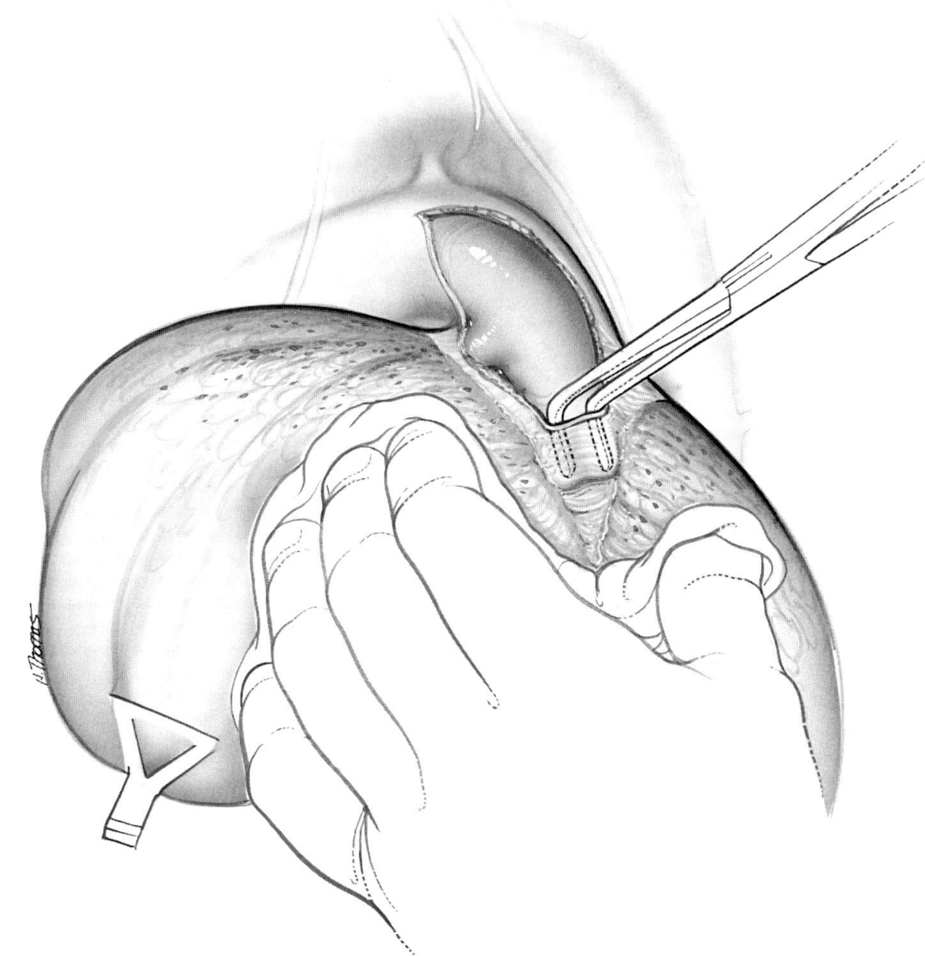

LEFT UPPER LOBECTOMY

EXPOSURE OF THE PULMONARY ARTERY BRANCHES

In this situation we have exposed the pulmonary artery and are exposing the branches to the left upper lobe. The number of branches to the left upper lobe is variable. Ordinarily there is one each to the apical segment, posterior segment, anterior segment, and lingula, but there may be more or fewer, and the surgeon must inspect carefully as dissection continues, to be certain that all of these branches are found.

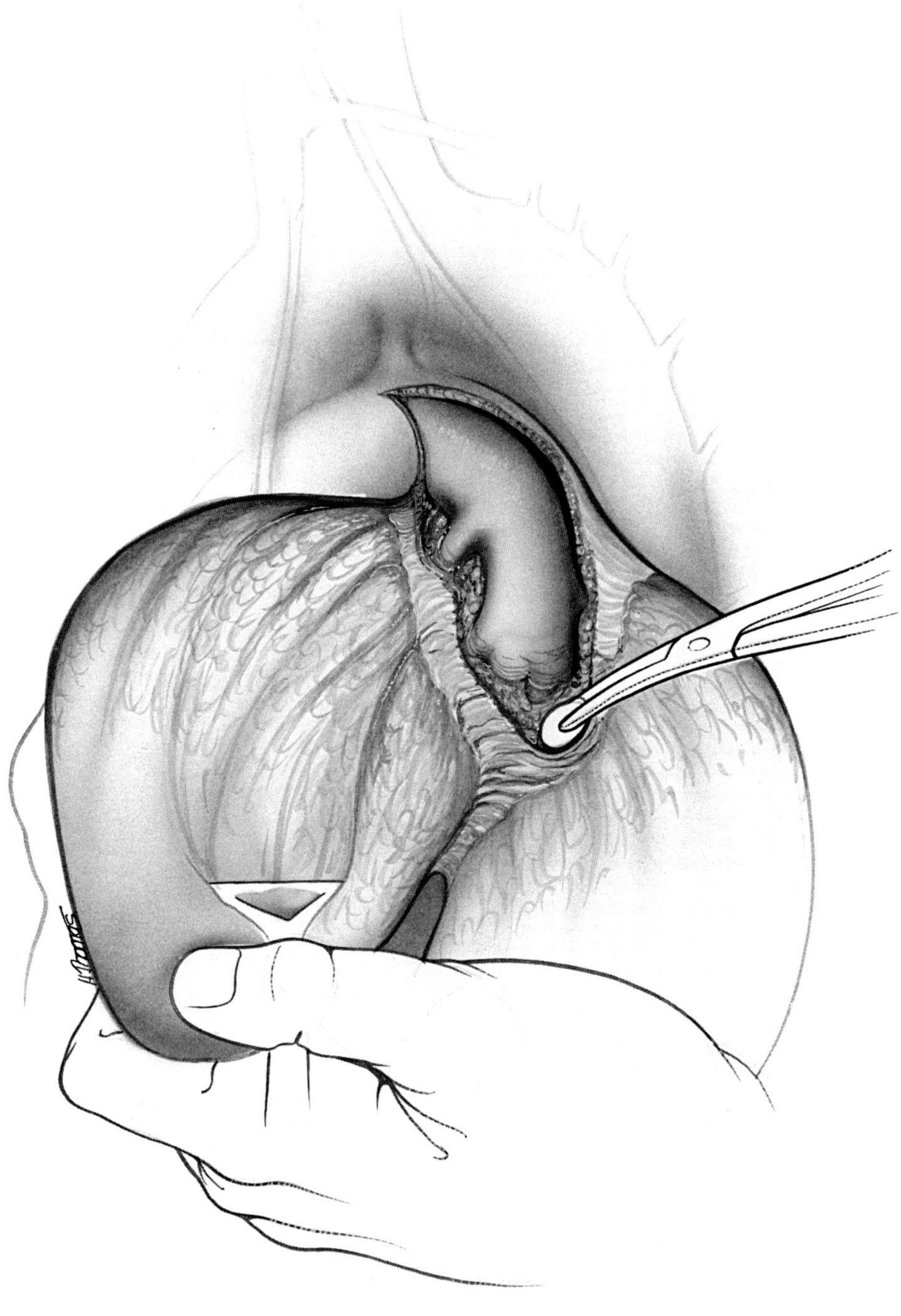

LEFT UPPER LOBECTOMY

CLOSURE OF THE PULMONARY ARTERY BRANCHES

In this view the upper and lower lobes are separated and one can see that there are three branches of the pulmonary artery to the left upper lobe that have been ligated. The first and highest branch is ligated, suture ligated, and distally ligated but has not been cut yet, whereas the second and third branches have been ligated proximal to the branches. The branches here will be cut distal to the bifurcation of the two branches in the middle artery depicted and distal to the three branches in the caudal artery depicted. In fact, the surgeon would probably complete the ligation and division of one branch before moving on to the second and third. The surgeon has the option of either beginning with the highest branch of the main pulmonary artery or beginning with the lingular branch and working cephalad. More commonly the highest branch is the most difficult to control. This would depend where the tumor was, and the surgeon would exercise appropriate judgment. At times the surgeon must divide the highest vein branch of the superior pulmonary vein to get adequate exposure of the highest or first pulmonary artery branch.

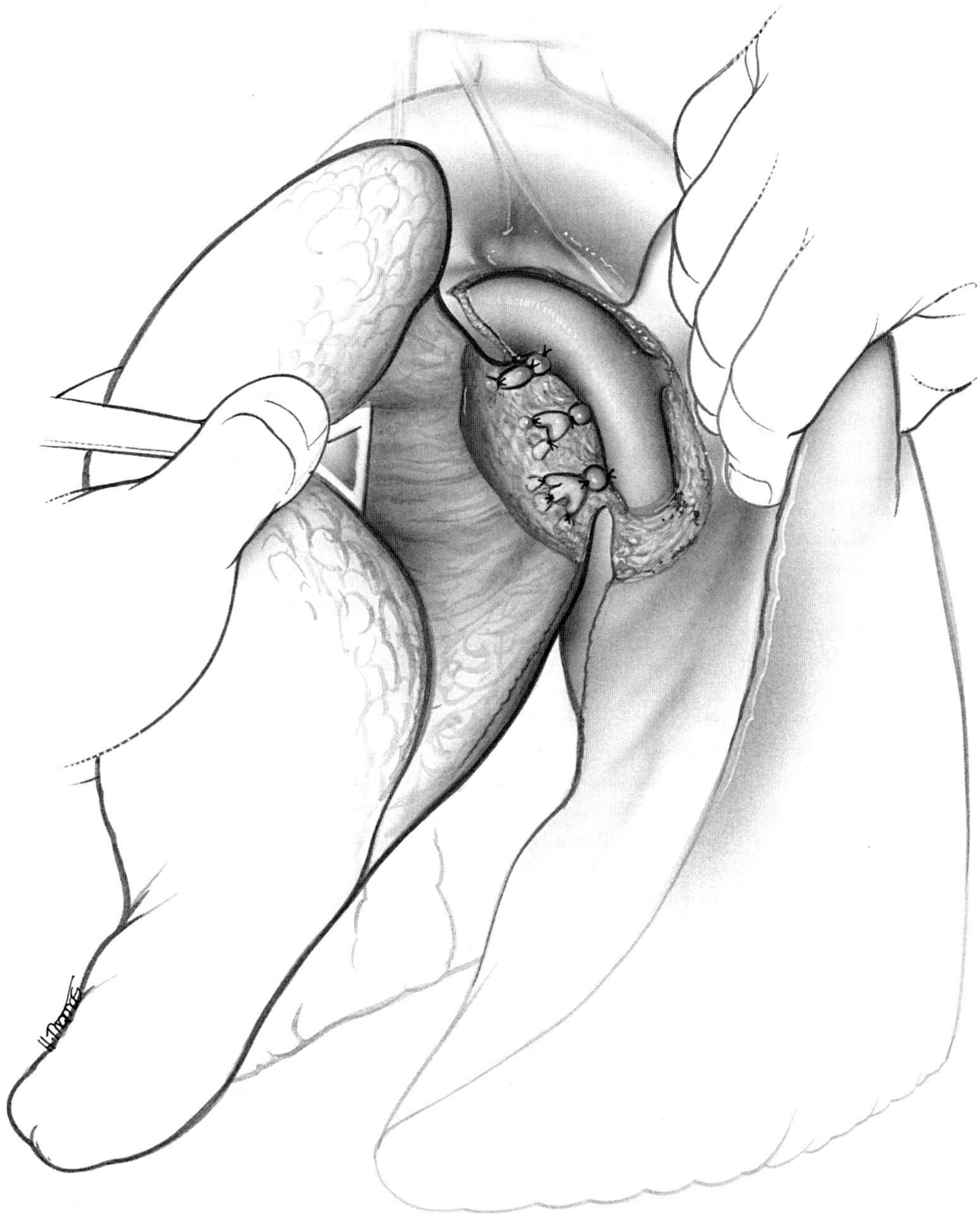

LEFT UPPER LOBECTOMY

EXPOSURE OF THE MAIN BRONCHUS

In this drawing the exposure is the same as in the previous drawing but we now can see that all three branches have been divided, showing the proximal stumps on the main pulmonary artery and the distal stumps on the specimen to be removed. This maneuver has now exposed the posterior of the left main bronchus where it is bifurcating into the left lower lobe bronchus going caudad to the left lower lobe and the left upper lobe bronchus heading toward the left upper lobe, where it soon branches, leaving the lingular bronchus going caudad. The superior division of the left upper lobe bronchus is running cephalad.

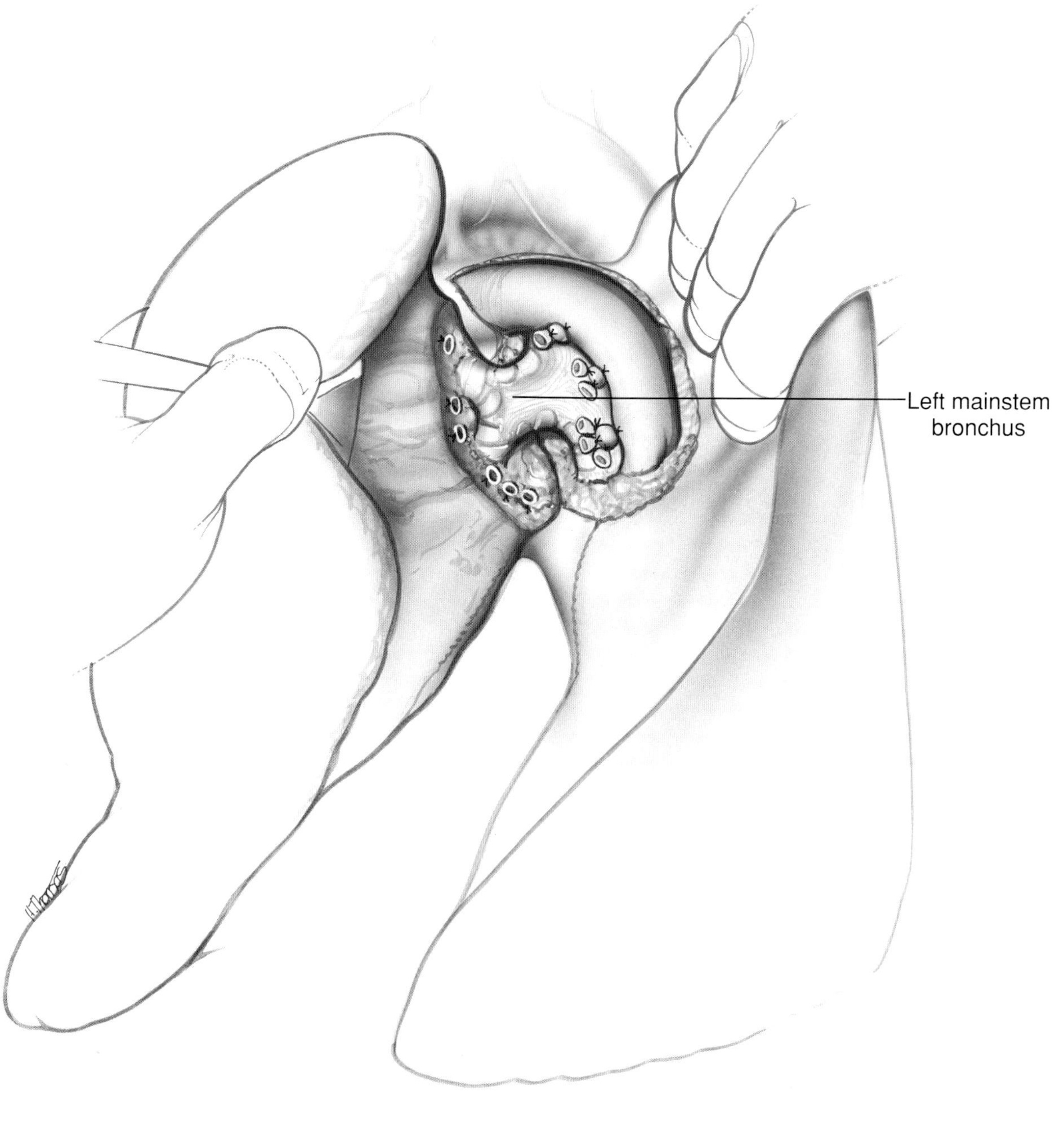

LEFT UPPER LOBECTOMY

CLOSURE OF THE SUPERIOR PULMONARY VEIN AND BRANCHES

In this view we are now looking at the front of the left upper lobe, which has been swung to the right toward the spine. We can see the superior pulmonary vein, which has a proximal tie. This would normally be done with a heavy silk such as 1-0 or its equivalent. The suture ligatures on the branches are distal to the trifurcation, and there are additional ties to prevent backbleeding from the vein. One should keep these ties as far apart as possible so that the stumps are as long as possible. An alternative to this technique would be to place the suture ligature distal to the first heavy tie and proximal to the trifurcation of the vein. We are showing this approach rather than using the stapler since at times there is not enough room for the stapler and the surgeon must be familiar with multiple ways to handle blood vessels.

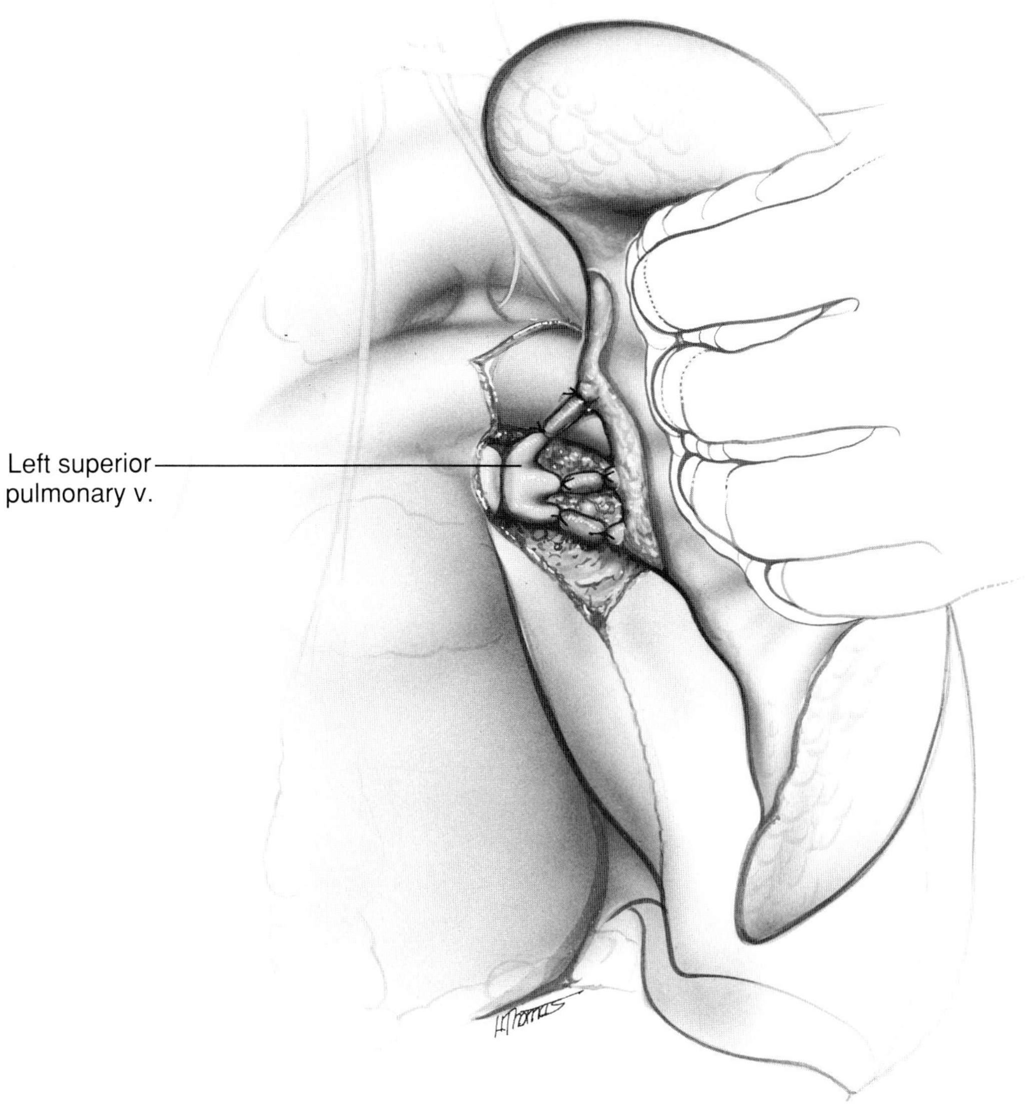

LEFT UPPER LOBECTOMY

REMOVAL OF THE UPPER LOBE

In this situation the left upper lobe specimen has been removed. We can see the hilum of the left upper lobe. Centrally is the stapled left upper lobe bronchial stump. Anteriorly is the ligated superior pulmonary vein with its three suture-ligated branches, and again on the main pulmonary artery we can see the three suture-ligated branches of the pulmonary artery to the left upper lobe.

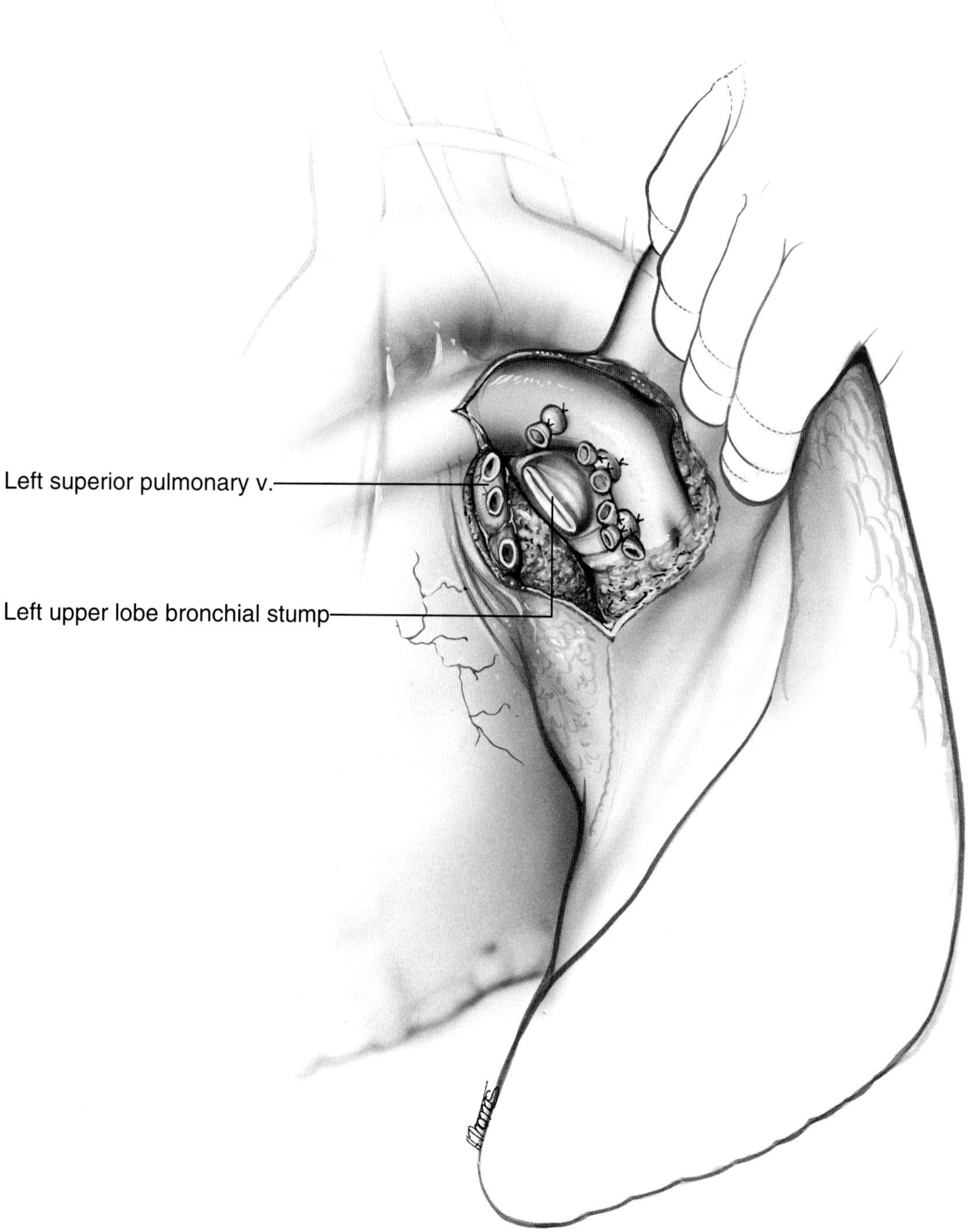

LINGULECTOMY

LIGATION OF THE LINGULAR ARTERY

Here the view is again in the longitudinal fissure with the left upper lobe to the viewer's left and the left lower lobe to the viewer's right. The fissure is opened. The visceral pleura over the inferior hilum has also been opened, and the dissection has been carried out. The pulmonary artery can be seen immediately in front of the fingers coursing down the fissure. The lingular artery, which in this case has three branches, has been ligated and the three branchs have been suture ligated as well as ligated distally. The artery has been divided, and the lingular bronchial branch is now visible just medial and slightly anterior to the artery branches.

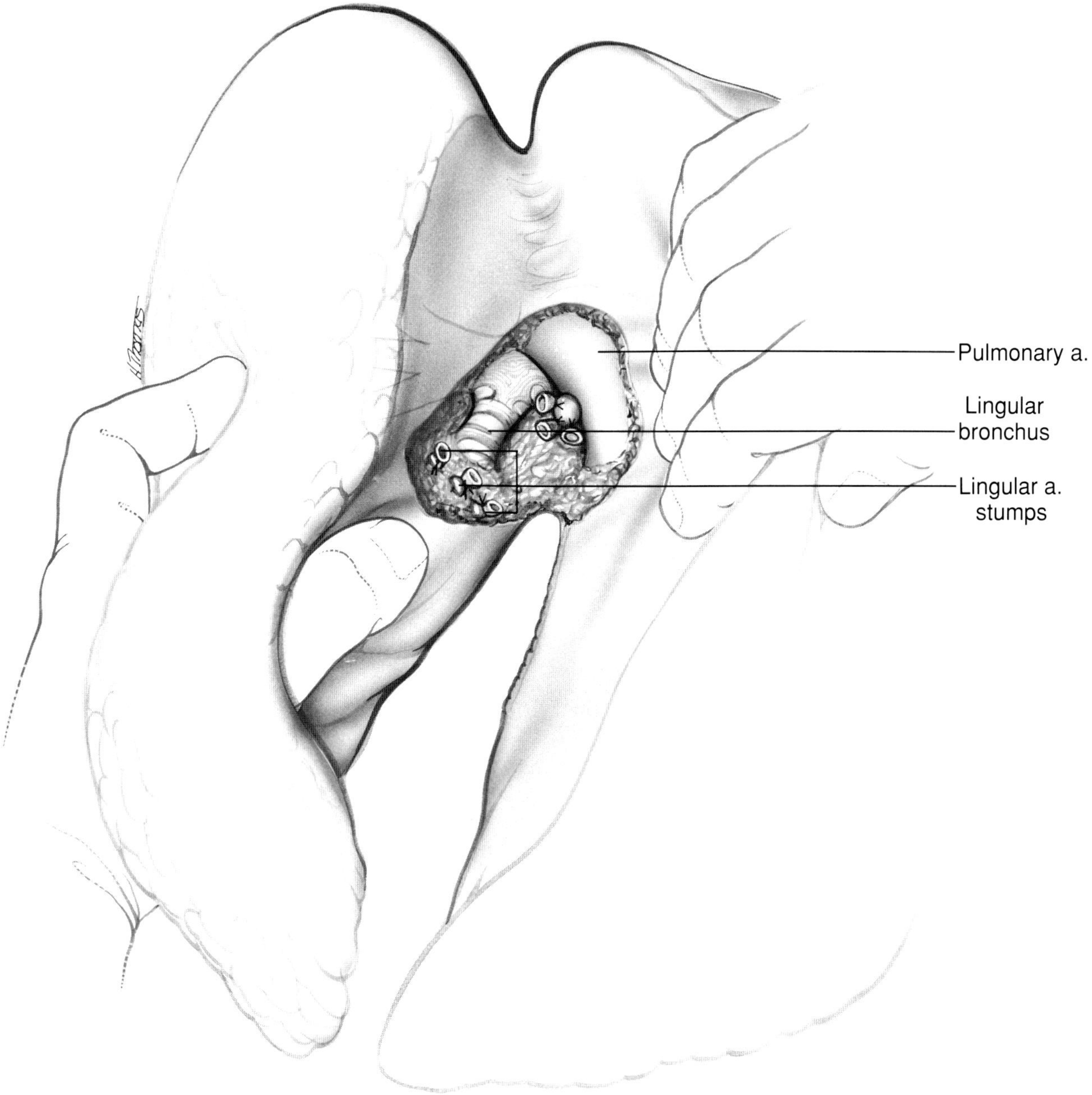

LINGULECTOMY

DISSECTION OF THE LINGULAR BRONCHUS

This is the same view as the previous drawing. Here the lingular bronchus has been dissected free. The small retractor is gently reflecting the vascular structures so that the stump of the lingular bronchus is better exposed. A decision has been made that the lingular bronchial stump will be sutured closed by hand rather than be stapled. In this view it is with poetic license cut and left open. If the entire lung is out of function with a double-lumen endotracheal tube, there will be no leak. A clamp has been placed on the distal bronchial stump because this is an important part of completing the lingulectomy.

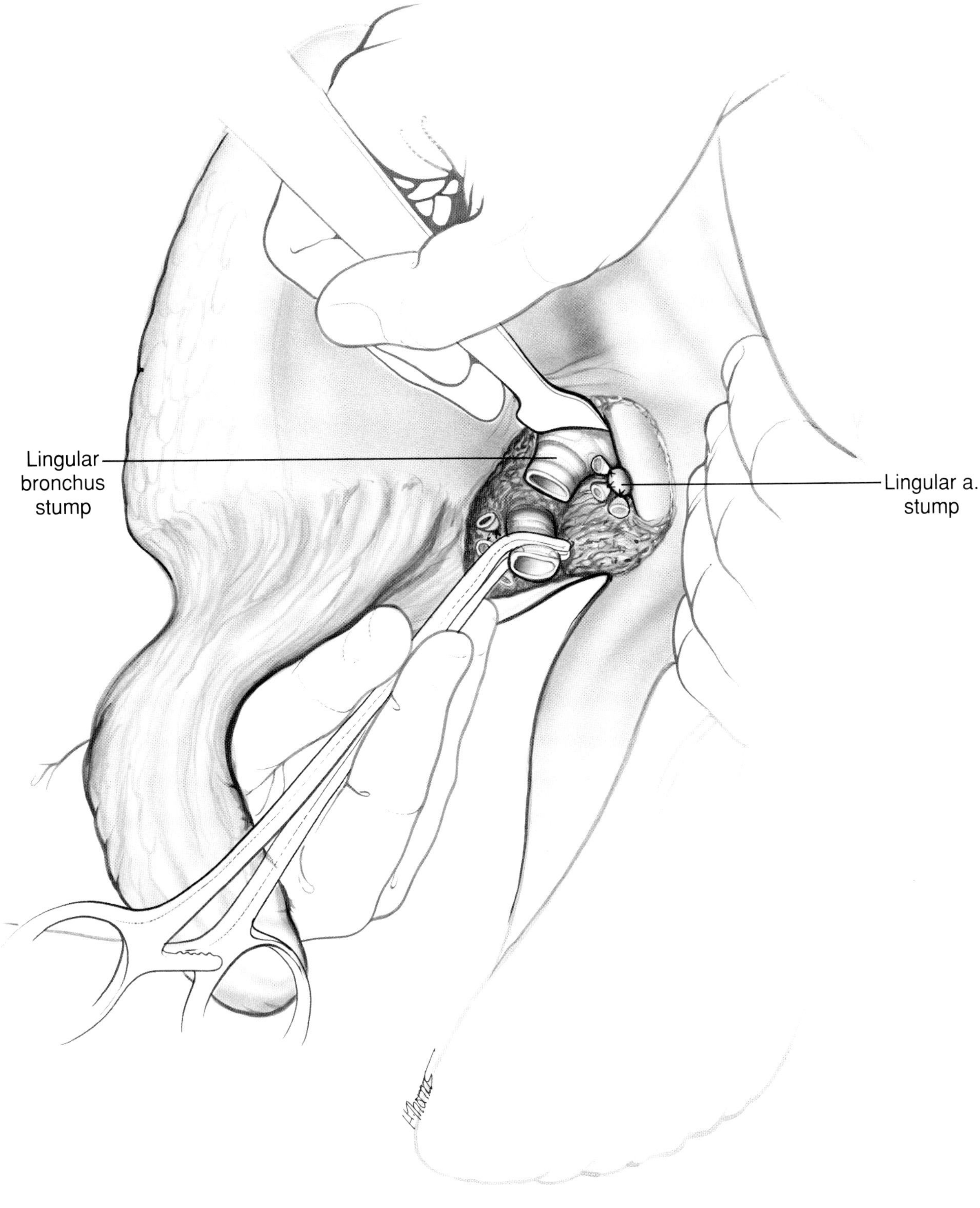

Lingular
bronchus
stump
Lingular a.
stump

LINGULECTOMY

FREEING OF THE LINGULA

This is the same view as the previous drawing. The lingular bronchus has in this case been closed with two interrupted sutures over the end, which have involved the distal cartilagenous ring. Since this is a rather small bronchus, normally two or three sutures will suffice as long as it is rendered airtight. At this point it is helpful if the left upper lobe is left inflated so that the operator can see the difference between the inflated residual upper lobe and the deflated lingula. The important landmark to the intersegmental plane is that there should be collecting veins that drain the lingula and the adjacent anterior segment toward the superior pulmonary vein in the hilum of the right upper lobe. Here the lingula is being gently pulled free and the electrocautery is controlling the bleeding that can ensue from this somewhat raw intersegmental plane. If there is no inflammation or tumor in this plane, it opens up readily. If necessary, venous bleeders can be ligated with fine silk. Air leaks can be clamped with a small hemostat and ligated.

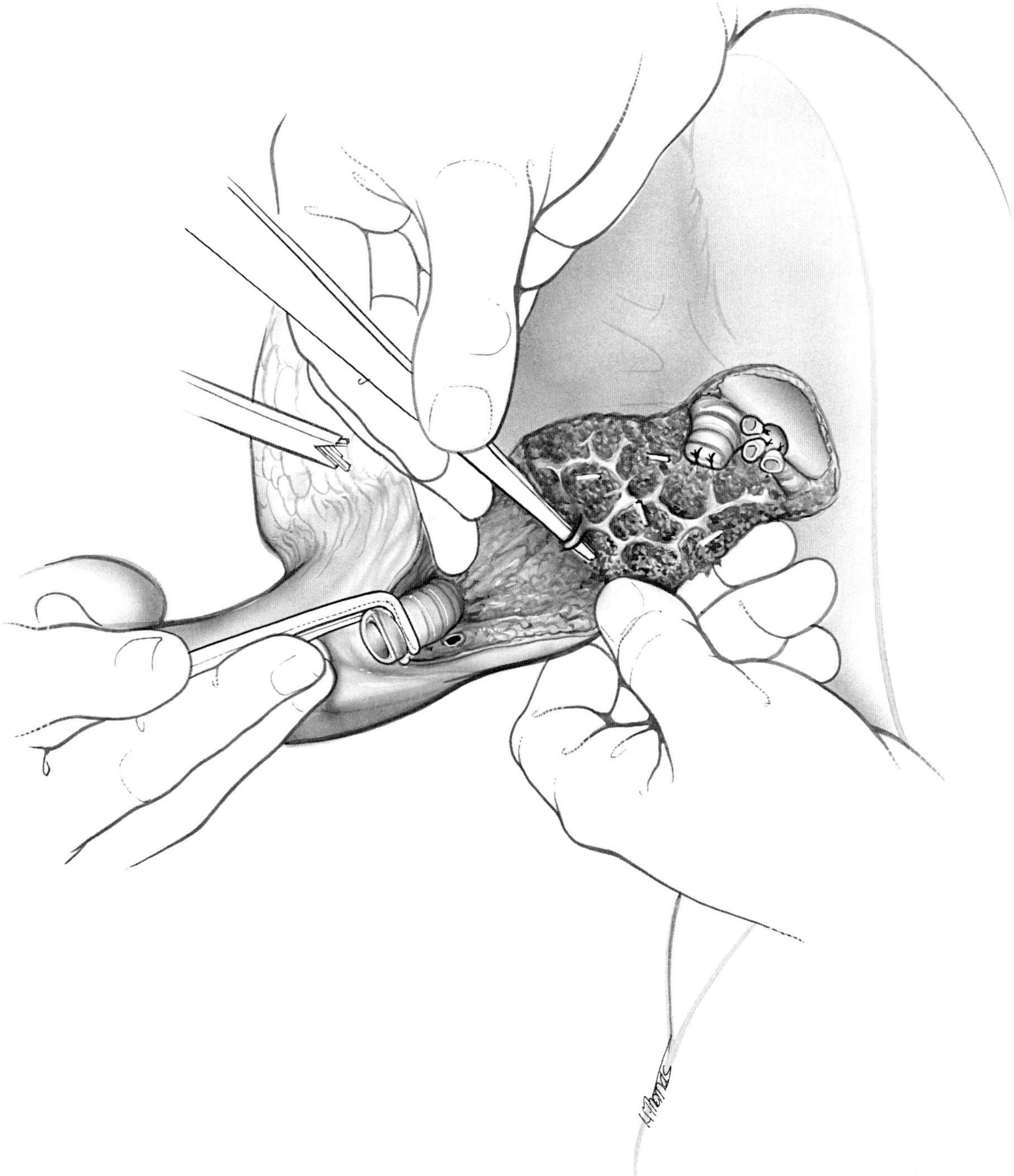

LINGULECTOMY

REMOVAL OF THE SPECIMEN

In this drawing the specimen has been removed. The hand is elevating the inflated residual upper lobe. It is carefully inspected to ensure that there are no bleeding points that need ligation, suturing, or cauterizing. In similar fashion, any significant air leak can be ligated, although these normally stop quite promptly if the true intersegmental plane is followed. An alternative to this technique would be to use the GIA stapler or other device to wedge off the lingula from the upper lobe. This lingulectomy is usually done for small tumors or unknown lesions in the lingula. The stapling device produces fewer air leaks, especially in emphysematous patients, but it has a disadvantage of preventing the residual upper lobe from inflating quite so much.

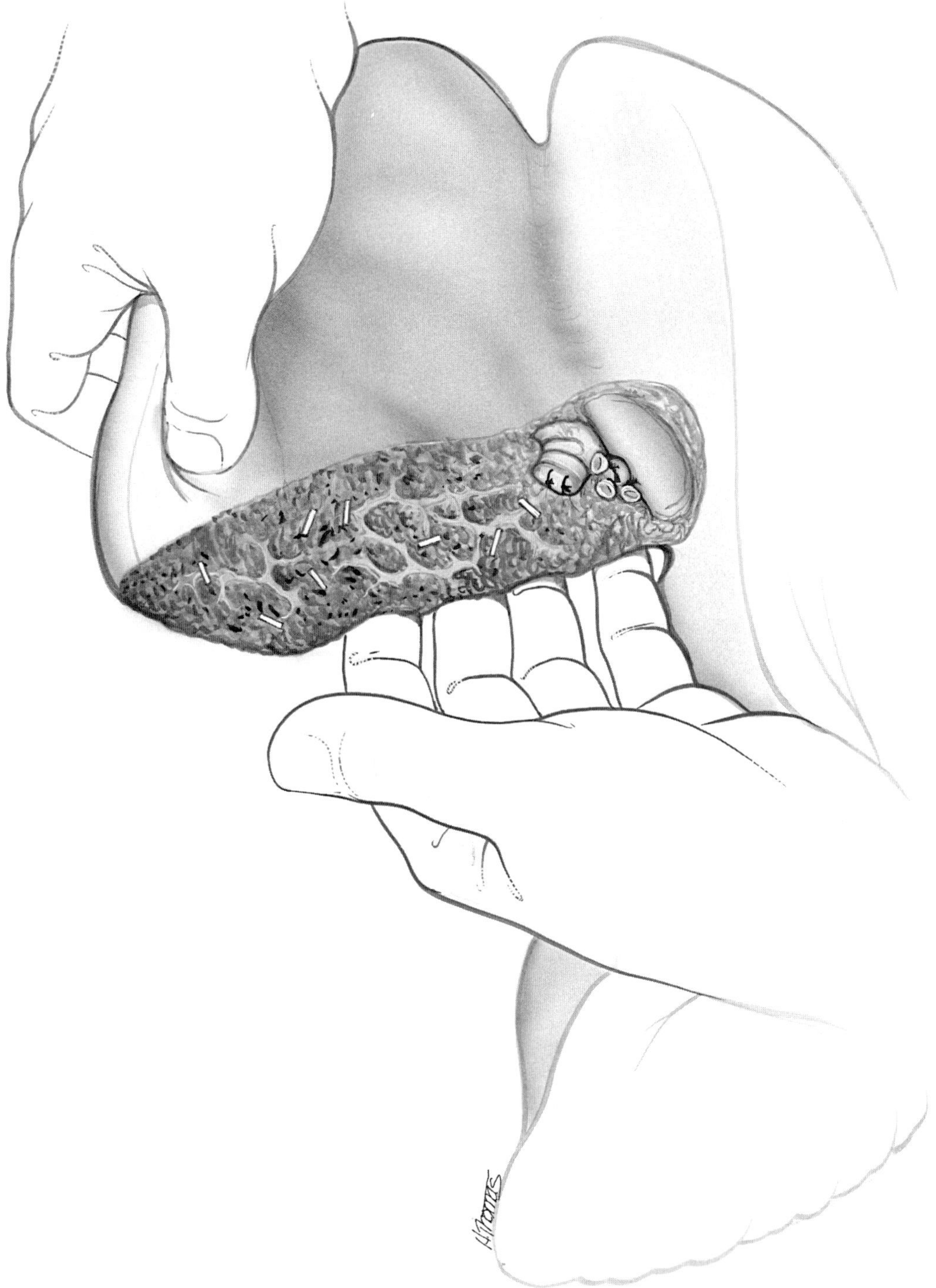

LEFT LOWER LOBECTOMY

EXPOSURE OF THE PULMONARY ARTERY BRANCHES

Here we are looking at the left lung laterally. The hand is drawing the left upper lobe anteriorly. The fissure has been opened. The sheath over the main pulmonary artery has been opened, and we can see some of the pulmonary artery branches. On the posterior side of the main pulmonary artery the first branch to the left lower lobe is the superior segmental branch. The artery continues on to the basal branches of the left lower lobe. The nondissected branches to the left upper lobe are seen. There is still some unopened fissure between the left upper and left lower lobes in the anterior-inferior area.

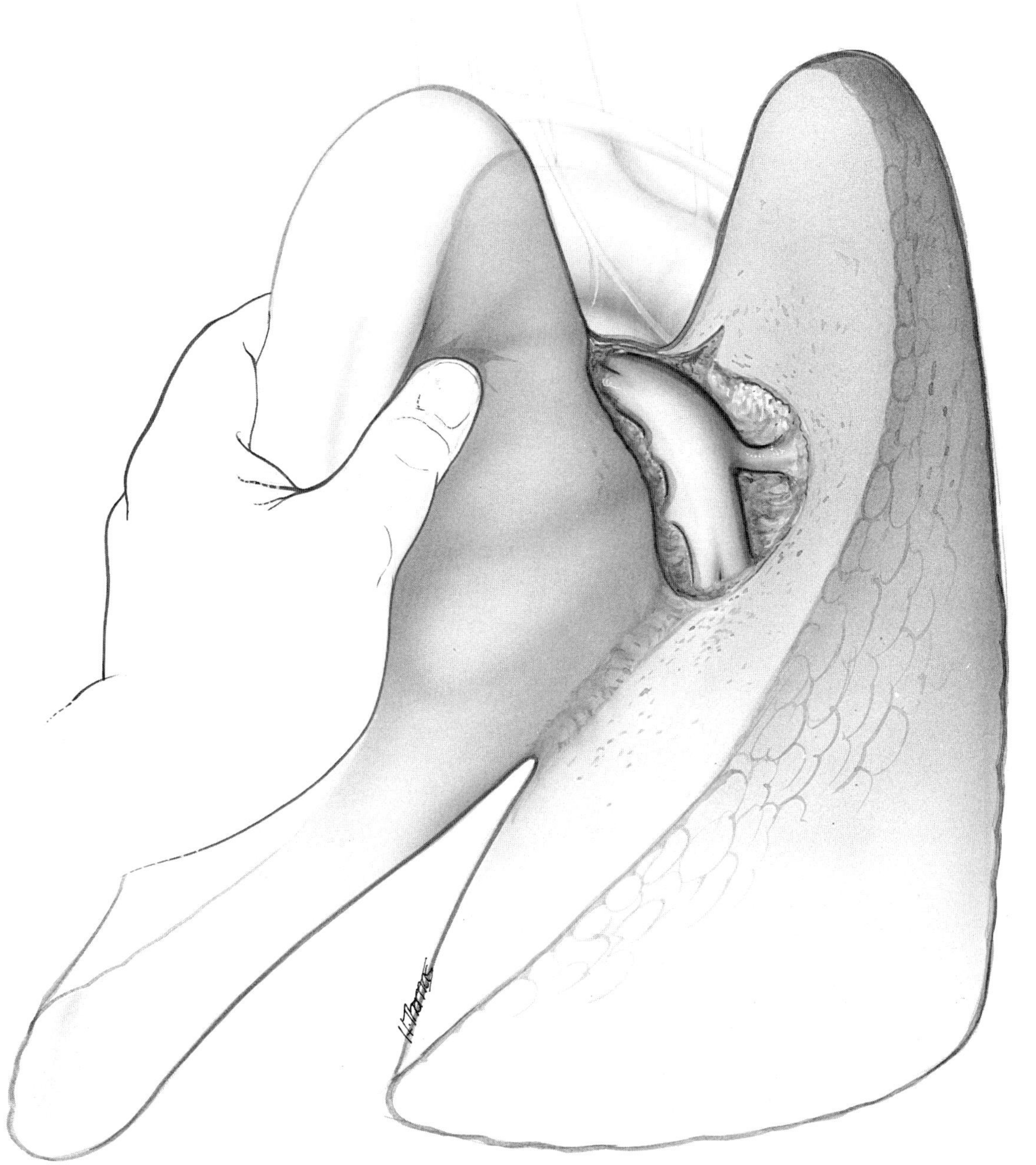

LEFT LOWER LOBECTOMY

DIVISION OF THE SUPERIOR SEGMENTAL ARTERIAL BRANCH

This is the same view in the longitudinal fissure. The superior segmental arterial branch has been ligated, suture ligatured, tied distally, and divided with an adequate stump. If the tumor does not prohibit the dissection, as already indicated it is better to preserve the bifurcation of the superior segmental artery so that the ties cannot slip off. The pulmonary artery branches to the basal segments have been controlled with a proximal tie and a proximal suture ligature. The two main distal branches have been ligated distally, and the branches have been cut, leaving the bifurcation attached to the main pulmonary artery. The pulmonary artery has been dissected freer than is necessary to show the anatomy of the bronchus. It is not easy to demonstrate the left main bronchus and its bifurcation into left upper and left lower branches unless the artery is divided and dissected away. The superior segmental bronchus comes off rather high. One has to assess each patient's anatomy. Sometimes it is not possible to staple one bronchial stump in doing a left lower lobe lobectomy without encroaching on the airway to the left upper lobe. In those circumstances one must have two bronchial stumps, namely the superior segmental stump and the basal segmental stump to the lower lobe. In the situation depicted here it was believed that adequate space was left with one bronchial stapler seen in later illustration of lower lobe removal.

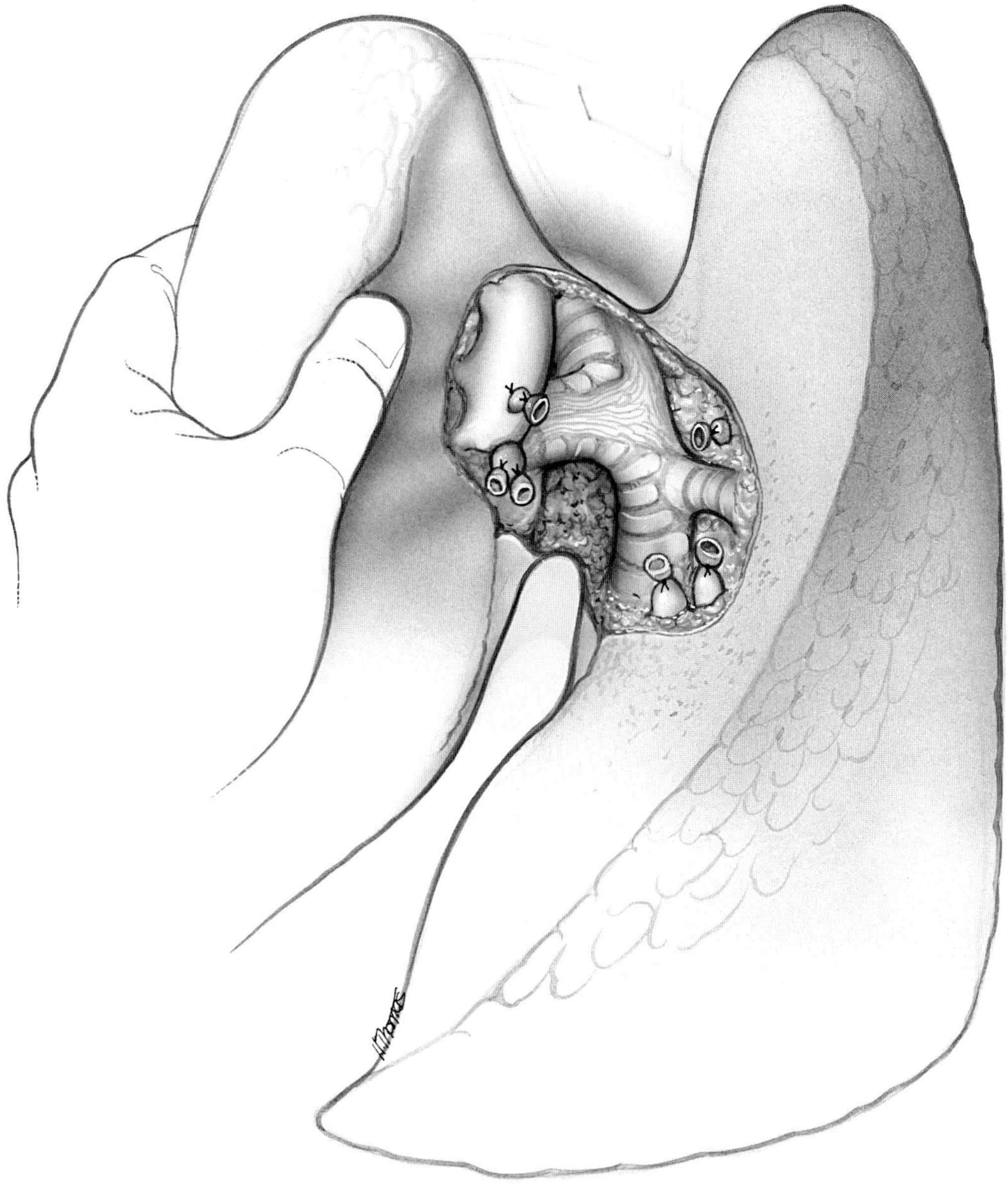

LEFT LOWER LOBECTOMY

PREPARATION FOR DIVIDING THE INFERIOR PULMONARY VEIN

The left lower lobe is being drawn anteriorly, demonstrating the residual attachment of the inferior pulmonary vein, which is located immediately caudad to and in the same plane as the mainstem bronchus. The inferior pulmonary ligament has been divided. The esophagus can be seen coursing down just in front of the descending aorta. The vagus nerve accompanies the esophagus. The recurrent nerve is drawn in as it goes under the aortic arch.

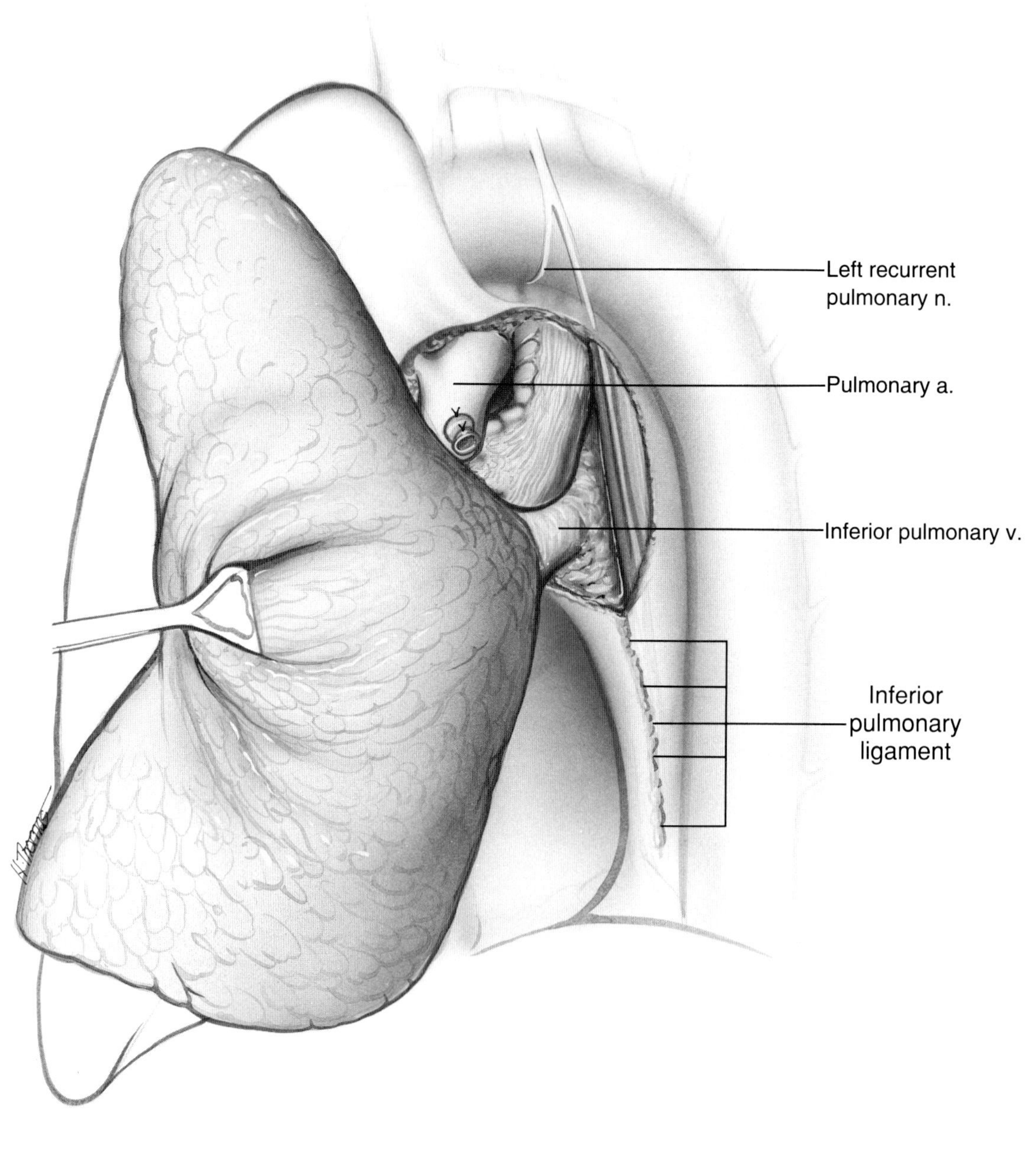

LEFT LOWER LOBECTOMY

REMOVAL OF LOWER LOBE

In this view we are again laterally looking into the fissure. The inferior pulmonary vein has been stapled and ligated distally and has been divided. The bronchus has been stapled. After the surgeon has placed the stapler and closed it appropriately, the anesthetist is requested to aspirate the left upper lobe and inflate the left upper lobe to ensure that there is no impairment in inflation. This has been done. There is only a little residual areolar tissue and visceral pleura attaching the left lower lobe to the hilum.

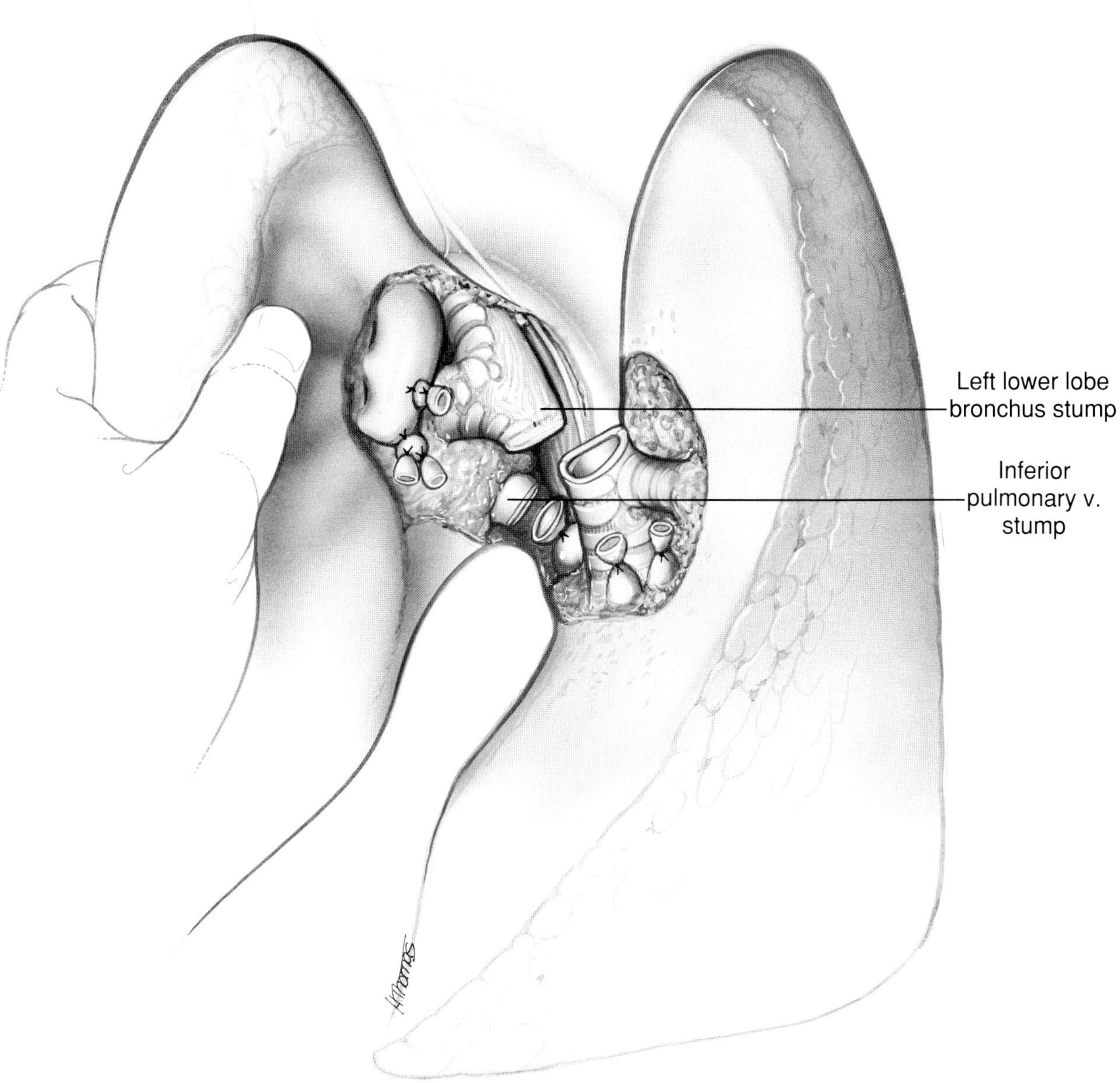

LEFT LOWER LOBECTOMY

REMOVAL OF LYMPH NODES

We are viewing the left upper lobe from the same location. The left lower lobe has been removed. The anatomy of the pulmonary artery stumps, bronchial stump, and inferior pulmonary vein is clearly visible. Again, all of the lymph nodes locally have been removed, but in fact the surgeon also is responsible for removal of the mediastinal lymph nodes on this side.

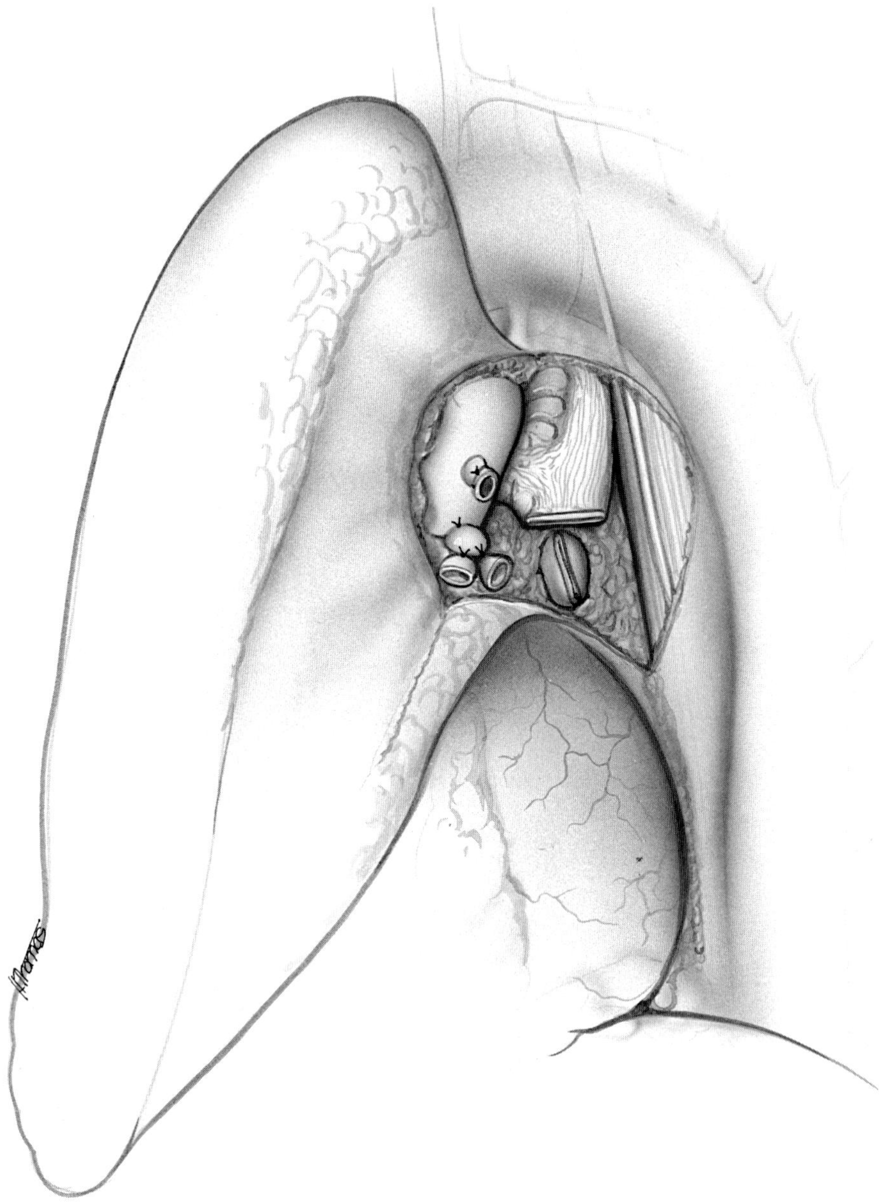

LEFT PNEUMONECTOMY

EXPOSURE OF THE MAIN PULMONARY ARTERY

The patient is in the right lateral position and the chest has been opened through a generous incision in the left fifth interspace. The lung has been palpated, and it has been decided that pneumonectomy should be done. The mediastinum has been palpated, and there are no contraindications to proceeding with the pneumonectomy. In this view the lung is being displaced caudad, the mediastinal pleura has been opened over the cephalic portion of the hilum in a transverse fashion, and the main pulmonary artery can be seen. The phrenic nerve will be coursing anterior to the hilum, and the vagus nerve will be coursing posterior to the hilum. By keeping the dissection close to the pulmonary artery, damage to the recurrent branch of the vagal nerve is prevented. The main pulmonary trunk has been exposed, and the first branch of the main pulmonary artery, usually to the apical portion of the left upper lobe, is seen. The superior pulmonary vein is immediately caudal to the pulmonary artery in this location and one has to be careful not to injure and to avoid or secure the cephalic branches of the superior pulmonary vein which come up onto the branches of the pulmonary artery. The bronchus is posterior and caudal to this main pulmonary trunk.

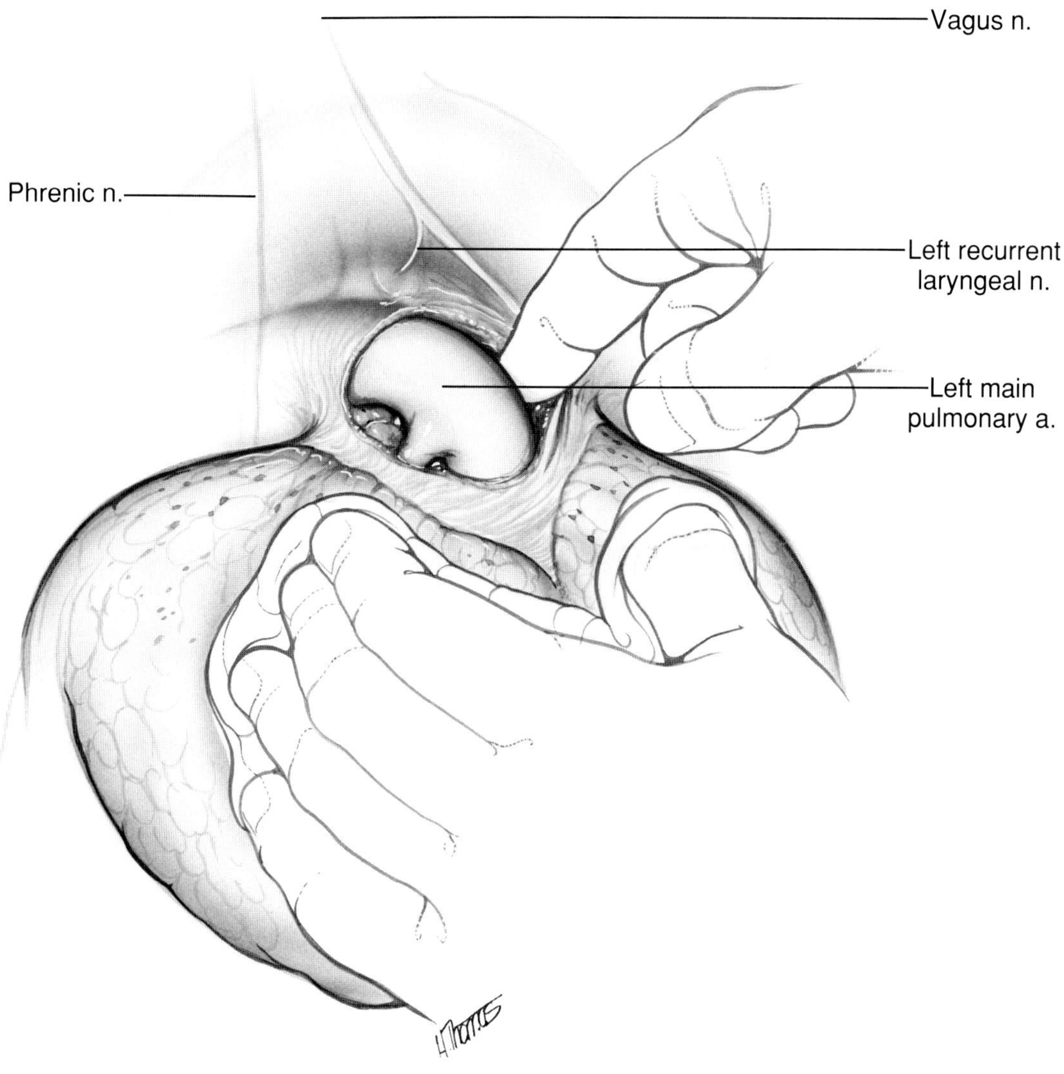

LEFT PNEUMONECTOMY

EXPOSURE OF THE ARTERIAL BRANCHES

In this view we are looking at the front of the left lung hilum. The mediastinal pleura, which had been opened cephalad, has been opened caudad around the hilum anteriorly. The inferior pulmonary ligament has been divided. The division of the mediastinal pleura has been continued up posteriorly behind the lung hilum and between the vagus nerve and the lung hilum. The right index finger of the surgeon is partially around the left main pulmonary artery. The branches here are dissected out and are more readily visible than if there were a hilar tumor. The superior pulmonary vein has been dissected free from the pulmonary artery and is immediately caudal to the finger. The inferior pulmonary vein has not yet been dissected free but is running in the inferior portion of the hilum. The mainstem bronchus is posterior to the finger and caudal to the finger, being located in this drawing mostly posterior to the superior pulmonary vein.

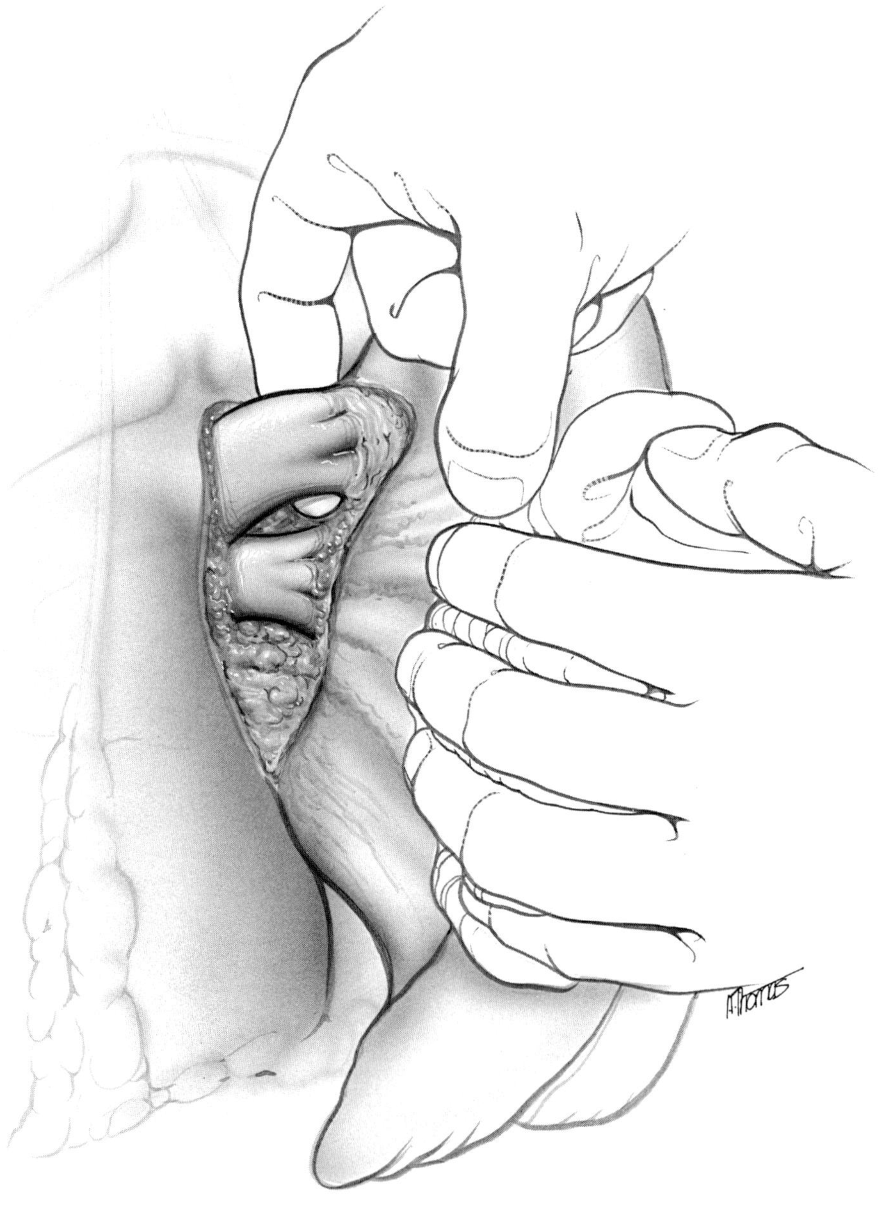

LEFT PNEUMONECTOMY

DIVISION OF THE PULMONARY ARTERY AND VEIN

In this view we are still looking at the front of the hilum of the left lung. The main pulmonary artery and the superior pulmonary vein have both been divided. The phrenic nerve is seen to be anterior to the hilum descending toward the anteromedial portion of the pericardium of the heart. The vagus nerve can be seen crossing the aortic arch running posterior to the hilum and is visible in the opened mediastinal pleura. The recurrent nerve has been ghosted in. It can be seen to branch at the upper aortic arch and run medial to the vagus nerve; it then hooks around caudad and posterior to the ligamentum arteriosum, which in turn runs from the concave side of the aortic arch to the bifurcation of the main pulmonary truncus. The distal pulmonary artery and superior pulmonary vein have been ligated. This is idealized in rather long condition because more frequently it is necessary to ligate two or three branches of these vessels distally. Proximally we have ordinarily handled these stumps with the stapling device, which does not require a suture. If one is not going to use a stapler, one would use a heavy braided 1 silk ligature reinforced distally with a suture ligature placed proximal to its branches.

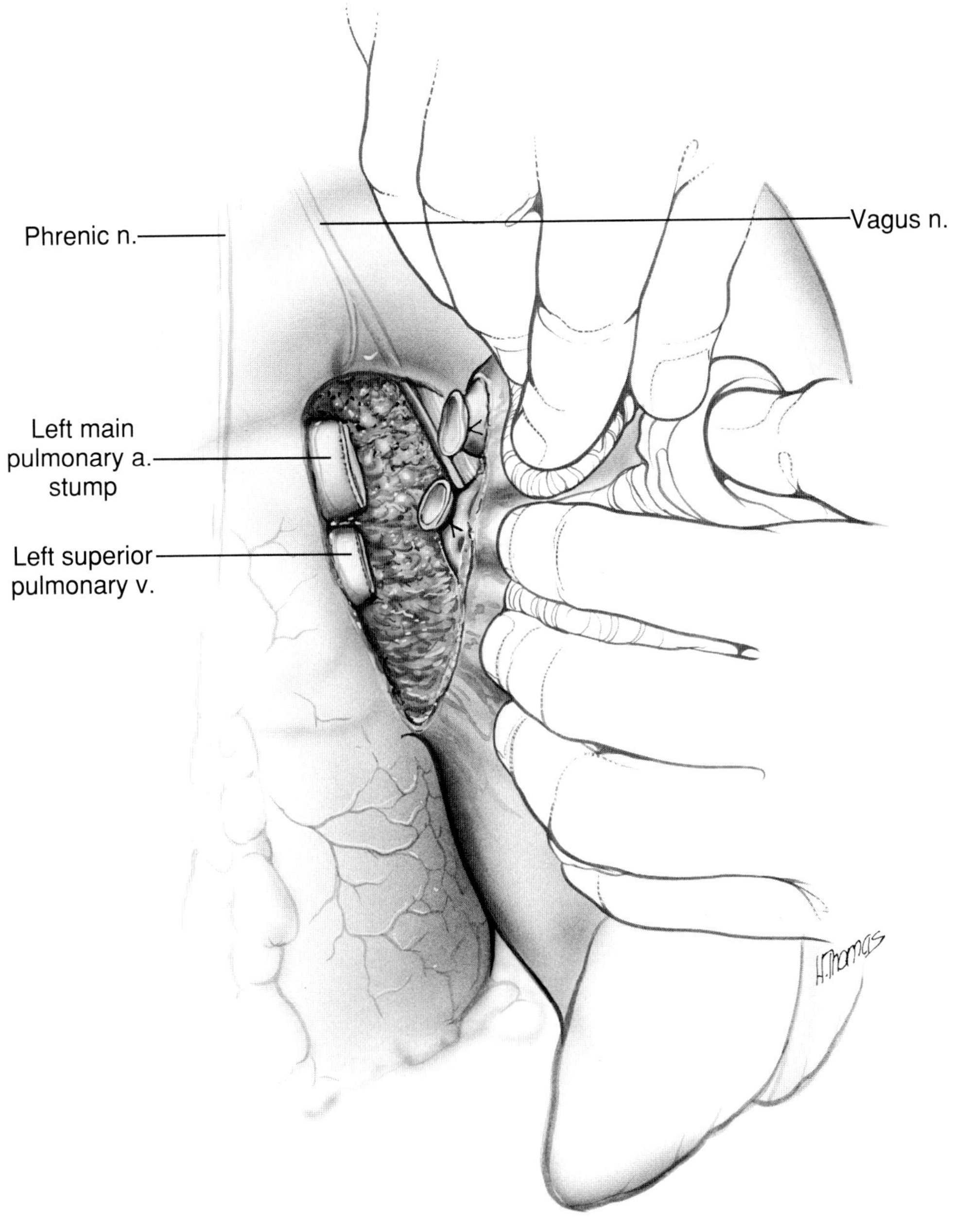

LEFT PNEUMONECTOMY

ANTERIOR DISPLACEMENT OF THE LUNG

In this view the lung is being displaced anteriorly and we are looking at the posterior mediastinum. We can see that the mediastinal pleura has been opened around to the level of the inferior pulmonary vein. The aortic arch, the esophagus with the vagus nerve going down it, is visible. The intact left mainstem bronchus is in the cephalic part of the picture and the inferior pulmonary vein in the caudal part. The plan here is next to encircle the inferior pulmonary vein and to staple the vein relatively close to its base with a distal ligature. The main pulmonary artery and superior pulmonary vein have already been divided.

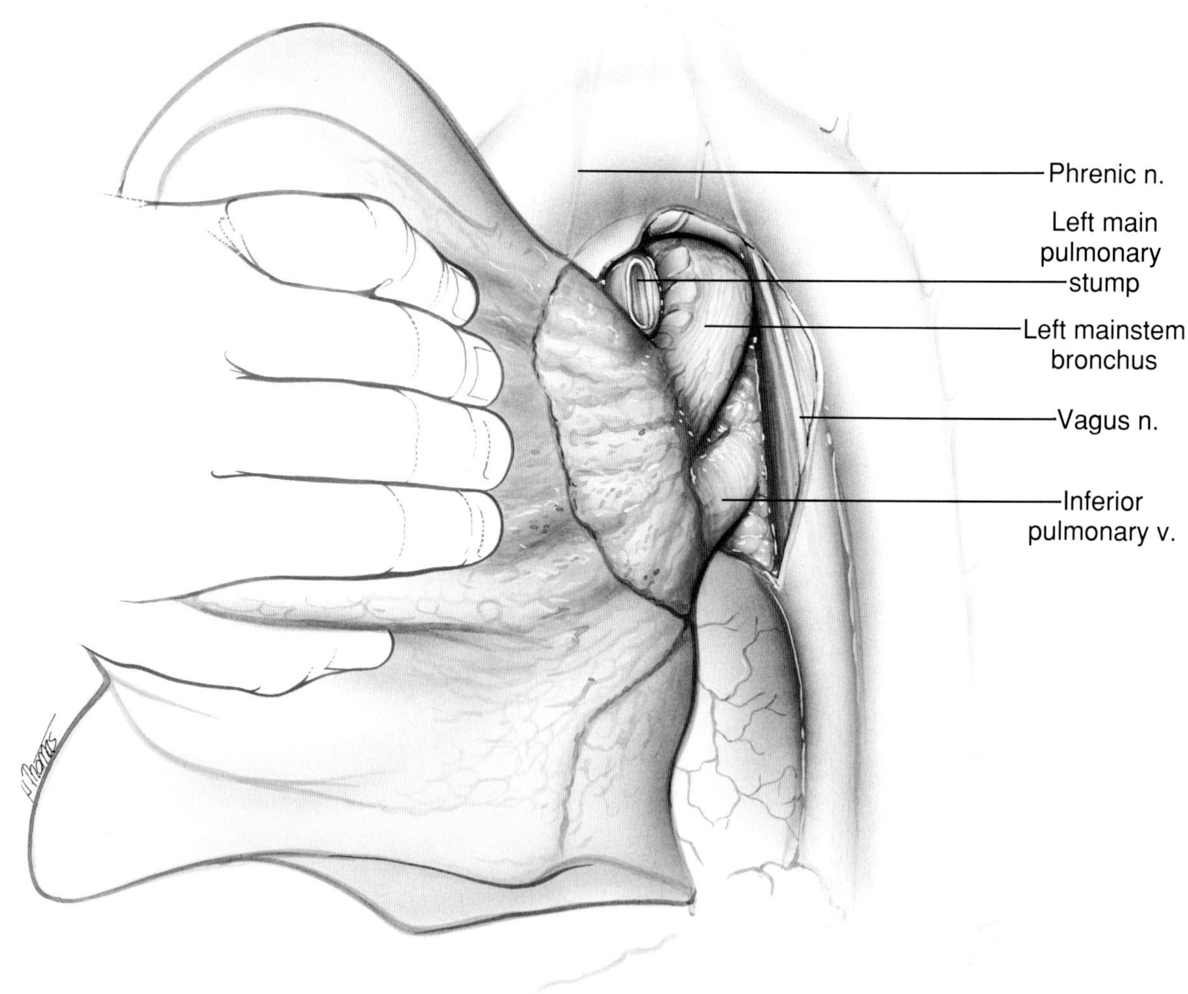

LEFT PNEUMONECTOMY

REMOVAL OF LUNG

In this view we are still looking at the posterior mediastinum with the lung drawn anteriorly. We can see the stump of the left main pulmonary artery above and to the left and the stapled stump of the inferior pulmonary vein caudal to the bronchus. The stapled and divided superior pulmonary vein is hidden by the bronchus. We are in the process of dissecting posteriorly to the carina. The retractor is displacing the esophagus posteriorly. We can still see some areolar tissue in the subcarinal space and posterior. It is important to remove all of the lymph nodes that we see in the inferior carinal space, which are position 7, and around the inferior pulmonary vein and the inferior pulmonary ligament which are positions 8 and 9. In fact we also would remove any lymph nodes in the aortic window, which is location 5.

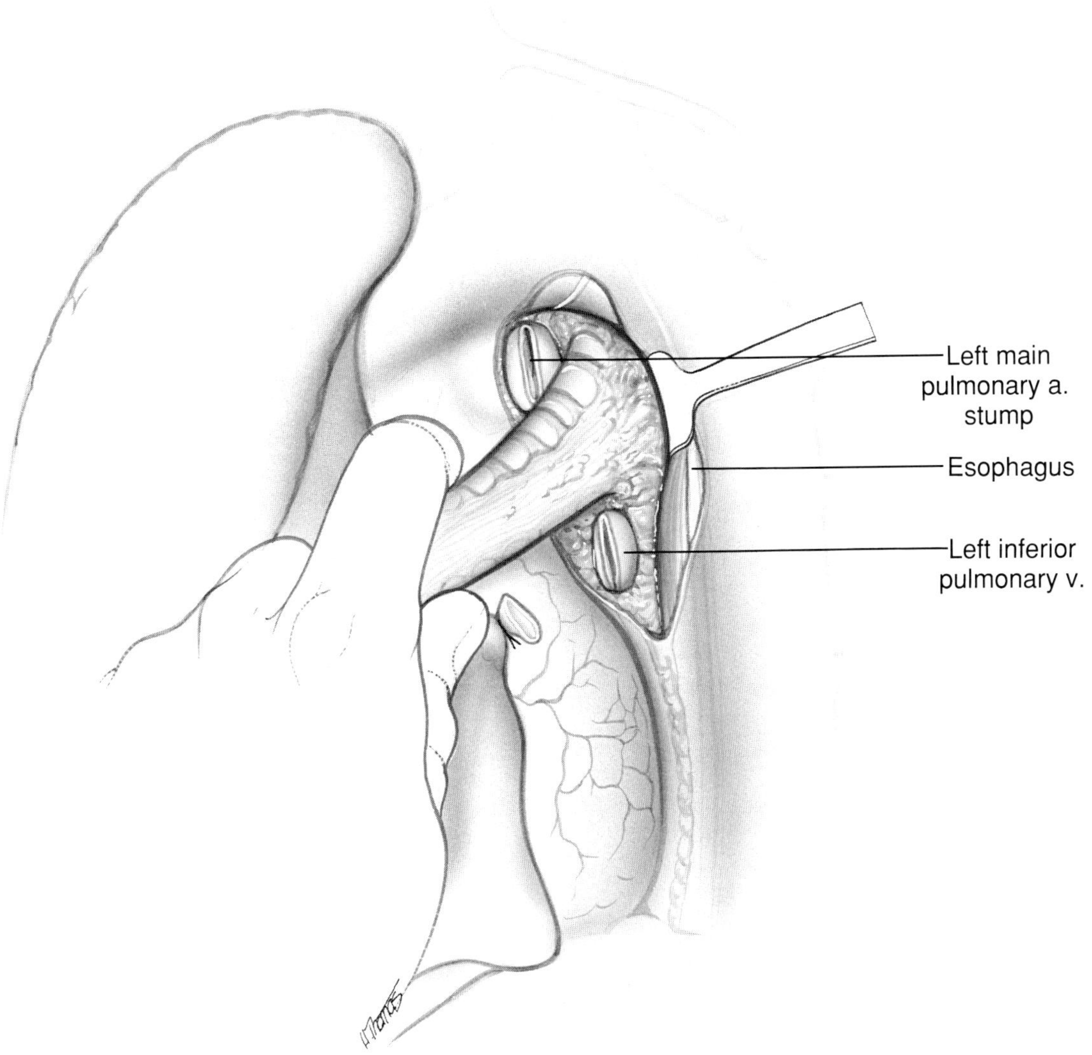

LEFT PNEUMONECTOMY

REMOVAL OF LYMPH NODES

In this view we are looking at the hilum of the left lung. We can see the pulmonary artery stump most cephalic. In the midportion anteriorly is the superior pulmonary vein, and in the midportion posteriorly is the left main bronchus. The most caudal structure is the stapled inferior pulmonary vein. Again, the vagus nerve can be seen on the esophagus. The recurrent nerve can be seen swinging posterior to and will go medial to the ligamentum arteriosus, which is sketched in here, as is the phrenic nerve anteriorly. It is important that the lymph nodes in the hilar region be removed for staging, sampling, and tumor control. In fact we would extend the mediastinal pleura upward onto and over the aortic arch since we would also want to sample the lymph nodes anterior to the hilum, position 5, and to ensure that we have removed any lymph nodes that were palpable in the supra-aortic area. If N-2 nodes were present, it would be important to do a mediastinal lymph node dissection. Ideally the available lymph nodes should be dissected free and removed with the specimen, but this is not always practical. Lymph nodes must be removed for staging purposes as well as treatment.

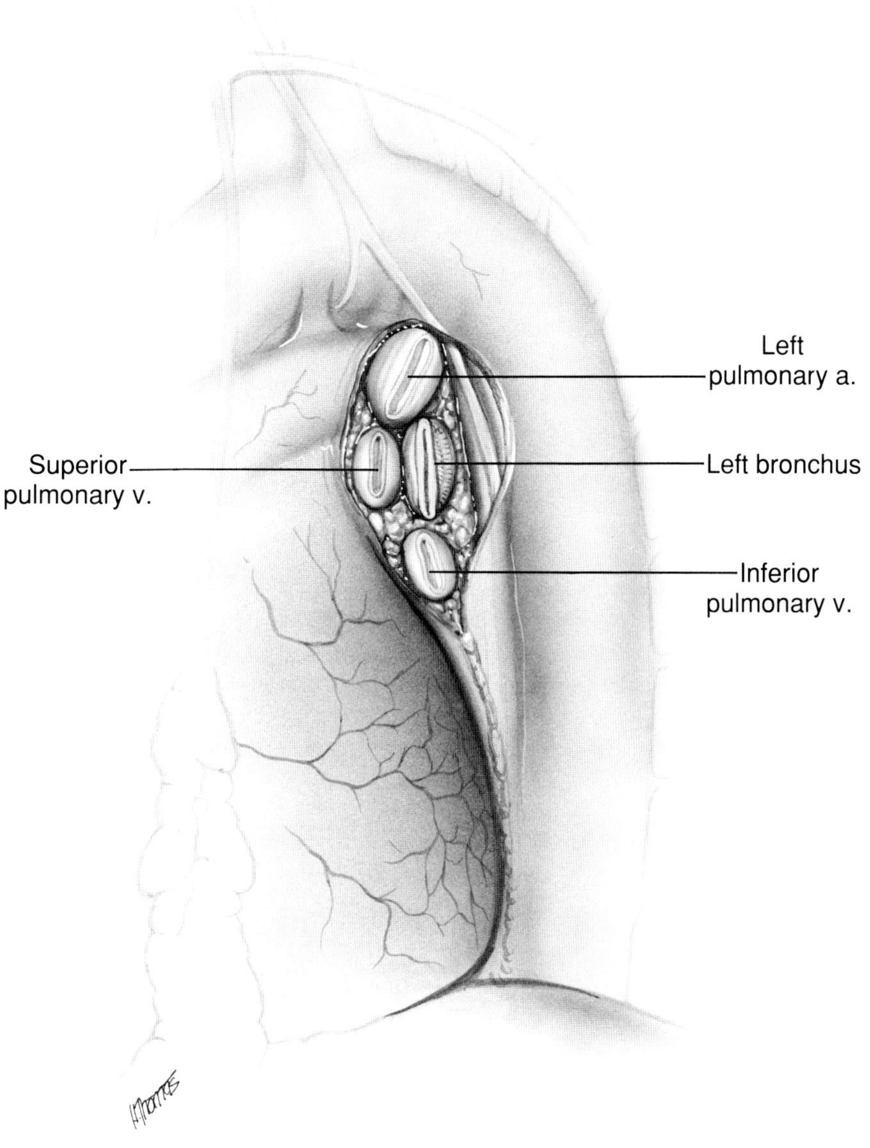

LEFT PNEUMONECTOMY, VARIATION

In this view we are looking at the left lung and mediastinum through a lateral incision. The lung is drawn posteriorly so that we can look at the anterior portion of the left lung and the mediastinum. In this instance the carcinoma in the left lung is flush with the pericardium, so that for a cancer resection it is not possible to ligate the pulmonary artery and the pulmonary veins outside the pericardium.

Before the surgeon is committed to a surgical resection, the pericardium must be opened sufficiently widely that the structures inside the pericardium can be explored. Attention must be directed to the main pulmonary artery to see whether the chest contains enough uninvolved pulmonary artery to divide it safely between its origin at the truncus and where it pierces the pericardium. Similarly, the superior and inferior pulmonary veins must be identified and there must be a clear surgical margin when the left atrium or the veins are occluded. The atrium or veins should have an adequate cuff for hand sewing with a two-row continuous 5-0 vascular suture material. Alternatively, there must be enough room to use a vascular stapler(s).

The phrenic nerve should be inspected carefully in these circumstances. The phrenic nerve runs directly anterior to the lung hilum. If it is involved by tumor or if it is so close to the tumor that it would leave tumor behind were the phrenic nerve to be spared, the surgeon has to make a decision about removing the phrenic nerve. Since in this circumstance the patient is having a pneumonectomy, and presumably it has been demonstrated preoperatively that the patient can live with one lung, it is reasonable to remove the phrenic nerve after the surgeon is convinced that the pneumonectomy is feasible.

In this drawing the phrenic nerve can be seen anterior to our pericardial incision. The mediastinal pleura has been incised directly in front of the hilum and the tumor, and the underlying pericardium has been opened relatively wide. The mediastinal pleura and pericardium are relatively fused over the pericardium so that it is not as simple to separate these two structures as would appear in this drawing. To show the anatomy clearly, the artist has drawn the pulmonary veins longer than normal. In this approach it is important to realize that the reflection of the pericardium goes quite high in the mediastinum. The ligamentum arteriosum can be seen coursing from the concave side of the aortic arch to the bifurcation of the pulmonary truncus.

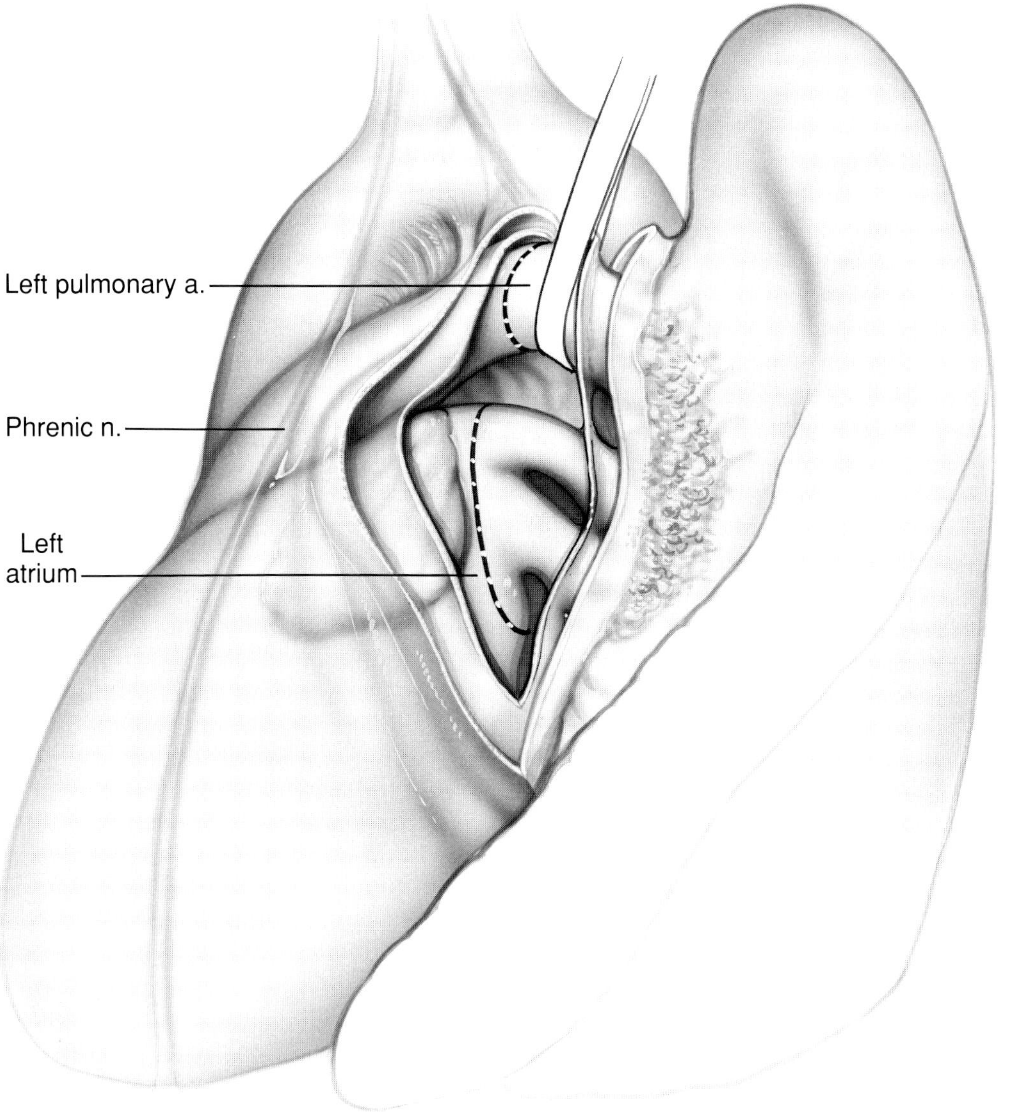

Left pulmonary a.
Phrenic n.
Left
atrium

RADIOTHERAPY

IMPLANTATION RADIOTHERAPY (BRACHYTHERAPY, ENDOCURIE THERAPY)

The implantation technique is indicated for treatable tumors that cannot be surgically excised. An example would be a patient with high-grade emphysema who cannot have excision of any lung tissue. If treated with chemotherapy and/or external radiotherapy alone, such individuals have a low control rate and a low cure rate.

In our experience control of T1 and T2 tumors by implantation technique has been approximately 80 percent of what was anticipated with resection. This would mean that if a T1, N0, M0 lung cancer was associated with an 85 percent 5-year survival rate with surgical excision, an implant treatment local to the "tumor" should give a "cure rate" of 80 percent × 85 percent, or approximately 65 percent.

The accompanying drawing shows a lateral-approach thoracotomy in which a tumor has been exposed in the right upper lobe. The radiation oncology consultant has placed a series of hollow needles about 1.0 cm apart and penetrating to the inner edge of the tumor. A special device is attached successively to each needle, through which is dropped I-125 pellets. The device attached to the hollow needle deposits one seed every centimeter as the needle is withdrawn. The aim of this technique is to place I-125 pellets at 1-cm intervals throughout the tumor.

The upper drawing shows the needles in position. The lower left drawing shows the needles penetrating to the bottom of the tumor. If there is undue bleeding, the needle is withdrawn until the bleeding stops to avoid placing the seed in a blood vessel. By feeling both sides of the lobe one can generally avoid the major vascular structures. The bottom right-hand drawing depicts the planned distribution of these seeds 1 cm in every dimension.

For precaution against radiation, it is preferable to complete all surgery and dissection before implantation. Wearing two pairs of surgical gloves is reasonable protection during implantation. Once the lung has been seeded, further manipulations inside the chest are avoided. Chest tubes are quickly placed and the chest closed.

A double-lumen endotracheal tube is placed. Occasionally bleeding enters the endotracheal tree, but should not be allowed to spread to the dependent lung. At the conclusion of the operation a bronchoscope is placed. The double-lumen catheter used while the patient is supine is replaced with a single-lumen endotracheal tube for the postoperative bronchoscopy. Any blood is removed.

Because the implant needles transgress the lung parenchyma, antibiotics are administered during surgery to prevent septicemia.

The implant technique provides a good way to monitor the primary tumor. As the radiation effect shrinks the tumor, a chest x-ray will show the seeds moving closer together. If the effect is inadequate and the tumor grows, the seeds move farther apart.

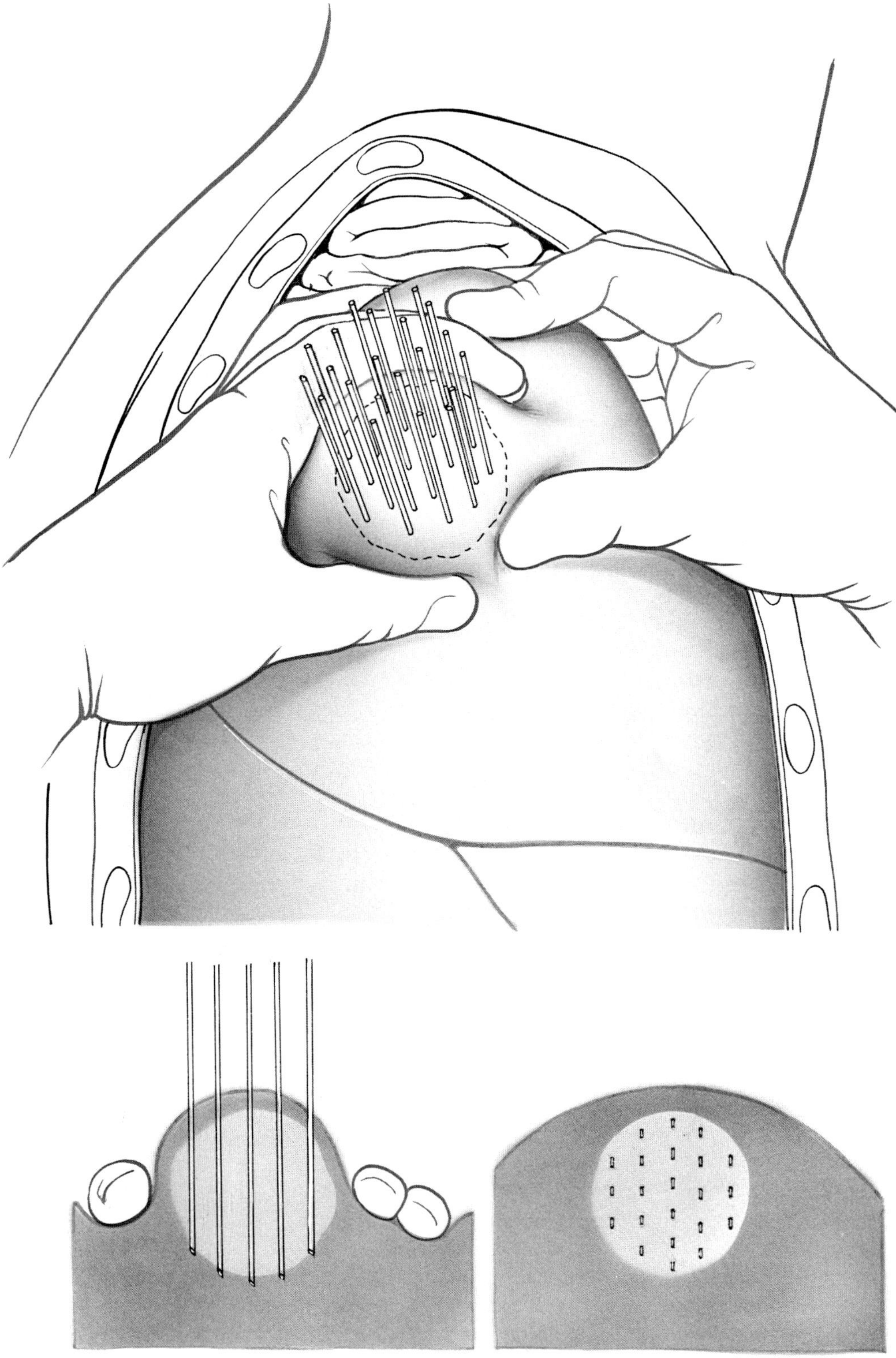

RADIOTHERAPY

AFTERLOADING TECHNIQUE

All too frequently in lung cancer patients the tumor has metastasized into the mediastinum, in particular the superior mediastinum, which is not amenable to block excision. Even with full external radiation therapy, it is difficult to sterilize these tumors. Internal afterloading offers a viable alternative.

The mediastinum is cleared of all removable metastatic lymph nodes. Ordinarily the azygos vein is divided. In this drawing, a right upper lobectomy has been completed, and the lymph nodes in the hilum cleared. Since cancer was found and presumably persists, five afterloading catheters are placed 1.0 to 1.5 cm apart. Spacing is determined by the radiation oncologist based on the strength of the isotope to be used. A hollow needle is passed into the chest cavity, and a small polyethylene catheter 3 mm in diameter and sealed at the end is inserted through the hollow needle and anchored in the chest at the appropriate location. This procedure is repeated until the appropriate number of catheters has been placed. Each catheter is secured in the chest by three absorbable catgut sutures. One suture is placed posteriorly near the spine and is tied tightly to the pleura with a loose loop around the catheter. Another suture is placed in the midmediastinum, and a third is placed in the anterior mediastinum. Where the catheter comes through the skin, a button is slipped on. This button is crimped to the catheter and sewn into the skin so that the catheter is held in position. Catheter placement poses problems in women with large breasts. To keep the catheters from being dislodged by a shifting breast, the needles are placed medial to the breast or in the inframammary crease. Catheters are spaced no closer than 1.5 cm from a bronchial or vascular stump. The lung is reinflated, everything is routinely checked, and the chest is closed. The patient is observed in the intensive care unit for a day or two. On the third or fourth day, providing the patient is doing well, the afterloading treatment is begun.

There are two afterloading techniques. One is to take the patient to the radiotherapy department twice daily for 2 or 3 days and to afterload the catheters with a relatively strong isotope for 10 to 20 minutes. By the sixth or seventh day, when the radiation is completed, the catheters are removed.

The second alternative is to move the patient into a shielded room and afterload the catheters with a lower-strength isotope for 48 to 72 hours. During this period, the patient does not receive intensive nursing care. After treatment is completed, the catheters are removed. The patient is ready to go home 8 to 9 days postsurgery.

An advantage of this technique is that the combination of I-125 seed implantation and afterloading radiotherapy makes thoracotomy a potential therapeutic event rather than a surgical exploration of a nonexcisable tumor.

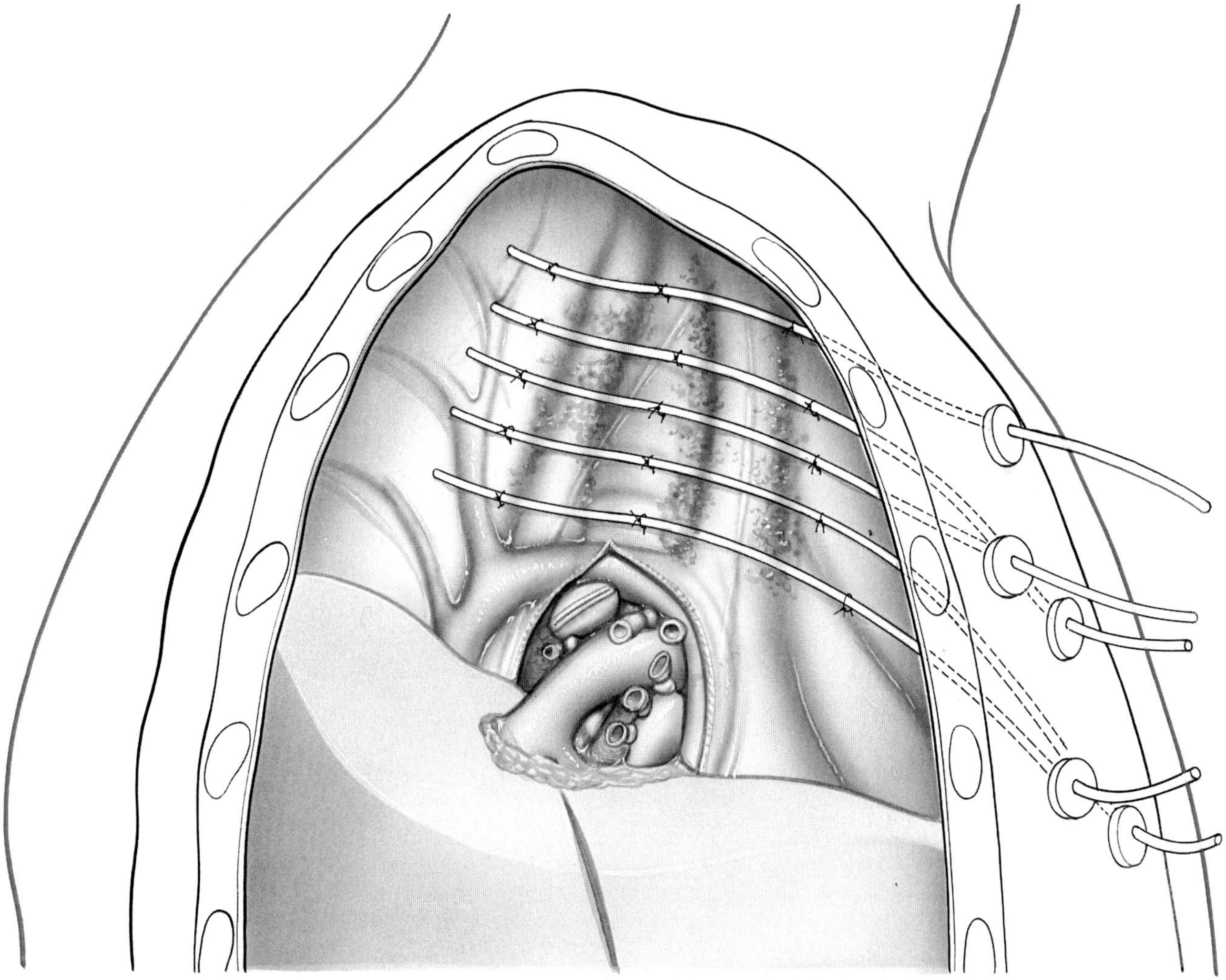

RADIOTHERAPY

SEEDING TECHNIQUE

In this view we are looking inside the right chest. A right lower-lobe lobectomy has been carried out. The right upper and right middle lobe are deflated and retracted anteriorly so that we can look at the mediastinum. The mediastinal pleura has been opened, and the esophagus is seen posteriorly. The carina, right mainstem bronchus, and a portion of the left mainstem bronchus can be seen. The superior vena cava can be seen running cephalad. In this situation we suspect that residual tumor is located between the anterior trachea and posterior superior vena cava, as well as anterior to the vena cava, and in the subcarinal space. Some years ago Hilaris devised a modification with I-125 seed sutures, whereby 10 seeds are incorporated in a thread, one seed every centimeter. With this technique one can take a suture containing 10 I-125 seeds and, with small bites of tissue, place the suture. Alternatively, one can lay the 10-seed suture in place and, with small bites of individual sutures between the seeds, hold them in place. It is important not to crush one of these seeds, as it would spill the radioisotope.

In this drawing one can see that there is a string of some 16 seeds in the pretracheal space, 20 seeds in the pre-superior vena caval space, and 10 seeds in the subcarinal space. The actual location of these seeds and the numbers used depend on the dose the radiation oncologist wishes to achieve and the strength of the seeds at the time of their placement. If higher doses are needed, more seeds are placed. These seeds can be used before or after external radiotherapy. The combination of internal radiotherapy with this seed technique plus the temporary afterloading technique followed by external radiotherapy permits our radiation oncologists to give very intense radiation only to the areas where it is needed with, hopefully, no undue damage to the more normal structures. A limiting factor in using permanent implants is the size of the tumor. The tumor must be under 6.0 cm in at least one dimension to avoid necrosis in the middle of the tumor from excessive irradiation.

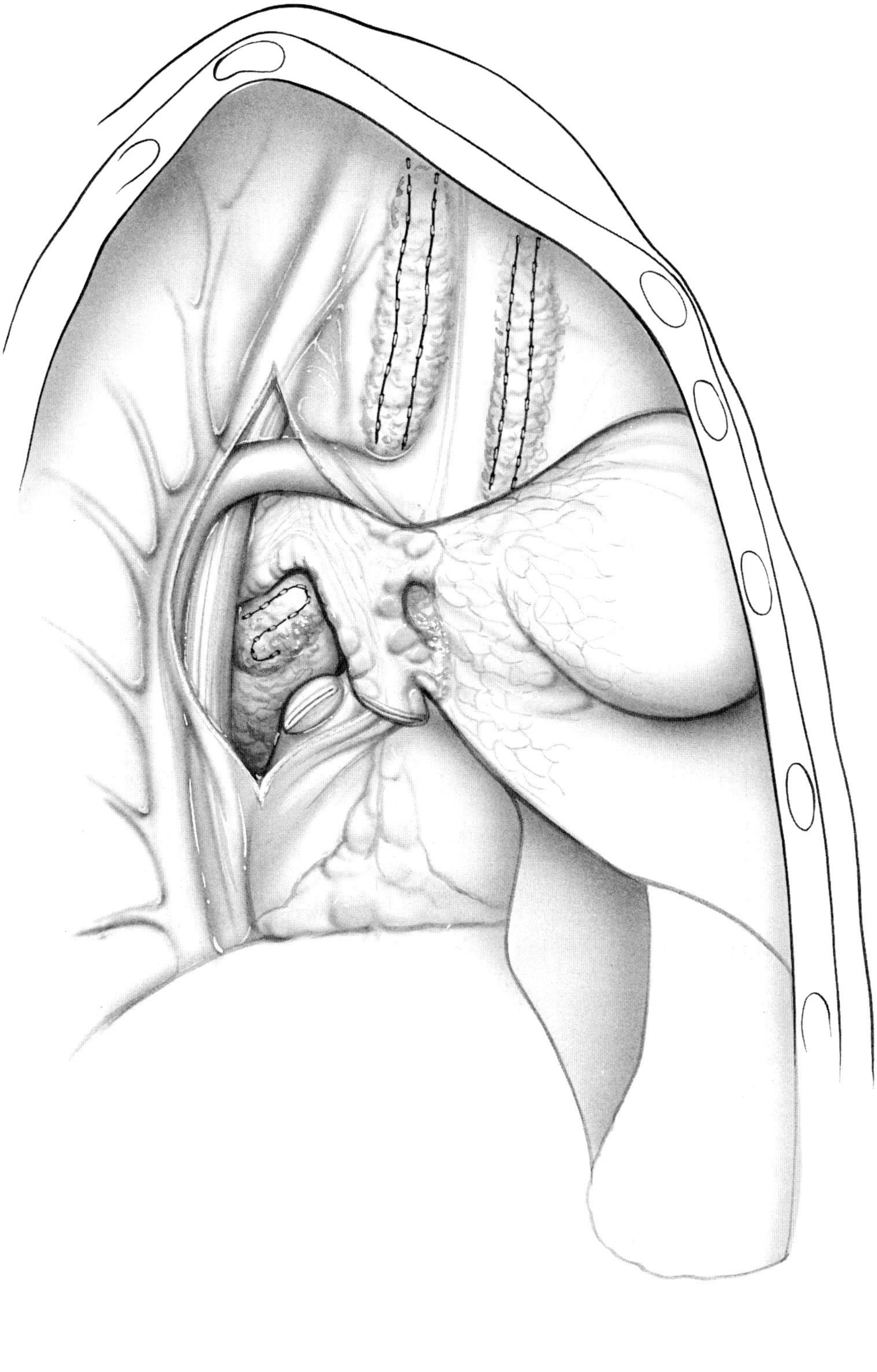

4

Esophagus

In North America and Western Europe the predominant risk factors for squamous cell carcinoma of the esophagus are alcohol ingestion and tobacco use. The risks increase with total consumption of alcoholic beverages and with concentration (distilled spirits carry greater risk than beer and wine). Tobacco, especially cigarette use, is the more important risk factor, but the combined use of alcohol and tobacco is a multiplicative risk.[1] Among urban blacks in the United States the risk is at least triple that among whites (14.0 versus 4.2 per 100,000), and the incidence among men in the United States is about quadruple that among women. Throughout most of the world, squamous cell carcinoma is associated with poverty and dietary difficiencies.[2]

Endemic areas, such as the Caspian littoral of Iran and certain mountainous and rural regions of China, have been characterized as arid lands with poor-soil quality whose inhabitants have monocereal diets of wheat or maize, deficient in calories, protein, fats, trace minerals, and vitamins.[3] During the past 50 years an epidemic of the disease has been described in South African blacks, especially in the Transkei. In South Africa, cigarette smoking and alcohol abuse play important roles, but studies in the Transkei have demonstrated that high-risk areas are found in association with soil of low agricultural potential, high alkalinity, trace-metal deficiency, and high levels of boron, similar to soils found in historic endemic areas. Areas of the Transkei where soils were derived from dolerite, rich in many minerals, including iron, magnesium, calcium, and phosphates, produced few cancers. It has also been noted in Africa that diets based on maize are associated with high risk whereas more traditional diets of sorghum, cassava, millet, and peanuts are associated with low risk.

Among specific food deficiencies associated with squamous cell carcinoma are milk, meat, fresh fruit and vegetables, vitamins (riboflavin, vitamin A, vitamin C), and minerals (zinc, iron, molybdenum). Specific exposures associated with esophageal cancer have included tobacco, snuff, betel quid, radiation, asbestos, bracken fern, solvents and dyes, nitrosamines, heavy metals, and thermal irritation associated with drinking "burning-hot" tea and coffee. Except for tobacco, these exposures are not important contributors in endemic areas, where information concerning principal carcinogens remains elusive. Plant pathogens invading kernels of weakened plants growing in the poor soil of endemic areas, *Alternaria alternata* on Iranian wheat and *Fusarium moniliforme* on corn in China and the Transkei, have been shown to enhance tumor growth in the nitrosamine model at levels lower than those occurring in the human diet in endemic areas.[4,5]

Except for an association with keratosis palmaris plantaris (tylosis), an autosomal dominant trait, familial association has been difficult to separate from environmental influences.[1] Risk factors of significance include damage to esophageal mucosa such as esophagitis; exposure to corrosives, especially lye, with cicatrix formation; and stasis associated with dismotility disorders. A history of squamous cell carcinoma at other sites is a risk factor for esophageal cancer, and there is a 25 percent risk of a second aerodigestive tumor developing within 5 years of treatment for esophageal carcinoma.[6]

Adenocarcinoma of the esophagus is a disease of increasing frequency in the United States. Older papers described adenocarcinoma as comprising as few as 2 percent of esophageal tumors, but in recent years the incidence has been markedly increasing. A recent 35-year review from a large health maintenance organization found 107 adenocarcinomas among 557 esophageal tumors, but the incidence rate increased from 0.12 to 0.53 per 100,000 patient-years during the years under review.[7] In many papers from Western Europe and in reports of recent trials conducted in the United States, the proportion approximates 50 percent.[8,9] Risk factors differ from those associated with squamous cell carcinoma in that white race is a very strong risk factor and male sex is an even stronger risk factor for adenocarcinoma than for squamous cell carcinoma.[7]

Columnar epithelium (Barrett's esophagus) is a known risk factor for development of adenocarcinoma, which is thought to be an acquired condition secondary to reflux esophagitis, but it remains unknown whether successful treatment of the esophagitis changes the risk. Once columnar metaplasia develops, the incidence rate of subsequent cancer is in the range of 1 per 300 patient-years. Studies involving multiple endoscopic biospies have demonstrated a very high risk of subsequent invasive adenocarcinoma among subjects with severe dysplasia. Some authorities have recommended esophagectomy for patients with severe dysplasia for this reason. The cost-effectiveness of endoscopic screening for Barrett's esophagus remains to be determined, however. Except for white race, male sex, and Barrett's esophagus risk factors for adenocarcinoma of the esophagus remain obscure.[10,11] Cigarette smoking and alcohol abuse have not been convincing risk factors in retrospective studies, and a case-control study investigating alcohol and tobacco as risk factors for development of adenocarcinoma among a Barrett's esophagus cohort found no strength of association.[12]

EARLY DETECTION AND DIAGNOSIS

In endemic areas early-detection programs involving mass-screening cytologic examination of the esophagus have proven efficacy. Studies in China have demonstrated the feasibility of finding early tumors through collection of cytologic samples such as on swallowed sponges, balloons, or brushes, and treatment of patients whose tumors were detected by screening programs has yielded excellent results.[13] These methods are too costly for routine use in areas of lower incidence, but there may be applications even in the United States for identified high-risk subjects. Most patients with esophageal cancer present with progressive dysphagia, often associated with weight loss. Pain is reported by approximately 30 percent of patients. Cough or hoarseness is unusual except when tumor is close to the airway, in which case its incidence may approach 20 percent. History will frequently reveal risk factors, such as smoking and alcohol abuse. The barium swallow will generally confirm mucosal abnormalities. However, esophagoscopy is used to obtain tissue for diagnosis and to search for other mucosal defects. Bronchoscopy is routinely used to assess airway invasion by cervical and upper thoracic tumors. Computed tomography (CT) is useful in assessing tumor dimensions, encroachment or invasion into neighboring structures, adenopathy, and spread to the lungs, liver, and adrenals. When clinical suspicions dictate, special studies such as bone scans, brain scans, and CT scans of the brain are helpful, but their use is not routine. Magnetic resonance imaging (MRI) may have advantages over CT in distinguishing metastatic disease from other adrenal abnormalities.[14,15] Esophageal ultrasonography can prove useful in estimating tumor dimensions and transmural spread.[16]

STAGING

Staging systems represent attempts to correlate the extent of disease with its prognosis. Some surgical scholars have accurately described shortcomings with TNM staging systems and suggested systems depending upon examination of the surgical specimen.[17] They have been able to demonstrate the value of systems similar to that of Dukes used for colorectal carcinoma, in that wall penetration and accurate assessment of nodal spread are most important prognostic indicators of local regional disease. It is not surprising that esophageal tumors should have prognostic indicators similar to those of other gastrointestinal tract tumors, but staging systems requiring study of the surgical specimen preclude easy comparison of results from patients treated nonsurgically or treated by other means prior to surgery. We recommend the use of the system proposed by the American Joint Commission on Cancer (AJCC, 1988) in cooperation with the Union Internationale Contre le Cancer (UICC).[18] In this system the esophagues is divided into four regions: cervical (from the cricoid cartilage to the suprasternal notch, approximately 18 cm from the incisors), upper thoracic (from the thoracic inlet to the bifurcation of the trachea, approximately 24 cm from the incisors), midthoracic (the proximal half of the esophagus distal to the tracheal bifurcation, approximately 32 cm from the incisors), and lower thoracic (the lower half of the esophagus distal to the bifurcation of the trachea, including the abdominal portion). The systems apply to squamous cell carcinomas and to adenocarcinomas because treatment options and outcomes are similar and no purpose is served in separating these two most common cell types. Other cell types are rare and are considered separately. A TNM system is used (Table 4-1). T designations describe the depth of invasion of the primary tumor, ranging from in situ (Tis) progressing to invasion of adjacent structures (T4). In this system the length of tumor or whether it is circumferential plays no part, acknowledging that these factors are not as important as depth of invasion extending through the four layers of the esophagus: mucosa, submucosa, muscularis, and adventitia. N designates regional lymph node involvement, with lymph node distributions designated as regional in relationship to the four anatomic regions of the esophagus or as metastatic if outside of these regional lymphatic drainage boundaries (Table 4-2). M designates metastatic

Table 4-2. Regional Lymph Node Involvement—TNM Staging System

Cervical esophagus[a]
Superior mediastinal
Internal jugular
Upper cervical
Cervical, NOS
Periesophageal
Supraclavicular
Intrathoracic esophagus (upper, middle)[b]
Internal jugular
Tracheobronchial
Peritracheal
Perigastric
Carinal
Hilar (pulmonary roots)
Posterior mediastinal
Periesophageal
Intrathoracic esophagus (lower)
Left gastric
Cardiac
Perigastric, NOS
Posterior mediastinal
Nodes of lesser curvature of stomach

Abbreviation: NOS, not otherwise specified.

[a] The cervical nodes including the supraclavicular lymph nodes.

[b] The mediastinal and perigastric lymph nodes, excluding the celiac nodes. Involvement of more distant nodes is considered distant metastasis.

(Adapted from Beahrs et al.,[18] with permission.)

Table 4-1. TNM Staging System

Stage	Description
Primary tumor (T)	
TX	Primary tumor cannot be assessed
T0	No evidence of primary tumor
Tis	Carcinoma in situ
T1	Tumor invades lamina propria or submucosa
T2	Tumor invades muscularis propria
T3	Tumor invades adventitia
T4	Tumor invades adjacent structures
Lymph node (N)	
NX	Regional lymph nodes cannot be assessed
N0	No regional lymph node metastasis
N1	Regional lymph node metasasis
Distant metastasis (M)	
MX	Presence of distant metastasis cannot be assessed
M0	No distant metastasis
M1	Distant metastasis

(Adapted from Beahrs et al.,[18] with permission.)

Table 4-3. TNM Stage Groupings

Stages			
0	Tis	N0	M0
I	T1	N0	M0
IIA	T2	N0	M0
	T3	N0	M0
IIB	T1	N1	M0
	T2	N1	M0
III	T3	N1	M0
	T4	Any N	M0
IV	Any T	Any N	M1

Histopathologic grade (G)
- GX Grade cannot be assessed
- G1 Well differentiated
- G2 Moderately well differentiated
- G3 Poorly differentiated
- G4 Undifferentiated

Histopathologic type
The staging classification applies to all squamous cell carcinomas, which are most common, and to the adenocarcinomas. Other histologic types are reported separately.

(Adapted from Beahrs et al.,[18] with permission.)

sites. TNM stage groupings are represented in Table 4-3. For purposes of clinical staging, routine radiography examinations, CT, MRI, ultrasonography, and biopsy of accessible nodes may be used. We recommend that surgical studies report results based upon clinical staging as well as pathologic staging so that comparison can be made between surgical series and those in which other forms of treatment were used instead of, or prior to, surgery. It is important to remember when comparing results of surgery with those of radiation therapy that there will be a bias in favor of surgery because pathologic staging usually results in "upstaging." In radiation therapy series, biases may be introduced by assuming most patients to be incurable and withholding curative attempts from all but the earliest staged tumors in the most fit patients.

PATHOLOGY

Grossly, esophageal tumors may be fungating, ulcerative, or infiltrating. The predominant cell type has been squamous cell carcinoma, mostly in the midesophagus, but there has been a tendency in recent years toward a predominance of adenocarcinomas of the distal esophagus. Tumors may spread via lymphatic channels coursing longitudinally in the submucosa, which may run considerable distances before penetrating muscle layers where cells may either be deposited in local lymph nodes or course through adventitial longitudinal lymphatics before depositing in more distant nodes. This longitudinal course explains why submucosal involvement is found as far as 10 cm from the primary mucosal tumor in about 5 percent of cases and also that involved nodes may be quite distant from the primary site with uninvolved nodes between them and the primary tumor.[19] Blood-borne metastases were described as uncommon in older clinical series in which failure of local control was prominent, but it is clear that most patients in the United States have disseminated disease at the time of diagnosis, even if detection is not possible by the techniques currently available.[20]

SURGERY

RESECTION

Our standard operation for esophageal cancer attempts to widely excise the organ and its lymphatic drainage with at least 10.0-cm margins. The patient is placed in a supine position and elevated 30 degrees on the right side, with the right arm prepped free, providing access to the right neck, right chest, and abdomen. We perform a midline abdominal incision for mobilization of the stomach. The left gastric artery is divided close to its origin so that lymph nodes along the lesser curve may be taken with the specimen. Care is taken to preserve the gastroepiploic arcade and right gastric artery. A pyloromyotomy or pyloroplasty is routine. After Kocher's maneuver the fundus of the stomach will always reach to the neck without tension. An anterolateral chest incision is performed through the fifth intercostal space, and the esophagus is mobilized widely to a point proximal to the divided azygos vein or up to the neck, if required, to come closer to the preferred 10.0-cm margin. The stomach is delivered through the widened hiatus into the thorax, and the specimen is excised by using the stapler device along the lesser curvature so that the specimen generally involves esophagus, periesophageal tissue, and nodes with portions of fundus, cardia, and lesser curve of the stomach and its regional nodes. The staple lines are reinforced with interrupted suture, and the anastomosis is generally accomplished with a circular anastomotic stapling device high in the thorax. If a neck incision is required for better margins, our anastomosis is performed in two layers of interrupted braided absorbable suture. A nasogastric tube is passed into the stomach at completion of the anastomosis (and sutured to the nose to prevent dislodgment prior to transporting the patient from the operating room). Anterior and posterior chest tubes are left in the thorax, and a feeding jejunostomy is performed prior to abdominal closure. Tube feedings are begun early in uncomplicated cases, and clear liquids are initiated on the eighth postoperative day if contrast studies confirm no leak and good gastric emptying.

Less extensive esophageal resections may be performed through the left chest and have been advocated for tumors of the distal esophagus and cardia. One objection to this approach is that submucosal tumor extension is occasionally quite proximal to the required margins estimated at endoscopy and it is difficult to extend the operation more proximally in the left chest. Nonetheless, admirable results have been obtained when this approach has been selected by some experts,[21] and we sometimes use it for tumors of the cardia and intra-abdominal esophagus.

Transhiatal blunt esophagectomy involves the standard abdominal mobilization of the stomach along with a neck incision to identify the esophagus. With neck and abdominal tension applied to the esophagus, the organ is bluntly dissected from mediastinal structures. Hemoclips may be applied through the hiatus to the small segmental vessels at the aorta, which may then be divided. The esophagus is gently dissected from the airway through the neck incision. When the organ is freed, it is divided at the neck, ligated on the specimen side, and withdrawn into the abdomen. The stapling device is applied along the lesser curvature as described for the standard operation. The fundus is then sutured to a rubber drain, which is passed from the neck. By gently pushing the stomach while pulling the drain, the fundus is delivered into the neck, where a two-layer anastomosis is performed. Cardiac rhythm disturbances or hypotension sometimes occurs while the surgeon's hand displaces the heart, but the operation can generally continue, allowing a recovery period to follow brief intervals of dissection. We position the patient the same way for this procedure as for our standard esophagectomy so that we have access to the right chest should the necessity arise for urgent thoracotomy or if palpation reveals a tumor too adherent for safe blunt dissection.

Akiyama et al. have described a radical operation in which special care is taken to dissect nodes from the posterior mediastinum, including tracheobronchial, paraesophageal, para-aortic, and pulmonary hilar nodes, along with an extensive abdominal node dissection.[22] They confirmed that even when tumor was located in the upper thoracic esophagus, abdominal node metastases were found in more than 30 percent of cases, and that with distal esophageal tumors, positive nodes were found in the superior mediastinum in about 10 percent. They concluded that regardless of tumor location, thoracic and abdominal esophagectomy is required along with extensive thoracic and abdominal lymphadenectomy. They did not remove the spleen and pericardium.

Skinner et al. have described a radical en block dissection that, in addition to providing 10.0-cm margins from the primary tumor, involves excision of all resectable tissue in the posterior mediastinum including both pleural surfaces, pericardium, thoracic duct, mediastinal nodes, and azygos vein. The abdominal portion of the specimen includes a 10.0-cm margin on the gastric side, spleen, a cuff of esophageal hiatus, and regional nodal tissue. Skinner et al. exclude patients with "unfavorable pathology," defined as those having both transmural tumor and more than four positive nodes.[17]

DeMeester et al.[23] extended the en bloc operation of Skinner et al. to include the proximal 75 percent of the stomach so that the specimen involved a tissue block of thoracic and abdominal esophagus, proximal stomach, and all potentially involved nodes. The operation was restricted to the middle and distal esophagus and excluded patients with unfavorable pathology as defined by Skinner et al. Colon interposition is used by DeMeester et al. to reestablish intestinal continuity.

ALTERNATIVE SURGICAL PROCEDURES

BYPASS

Retrosternal bypass using the stomach or colon has been employed for palliation of advanced esophageal tumors. The procedure is conceptually attractive, but results have been disappointing because of the high mortality rate and brief survival.[24] An occasional patient such as one with an early airway fistula may benefit, but most will not. We have found the procedure futile in patients whose tracheaesophageal fistulas present as part of an extensive disease process or in whom pulmonary sepsis is already established.[25]

GASTROSTOMY AND JEJUNOSTOMY

These procedures do not palliate esophageal cancer patients, because if they are not tormented by aspiration they can usually swallow. Palliative attempts must be directed toward dysphagia rather than nutrition alone.

ENDOPROSTHESIS

Patients with a brief life expectancy may have an endoprosthesis inserted perorally over a wire introduced after dilatation, endoscopic laser therapy, or bipolar electrocoagulation. These devices may be kept patent for passage of saliva and liquids, eliminating the most distressing symptoms of the disease.[26,27] Insertions requiring laparotomy are sometimes performed when unexpected operative findings preclude a resection, but we prefer peroral insertions when elective intubation is planned, in order to avoid the increased morbidity and mortality associated with a laporatomy in these patients.

POSTOPERATIVE CARE

Because esophageal surgery may involve entry into three body cavities, namely the neck, thorax, and abdomen, the patient has a relatively large area of trauma and develops a so-called "third space." To correct this condition, large volumes of fluids are required. For the first 48 hours it is usually necessary to overtransfuse the patient and carefully monitor the replacement of electrolytes. On about the third day the third space mobilizes, if all is well, and the patient begins diuresis.

If a pleural cavity has been entered during surgery, it should be drained. Even if entry is only suspected, drainage of the pleural spaces should be undertaken as a precaution. Jejunostomy is routinely performed as a preferred method of postoperative fluid, electrolyte, and colloid administration, eliminating the need for prolonged parenteral nutrition. The nasogastric tube can be placed on free drainage since the main concern is that the stomach does not become distended. It is important that the patient cough well. There should be no blind nasotracheal aspiration, because it might injure the esophagogastric anastomosis. The cervical drainage should be minimal and saliva free.

Many of the patients undergoing esophagectomy have impaired cardiovascular systems and are elderly. They must be monitored carefully. Intake and output must be recorded on a daily basis. Flow sheets should be kept, trend lines noted, and weight monitored daily. On the seventh day a gastrografin swallow is given to the patient in the upright position to ascertain that the fluid goes down the esophagus, through the stomach, and into the duodenum without delay or leak. Provided this is so, the nasogastric tube can be removed. Feeding by mouth begins with sips of clear liquid. Daily radiographs are taken as feedings are started to ascertain that the stomach is emptying and is not distended. If the patient tolerates sips of fluids, 4 oz of clear liquids are given per hour, followed by full liquids and then by a mechanical soft diet. The patient is ready for discharge about 12 days postoperatively.

Throughout postoperative care and for life, the patient must sleep with the head up, since there can be free regurgitation. Frequent small meals should be taken.

RESULTS

Müller and colleagues reviewed all publications on surgical treatment of esophageal carcinoma appearing in the interval from 1980 to 1988 if they contained at least a summary in a Western European language.[28] After excluding editorials, reviews, case reports, papers dealing primarily with head and neck tumors, papers dealing primarily with adenocarcinomas of the cardia, and republication of the same material, they were left with 130 papers describing 76,911 patients that they were able to compare with an earlier review of tumors reported in the interval from 1953 to 1978[29] (Table 4-4).

The authors point out that operability (the fitness of the patient to tolerate the procedure) and resectability (whether the removal of the tumor is technically feasible and reasonable) depend upon the policy and philosophy of institutions or surgeons, rather than on measurable differences in the extent of disease. For aggressive surgeons such as Ellis,[21] who believed in the value of palliative or incomplete resections, resectability was in the neighborhood of 90 percent. The majority of surgeons did not resect in situations of extensive

Table 4-4. Results for Esophageal Cancers Resected between 1980 and 1988 Compared with Those Resected between 1953 and 1978

Parameter	1980–1988[28]	1953–1978[29]
Resected	56	39
Operative mortality	13	29
1-year survival	48	45
2-year survival	21	20
5-year survival	18	12

local invasion or involvement of major abdominal organs or distant organ metastases. Mortality rates were not significantly different for series reporting squamous cell carcinomas and those mixing squamous cell carcinomas and adenocarcinomas, nor were differences discovered to be related to the tumor level. The mortality rate for "curative" resections was lower than that for palliative resections, 11 ± 7 percent versus 19 ± 8 percent. Transthoracic resection by either the right or left approach had similar mortality rates when the anastomoses were performed in the chest (median 13 versus 14 percent), but cervical anastomosis reduced the mortality rate to a median of 10 percent. A lower mortality rate (median, 8 percent) was achieved with transhiatal blunt esophagectomy, but Müller et al. caution that since this operation has only recently been introduced in most centers, improved mortality rates may represent recent improvements in postoperative care rather than a truly less morbid operation. The lowest operative mortality rates were published by surgeons with greater personal experience in resection, and a learning curve was demonstrated by the fact that improved results were demonstrated by surgeons publishing in both eras (e.g., Ellis with 20 percent mortality in 1960 and 2 percent in 1985). There is a difference in hospital mortality and in overall long-term survival depending upon the country of origin, with Japanese reports demonstrating considerably lower mortality rates (6 percent) than those from other countries. Orringer has pointed out that Japanese studies have addressed earlier disease with more superficial tumors and fewer positive nodes, whereas U.S. studies addressed tumors that more often have deeper penetration into (or through) the esophageal wall and positive lymph nodes so that better results may reflect biologic variation rather than surgical triumph.[30] Table 4-5 compares the data of Müller et al. with the results of a large Japanese study.[31]

There are no data to prove the superiority of any operative technique. No differences in survival have been demonstrated between approaches from the chest and transhiatal resections, nor have efforts to systematically perform extensive node dissections resulted in improved survival when a lower proportion of advanced disease is taken into account.[28] Abe et al.[32] have found that extensive en block resection, such as described by Akiyama et al.,[22] failed to result in 5-year survival if more than one node was positive; they contend that when the number of nodes per patient and number of nodes positive per patient were compared in their study and that of Akiyama et al., they were similar. Abe et al. report a 50.9 percent 5-year survival if no or one node is positive but no 5-year survival if two or more nodes are positive. They argue that radical en block resection should be very selectively used if it benefits so few patients.

The results of DeMeester et al. for radical en bloc resection have been reported for only 14 patients, with one perioperative death and only one patient available for 5-year follow-up.[23] An actuarial survival of 66 percent at 2 years with only two patients evaluable at 2 years for the 14 highly selected patients of DeMeester et al. is not significantly different from the 50 percent 2-year survival reported by Orringer for 15 stage I and stage II patients treated by transhiatal esophagectomy.[33] It has been noted that a statistical analysis of the results of DeMeester et al. showing improved survival of patients undergoing radical en bloc resection compared with their other patients does demonstrate an improvement that is unlikely to be due to chance, but it is unproven that their better outcome is due to the different operation rather than to selection factors.[34] At present, convincing answers to whether a more radical than conventional operation improves outcome or whether a less extensive operation such as transhiatal esophagectomy is as good remain to be obtained. Transhiatal esophagec-

Table 4-5. Five-Year Survival by Stage of Disease: A Large Collective Review Compared with a Large Japanese Study

Stage	Müller et al.[28] (6,718 total)	Iizuka et al.[31] (5,506 total)
I	70	64.2
II	38	—
IIA	—	40.9
IIB	—	24.7
III	15	17.2
IV	6	5.4

tomy has been criticized as less safe and theoretically less effective as a cancer operation, but experienced surgeons report few intraoperative problems, and long-term survival has been comparable to that obtained by operations performed under direct vision.[35]

We perform resection for palliation in low-risk patients because survival is as good as with other means of treatment (about 20 percent 1-year survival)[7,35,36] and relief of aspiration and dysphagia are superior. In addition, resection and reconstruction will prevent fistulization, abscess formation, and bleeding.[37] Other modes such as laser therapy, palliative radiation, chemotherapy, and attempts to maintain patent lumen with a combination of laser therapy, dilations, and endoprostheses are preferable for incurable patients with poor performance status.[7,35,36]

COMPLICATIONS

The comprehensive review by Müller et al. found an average complication rate of 36 percent, but they speculated that this was a low estimate because authors tended to focus upon only the most serious problems or upon those associated with technique.[28] The most frequent serious or lethal problems in Western series[38] have been related to anastomotic leaks, pneumonia, respiratory failure, and myocardial infarction (Table 4-6).

Table 4-6. Major Complications of Esophagectomy

Pulmonary
Pneumonia
Atelectasis
Respiratory failure
Cardiac
Arrhythmias
Myocardial infarction
Anastomotic
Leak
Stricture
Infections
Wound
Mediastinitis
Empyema
Urinary tract
Hoarseness
Chylothorax

Müller et al.[28] found that pneumonia and atelectasis were less frequent among transhiatal esophagectomy patients than among open thoracotomy patients, and respiratory failure was halved (13 versus 27 percent). Even very experienced esophageal surgeons report an incidence of pulmonary complications greater than 12 percent, with pneumonia and respiratory failure being major causes of perioperative mortality. Fan and colleagues found that age greater than 65, arterial PO_2 less than 10 kPa (normal range, 11 to 14.4 kPa), serum albumin less than 39 g/L (normal range, 35 to 50 g/L), peak expiratory flow rate less than 65 percent predicted, and a procedure requiring three surgical wounds were incremental risk factors for postoperative pulmonary mobidity.[39] Myocardial infarction has been reported in 2 to 5 percent of recent series. Atrial fibrillation and premature ventricular contractions are common minor complications but occasionally are major management problems.[28,39]

Anastomotic leaks complicate 10 percent of esophageal reconstructions. The leak rate is similar for anastomoses in the neck or the chest, but fatal complications are less common if the anastomosis is performed in the neck. Leakage rates are similar with one-layer and two-layer anastomoses and with hand-sutured and stapled anastomoses. The leakage rate is lower with absorbable than with nonabsorbable sutures (7 versus 11 percent).[28] Fan et al. have found that 62 percent of esophageal fistulas will heal with conservative measures (total parental nutrition and adequate drainage) within 4 weeks in the absence of extensive sepsis, intestinal discontinuity, distal obstruction, or epithelialization of the fistulous tract.[40] They found that incomplete resections or low preoperative albumin levels were associated with a high risk of failure to close spontaneously. They advise surgical repair in cases of nonclosure within 4 weeks and early repair in cases of low albumin or residual disease. One-third of the patients who failed to close their fistulas within 4 weeks died of sepsis.[40]

Hoarseness complicates 2 to 10 percent of esophageal resections but is most often temporary.[41] Chylothorax is an infrequent complication of esophagectomy but is accompanied by a high mortality rate (up to 50 percent in some series). If a brief conservative management with drainage and total parenteral nutrition fails, better outcomes result from thoracic duct ligation. Reoperation should be performed on the previously operated side so that leaking vessels may be identified and individually ligated because thoracic duct ligation alone has not been uniformly successful.[42,43]

RADIOTHERAPY

Doses of 6,000 to 7,000 cGy in fractions of 180 to 200 cGy/day, 5 days a week, are required to control gross tumors; lesser doses suffice for subclinical disease. The fields usually include generous margins, taking into account the propensity for wide drainage within the muscular walls of the esophagus. In addition to treatment directed toward the esophagus, external-beam fields may include nodal areas from the supraclavicular down to the celiac. Many patients referred for radiation therapy are known to have advanced disease with such poor performance status that a full treatment course cannot be planned.[44] In these cases we have found it useful to perform a short course of intensive intracavitary radiation delivered via a nasogastric tube at either a low dose rate (cesium 137 [Cs-137] source, 160 to 170 cGy/h, for a total dose of 2,000 cGy delivered in three sections over 1 week) or a high dose rate (iridium 192 [Ir-192] source, 200 cGy/min, for a total dose of 1,250 cGy delivered in one session).[45,46]

Preoperative radiotherapy has been delivered by a variety of methods with the expectation that it would decrease tumor bulk and improve resectability, reduce metastases induced by operative manipulation, and destroy residual tumor left following resection.[47] Postoperative radiation has also been given in the hope of destroying residual tumor in the operative field.[48]

RESULTS

In retrospective studies reported from the Southern California Permanente Medical Group, radiotherapy had survival rates similar to surgery, with up to 20 percent 5-year survival among those treated for cure but less than 20 percent 1-year survival among patients treated for palliation,[7,35,36] Palliative treatment was provided to the majority of patients. Selection criteria excluding so many radiotherapy patients from curative attempts were difficult to determine in a retrospective study, but there may be an assumption of futility on the part of some treating therapists, and there is a high attrition rate among patients in whom more treatment was planned than was completed.[49] If only the most fit and motivated patients with early disease are given radical treatment, the true potential for cure will not be tested or fairly compared with surgery. On the other hand, it is difficult to compare radiotherapy with studies in which advanced disease was determined only at surgery (upstaging), so that a bias in favor of surgical results will be introduced. Nonetheless, there are several studies demonstrating that cure rates are similar for radiotherapy and resection. Survival with palliative radiation is as good as with palliative resection,[7,35,36] but for the patient with good performance status relief of symptoms of dysphagia may be improved and prolonged with resection.[37] For patients in whom advanced disease precludes cure and whose performance status makes them prohibitive surgical risks, we have reported that 12-hour intracavitary treatment with up to a 2,000-cGy total dose provides significant improvement in dysphagia to the extent that most patients retain or regain their ability to swallow solid foods until death from distant disease.[45] More recently we have used high-dose-rate intracavitary treatment at a rate of 150 cGy/min for less than 10 min with early results equally satisfactory. This expeditious, efficient, and uncomplicated mode of delivery is especially useful for the very sick patient who would otherwise have only intubation or hospice care as options.[46] We would advise consideration of intracavitary radiotherapy for use in cases of microscopic positive margins following esophagectomy and have also used it in ongoing multidisciplinary protocols, but our experiences with these problems are too early to report.

COMPLICATIONS

Short-term complications of radiotherapy for carcinomaa of the esophagus are frequent and include esophagitis, pneumonitis, pericarditis, skin changes and hair loss, transient myelosuppression, gastrointestinal complaints (including nausea, vomiting, anorexia, and weight loss), and fatigue. Perforation with fistulization or hemorrhage are often listed but should truly be considered complications of the disease rather than its treatment since radiation only precipitates the inevitable by killing tumor cells already invading the airway or aorta.[49]

Longer-term complications include stricture, pulmonary fibrosis, pericardial constriction, myocarditis, bone necrosis, and transverse myelitis.

Transient dysphagia is common, but fibrous strictures take approximately 3 months to develop. Occasionally strictures are refractory to dilatation and may require resection for that reason and also to resolve questions of residual or recurring tumor.

CHEMOTHERAPY

Disseminated disease is present in the majority of esophageal cancer patients at the time of diagnosis, even among those believed resectable for cure. This is verified by autopsy observations and also by life history studies demonstrating that most patients die of distant disease even when local control has been achieved by radiotherapy or by surgery.[50] Consequently, there has been much interest in discovering combinations of drugs effective against this tumor. Pioneering efforts in this search for effective combinations against squamous cell carcinoma of the esophagus were carried out by investigators at Memorial Sloan Kettering Cancer Center initially using combinations of drugs that had demonstrated effects against head and neck tumors (cisplatin and bleomycin). When these drugs were used prior to surgery in patients with local-regional disease (LRD), half of the patients experienced subjective improvement in swallowing even though only 14 percent had objective partial responses. Similar objective response rates were documented among patients with extensive disease (ED). The later addition of the vinca alkyloid vindesine improved survival in a subsequent cohort of LRD patients treated prior to surgery and improved the partial response rate among ED patients.[51] When Kelson et al.[52] performed a randomized prospective trial comparing cisplatin-bleomycin-vindesine chemotherapy with preoperative external-beam radiotherapy at 5,500 cGy, similar objective responses and survival were found in the cohorts. They concluded that chemotherapy was as good as radiotherapy for local control of squamous cell carcinoma.[52] Other drugs have been effective in combination with cisplatin, especially mitoguazone, originally substituted for bleomycin in an attempt to avoid the pulmonary toxicity of belomycin, mitomycin C, which may have similar toxicity to bleomycin, methotrexate with folinic acid rescue, and 5-fluorouracil (5-FU). In the hands of experienced medical oncologists a variety of combinations, doses, and schedules have produced objective responses including complete response rates above 20 percent documented by study of surgical specimens. Others have verified the observation of Kelson et al. that even modest objective responses may result in significant relief of dysphagia among ED patients. Several combinations have been found useful, either alone or in combination with other palliative efforts (dilatation, endoprostheses) in relieving dysphagia in patients too ill to withstand standard radiation or surgery.[53]

Cisplatin plays a key role in modern protocols for chemotherapy of carcinoma of the esophagus. There are now several reports of cisplatin-based chemotherapy combinations resulting in response rates of greater than 50 percent for squamous cell carcinomas and also for adenocarcinomas. Muggia has described several areas that may become clinically important in expanding the use of cisplatin. Sodium thiosulfate has been shown to permit intensive high doses of cisplatin with diminished nephrotoxicity, neurotoxicity, and anemia. Circadian dosing strategies may improve efficacy, as has been reported for evening doses in treating gynecologic cancers. Prediction of response may be feasible from studies of the ability of tissues to retain platinum-DNA adducts prior to drug administration. Since enhanced repair of platinum-DNA adducts has been implicated in tumor resistance, there may be a role for pretreatment study to predict resistance and also a clinical application of drugs that inhibit DNA repair to enhance cytotoxicity. Hyperthermia may increase the uptake of cisplatin and DNA damage even among resistant cells.[54]

COMBINATION THERAPY

CHEMOTHERAPY AND SURGERY

Kelson et al.[52] have recently published results of their prospective trial for squamous cell carcinoma comparing preoperative radiotherapy with preoperative chemotherapy consisting of two courses of cisplatin, vindesine, and bleomycin. Radiation was delivered at 4,500 cGy to the primary tumor with 5-cm proximal and distal margins and regional nodes, followed by a boost to 5,500 cGy to the primary tumor with a 2-cm margin. Patients in the chemotherapy limb of the study received cisplatin, 120 mg/m^2, on days 1 and 29; vindesin, 3 mg/m^2, on days 1, 8, 15 22, 29, 38, and 43; and bleomycin, 10 U/m^2 intravenous bolus followed by a 4-day continuous infusion at 10 U/m^2 per day beginning on day 3 and ending on day 7 and beginning on day 31 and ending day 36. There were no deaths attributed to the induction therapy. Surgery was performed during the eighth week following initiation of therapy. Patients who had complete resection of T1–2, N0, M0 tumors were considered to have curative resections and received no further treatment. Resections were considered palliative if margins were microscopically positive, lymph nodes were positive, or tumor had penetrated into periesophageal tissue. These patients received postoperative radiotherapy if initially on the chemotherapy limb and vice versa. Most (75 percent) of the chemotherapy patients were operable and 58 percent were resectable with an operative mortality of 11 percent. The median survival of patients with resectable tumor was 16 months, but that for responders was 26.6 months. Kelson et al. concluded that the results with preoperative radiotherapy and with chemotherapy were similar but the impact on survival, even with all three modes (because of the crossover design of the study) was poor and not better than results with surgery alone. They mentioned that the phenomenon of "responders" doing better than "nonresponders" may not be a causal relationship. They concluded that more effective chemotherapy combinations remain to be discovered and that surgery remains standard care outside of carefully designed clinical trials.

Adjani et al.[55] at the M.D. Anderson Cancer Center evaluated prolonged perioperative courses of etoposide, 5-FU, and cisplatin (EFP) for adenocarcinoma of the esophagus or gastroesophageal junction. They planned a total of six courses, two preoperatively and four postoperatively, and a median of five courses were actually administered, with a 77 percent major response rate. There was modest toxicity associated with the protocol but no deaths attributable to complications of chemotherapy. This study showed complete resection to be associated with improved survival and demonstrated that up to six courses of platinin-based chemotherapy could be provided, but they could not conclude that EFP imparted survival benefit in this pilot study.

CHEMORADIATION

Laboratory data have demonstrated the ability of 5-FU, cisplatin, and other agents to potentiate tissue radiation sensitivity, and Leichman et al.[53] have stated that all future trials involving radiotherapy should also include chemotherapy. Leichman et al. reported results of trials demonstrating improved survival of patients treated with chemoradiation compared with radiation alone and of chemoradiation followed by surgery compared with radiation followed by surgery. Investigations are in progress to attempt to improve the therapeutic ratio of chemoradiation, especially to decrease the toxicity sometimes observed with simultaneous chemoradiation. When radiation is administered following the planned dose of chemotherapy the reduction in toxicity is thought to be accompanied by a reduced intensity of treatment. Looney and Hopkins have demonstrated that a strategy of alternating intensive doses of chemotherapy with radiation allows delivery of both treatments at initiation of induction therapy.[56] They believe that alternating dosing reduces toxicity while minimizing buildup of resistance of tumor cells to either technique and, of course, provides early chemotherapy for micrometastases. Vikram et al. have reported early success with this "sandwich" technique in locally advanced tumors of the hypopharynx and proximal esophagus.[57]

Coia et al. have reported superior results of 5-FU and mitomycin C chemotherapy combined with external radiation therapy when compared with external radiation therapy alone.[58] Among their combined-therapy cohort, the local failure rate was halved compared with that in a radiation-only group (37 versus 76 percent local failures). The superiority of local control achieved by modern chemotherapy has demonstrated the efficacy of several treatment combinations, but the fact that so many patients whose local control has been achieved still die of distant disease emphasizes the need for better protocols to control systemic disease.

CHEMORADIATION AND SURGERY

Orringer et al.[59] have recently reported their results of a prospective multidisciplinary protocol involving an intensive in-hospital chemoradiation protocol followed by transhiatal esophagectomy. External-beam radiotherapy was administered at 150 cGy twice daily for 5 days per week to a dose of 4,500 cGy simultaneously with cisplatin (20 mg/m^2/day) by continuous infusion on days 1 through 5 and 17 through 21, vinblastine (1 mg/m^2/day) by intravenous bolus on days 1 through 4 and 17 through 20; and 5-FU (300 mg/m^2/day) by continuous infusion for the entire 21 days. Transhiatal esophagectomy was scheduled after a 3-week rest. Two patients died of sepsis due to bone marrow suppression. The overall operability was 95 percent, with complete resection thought accomplished in all but 1 of 39 patients operated upon. There was a single operative death (2 percent). Median survival was 29 months overall but has not yet been reached for adenocarcinomas. Orringer et al. concluded that the 2-year survival of 60 percent among this study cohort compared with 32 percent for historical controls treated by transhiatal esophagectomy alone suggests a benefit of combined therapy. They noted that prospective trials are in progress to verify the benefits of combined therapy.

The Southern California Permanente Medical Group is conducting a study involving preoperative 5-FU and cisplatin followed by high-dose intraluminal radiation therapy of 1,250 cGy in one fraction. After a 3-week rest, either transhiatal esophagectomy or conventional esophagectomy may be performed at the discretion of the operating surgeon. Results are too early to evaluate in detail, but there was a preoperative death due to sepsis and bone marrow toxicity. There have been no perioperative deaths in our early experience, and actuarial 2-year survival is approximately 50 percent. There is a cost advantage to this protocol compared with that of Orringer et al. in that it may be given mostly on an outpatient basis.

Although resection or radiotherapy remains standard care in curative attempts for esophageal cancer, we believe the future efforts should be multidisciplinary. Chemotherapy combinations are known to have an effect upon LRD and are presumed to be effective against undetected distant disease. A remaining future challenge in chemotherapy is the discovery of combinations, doses, or schedules that can be given in a cost-efficient manner with reduced toxicity. Optimal timing, dosimetry, and method of delivery of radiotherapy in a multidisciplinary setting also remain to be determined. The timing of surgery, the type of operation, and even the value of routine esophagectomy in a multidisciplinary setting are legitimate topics of debate. Prospective randomized trials involving multiple centers are required to answer these questions.

REFERENCES

1. Day NE, Munoz N: Esophagus. p. 596. In Schottenfeld D, Fraumeni JF (eds): Cancer Epidemiology and Prevention. WB Saunders, Philadelphia, 1982
2. Blot WJ: Epidemiology of esophageal cancer. p. 295. In Roth JA, Ruckdeschel JC, Weisenburger TH (eds): Thoracic Oncology. WB Saunders, Philadelphia, 1989
3. VanRensburg SJ: Oesophageal cancer. Risk factors common to endemic regions. S Afr Med J, suppl. 70:9, 1987
4. VanRensburg SJ: Epidemiologic and dietary evidence for a specific nutritional predisposition to esophageal cancer. JNCI 67:243, 1981
5. Warwick GP: Some aspects of the epidemiology and etiology of oesophageal cancer with particular emphasis on the Transkei, South Africa. Cancer Res 17:81, 1973
6. Vikram B, Strong EW, Shah JP, Spiro R: Second malignant neoplasm in patients successfully treated with multi-modality treatment for advanced head and neck cancer. Head Neck Surg 6:734, 1984
7. Harvey JC, Kagan AR, Ahn C: Adenocarcinoma of the esophagus: a survival study. J Surg Oncol 45:29, 1990
8. Desa L, Raghunath AG, Chawla SL et al: Treatment policy for the management of carcinoma of the esophagus. Bri J Surg 73:275, 1988
9. Forastiere AA, Orringer MB, Perez-Tamayo C et al: Concurrent chemotherapy and radiation therapy followed by transhiatal eosphagectomy for local-regional cancer of the esophagus. J Clin Oncol 8:119, 1990
10. Reid BJ, Weinstein WM: Barrett's esophagus and adenocarcinoma. Annu Rev Med 38:477, 1987
11. Harvey JC, Kagan AR, Hause D et al: Adenocarcinoma arising in Barrett's esophagus. J Surg Oncol 45:162, 1990
12. Levi F, Ollyo JB, LaVecchia C: The consumption of tobacco, alcohol and the risk of adenocarcinoma in Barrett's esophagus. Int J Cancer 45:852, 1990
13. Shaw LF, Gao ZG, Yung NP et al: Results of surgical treatment in 6123 cases of carcinoma of the esophagus and gastric cardia. J Surg Oncol 42:170, 1989
14. Sharma OP, Subnani S: Role of computerized tomography imaging in staging oesophageal carcinoma. Semin Surg Oncol 5:355, 1989
15. Sutton D: The adrenals. p. 1033. In Sutton D (ed): Textbook of Radiology and Imaging. 4th Ed. Churchill Livingstone, New York, 1987
16. Takemoto T, Ito T, Okita K: Endoscopic ultrasonography in the diagnosis of esophageal carcinoma with particular regard to staging it for operability. Endoscopy 18 (suppl. 3):22, 1986
17. Skinner DB, Ferguson MK, Soriano A et al: Selection of operation for esophageal cancer based on staging. Ann Surg 204:391, 1986
18. Beahrs OH, Henson DE, Hutter RVP, Myers MH (American Joint Committee on Cancer) (eds): Manual for Staging of Cancer. 3rd Ed. p. 63. JP Lippincott, Philadelphia, 1988
19. delRegato JA, Spjut HJ, Cox JD (ed): Cancer: Diagnosis, Treatment and Prognosis. 6th Ed. p. 464. CV Mosby, St. Louis, 1985
20. Anderson I, Lad T: Autopsy findings in squamous cell carcinoma of the esophagus. Cancer 50:1587, 1982
21. Ellis FH: Treatment of carcinoma of the esophagus and cardia. Mayo Clin Proc 64:945, 1989
22. Akiyama H, Tsurumaru M, Kamamara T, Ono Y:

Principles of surgical treatment for carcinoma of the esophagus. Ann Surg 194:438, 1981
23. DeMeester TR, Zaninotto G, Johansson K-E: Selective therapeutic approach to cancers of the lower esophagus and cardia. J Thorac Cardiovasc Surg 95:42, 1988
24. Orringer MB: Substernal bypass of excluded thoracic esophagus—results of an ill-advised operation. Surgery 96:467, 1984
25. Hause DW, Kagan AR, Fleischman E, Harvey JC: Tracheoesophageal fistula complicating carcinoma of the esophagus. Am Surg (in press)
26. Gasparri G, Casalagno PA, Camandona M et al: Endoscopic insertion of 248 prostheses in inoperable carcinoma of the esophagus and cardia: short-term and long-term results. Gastrointest Endosc 33:354, 1987
27. Santhi SV, Desai PB: Palliative management of esophageal cancer. Semin Surg Oncol 5:373, 1989
28. Müller JM, Erasmi H, Stelzner M et al: Surgical therapy of esophageal carcinoma. Br J Surg 77:845, 1990
29. Earlam R, Cunha-Melo JR: Oesophageal squamous cell carcinoma: a critical review of surgery. Br J Surg 67:381, 1980
30. Orringer MB: Ten year survival after esophagectomy for carcinoma: surgical triumph or biologic variation? Chest 96:970, 1989
31. Iizuka T, Isono K, Kakegawa T, Watanabe H: Parameters linked to 10-year survival in Japan of selected esophageal carcinoma. Chest 96:1005, 1989
32. Abe S, Tachibana M, Shiraishi M, Nakamura T: Lymph node metastases in resectable esophageal cancer. J Thora Cardiovasc Surg 100:287, 1990
33. Orringer MB: Transhiatal esophagectomy without thoracotomy for carcinoma of the thoracic esophagus. Ann Surg 200:282, 1984
34. Kirklin JW, Blackstone EH: The DeMeester paper on carcinoma of the esophagus. J Thorac Cardiovasc Surg 100:456, 1990
35. Harvey JC, Kagan AR, Frankl H et al: Squamous carcinoma of the distal esophagus: a survival study. J Surg Oncol 46:97, 1991
36. Harvey JC, Davidson W, Frankl H et al: Squamous carcinoma of the mid-esophagus: a survival study. Am Surg 57:615, 1992
37. Belsey R, Hiebert CA: An exclusive right thoracic approach for cancer of the middle third of the esophagus. Ann Thorac Surg 18:1, 1974
38. King RM, Pairolaro PL, Trastek VF et al: Ivor Lewis esophagogastrectomy for carcinoma of the esophagus: early and late functional results. Ann Thorac Surg 44:119, 1987
39. Fan ST, Lau WY, Yip WC et al: Prediction of postoperative pulmonary complications in oesophagogastric cancer surgery. Br J Surg 74:408, 1987
40. Fan ST, Lau WY, Yip WC et al: Healing of esophageal fistulas after surgical treatment for carcinoma of the esophagus and upper part of the stomach. Surg Gynecol Obstet 166:307, 1988
41. Hankins JR, Miller JE, Attar S, McLaughlin JS: Transhiatral esophagectomy for carcinoma of the esophagus: experience with 26 patients. Ann Thorac Surg 44:123, 1987
42. Robinson CLN: The management of chylothorax. Ann Thorac Surg 39:90, 1985
43. Ferguson MK, Little AG, Skinner DB: Current concepts in the management of chylothorax. Ann Thorac Surg 40:542, 1985
44. Fisher SA, Frady LW: Carcinoma of the esophagus. p. 700. In Perez CA, Brady LW (eds): Principles and Practice of Radiation Oncology. JP Lippincott, Philadelphia, 1987
45. Fleischman EH, Kagan AR, Bellotti JE et al: Effective palliation for inoperable esophageal cancer with intensive intracavitary radiation. Gen Surg Oncol 44:234, 1990
46. Fleischman EH, Anderson P, Bellotti JE: Intracavitary radiation in the treatment of advanced esophageal carcinoma: a trial of high vs low dose brachytherapy. Radiother Oncol (in press)
47. Gignoux M, Roussel A, Paillot B, Gillet M: The value of preoperative radiotherapy in esophageal cancer: results of a study of the EORTC. World J Surg 11:426, 1987
48. Iizuka T, Ide H, Kagegawa T, Sasaki K: Preoperative radioactive therapy for esophageal carcinoma. Chest 93:1055, 1983
49. Earlam R, Cunha-Melo JR: Oesophageal squamous cell carcinoma. II. A critical review of radiotherapy. Br J Surg 67:457, 1980
50. Kelson D: Neoadjuvant therapy of esophageal cancer. Can J Surg 32:410, 1989
51. Kelson DP, Bains M, Hilaris B et al: Combined modality therapy of esophageal cancer. Semin Oncol 11:169, 1984
52. Kelson DP, Minsky B, Smith M et al: Preoperative therapy for esophageal cancer: a randomized comparison for chemotherapy vs. radiation therapy. J Clin Oncol 8:1352, 1990
53. Leichman L, Berry BT: Experience with cisplatin in treatment regimens for esophageal cancer. Semin Oncol 18:64, 1991
54. Muggia F: Cisplatin update. Semin Oncol 18:1, 1991
55. Ajani JA, Roth JF, Ryan B et al: Evaluation of pre- and postoperative chemotherapy for resectable adenocarcinoma of the esophagus or gastroesophageal junction. J Clin Oncol 8:1231, 1990
56. Looney WB, Hopkins HA: Rationale for a different chemotherapeutic and radiation therapy strategies in cancer management. Cancer 67:1471, 1991
57. Vikram B, Malamud S, Gold J et al: Chemotherapy rapidly alternating with accelerated radiotherapy

for advanced carcinomas of the hypopharynx and upper esophagus: a feasibility study. Head Neck (in press)

58. Coia LR, Engstrom PF, Paul AR et al: Long term results of infusional 5-FU, mitomycin-C, and radiation as primary management of esophageal carcinoma. Int J Radiat Oncol Biol Phys 20:29, 1991
59. Orringer MB, Forastiere AA, Perez-Tamayo C et al: Chemotherapy and radiation therapy for transhiatal esophagectomy for esophageal carcinoma. Ann Thorac Surg 49:348, 1990

ATLAS OF ESOPHAGEAL SURGERY

SURGICAL ANATOMY AND BASIC TECHNIQUES

The esophagus is the muscular tube connecting the pharynx to the stomach. It is lined with stratified squamous epithelium, a submucosal layer, and an inner circular muscle layer. It has an outer coat of longitudinal muscle. There is no serosa.

The esophagus begins in the midline in the lower neck with the cricopharyngeus sphincter opening into the esophagus, which is directly behind and caudal to the glottis. The esophagus enters the thorax usually in the midline between the trachea and the anterior border of the spine, but as it enters the chest it moves to the right and descends mostly in the right thorax on the anterolateral border of the spine until it reaches the lower quarter of the chest. It then swings to the left and pierces the diaphragm anterolateral to the spine through the esophageal hiatus. The esophagus continues onward for 2 to 3 cm along the left side of the liver, where it joins with the cardiac sphincter and the stomach.

It is important to remember that in the top half of the thorax the esophagus is either contiguous with the membranous portion of the trachea or the membranous portion of the right mainstem bronchus. The vagus nerves run in the posterior carotid sheaths and enter the thorax posterior to the carotid vessels but swing posteriorly so that the right vagus nerve runs along the right lateral surface of the esophagus down the right chest. The left vagus nerve, in similar fashion, comes toward the esophagus but crosses the arch of the aorta laterally; at about the level of the aortic arch it gives off a branch, namely the recurrent nerve, which courses medially toward the caudal esophagus and loops under the ligamentum arteriosum medially. The left recurrent nerve runs in the groove between the left side of the esophagus and the trachea cephalad into the neck, where it is the motor nerve to the left vocal cord. The left vagus nerve joins the esophagus and runs down the left side of the esophagus into the abdomen, where it then swings somewhat anteriorly and comes to the anterior surface of the esophagogastric junction. In turn the right vagus nerve, rotating slightly posteriorly, comes through the esophahgeal hiatus and lies on the posterior surface of the esophagogastric junction. Both vagal nerves give off numerous branches in the thorax.

On the right side, the right recurrent laryngeal nerve branches from the vagus trunk at the apex of the thorax and runs posteriorly to the subclavian branch of the right innominate artery; from this location it runs medially and cephalad again in the tracheoesophageal groove up to the larynx, where it is the motor nerve to the right vocal cord.

The blood supply to the esophagus comes from branches of the inferior thyroid arteries, from direct branches from the aorta itself (since the esophagus is in close proximity to the descending aorta along the caudal two-thirds of the thorax), and from the left gastric artery and left inferior phrenic artery. It is important to remember that the thoracic duct lies posterior to the esophagus near the aorta on the anterior portion of the spine and runs up in this region just anterior to the spine, tending toward the left side as it reaches the upper thorax and rises into the neck, where it swings anteriorly and ultimately inserts into the venous system at the junction of the left subclavian vein and the right internal jugular vein. There are numerous lymphatic branches running in the mediastinum along with the lymph nodes of the mediastinum. Usually dividing these is no problem unless one is dealing with a major branch of the thoracic duct. Occasionally after esophageal surgery, but more usually after aortic surgery, such as coarctation operations and patent ductus arteriosus divisions, a leaking lymphatic may prove troublesome and will require reoperation for ligature.

ANASTOMOSIS

The surgical approach is determined by which portion of the esophagus is involved with tumor and which portion the surgeon wishes to resect. However, in the case of the esophagus one cannot resect a central piece, mobilize the ends, and carry out a primary anastomosis. This is because the esophagus is not vertically elastic (although it is quite distensible laterally), and one cannot preserve its blood supply if it has been completely mobilized. Therefore, if one resects a segment of esophagus it is necessary to bridge this defect, and the most satisfactory bridge currently available is the stomach. If the stomach is moved cephalad, with no tension, the esophagus can be anastomosed to the stomach at any level. A surgical problem arises, however, if there is insufficient stomach for this to be done. Probably the second best choice under these circumstances is to use a colon interposition. Our preference, if anatomically feasible, is to use the transverse colon in an isoperistolic fashion. A colon segment will reach proximally from the cervical esophagus and distally to the gastric remnant. A third choice is to use an appropriate limb of the small intestine. Jejunum can be mobilized and brought up into the chest as well, but in our experience it has been difficult to get the jejunal loop high into the thorax and neck. The next alternative, if the surgical team is sufficiently skilled, is a free microvascular graft of a jejunal segment where the arterial and venous supply of the segment is anastomosed to appropriate vessels such as thyroid vessels or internal mammary vessels. This technique, if it works, is excellent, but there is a chance that the graft will not survive. Finally, one can leave a cervical esophagostomy and gastrostomy with no connection or later create a lined skin tube connection. Neither of these approaches is very satisfactory.

If one plans to resect the cervical esophagus or the esophagus in the region of the sternal notch, almost the entire esophagus may be removed and the stomach brought up into the neck for anastomosis either to the stump of the cervical esophagus or to the pharynx. To carry out this operation, also known as the gastric pullthrough, it is customary for the patient to be supine and for the neck, chest, and abdomen to be prepared and draped. A laporatomy is carried out for evaluation and mobilization of the stomach. The neck is explored to ensure that the tumor is removable and to ascertain the extent of tumor resection required. Not infrequently, in more advanced cases, this must be accompanied by a laryngectomy and permanent tracheostomy. The thoracic part of the operation consists of blunt dissection from the abdomen and neck to mobilize the esophagus so that the stomach can be drawn up through the posterior mediastinum and anastomosed in the neck.

THORACOTOMY

For tumors located around the cardia of the esophagus or gastric tumors growing up into the distal esophagus, it is our custom to operate through a left thoracotomy. This can be done with the patient in the straight lateral approach with preparation and draping of the left chest and upper abdomen. Usually a seventh-interspace incision will permit the surgeon to mobilize the distal esophagus. An appropriate incision can be made in the diaphragm to avoid denervating a major portion of the diaphragm and the stomach can be readily reached, prepared, and mobilized through the left chest. After a proper resection of the esophagus and stomach, the esophagogastrostomy can be carried out, usually with a stapling device, with the anastomosis below the aortic arch.

For the other operations on the esophagus (such as surgery for tumors in the esophagus above the cardia and in particularly at the level of the tracheal carina) when it is believed that there is adequate normal esophagus at the top of the right chest, we prefer a combination laporatomy and right thoracotomy.

ESOPHAGOGASTRECTOMY

PATIENT POSITIONING

The approach, as depicted, involves placing the patient on the operating table with the right side of the torso rotated upward about 15 to 20 degrees. The position is maintained by support under the right buttocks. The right arm is prepared in a sterile fashion so that the right neck, chest, and abdomen can be prepared and draped. With this approach a midline laporatomy permits the surgeon to explore the abdomen to ensure resectability.

The right neck can be explored and the cervical esophagus mobilized. This combined approach permits the surgeon to mobilize the esophagus with its tumor before the esophagus is transected above or the stomach is transected below. The thoracic esophagus is mobilized by a hand in the neck reaching down into the thorax and a hand in the abdomen reaching up into the thorax.

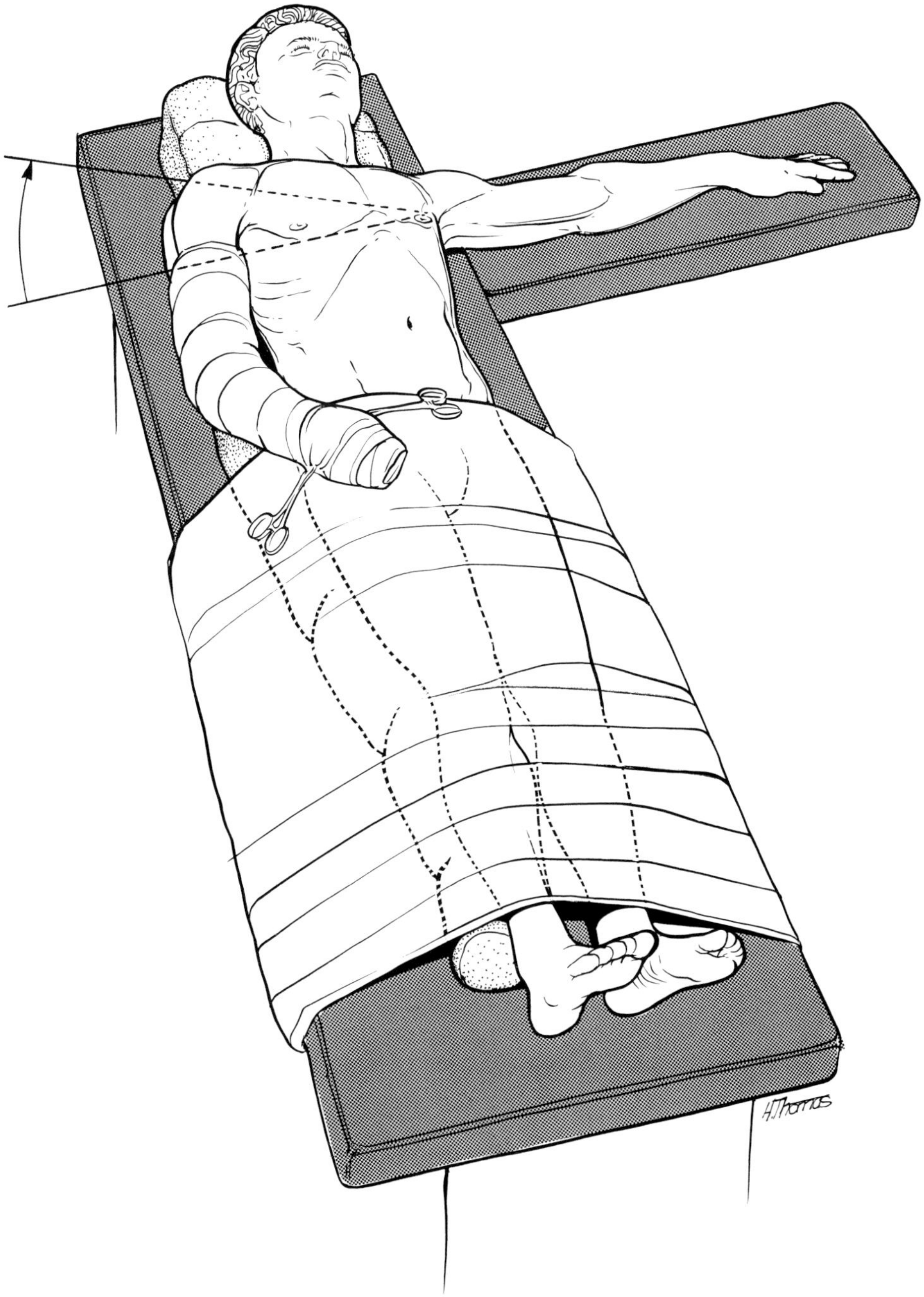

ESOPHAGOGASTRECTOMY

ANATOMIC ORIENTATION

In this drawing the esophagus is seen behind the tracheobronchial tree as it descends through the thorax. Depicted are arterial branches from the aorta providing the blood supply to the esophagus. The esophagus curves to the left as it enters the abdomen and connects with the upper stomach. The left lobe of the liver obscures the next essential part of the anatomy. The ligamentous adhesions of the left lobe of the liver to the under surface of the diaphragm usually must be divided so that the left lobe of the liver can be folded forward out of the way. One must be careful not to injure the liver during this maneuver and to remember that the inferior vena cava is in the anterior portion of the diaphragm and liver to the right of the midline.

With this exposure one then can find and visualize the celiac axis. The artist shows here the left gastric artery, which must be divided to permit mobilization of the stomach. The splenic artery courses posteriorly to the stomach and enters the hilum of the spleen. Branches are given off as short gastric vessels, and the left gastroepiploic artery originates here. The hepatic artery is coursing to the right and will give off the right gastric artery and most especially the right gastroepiploic artery, which will pass behind the region of the pylorus and provides the anastomotic arcades that will course around the greater curvature of the stomach. It is mandatory that the surgeon be aware of and preserve the possible arcades of the greater curvature and lesser curvature while mobilizing the stomach. Under no circumstance should the right gastric artery or right gastroepiploic artery be injured. The relationship with the omentum is also shown, and it must be remembered that the superior mesenteric artery supplying the small intestine and colon will be behind the stomach coming out of the inferior edge of the pancreas as a direct branch off the aorta.

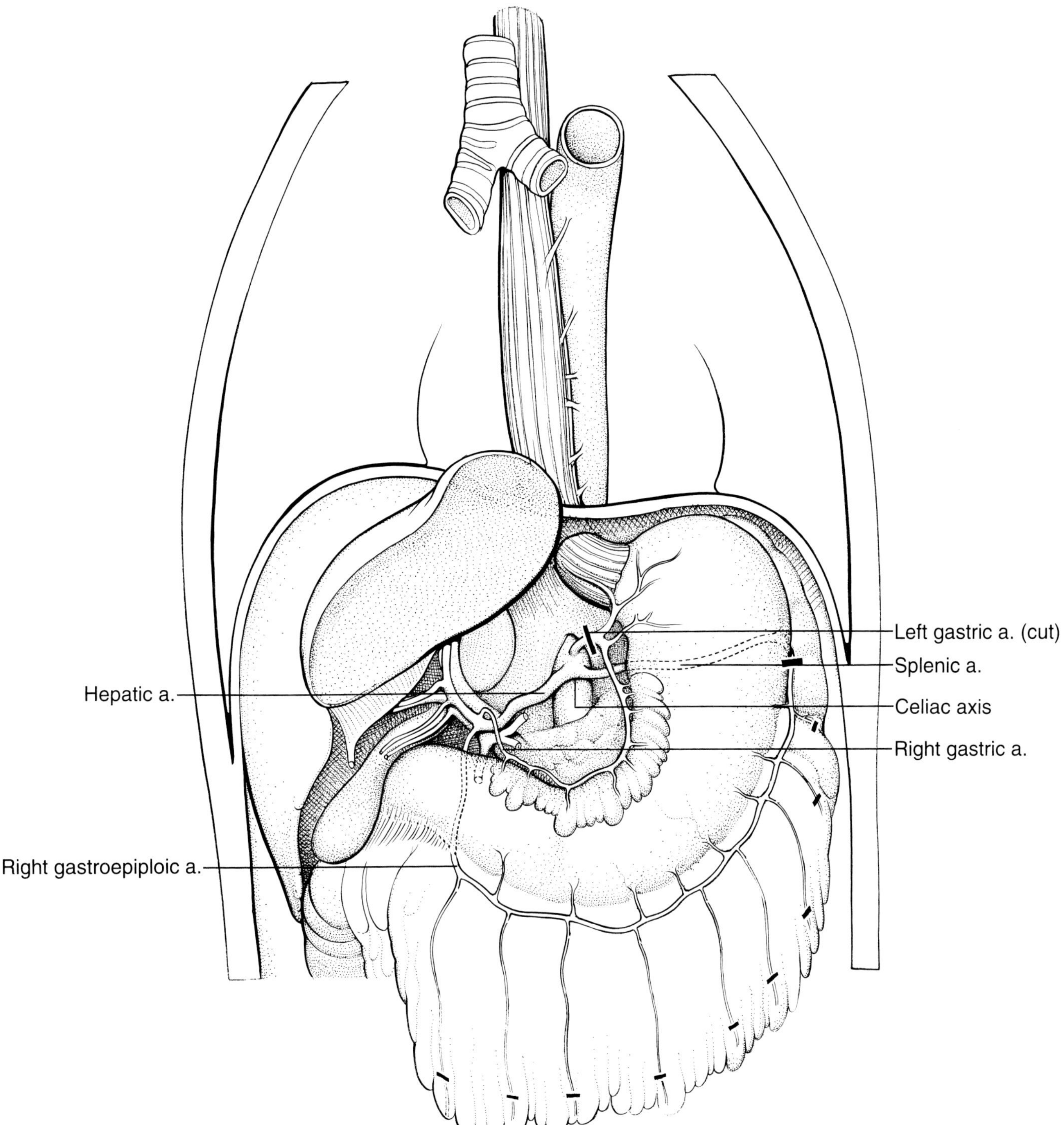
Left gastric a. (cut)
Splenic a.
Hepatic a.
Celiac axis
Right gastric a.
Right gastroepiploic a.

ESOPHAGOGASTRECTOMY

MOBILIZING THE STOMACH

The first step in the procedure of mobilizing the stomach consists of lifting up the omentum and the transverse colon. The surgeon then enters the lesser omental space by going through the outer layer of the omentum while preserving the vascular arcades along the greater curvature of the stomach and being careful to avoid the mesentery of the transverse colon with its middle colic artery. Once this space is identified, the greater curvature of the stomach should be mobilized by dividing the omentum below the appropriate vascular arcades, from the pylorus all the way to the short gastric vessels. Great care and good exposure are necessary to separate the stomach from the spleen by ligating and dividing the short gastric vessels.

Once the left lobe of the liver has been moved to the right, a retracting device may be used to elevate the left and right costal arches while the fundus of the stomach is being mobilized. As the greater curvature is mobilized, it is helpful to identify the intra-abdominal esophagus. This is exposed by opening the peritoneum reflections. Having a nasogastric tube in the stomach is also useful. When the esophagus is freed, it is customary to pass a Penrose drain around it. Traction on the Penrose drain improves exposure.

In this drawing the splenic flexure and spleen are seen. The surgeon's hand is seen being placed into the posterior mediastinum behind the esophagus, which indicates that the lowest esophageal arterial branch from the aorta has been clipped. If the sternum is lifted well and the esophagus is displaced forward, the surgeon has visual access into the thorax and can see or feel some of the vessels. An attempt should be made to maintain hemostasis by using clips or cautery.

It is important that the surgeon, working from below, mobilize upward as much as possible for the esophagus. It is wise to remember that the blood supply to the esophagus comes from the aorta and that more care has to be used in the separation of the esophagus from the aorta than any other aspect of mobilization. The surgeon must be careful to avoid undue compression of the heart. Since the hand is in the posterior mediastinum, it is easy to compress the heart against the sternum. This decreases cardiac filling and cardiac output, with resultant lower blood pressure. The anesthetist should be warned to watch the circulation carefully so that with any undue cardiovascular effect the surgeon can promptly remove his hand. Early use of an "upper-hand" retractor facilitates dissection at the hiatus and in the mediastinum by elevating the sternum, thus increasing the anterioposterior space.

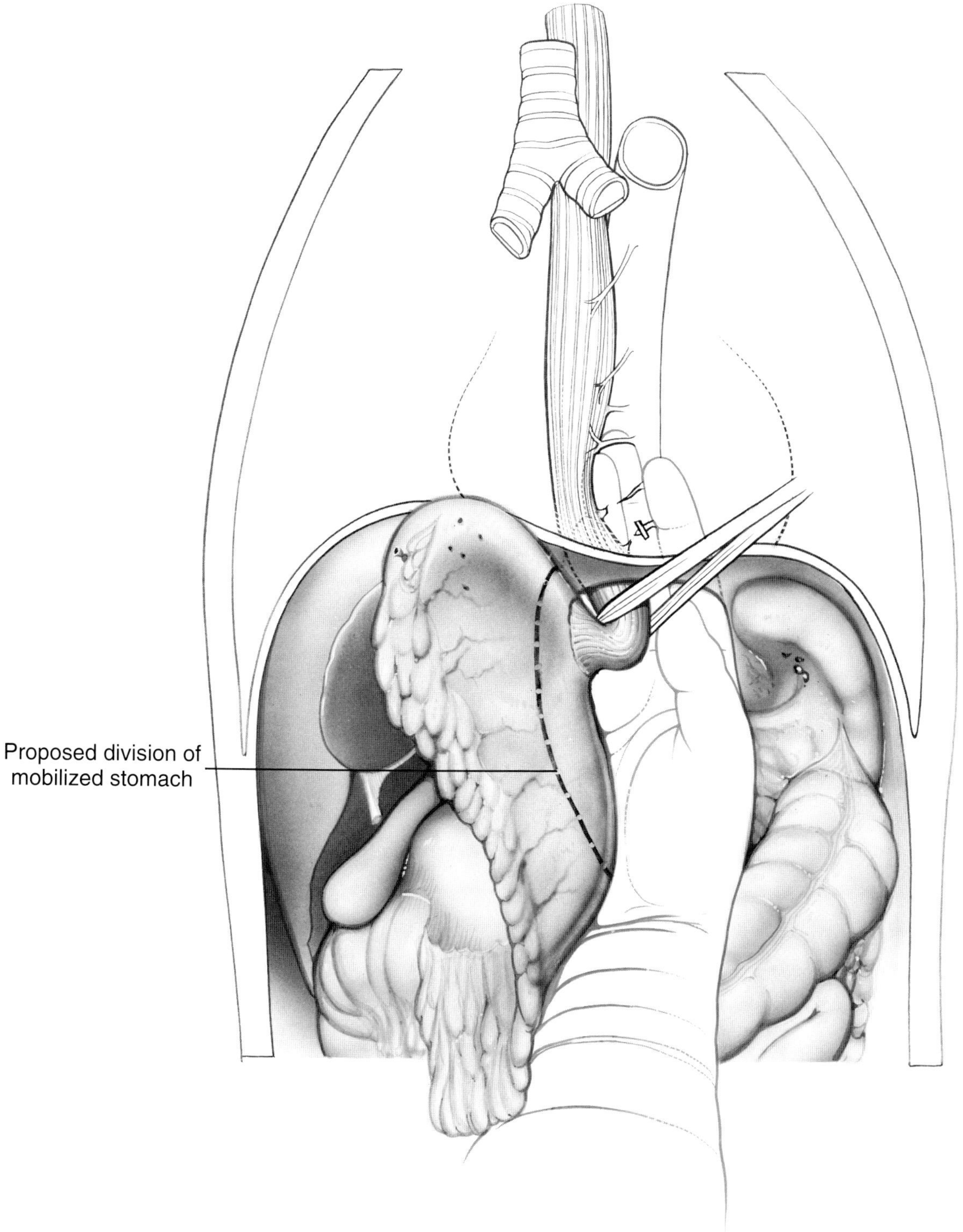
Proposed division of
mobilized stomach

ESOPHAGOGASTRECTOMY

RELEASE OF THE DUODENUM

In this drawing the stomach has been completely mobilized. The left gastric artery has been identified and divided close to where it comes off the celiac axis. Any lymph nodes in the vicinity of the celiac axis should be dissected free for frozen section and for pathologic examination. The lesser curvature should be divided down toward the pylorus, but care must be taken to identify the hepatic artery, gallbladder, and common duct. The dissection should continue close to the pylorus, but under no circumstance should the right gastric artery or any of the hepatic hilar structures be injured. A Kocher maneuver should be done to release the duodenum. Since a complete vagotomy will ensue with the removal of the whole esophagus, it is customary to do a pyloroplasty.

If there has never been any antral or pyloric disease, it is permissible to do a muscle-cutting pyloroplasty, ensuring that the entire pylorus muscle is divided so that there is a gap, and a loose one-finger aperture through the pylorus can be felt. The other conventional pyloroplasty is where the distal antrum, pylorus, and proximal duodenum are opened longitudinally through all layers and the incision is closed transversely in two layers, with an inner continuous chromic catgut layer and an outer interrupted silk suture layer.

After this has been done, the surgeon exerts traction on the esophagus and, with his hand, frees the esophagus in the esophageal hiatus of the diaphragm.

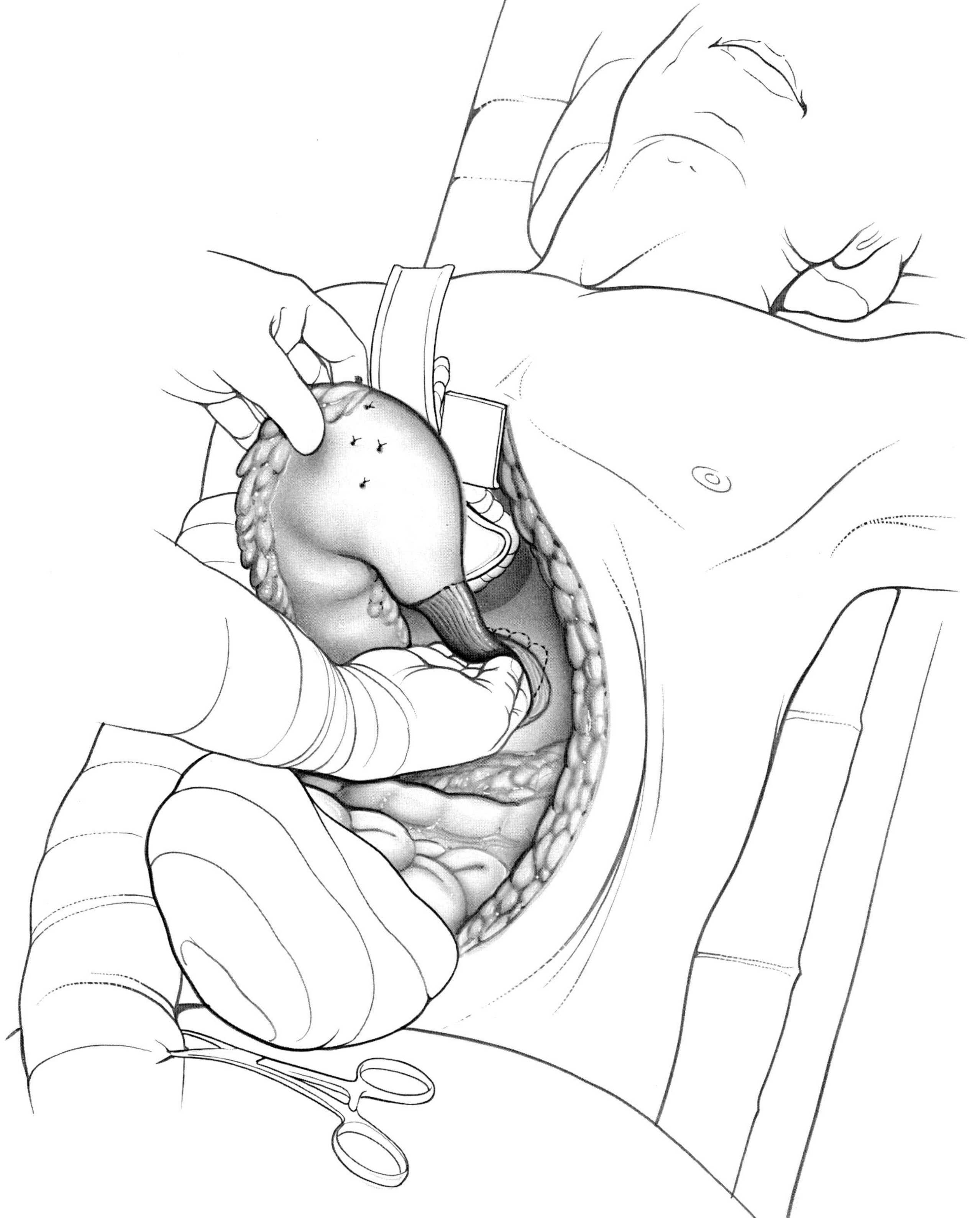

ESOPHAGOGASTRECTOMY

CERVICAL INCISION

In this view we are switching our focus to the patient's neck. There should be some elevation behind the shoulders so that this area becomes prominent. One can use a transverse incision, as depicted here, or an incision along the anterior border of the sternocleidomastoid muscle. After the platysma muscle has been divided, the surgeon should palpate and ascertain the medial location of the carotid artery and internal jugular vein along with the accompanying vagus nerve. A nasogastric tube in the esophagus makes it relatively easy to palpate the location of the esophagus. The sternocleidomastoid muscle is retracted laterally. Here the finger gently mobilizes the esophagus from the spine, which is immediately behind the esophagus. One has to be careful in separating the anterior portion of the esophagus, which is immediately behind the membranous portion of the larynx and the trachea. The artist has shown the course of the right recurrent laryngeal nerve. This branch of the right vagus nerve returns to the neck posterior to the subclavian artery and runs in the tracheoesophageal groove to the upper larynx.

The most difficult part of this mobilization is the avoidance of injury to the right and especially the left recurrent nerve. The vagus nerve gives off the left recurrent nerve at about the level of the aortic arch. The nerve courses posteriorly and medially under and behind the ligamentum arteriosum and joins the tracheoesophageal groove on the left side running up to innervate the left vocal cord. The surgeon must be aware of these nerve structures and safeguard against their injury during the freeing of the esophagus. It is best to do this dissection with the finger and blunt dissecting sponges hugging (but not injuring) the muscularis of the esophagus. Here experience is extremely helpful. Once the esophagus has been mobilized, a Penrose drain is usually passed around it for traction. One dissects far enough cephalad to be certain of adequate proximal length of cervical esophagus to carry out the planned anastomosis to the stomach at this level. This should be a relatively bloodless dissection.

All patients with cancer of the esophagus in the midchest and cephalad must have preliminary bronchoscopy to ensure that the membranous trachea is not involved. Injury to the membranous trachea can occur when the esophagus is mobilized. The stomach is drawn up into the neck and is anastomosed to the cervical esophagus, so that it lies behind the tracheobronchial tree. The stomach's serous covering will adhere and form a closure of any defect in the membraneous portion of the trachea.

Correct postoperative care is essential. To ensure good drainage of both pleural cavities, one or two chest tubes are inserted in each pleural cavity and drainage established by water seal and some suction. It is essential that the patient breathe spontaneously rather than being on positive-pressure anesthesia if there is injury to the membranous trachea. A jet respirator is useful if necessary since it can effect respiration with an open system.

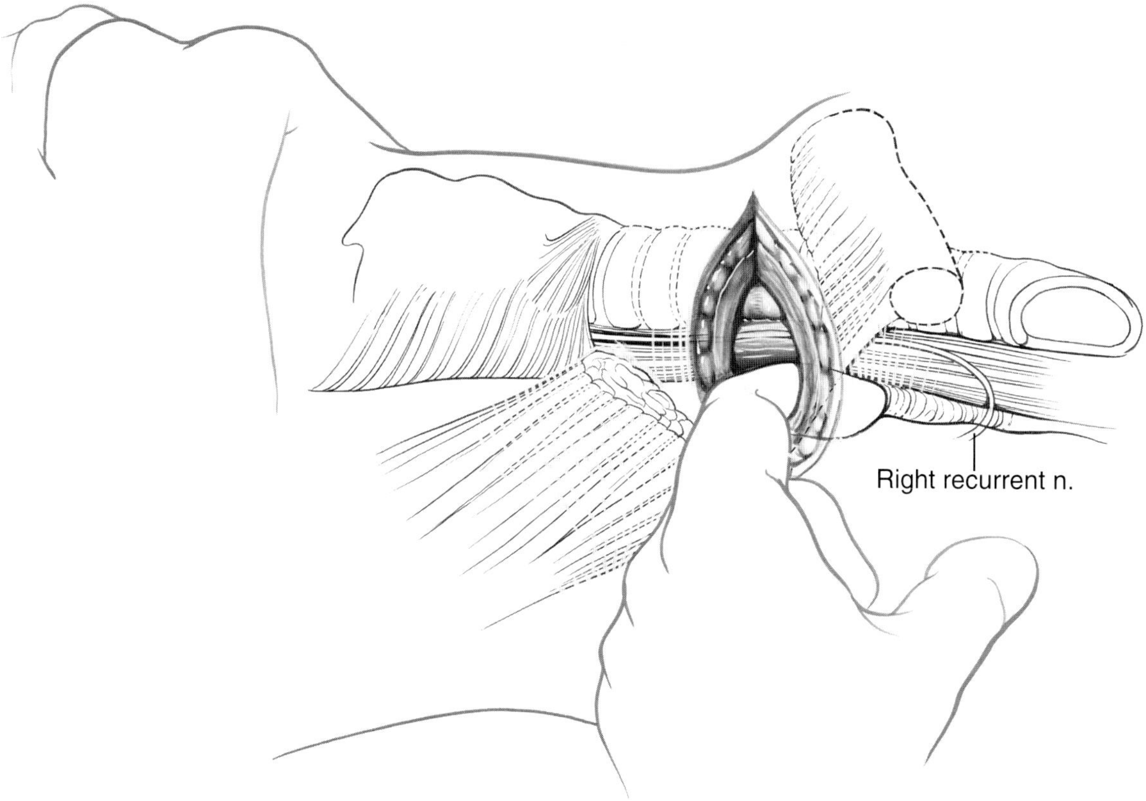
Right recurrent n.

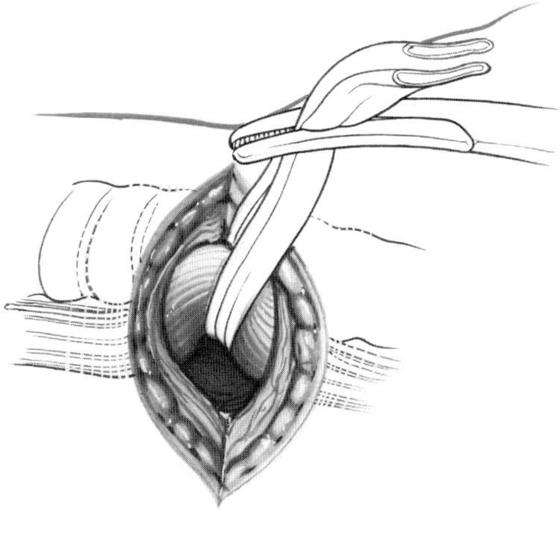

ESOPHAGOGASTRECTOMY

MOBILIZING THE ESOPHAGUS

In this lateral projection, the surgeon's right hand is seen in the posterior mediastinum behind the esophagus and is working from the lower thorax upward, while a finger of the left hand is working from the cervical incision downward. This dissection should continue until the fingers meet. Again one must remember that the branches of aorta can bleed, and to the greatest extent possible, hemostasis should be maintained. The dissection should be close to the esophagus. The surgeon dissects in a blunt fashion working directly on the wall of the esophagus and tumor. The vagus nerves join the esophagus after the right recurrent branch; one must continue to be careful of the recurrent nerves. Only rarely is it necessary to do a thoracotomy to control bleeding or to assist in tumor mobilization. However, opened pleural cavities should be drained and drainage monitored.

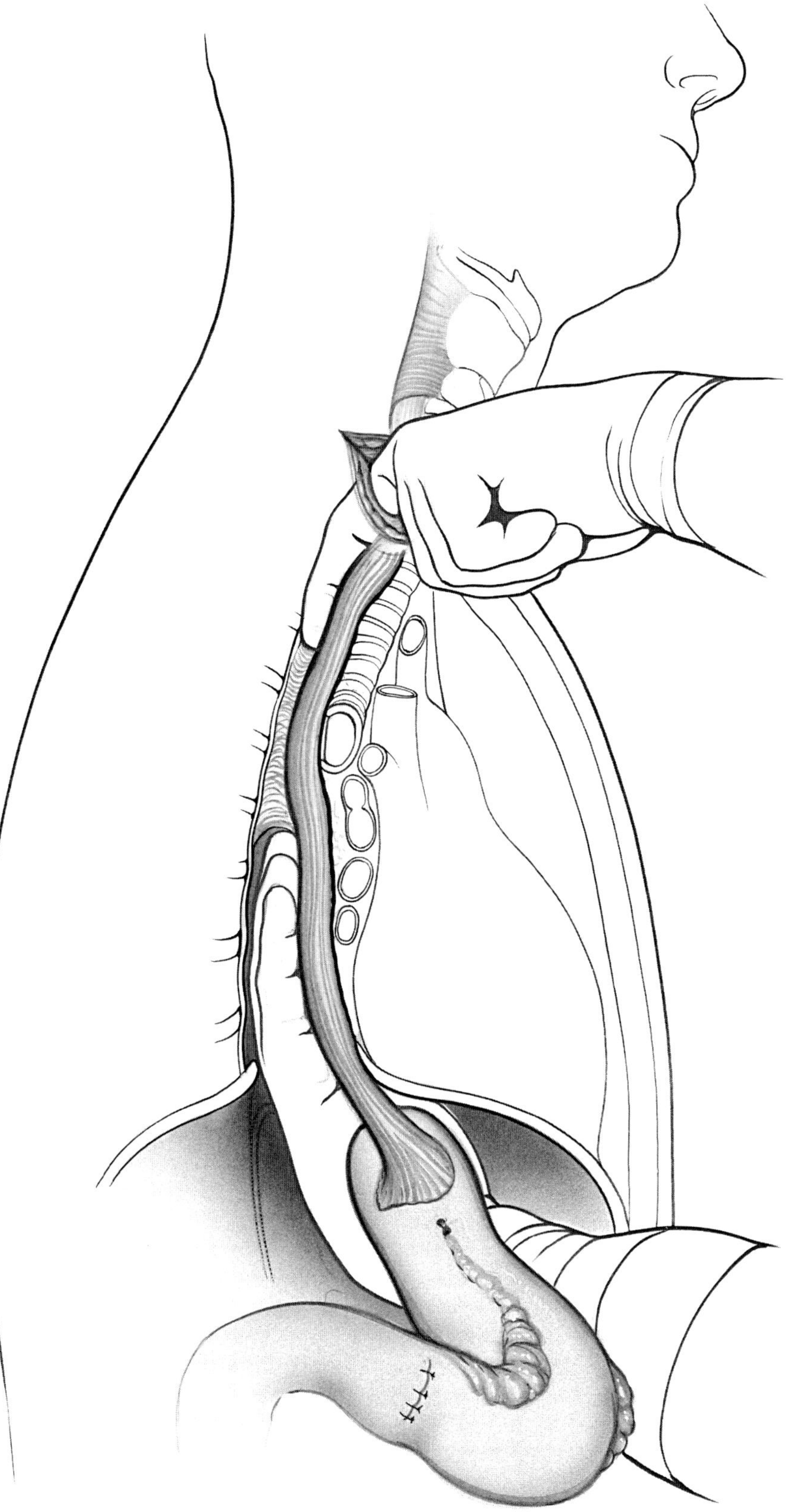

ESOPHAGOGASTRECTOMY

EXCISING THE ESOPHAGUS FROM THE STOMACH

In this stage of the procedure the entire esophagus has been freed, the surgeon is convinced that the operation is completely feasible, and the patient's condition is stable enough to complete the operation. The stapler has been used to excise the distal esophagus free from the stomach. Since there tends to be oozing through the staples on the stomach side, a row of absorbable braided sutures of 3-0 weight has closed the stomach over this staple line. The cervical esophagus has been divided with an adequate stump left for future anastomosis. The divided specimen has then been removed. As depicted here, a Penrose drain has been sewn to the fundus of the stomach and an available catheter has been placed in the posterior mediastinum. One end of the catheter has been attached to the Penrose drain on the stomach, and a hemostat is prepared to draw the catheter, Penrose drain, and stomach upward into the posterior mediastinum.

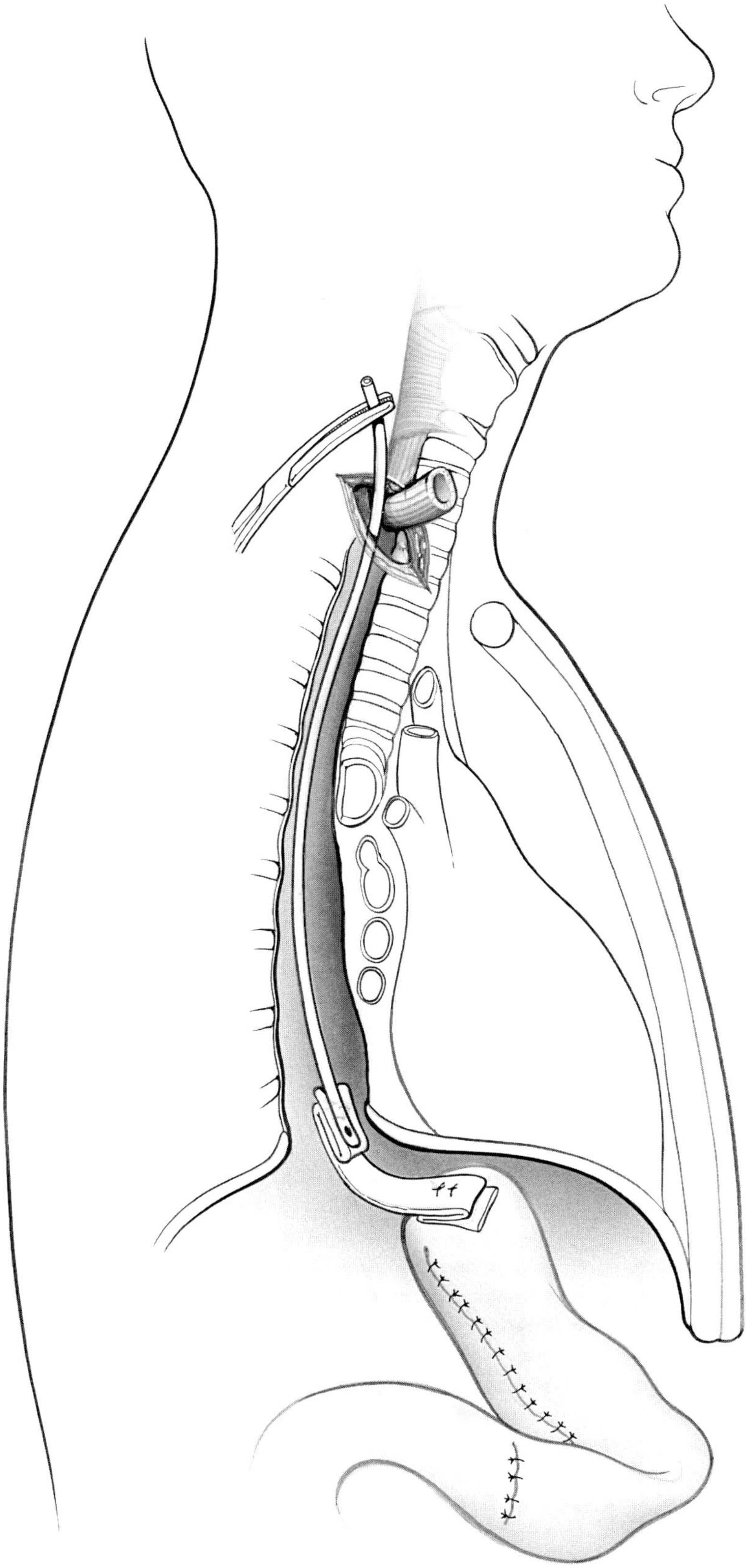

ESOPHAGOGASTRECTOMY

ADVANCING THE STOMACH

As seen here, the stomach is being passed up the posterior mediastinum into the neck. It cannot be stressed enough that the passage of stomach upward is done by pushing rather than pulling. The catheter is primarily a guide applying gentle traction as the hand in the posterior mediastinum advances the stomach. It is of the utmost importance that the opening in the esophageal hiatus be sufficiently large to accommodate the stomach, which is larger than was the esophagus. The esophageal hiatus can be manually stretched, or a stapling device can make a stapled "V" incision in the esophageal hiatus toward the right. The esophageal hiatus must be able to admit four fingers comfortably to be certain there is room for the stomach.

The stomach must be advanced and passed up the mediastinum into the neck with absolutely no rotation. The surgeon must be careful to see exactly where the lesser curvature and greater curvatures are so that as the stomach advances up the chest into the neck, the lesser curvature is kept exactly to the right and the greater curvature exactly to the left.

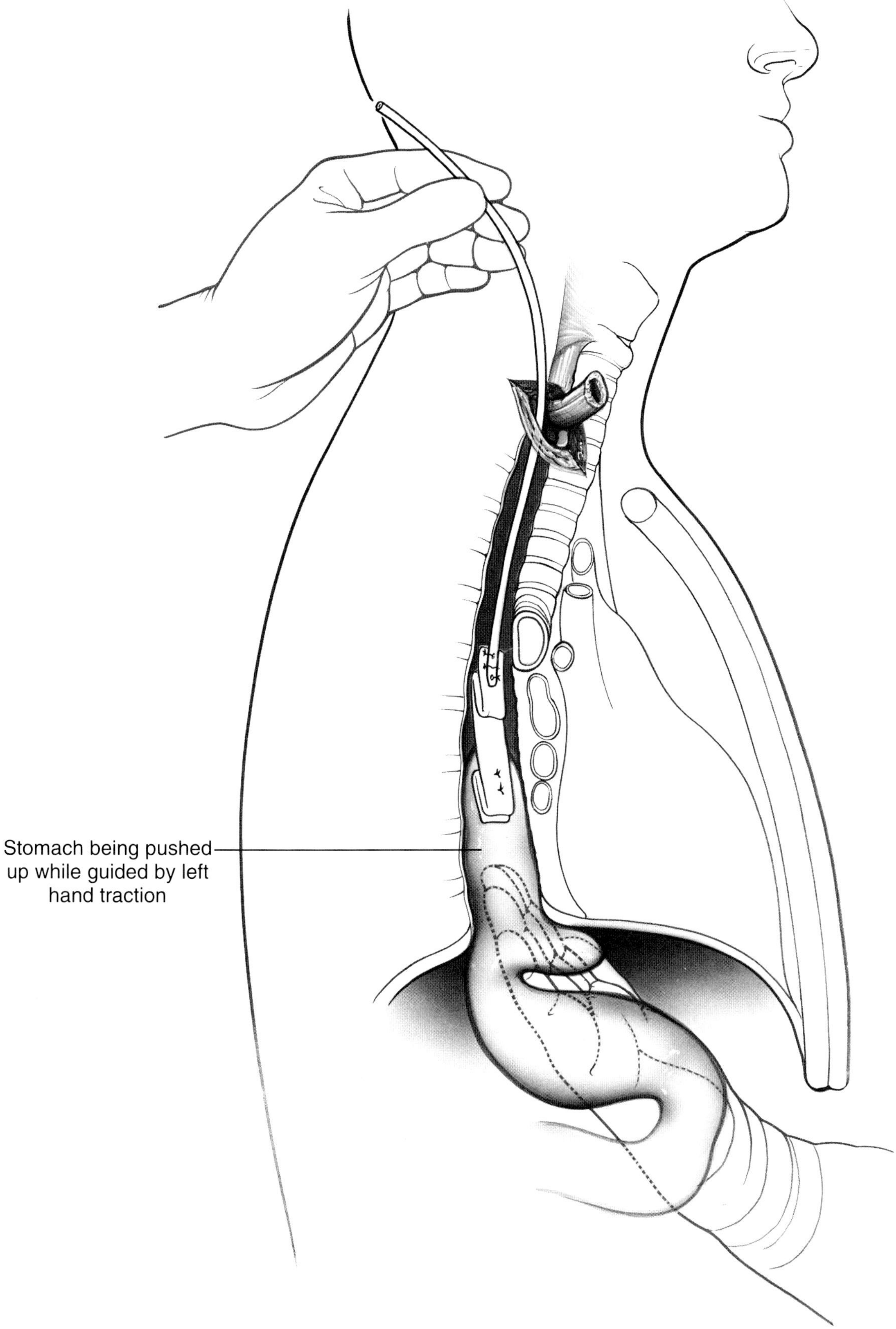
Stomach being pushed up while guided by left hand traction

ESOPHAGOGASTRECTOMY

ANASTOMOSIS

Again we are looking at this operation in its lateral aspect. The stomach has been passed upward far enough that the fundus can be gently drawn outside the cervical incision, as is shown in the inserted drawing. In similar fashion the esophageal cervical stump is long enough that it, to, can be drawn outside the cervical incision. The appropriate-sized opening has been made in the fundus of the stomach away from the lesser curvature closure. The sewn Penrose drain area is removed. The opening in the stomach matches the spread esophageal opening above. In this drawing a one-layer anastomosis is being made. Usually we place the two-angle sutures, followed by a posterior layer of interrupted sutures through all layers. All the sutures are placed before any of the knots are tied. After the sutures have been placed they are tied successively. There must be good mucosa-to-mucosa coaptation. After the posterior row has been placed, a continuing series of interrupted all-layer sutures is placed anteriorly. Silk sutures were previously used, but absorbable braided sutures do better.

An alternative technique is to use a two-layer anastomosis. The posterior row angle sutures are placed first, catching the muscularis and submucosa of the esophagus to the serosa and muscular layer of the stomach. They are completed, tied, and cut. An inner posterior mucosal row is placed next by using interrupted sutures. They are tied and cut. The anterior mucosal row is placed. The anterior outer row is placed last.

After the completion of the anastomosis, the anastomosis is replaced in the mediastinum. The nasogastric tube, which had been drawn up into the cervical esophagus before esophagectomy, should be passed down into the stomach after the posterior row of the anastomosis is done. It is important to drain the neck. A counterincision is made laterally, and a Penrose drain is passed into the posterior mediastinum. Following this the incision is closed anteriorly.

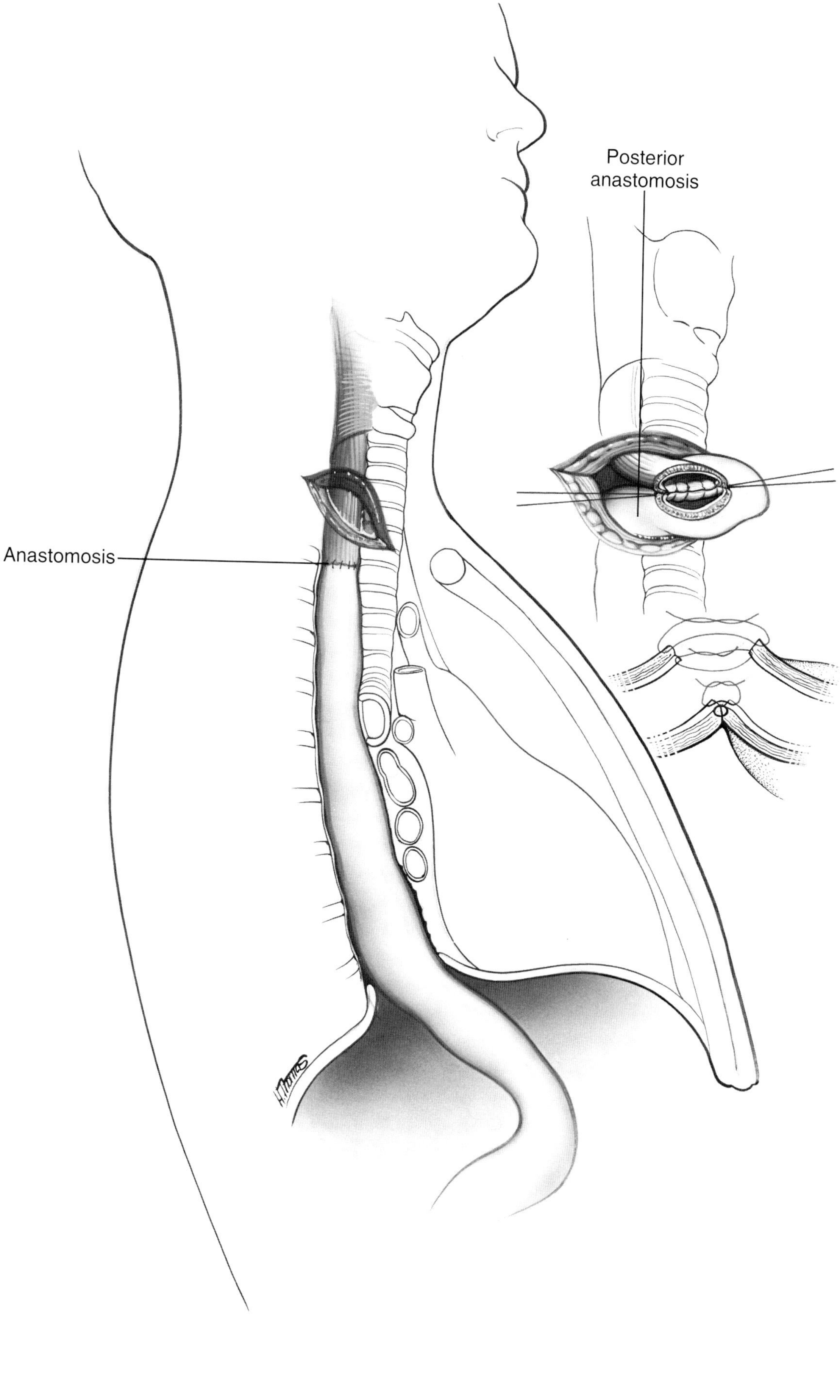
Posterior
anastomosis
Anastomosis

LESIONS IN THE LOWER ESOPHAGUS

Lesions around the lower esophagus, the cardia, or the fundus of the stomach extending upward into the distal esophagus can be satisfactorily handled through the left chest. The classic approach is a left lateral thoracotomy with the incision at about the seventh interspace in a standard-sized man. This permits good exposure of the thoracic esophagus from the diaphragm to the aortic arch. The aortic arch is somewhat of a limiting factor because it is relatively immobile. If the surgeon believes that the resulting anastomosis of the esophagus to the stomach can be satisfactorily done at the level of the aortic arch and slightly below, the left side has many advantages.

The left thoracotomy in the seventh interspace combined with an incision through the diaphragm readily exposes the stomach and gives relatively good access to the upper abdomen. If one has reason to believe that this will not provide adequate exposure of the stomach, one can always make a counterlaporatomy incision in the abdomen. Here one can use a midline laporatomy. If necessary one can cut across the costal arch and combine a thoracotomy with midline laporatomy, giving outstanding exposure of the left chest and most of the upper abdomen. The disadvantages of this approach are that the chest is less stable and that one has to remember the course of the phrenic nerve. The phrenic nerve enters the chest crossing anteriorly to the anterior scalene muscle, and as it comes into the chest along the innominate veins, it descends in the thorax and comes to lie directly anterior to the lung hila. It then descends along the lateral wall of the pericardium and innervates the anteromedial portion of the diaphragm. From this location the fibers arc and stream laterally and posteriorly. In consequence, if one makes an incision from the esophageal hiatus on the left to the costal arch anteriorly close to the pericardium, most of the diaphragm will be denervated. To avoid this, one can carry a curved incision from the esophageal hiatus around the chest wall laterally so that a small rim of diaphragm is left attached to the thoracic wall, but the major part of the diaphragm is well innervated from the anteromedial phrenic location.

ESOPHAGEAL MOBILIZATION IN LEFT THORACOTOMY

EXPOSURE

In this view we are looking at the mediastinum through a lateral thoracotomy in the seventh interspace. The lung is being retracted anteriorly. The diaphragm is retracted somewhat caudad. The aorta can be seen lying anterior and lateral to the spine. The mediastinal pleura between the lung and aorta has been opened. Two stay sutures are in position to visualize the underlying esophagus, with the left vagus nerve lying on the esophagus.

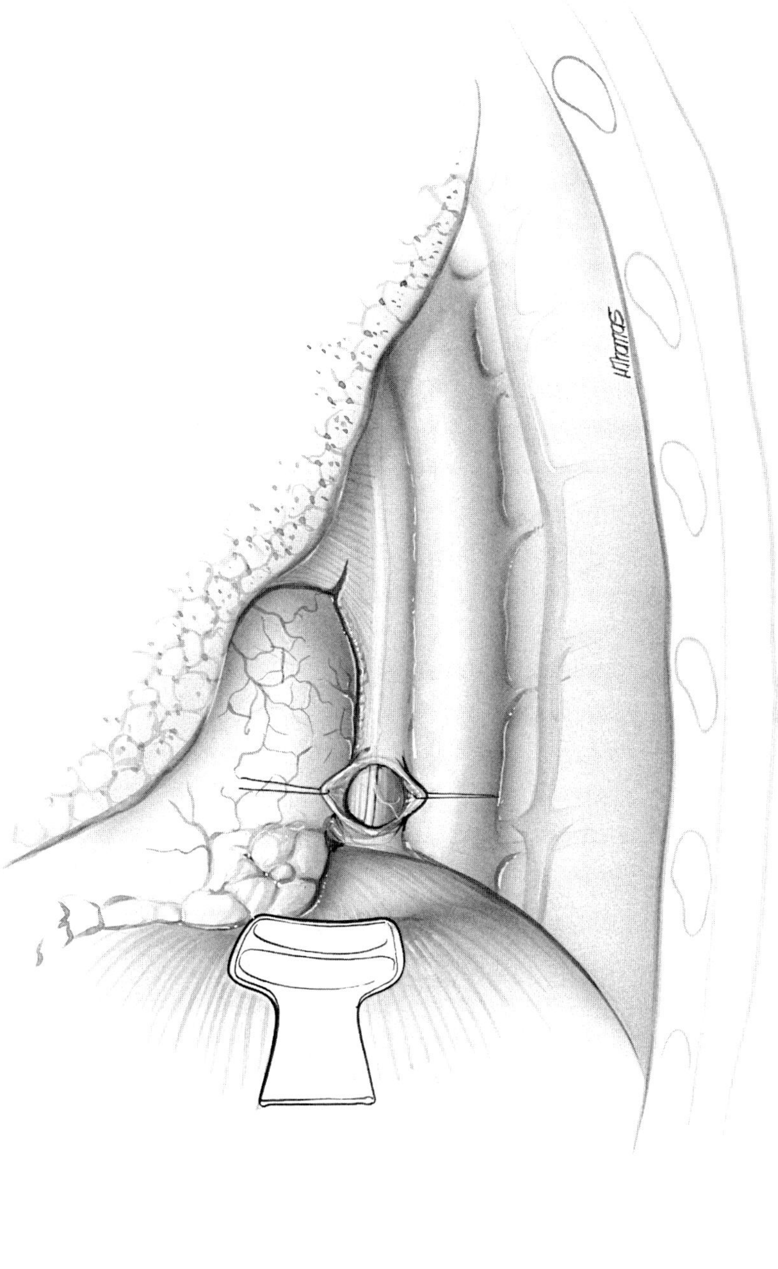

ESOPHAGEAL MOBILIZATION IN LEFT THORACOTOMY

RETRACTING THE ESOPHAGUS

In this view we are looking at the posterior mediastinum through a left lateral thoracotomy. The esophagus has been mobilized in the lower thorax below the aortic arch. An incision can be seen in the mediastinal pleura. The esophagus is being retracted with a Penrose drain. The vagus nerve can be seen running along its left side. The aorta is posterior to the right, and two branches from the aorta to the esophagus are visible at this level. An incision has been made posterolaterally in the diaphragm, and two suture ligatures have been placed both for traction exposure and to control bleeding. The hemostat has been placed in the abdomen under the diaphragm and is being brought out adjacent to the esophagus in its left lateral side. It is important that when this is done an exploring finger makes sure that the undersurface of the diaphragm is free and no injury is made to the underlying spleen, stomach, kidney, or whatever might inadvertently be approached. The planned incision here in the diaphragm is going to be in a posterolateral direction to preserve the innervation of the anterior portion of the diaphragm as discussed above. If this exposure were not adequate we could continue the most lateral portion of this incision around anteriorly, leaving a rim of attached diaphragm inside the chest wall.

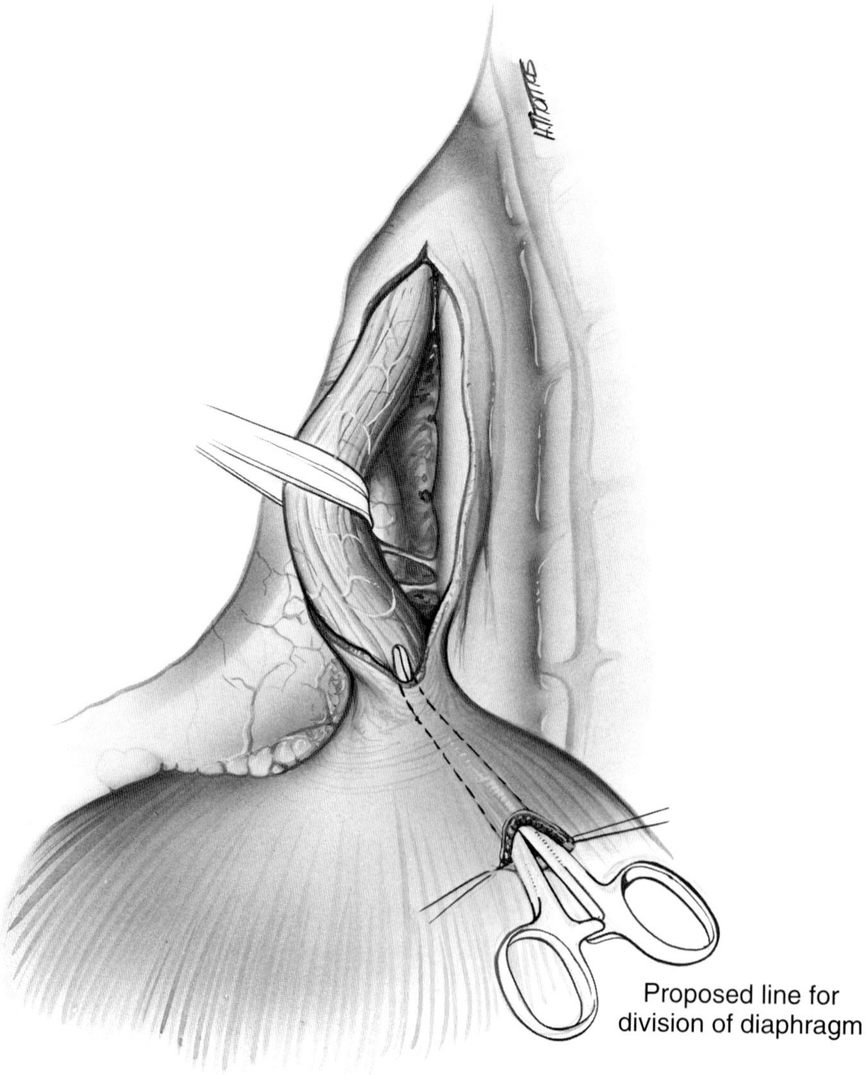

ESOPHAGEAL MOBILIZATION IN LEFT THORACOTOMY

OPENING THE DIAPHRAGM

In this drawing we have the same approach and view as the last drawing. The diaphragm has been opened. This can be done in one of two ways. A relatively easy way is to take a large stapling device of 90 mm and one with one or two passes open the diaphragm. The other alternative is to open it with scissors and clamp the blood vessels as one goes. Then the surgeon places mattress sutures with a hemostat tag so that the weight of the hemostat and the suture will retract and fold the divided leaf of the diaphragm out of the surgeon's way.

In this drawing we are now looking at the stomach from above with the spleen posteriorly and laterally to the left of the stomach but protruding through this incision. The cardia of the stomach is still attached and bound to the medial portion of this esophageal hiatus with peritoneum reflected around it.

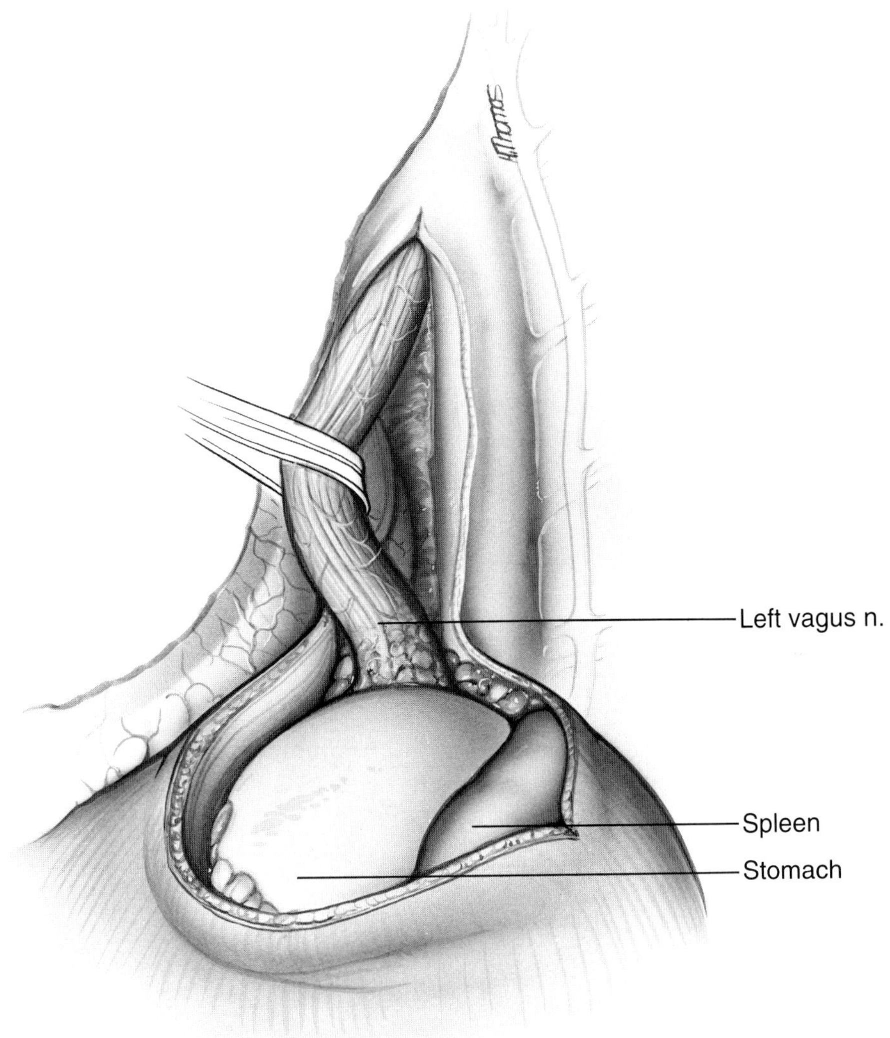

ESOPHAGEAL MOBILIZATION IN LEFT THORACOTOMY

MOBILIZING THE ESOPHAGUS AND STOMACH

Here the artist has drawn what we plan to do in esophageal mobilization to treat this cancer located at the cardia involving the contiguous stomach and the lower esophagus. Our first approach is to mobilize the esophagus from the esophageal hiatus and to mobilize the stomach as widely as necessary to remove all of the tumor. Again it is important to maintain as much of the gastric blood supply as possible. The short gastric vessels have to be divided. The left gastroepiploic vessels will have to be divided high on the greater curvature. Some mobilization of the lesser curvature will be necessary. The surgeon enters the lesser omental space and preserves the gastroepiploic arcades, avoiding the blood supply to the transverse colon. The left gastric artery must be ligated close to the celiac axis and the arcades along the lesser curvature preserved. The right gastric artery is preserved. Care is taken to protect the biliary structures and blood vessels. Any lymph nodes found along the lesser curvature should be removed with the specimen if possible. Other available lymph nodes of the specimen to be removed should be included. The artist has drawn a proposed line of stomach resection. This is done with a stapling device after the specimen has been mobilized. We close the stomach over the staple line with interrupted sutures to minimize oozing. Next the esophagus is divided and the specimen is sent to the pathology department for frozen-section examination of the surgical margins. Carcinoma can have "skip areas" in the esophagus.

There has been controversy about how radical to be in resecting the thoracic esophagus for carcinoma. Opinions vary from the extremes of gastric pullthrough, with no attempt to remove any thoracic lymph nodes, to extensive meticulous lymph node dissection with en bloc operations. Our policy when we are directly freeing the esophagus is to remove all visible lymph nodes with appropriate labeling and staging. If residual tumor is found in the mediastinum or abdomen that is not amenable to surgical removal, internal radiotherapy with Iodine-125 (I-125) seed implantation or I-125 seed suture placement can be used, or catheters can be left for afterloading of internal radiotherapy.

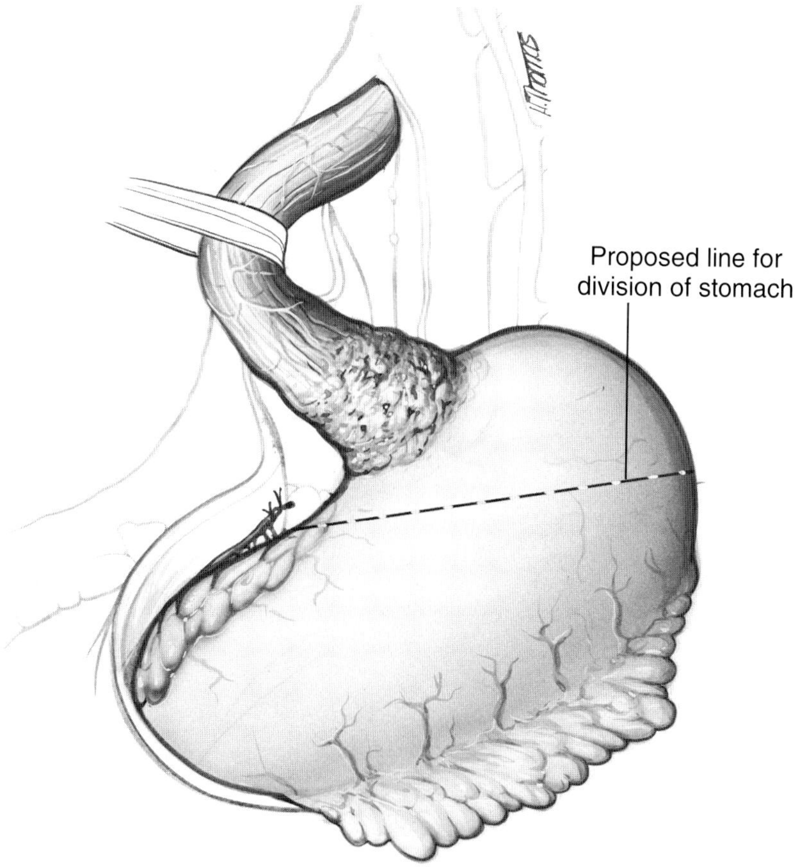

ESOPHAGEAL MOBILIZATION IN LEFT THORACOTOMY

ANASTOMOSIS

In this view we see the mediastinum through a left thoracotomy. The mobilized stomach is in the thorax. The lesser curvature of the stomach is kept in a position of nonrotation so that it faces the mediastinum. The greater curvature, with its arcades and some of the omental apron fat, is lateral. A small incision is made in the anterior surface of the stomach in a location with good blood supply not too close to any of the arcades. The stapling device with its pointer attachment protruding from the anvil is inserted into the stomach and brought through the fundus cephalic to the suture line or blood vessels. The touch of an electrocautery on the pointerhead may ease its perforation of the stomach wall. The pointer head is removed and the hammer portion of the device with its supporting rod inserted.

For easier handling the esophagus is dilated. To dilate the esophagus a pursestring suture is placed and the esophagus is divided in a transverse fashion. Three long Allis clamps can be used to grasp and triangulate the esophagus with gentle traction. A Foley catheter is placed in the esophagus, and the balloon is inflated. The inflating balloon gently dilates the esophagus. The detachable hammer makes it easier to place as large a device as possible. The hammer is "rocked" into place. The pursestring is ligated to ensure that it is firmly in place with esophagus around it.

In this drawing the esophagus has been prepared with a pursestring suture that is untied. An Allis clamp is holding a portion of the esophagus as the anvil portion of the device is inserted. The esophagus should fit snugly about the rod of the stapling device between the hammer and anvil. The stomach also fits closely on the same rod.

Once the stomach is in the chest with no tension, the instrument in place, and the hammer portion covered by esophagus, the screw device brings the esophagus and stomach together. The hammer abuts the anvil. There are appropriate marks on the stapler that indicate when the appropriate amount of compression of the stomach and esophagus has occurred. The surgeon should palpate the junction of the hammer and anvil to ensure there is no soft tissue or foreign material in the way. Without rotating the esophagus or stomach, the stapler is firmly fired. This places the two concentric rows of staples and at the same time cuts away two "donuts" of stomach and esophagus. With the stapler still closed, the surgeon gently turns the stapler to free it. The device is withdrawn and disassembled so that the two donuts of tissue can be inspected. Less than a complete circle indicates that the anastomosis may be incomplete. The anastomosis is inspected to ensure that there is good approximation between the stomach and esophagus. In stapling the anastomosis there is a chance of stricture, especially in small anastomoses. It is therefore important to monitor these patients postoperatively and, if necessary, initiate early dilatation. Usually one or two dilatations will remedy early stricture formation. The defect in the anterior stomach through which the device was inserted is closed. The diaphragm is closed to permit passage of the stomach plus insertion of two fingers. Usually we attach the stomach to the diaphragm opening with a few sutures. A nasogastric tube is advanced into the stomach after the anastomosis is complete. While the specimen is being removed, the nasogastric tube is pulled up into the esophagus. Two chest tubes are placed to water-seal drainage. One tube is low and posterior for drainage; the other tube is anterior and higher for air leaks. The chest is closed in the usual fashion. If the right pleural space has been entered, a right chest tube is placed for drainage.

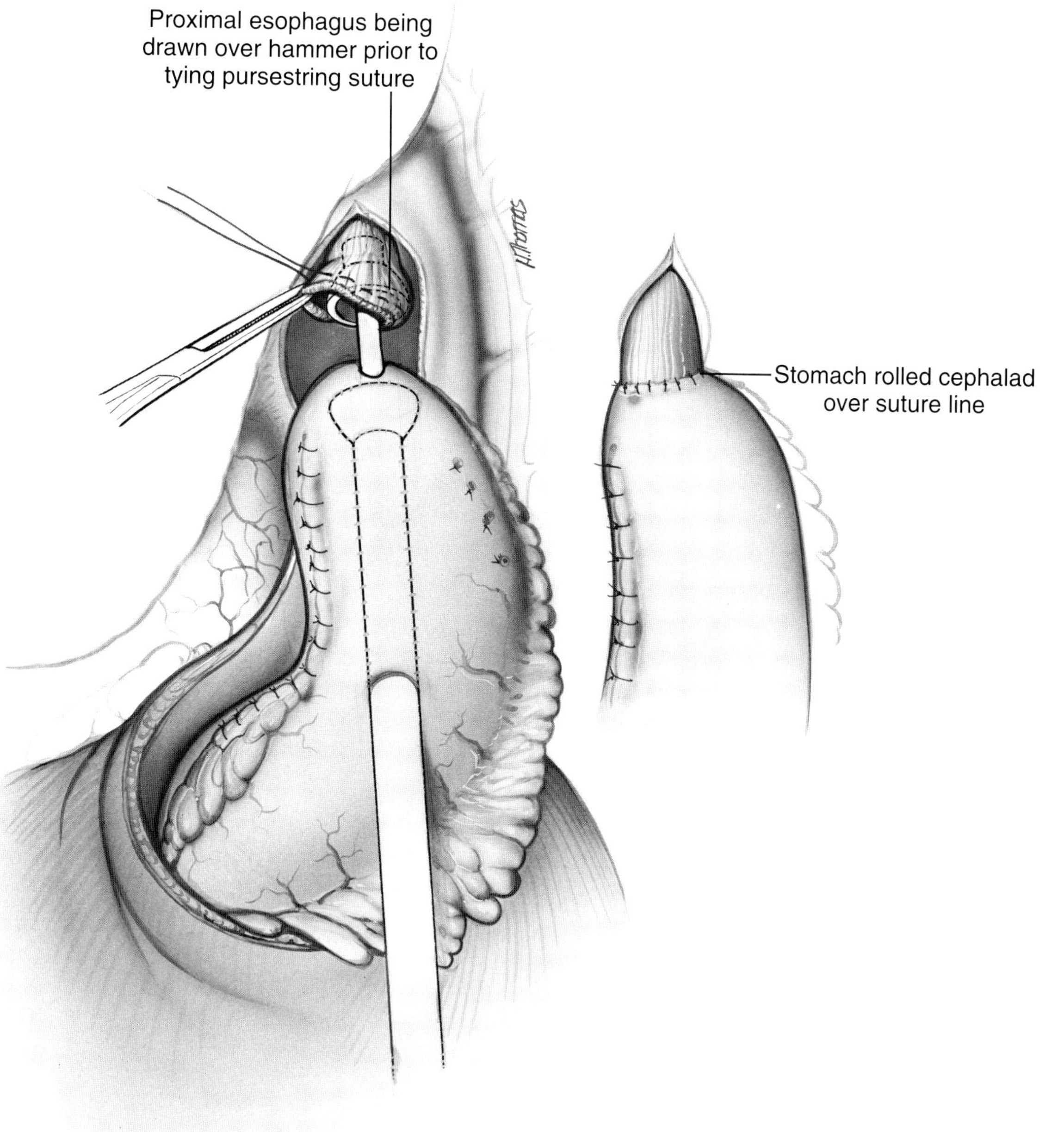

Proximal esophagus being drawn over hammer prior to tying pursestring suture
Stomach rolled cephalad over suture line

ESOPHAGEAL MOBILIZATION IN RIGHT THORACOTOMY

If the esophagus to be removed is above the cardia but well below the sternal notch, we prefer a laporatomy and right thoracotomy with the anastomosis of the esophagus to the stomach high in the right chest. The inferior vena cava on the right side prevents a right thoracotomy from giving the exposure that one can get on the left. This right operation can be done in two ways. One is to place the patient in an anterolateral position by elevating the buttocks, usually with use of the so-called "bean bag" mattress. This mattress, when evacuated of air, becomes firm in whatever shape it had before the air was evacuated. With the patient in an anterolateral position the operating table can be rotated to the right so that the patient is more supine or the table can be rotated to the left so the patient is more lateral. If this position is not precise, the surgeon will find it is difficult to operate. The advantage of this approach is that one can do a laporatomy first and ensure that there are no contraindications to surgery and that all is resectable before carrying out any irreversible steps. The chest as far back as the spine and anteriorly to the sternum plus the entire abdomen must be prepped and available.

The alternative to this approach is to put the patient in a supine position, prepare the abdomen, and carry out a midline laporatomy. The surgeon explores the abdomen to ensure that there are no contraindications and proceeds to mobilize the stomach. This has already been described in our previous illustrations (see figures on pp. 205, 207, and 209). After the stomach has been mobilized, one can enlarge the esophageal hiatus with a stapling device to permit the stomach's placement. The abdomen is then closed. The patient is repositioned in a straight lateral position, reprepared, and redraped and the operation continues as part two. A right thoracotomy is carried out. The esophagus is mobilized. The mobilized stomach can be drawn up gently into the chest as high as necessary. The esophagus is resected, and then the esophagogastrectomy is performed. The right chest is then closed in routine fashion.

EXPOSURE

In this view we are looking at the right chest and right mediastinum from the right thoracotomy. The chest is opened widely. The right lung is being retracted anteriorly, and an incision has been made over the mediastinum in the vicinity of the azygos vein. The azygos vein can be seen coursing anteriorly to join the superior vena cava. The azygos vein is seen both coming up the anterolateral surface of the lower spine and descending the anterolateral surface of the upper spine. It will have to be divided to give a clear view of the mediastinum. It should be ligated near the superior vena cava and a suture ligature placed to reinforce this ligature. Posteriorly one can ligate the descending and ascending azygos veins so that there is no possibility of slippage and no suture ligature is needed.

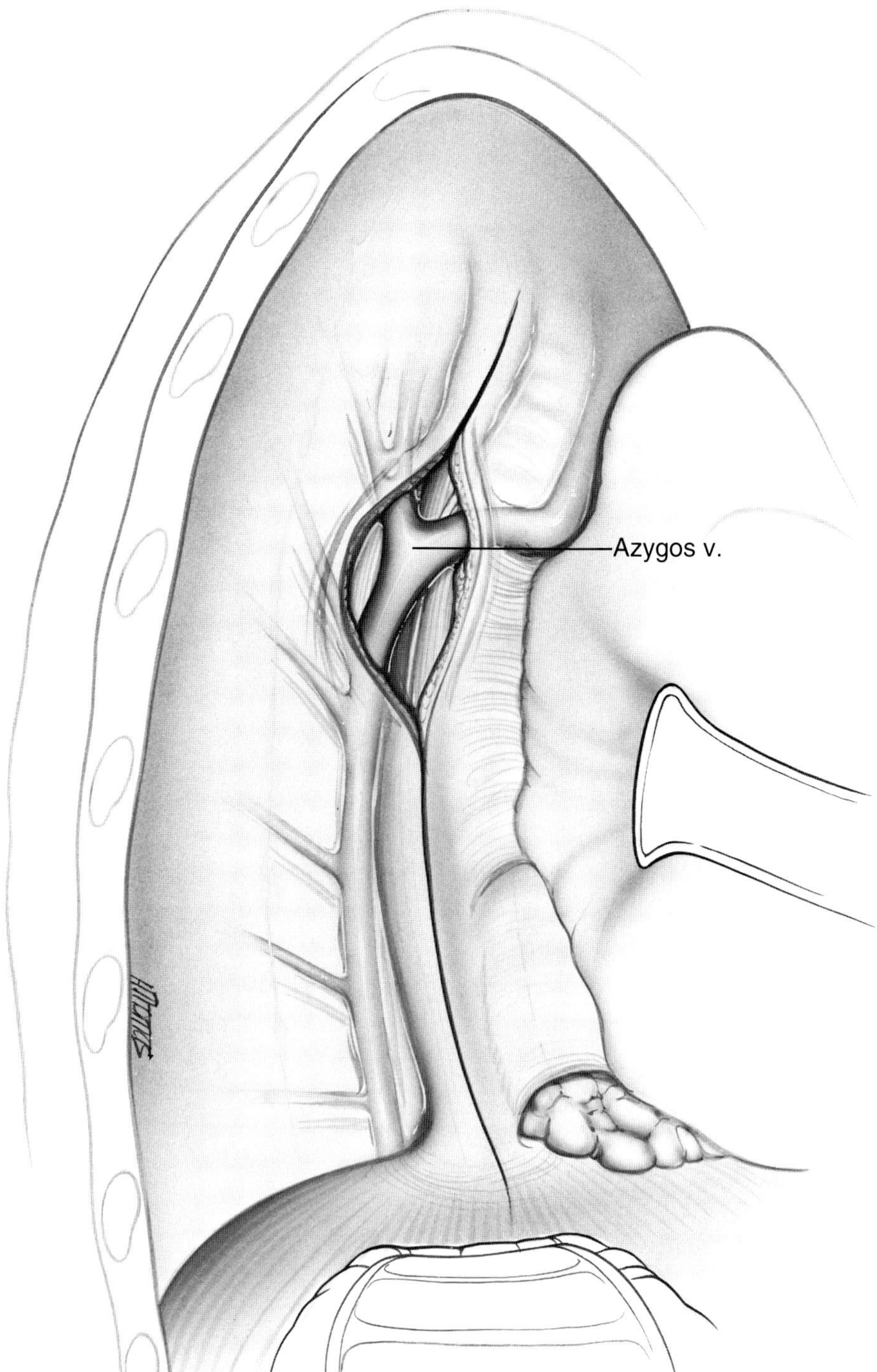
Azygos v.

ESOPHAGEAL MOBILIZATION IN RIGHT THORACOTOMY

FREEING THE ESOPHAGUS

In this view the mediastinal pleura has been opened widely from the diaphragm to the apex of the chest. The azygos vein has been ligated and suture ligated posteriorly. One can see the esophagus with the tumor below the bifurcation of the trachea. The right vagus nerve can be seen, and one can glimpse the left vagus nerve behind the freed esophagus. The posterior portion of the trachea and the right mainstem bronchus are visible. For a tumor in this location the lymph nodes from the esophageal hiatus up to the subcarinal area must be removed with the specimen. Whether or not one would remove a portion of the left pleura and pericardium would depend on whether tumor was thought to involve these structures. It is our practice to look for the vessels supplying the esophagus and to ligate them close to the aorta with 3-0 ties. Usually two small clips will suffice. If the tumor is higher in the chest, it is essential that bronchoscopy be done in advance. One must be careful not to injure the membranous portion of the tracheobronchial tree. One must remember the location of the right recurrent nerve high near the subclavian artery. The left recurrent nerve will travel with the left vagus nerve until it crosses the ligamentum arteriosum to ascend in the tracheoesophageal groove on the left side.

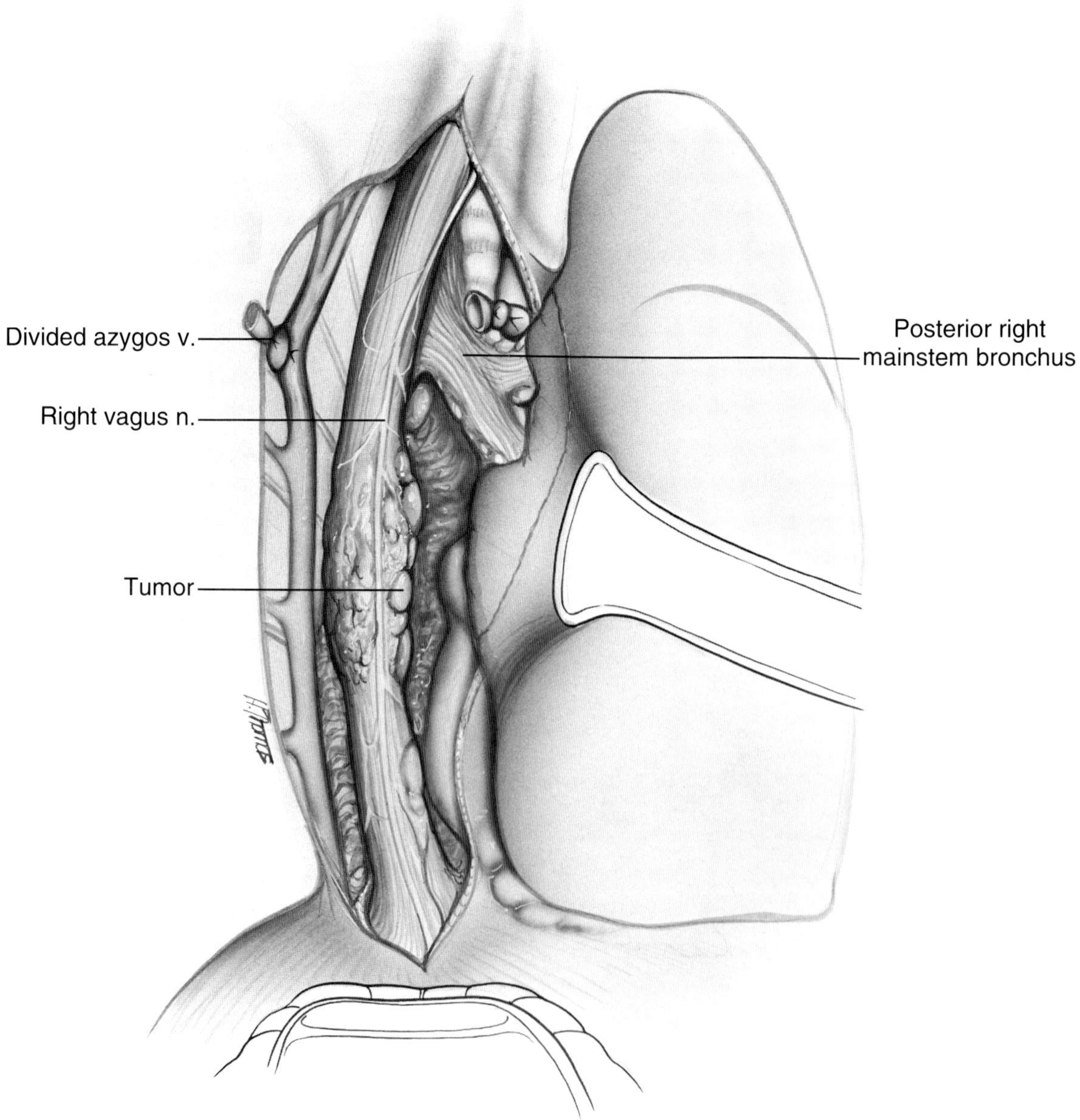

ESOPHAGEAL MOBILIZATION IN RIGHT THORACOTOMY

ADVANCING THE STOMACH

Dissection of the esophagus has been completed. The esophagus is free well above the tumor in the upper chest. The aorta can be seen quite plainly. Branches of the aorta crossing the spine as right intercostal arteries are clearly visible. The mobilized stomach has now been drawn through the enlarged esophageal hiatus into the chest. Care has been taken to ensure that the lesser curvature faces the right and the greater curvature faces the left so that there is no rotation of the stomach. Care must also be taken that there is no rotation of the esophagus. The trachea can be seen. The subcarinal lymph node packet should be removed.

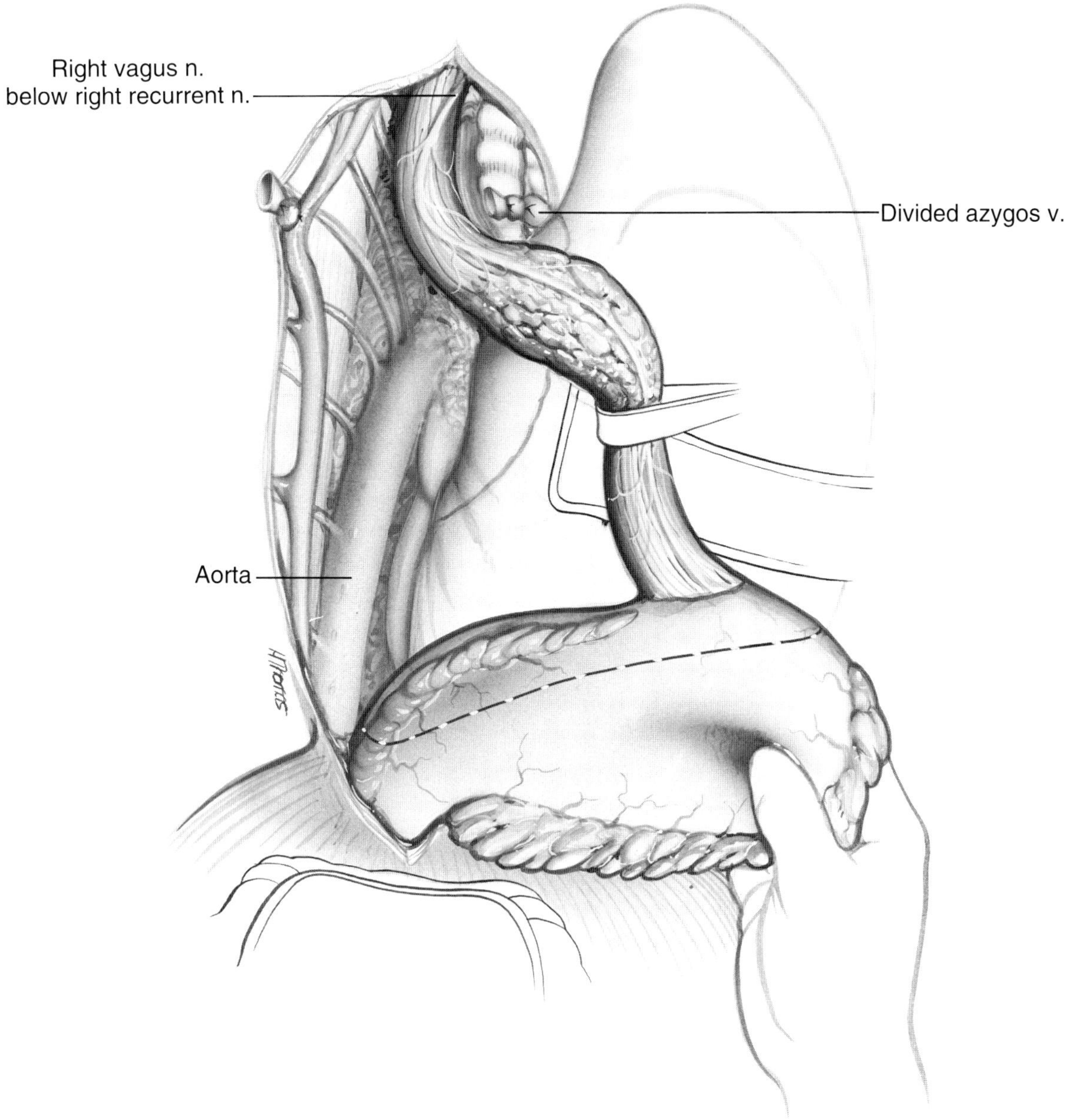

ESOPHAGEAL MOBILIZATION IN RIGHT THORACOTOMY

ANASTOMOSIS

Again we are looking into the right thoracotomy. The stomach is seen anastomosed to the esophagus. In this case it is about half way up from the carina. The stump of the right vagus nerve is seen. The lesser curvature of the stomach faces us. The stomach specimen has been amputated with the stapler. Interrupted sutures covering the staple line are seen. The surgeon has checked that the esophageal hiatus is not too tight. Two fingers should comfortably fit in the esophageal hiatus. There should be no tension, and we do not ordinarily sew the stomach to the hiatus at this point. This is an option. The nasogastric tube was withdrawn when the esophagus was excised, and it has been advanced down into the stomach for gastric drainage after we have completed the anastomosis. All the precautions and techniques mentioned about the use of the stapler have been applied. Not visible but present is a small anterior gastrotomy through which the stapling device had been passed into the stomach and up into the esophagus.

Two chest tubes will be placed for drainage, and the thoracotomy incision will be closed. If the left pleural cavity has been opened, a left chest tube should be placed. A chest x-ray is taken. If there is any suggestion of air, fluid, or blunting of the left costophrenic angle, a chest tube is placed in the left chest.

We ordinarily do the anastomosis as high in the right chest as possible. If placed high, the stomach can be sutured to the chest apex where the esophagus enters the chest. This affords less chance of an esophageal leak into the chest since the stomach will seal the thorax.

It is our routine after thoracotomy to wash out the thoracic cavity with tepid distilled water to remove all debris. This is also a means of detecting any air leak or bleeding. If the other pleural cavity has been opened, it should be drained. Blood loss must be accurately measured in all these procedures.

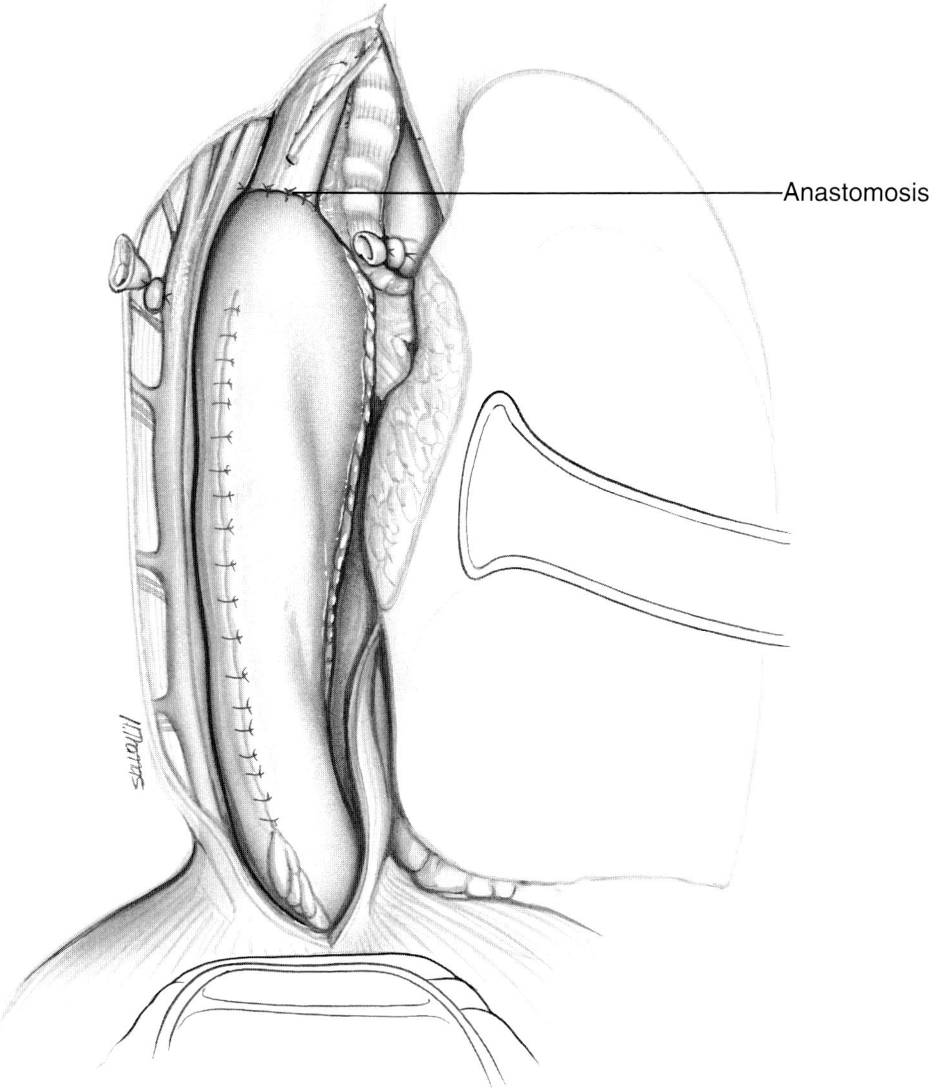
Anastomosis

ESOPHAGEAL MOBILIZATION IN RIGHT THORACOTOMY

COLON SEGMENT ANASTOMOSIS

A colon segment may be used to replace the esophagus when there is no option to use the stomach. This may be the case when there has been a previous gastrectomy.

The colon is mobilized. The omentum is retracted and the lesser omental bursa opened between the stomach and the transverse colon. Care is taken to avoid injuring the colon blood supply. When the hepatic and splenic flexures of the colon have been mobilized, the colon is lifted out of the abdomen and transilluminated to examine the anatomy of its blood supply. One must be certain there is a marginal artery arcade running from the cecum, around the ascending, transverse, and descending colon.

The colon segment should be long enough to stretch comfortably from the stomach to where it is to be anastomosed. It should have no redundant loops. As the "colon esophagus" is a gravity feed mechanism, redundant loops impair the passage of food.

An isoperistaltic segment of colon is preferred, but an antiperistaltic segment will also work. The cecum can be used as the proximal end in the neck, but it is bulky. The ideal segment is the transverse colon with the blood supply based on the middle colic artery.

Noncrushing vascular clamps are applied to all vessels that must be divided to free the selected segment. The marginal artery, both proximal and distal, must be occluded. A noncrushing clamp, such as a Satinsky clamp, should gently occlude the bowel at the levels of proposed bowel division. Thus the entire segment is isolated except for the major arterovenous branch nourishing the graft. The bowel is positioned comfortably and covered with moist laporatomy pads.

The colon segment is placed substernally. The distal retrosternal space is entered anterior to the diaphragm between the two parietal pleuras using a blunt dissection. The sternum is lifted up without unduly compressing the heart. An incision is made in the neck, and the esophagus is mobilized. The retrosternal space is entered and, working downward, a tunnel is opened. At the proximal end of the tunnel, a width of four fingers ensures adequate room for the anatomosis. One can divide the strap muscles or other muscles if necessary. It is important to avoid injuring the vessels in the anterior mediastinum as well as the vagus and phrenic nerve branches.

A window is made in the gastrohepatic omentum. From below, the prepared colon is passed behind the stomach through this window so that the vessels supplying the colon transplant are cephalic to the stomach. If this is not done, dilatation of the stomach could cause obstruction to the blood supply of the transplanted colon. While advancing the colon, the lesser curvature arcades of the stomach and the gastric vessels should be protected from injury. The drawing shows the proper position of the opening in the gastrohepatic omentum. The superior mesenteric artery coming from under the pancreas is seen with the middle colic branch going to the proximal portion of the colon. The colon is passed into the neck through the substernal tunnel. A pursestring suture is placed at the end of the segment. A catheter is passed from the neck to the abdomen and is tied to the colon by the ends of the pursestring suture. This catheter serves as a guide while the hand gently pushes the colon into the neck. The mesenteric blood supply of the colon must continue to face the right side of the patient throughout the advance. There must be no rotation, distortion, or kinking of the colon segment. Once settled in the substernal space, the colon must be straight. Excessive colon can be trimmed. The cervical esophagus is divided. If the thoracic esophagus is to be left in place, the thoracic esophageal end is stapled closed and placed in the thorax. The proximal cervical esophagus is anastomosed to the prepared colon segment by the hand-sewn technique depicted in previous drawings. The distal end of the colon transplant is anastomosed to the anterior surface of the stomach. The remaining abdominal colon is reanastomosed end to end.

A nasogastric tube is passed into the colon loop before the cervical anastomosis is complete. A nasogastric tube with many holes allows drainage in both the colon transplant and the stomach. This ensures there is distention of neither the colon loop or the stomach. The neck is drained. If either pleural cavity has been entered, chest tubes are placed for drainage.

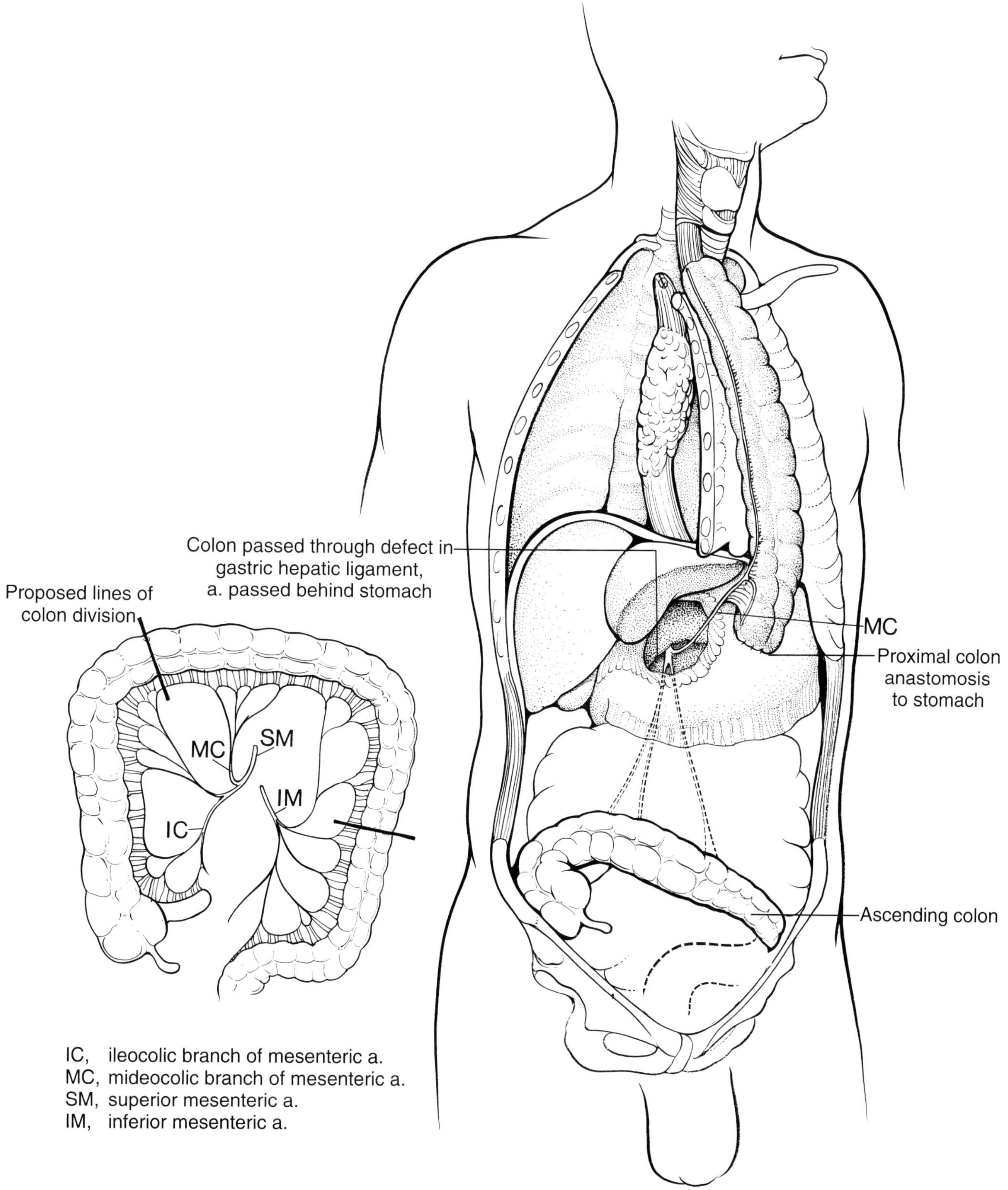

IC, ileocolic branch of mesenteric a.
MC, mideocolic branch of mesenteric a.
SM, superior mesenteric a.
IM, inferior mesenteric a.

5

Tumors of the Mediastinum

ANATOMY OF THE MEDIASTINUM

The mediastinum is defined laterally by the two pleural cavities, superiorly by the bony structures of the thoracic inlet and inferiorly by the diaphragm. The anterosuperior mediastinum is bounded by the sternum, the thoracic inlet, the diaphragm, and posteriorly by the pericardium and the bodies of the first four thoracic vertebrae. This compartment contains the thymus gland, the aortic arch and its major branches, the innominate veins, and lymphatic and areolar tissue. The middle mediastinum is bounded by the pericardial sac and superiorly extends to the fourth thoracic vertebra. It contains the heart and pericardium, the trachea, the hilum of each lung, and tracheobronchial lymph nodes. The posterior mediastinum lies between the pericardium and the vertebral column and extends superiorly to the anterior mediastinum. The esophagus, vagus nerves, sympathetic nerve chains, thoracic duct, descending aorta, azygos and hemiazygos venous systems, paravertebral lymph nodes, and areolar tissue all fall within the boundaries of the posterior mediastinum (Fig. 5-1).

Although lesions that arise in the mediastinum occur predominantly in one of the anatomic divisions, there is an overlap in their distributions (Table 5-1). The most constant relationships are the thyroid masses, teratomas, and thymomas, which are located in the anterosuperior mediastinum, and the neurogenic tumors, which are located in the posterior mediastinum.

In classifying mediastinal lesions by anatomic compartments, several schemes have been proposed. The major variation between the different proposals centers on the definition of a superior mediastinum in lieu of its incorporation wholly into the anterior mediastinum or into the other three compartments (anterior, middle, and posterior). Because the majority of the tumors that arise in the superior mediastinum are also found in the anterior mediastinum and because lesions that frequently arise in this region (the thoracic inlet) extend down into the chest and also occupy the anterior mediastinum, we prefer to combine these two into one compartment.

Overall the rate of malignancy of mediastinal masses is approximately 40 percent. In a large collective review of mediastinal tumors, neurogenic tumors and thymomas accounted for 20 percent each of all tumors in adults, with the former predominant in children (40 percent)[1] (Table 5-2).

Only 1 of 206 patients with thymoma in the Mayo Clinic series was younger than 20 years.[2] The incidence of thymomas in the adult population has risen in the past several decades as a result of a more determined effort to identify these lesions in persons with myasthenia gravis and autoimmune disorders. The advent of computed tomography (CT) and magnetic resonance imaging (MRI) of the chest has enhanced our ability to identify these tumors in patients in whom they had previously been unrecognized.

The third most common tumors in the mediastinum are the primary mediastinal lymphomas. Not all lymphomas with mediastinal involvement qualify as primary mediastinal neoplasms, and in some series the incidence of these malignancies has been overestimated.

DIAGNOSIS

The majority of patients who are asymptomatic on presentation have benign lesions. In the Duke University series[3] symptoms were present in 62

Table 5-1. Most Common Tumors of the Mediastinum by Compartment

Anterior	Middle	Posterior
Thymoma	Lymph node metastasis	Schwannoma
Teratoma	Foregut duplication cyst	Neurolemmoma
Thyroid	Vagal tumor	Ganglioneuroma
Pericardial cyst	Phrenic tumors	Neurofibroma
Germ cell tumor	Esophageal tumor	Neuroepithelioma
Lipoma	Hiatus hernia	Thymoma
Lymphangioma		
Metastatic carcinoma		

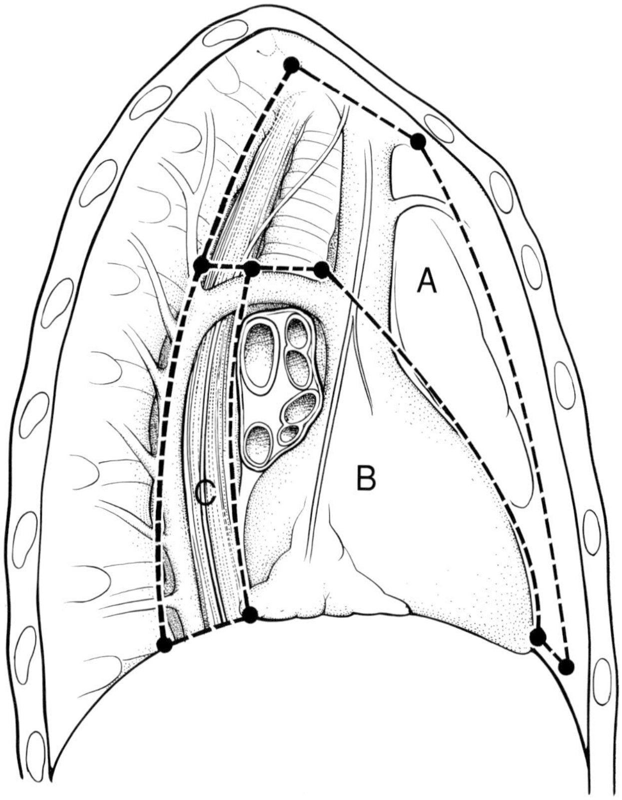

Fig. 5-1. Lateral view of the chest dividing the mediastinum into the **(A)** anterosuperior, **(B)** middle, and **(C)** posterior mediastinum.

Table 5-2. Relative Frequency of Various Primary Mediastinal Tumors and Cysts in 1,950 Adult Patients and 437 Children

	Adults		Children	
Tumor or Cyst	No.	Percent	No.	Percent
Neurogenic tumor	411	21	176	40
Thymoma	365	19	0	0
Lymphoma	246	13	80	18
Germ cell	207	11	47	11
Mesenchymal tumor	138	7	38	9
Endocrine tumor	125	6	0	0
Primary carcinoma	57	3	16	4
Cyst	401	20	80	18
Total	1,950	100	437	100

(Data from Silverman and Sabiston.[1])

percent of all patients and included chest pain (30 percent), dyspnea (16 percent), fever and chills (20 percent), and cough (16 percent). Of the lesions found on routine chest x-rays, 83 percent were benign. In contrast, 57 percent of the lesions in symptomatic patients were malignant. Less often, dysphagia, superior venal caval obstruction, vocal cord paralysis, Horner's syndrome, or spinal cord compression is noted. An interesting group of patients have primary mediastinal tumors or cysts that impinge upon the heart or great vessels, impede cardiac performance, and produce symptoms simulating primary cardiac disease.[4]

Another group of patients manifest systemic symptoms, which may be due to endocrine secretions by the tumor (such as hypercalcemia secondary to a parathyroid adenoma, systemic hypertension due to a neurogenic tumor, or thyrotoxicosis secondary to an intrathoracic goiter). In addition, association of the symptoms of myasthenia gravis with thymomas, opsomyoclonis with neuroblastomas, and fever of unknown origin with lymphomas are common.

The majority of the tumors arising in the mediastinum can be defined by routine posteroanterior and lateral views of the chest. The shape, size, and location in the appropriate mediastinal compartment can be readily determined. The value of routine chest x-rays in the early detection of these lesions can be inferred from a report by Fontenelle et al.[5] In a series of military personnel screened at regular intervals, they identified all benign lesions and 72 percent of all malignant lesions before they became symptomatic. This differs from the Mayo Clinic experience, in which it was reported that 50 percent of all malignant lesions of the mediastinum and 10 percent of the benign lesions were symptomatic (Fig. 5-2).

Prior to the advent of CT scanning, a variety of techniques were used to better define the extent of involvement of the mediastinal tumors. Coned-down views, tomography, barium contrast studies, fluoroscopy, aortograms, venograms, myelography, various nuclide imaging procedures, and other more exotic procedures have all been supplanted by CT scanning. The cross-sectional anatomy visualized allowed precise definition of the margins between the tumor and adjacent anatomic structures and has simplified the workup of these lesions (Figs. 5-3 and 5-4).

The role of MRI has not been clearly defined as yet. Vascular structures can be clearly identified without contrast, but this technique has the disadvantage of requiring longer scanning times and greater expense (Fig. 5-5). Studies comparing CT scans and MRI scans in the evaluation of mediastinal masses show a similar quality of imaging.[6]

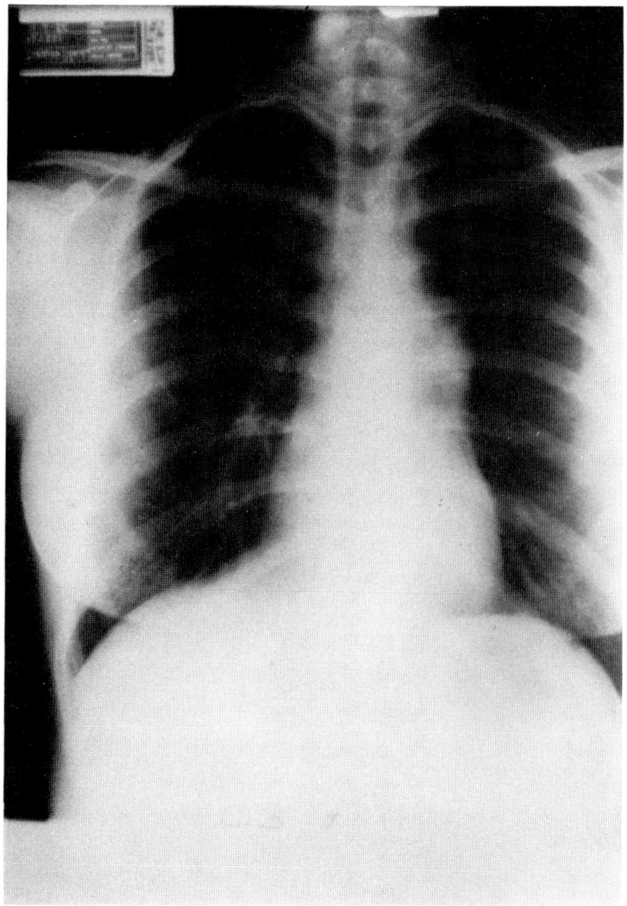

Fig. 5-2. Chest x-ray depicting an anterior mediastinal lesion in an asymptomatic while female.

NEOPLASMS OF THE ANTEROSUPERIOR MEDIASTINUM

THYMUS

Embryologically the thyroid gland originates from the endoderm as epithelial outgrowths of the lower portion of the third pharyngeal pouches on each side. The third pharyngeal pouches also give rise to the parathyroid glands, which migrate into the neck, while the right and left thymic outgrowths descend into the mediastinum to become a bilobed glandular structure. The epithelial cells arising in this anlagen spread out to form a reticulum with lymphocytes ultimately populating the spaces between these reticular epithelial cells. These lymphocytes arise in the bone marrow and migate to the thymus. The process of lymphoblastic differentiation into thymocytes takes place in fetal and early postnatal life. Congenital absence of the thymus, the DiGeorge syndrome, or removal of the thymus early in life results in a deficiency of cellular immune function. Thymectomy in the adult will also result in a decrease in immunologic competence. Measurements of T-cell function post-thymectomy revealed a gradual diminution of the total T-cell population owing to the loss of these thymus-derived cells.

The most common tumor found in the thymus gland is the thymoma. In a review of 598 thymoma patients found in the literature and 146 from the Mayo Clinic, 422 (71 percent) suffered from other diseases suspected of being associated with thymoma.[7] The disorders of immunity included among others, myasthenia gravis (44 percent), cytopenias (21 percent), cancer (17 percent), hypogammaglobulinemia (6 percent), polymyositis (5 percent), and systemic lupus erythematosus (2 percent). Other diseases reported to be associated with thymomas are listed in Table 5-3.

The pathologists at the Mayo Clinic first classified these lesions into four types: lymphocytic, epithelial, mixed, and spindle cell; the last is considered a variant of epithelial thymomas. The epithelial thymomas have tended to be more aggressive.[8] There is little association between the histologic features of the tumors and their invasive potential, as the majority of the tumors have few mitotic figures. Thus the malignancy of a thymoma is characterized more by whether it is well encapsulated. In most series approximately 25

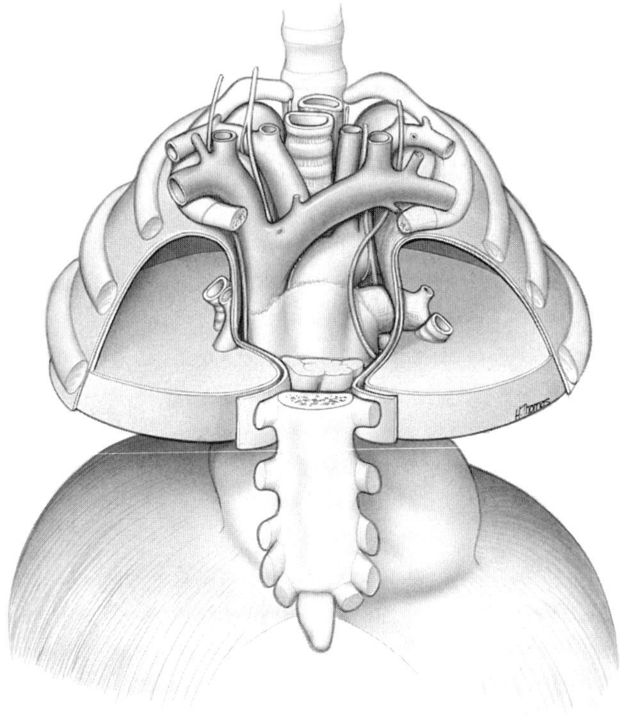

Fig. 5-3. Cross-sectional representation of the mediastinum at the level of the aortic arch. The relationship of the trachea to the innominate vessels and the recurrent laryngeal and vagus nerves to the aortic arch is clearly demonstrated.

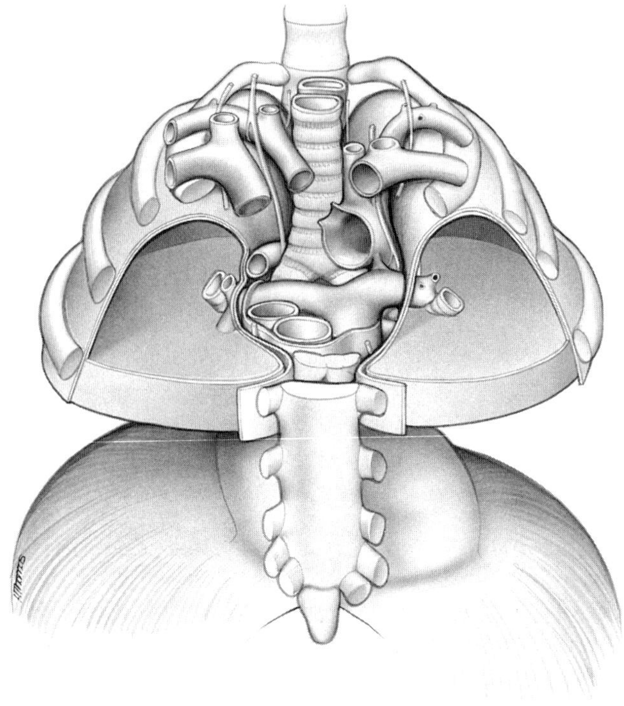

Fig. 5-4. Cross-sectional view at the level of the bifurcation of the carina.

Table 5-3. Syndromes and Diseases Associated with Thymomas

Immunologic Diseases	Severe Infections
Myasthenia gravis	Tuberculosis
Cytopenias	Syphilis
Hypogammaglobulinemia	Parasitic diseases
Polymyositis	Mycosis
Systemic lupus erythematosus	Cytomegalovirus infections
Rheumatoid arthritis	Staphylococcal sepsis
Thyroiditis	
Sjögren's syndrome	
Chronic ulcerative colitis	
Pernicious anemia	
Raynaud's disease	
Regional enteritis	
Rheumatic endocarditis	
Sarcoid	
Dermatomyositis	
Scleroderma	
Takayasu syndrome	

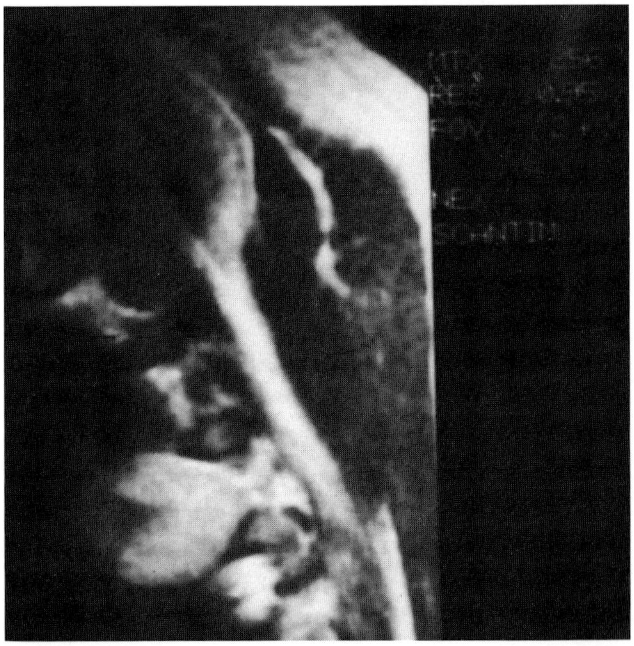

Fig. 5-5. MRI scan demonstrating a posterior mediastinal neurolemmoma.

percent of all thymomas have a fully malignant course, with the majority of those cases occurring in the nonencapsulated or invasive group. Nonetheless, there are well-encapsulated lesions that have full a malignant potential, and therefore it is prudent to assume that all thymomas are malignant (Fig. 5-6).

TREATMENT

Surgical Resection

Surgical resection of these tumors is the most effective therapy. If the thymoma is well encapsulated and a complete resection is performed, there is only a 2 percent incidence of local recurrence (Figs. 5-7, 5-8). These take the form of pleural, pericardial, or diaphragmatic implants or of a localized mediastinal recurrence. Poor prognosis is associated with an invasive tumor, for which the local recurrence rate approaches 20 percent. Two staging systems for thymomas are widely used: the Bergh and Japanese systems (Tables 5-4 and 5-5). An associated syndrome such as myasthenia gravis, which is present in a significant percentage of these cases, has also been associated with a poorer prognosis. With better control of the other sequelae of myasthenia gravis, the survival following resection for well-encapsulated tumors in these patients is now reported to be as good as that for well-encapsulated tumors resected in patients without myasthenia gravis.[9]

Invasive tumors may require a more aggressive surgical approach. A median sternotomy may be combined with a thoracotomy with resection of involved pleura, pericardium, phrenic nerve, lung parenchyma, or diaphragm. Resection of the innominate vein and portions or all of the superior vena cava has been reported.[10] When the tumor is not resectable because of involvement of adjacent structures, radiotherapy may play an important role.

Radiotherapy

Radiotherapy plays an important role as an adjuvant therapy for the primary treatment of thymoma. For the well-encapsulated lesion completely excised by surgery, adjuvant radiotherapy should be deferred because of the low incidence of recurrence. Verley and Hollmann advocate radiotherapy

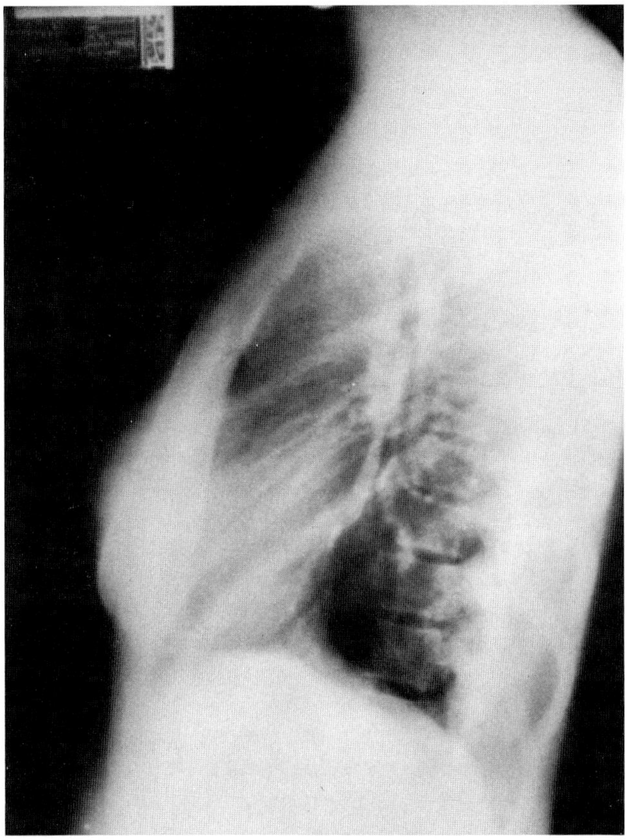

Fig. 5-6. Lateral chest x-ray demonstrating a thymoma of the anterior mediastinum.

Table 5-4. Bergh Staging System for Thymoma

Stage	Definition	Percent
I	Intact capsule	40
II	Pericapsular growth into the mediastinal fat tissue	19
III	Invasive growth into the surrounding organs and/or intrathoracic metastasis	41

Table 5-5. Japanese Staging System for Thymomas

Stage	Definition	Percent
I	Macroscopically completely encapsulated and microscopically no capsular invasion	40
IIa	Macroscopic invasion into surrounding fatty tissues or mediastinal pleura	14
IIb	Microscopic invasion into the capsule	
III	Macroscopic invasion into a neighboring organ (great vessels or lung)	34
IVa	Pleural or pericardial dissemination	3
IVb	Lymphogenous or hematogenous metastasis	9

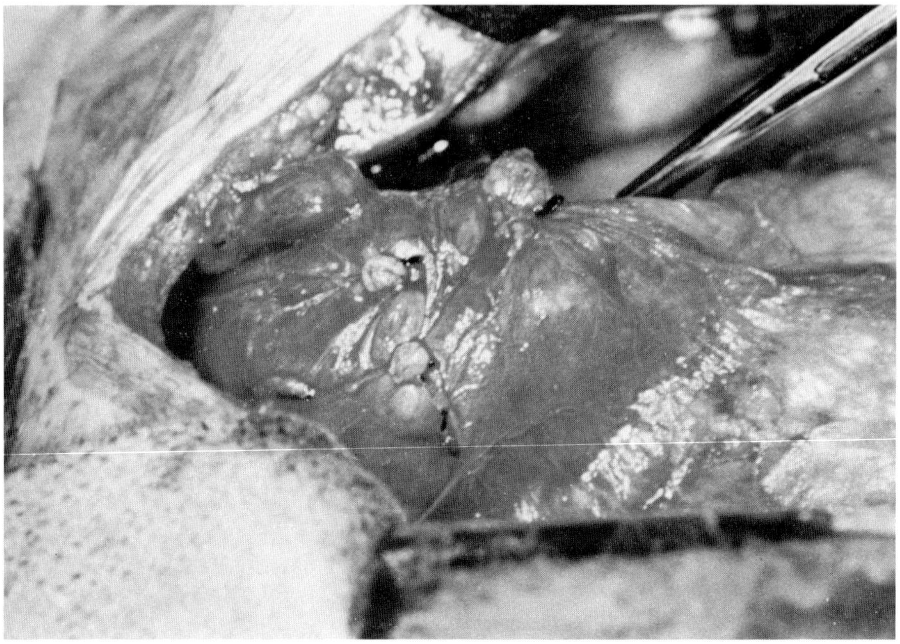

Fig. 5-7. Through a median sternotomy incision, the thymoma is mobilized off the underlying great vessels.

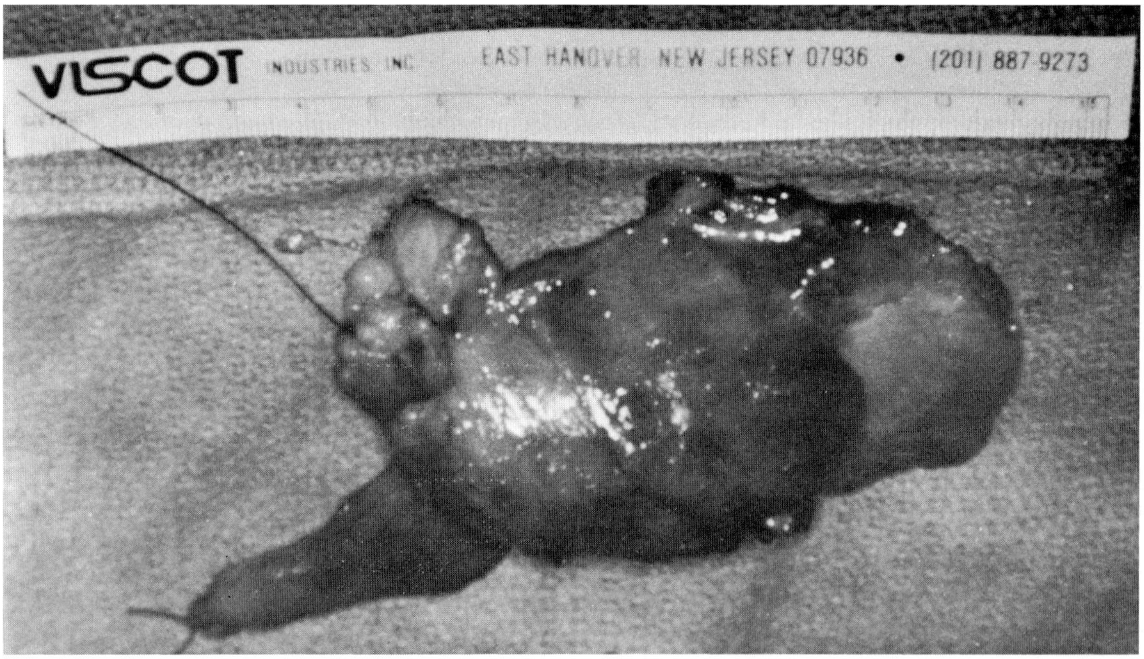

Fig. 5-8. The resected thymoma.

in all cases because of the inability to determine which cases will have a malignant potential.[11]

Radiotherapy as adjuvant therapy for invasive tumors, recurrences, or unresectable primary lesions has been reported to consist of dosages of 3,500 to 4,500 rads.[12] Penn and Hope-Stone recommend two large anterior oblique wedge fields with a total dosage of 4,500 rads over 6 weeks.[13] Skeggs used a single anterior and two posterior oblique fields.[14] Marks et al. recommend a dose of 4,000 rads to the tumor bed in 4 to 5 weeks if the invasive thymoma is completely removed.[15] For unresectable or partially resectable disease, a dose of 4,500 rads is recommended, with shrinking fields if the tumor responds.

It is important that the dosage not exceed 4,500 rads in order to reduce the incidence of radiation pneumonitis, which is reported to be as high as 40 percent. Other complications include mediastinitis, pericarditis, and myocarditis. It is also important to use oblique techniques to spare the spinal column. Recently the use of afterloading techniques has provided an additional means of delivery of an appropriate radiation dosage to the surgical bed. In addition, because the pleura is involved in many advanced cases, Batata et al. recommended postoperative intrapleural phosphorus 32 (P-32) instillation on the predominant side of the tumor. Fifteen millicuries of colloidal radioactive phosphorus diluted in 150 ml of saline is instilled prior to removal of the chest tubes.[16]

Chemotherapy

Chemotherapy has a limited role in the management of invasive thymomas. Corticosteroids have been used in advanced disease with limited results, as well as combined with single agents such as *cis*-platinum,[17] and doxorubicin.[18] Daugaard et al.[19] reported complete responses which lasted a median of 37 months in four of nine patients treated with vincristine, cyclophosphamide, lomustine, and prednisone. Other favorable results have been reported when using combination chemotherapy which has had success in lymphomas. Chahinian and associates observed five partial remissions and one complete response in patients treated with *cis*-platinum, bleomycin, doxorubicin, and prednisone.[20] Since this first report of a combination of drugs including *cis*-platinum, 33 patients have been treated with a variety of *cis*-platinum combination regimens resulting in 9 complete and 19 partial remissions.[21–25]

Although the relatively high response rates observed in the initial trials of combination chemotherapy suggest that invasive thymomas may be relatively sensitive to chemotherapy, more information is needed to define the role of chemotherapy.

GERM CELL TUMORS

Germ cell tumors that originate in the mediastinum are histologically identical to those that originate in the genital organs. It is relatively uncommon for germ cell tumors of testicular origin to metastasize exclusively to the mediastinum.[26] They usually metastasize to retroperitoneal lymph nodes, often bypassing the mediastinum via the thoracic duct.[27,28] In two large autopsy series, metastases to the anterior mediastinum were not found in a total of 30 patients with testicular germ cell neoplasm. Rarely, generalized metastases of a testicular neoplasm are found without a viable or identifiable primary source in the genital organs. In such cases the metastases are not confined to the mediastinum. When a germ cell tumor presents in the mediastinum in the absence of a detectable testicular primary neoplasm and in the absence of metastatic disease in the retroperitoneal lymph nodes, one may justifiably consider it a primary mediastinal tumor.

BENIGN TERATOMAS

The mediastinum is second only to the gonads in adults and the sacrococcygeal area in children as the primary location of germ cell tumors. The most common germ cell tumor is the teratoma. It occurs equally in males and females has no predisposing conditions or associated abnormalities. The pathologic appearance is identical to that of the benign teratoma arising in the ovary. Mature tissues from ectodermal, mesodermal, and endodermal layers are all present, but the ectodermal component usually predominates.

The classic radiographic finding of a tooth in the lesion occurs in these mediastinal lesions occasionally. Calcifications of a more nonspecific nature can occur in 25 percent of all cases.[29,30]

Although these lesions are benign histologically, they can be locally invasive in as many as 15 percent of the cases requiring more extensive surgery. Local recurrences are rare if a complete surgical excision is performed.

MALIGNANT SEMINOMAS

The malignant mediastinal germ cell tumors account for 5 to 10 percent of all mediastinal lesions. They occur in patients aged 2 to 70 years with a peak incidence between 20 and 35 years of age. There is a male predominance for this disease, but cases which occur in females are histologically identical.

These tumors are histologically identical to germ cell tumors that arise in the testis, and all histological subtypes seen in testicular tumors have been identified in the mediastinum. Pure seminomas account for approximately 35 percent of all lesions. Nonseminomatous lesions include the teratocarcinoma, embryonal carcinoma, choriocarcinoma, and endodermal sinus tumor in decreasing frequency. These account for 55 percent of all lesions, with the remainder being mixed tumors.

Although the etiology of these mediastinal tumors is unknown, there are several unproven hypotheses about their origin. These include totipotential cells that have become detached from the blastula or morula and primitive cells arising from the endoderm of the yolk sac or the urogenital ridge.[31]

There is a known association of these tumors with Klinefelter syndrome,[32] as well as an association with second hematologic malignancies unrelated to the aggressive chemotherapy used to treat this disease.[33]

The seminomas are the most common of the mediastinal germ cell tumors. Their symptoms, diagnosis, and radiologic features are characteristic of most anterior mediastinal tumors. Approximately 10 percent of seminomas are associated with elevated α-fetoprotein (AFP) or human chorionic gonadotropin (hCG) levels, the former occurring only in tumors that have nonseminomatous elements. In a recently reported series, the serum lactic dehydrogenase (LDH) level is elevated in the majority of patients.[34]

Most patients with mediastinal seminomas have extensive involvement of the great vessels when they are first seen. Only 20 percent of the tumors could be completely excised in the patients reported by Martini et al.[35] Because the tumor is extremely radiosensitive, local disease can usually be well controlled. The excellent response of seminomas to radiotherapy is in marked contrast to the response of nonseminomatous germ cell lesions.[36] A recent review of the contribution of radiotherapy to the management of primary malignant mediastinal germ cell tumors revealed an actuarial survival of 100 percent at 5 years. Actuarial survival at 10 years was reported by Bush et al. to be 69 percent.[37]

Treatment

The recommended radiotherapy for a mediastinal seminoma is a Y-shaped mediastinal field with supraclavicular and neck radiation to a midplane dose of approximately 4,500 to 5,000 rads over 6 weeks. The axilla should be included if cervical adenopathy is present because of the possible extension of disease to the next contiguous nodal group. The dose recommended is greater than that used routinely for gonadal seminoma because primary mediastinum lesions are almost always massive compared with a gonadal primary.

Surgery should be reserved for the primary treatment of small lesions that are completely resectable. The role of surgical debulking prior to definitive radiotherapy has not proven to be of benefit.

In recent years systemic chemotherapy with intensive *cis*-platinum-based combination regimens has shown a high degree of success in locally advanced and metastatic seminomas.

Jain et al. reported a complete response in 10 patients receiving predominately the VAB-6 regimen as primary therapy for nonresectable mediastinal disease.[34] In addition, Hainsworth et al.[38] and Daugaard et al.[39] reported on the efficacy of PVB (*cis*-platinum, vinblastine, and bleomycin) as salvage therapy in three of four patients who had previously undergone and failed radiotherapy.

In summary, seminomas are highly curable lesions when discovered. Surgical excision where feasible followed by radiotherapy (3,500 to 4,000 rads) is the treatment of choice for the early lesions. Advanced mediastinal lesions can be treated with radiotherapy, with approximately 60 percent of all lesions being cured. Those that fail radiotherapy can be salvaged with platinum-containing regimens. The latter can be used initially in patients with distant metastases as well.

MALIGNANT NONSEMINATOUS LESIONS

The nonseminatous lesions include the teratocarcinomas, embryonal lesions, and choriocarcinomas. Very few of these patients are asymptomatic at diagnosis, and the majority of the tumors are metastatic at presentation. The most common sites of metastasis include the lung pleura, supraclavicular and retroperitoneal lymph nodes, and liver. These lesions rarely metastasize to the bone, brain, or kidneys.

The majority of these lesions are associated with elevated AFP or hCG levels. In a series of 32 patients by Hainsworth et al.,[38] only 25 percent of the lesions contained neither of these two markers. The choriocarcinomas all had elevated hCG levels, and six of seven teratocarcinomas had elevated AFP levels. If these markers are present, they are useful as indicators of response to therapy. Another marker consistently elevated in these lesions is LDH.[40]

It has been reported that the CT scan can differentiate between the seminoma and nonseminomatous germ cell lesions. The latter are more inhomogeneous, with multiple areas of decreased attenuation representing necrosis and hemorrhage.[41]

Table 5-6. Nonseminomatous Mediastinal Germ Cell Tumors Treated with Cisplatin-Based Combination Chemotherapy

Series	No.	Chemotherapy	Complete Responses	Long-Term Disease-Free Survival
Fune et al.[42]	13	PVB	6	5
Hainsworth et al.[38]	12	PVB+A	7	7
Daugaard et al.[39]	5	PVB	1	1
Israel et al.[40]	29	VAB-3 (12 patients) VAB-5 (6 patients) VAB-6 (11 patients)	12	5
Total	59		26(44%)	18(32%)

Abbreviations: P, platinum; V, vincristine; B, bleomycin; A, adriamycin.

Because the majority of these patients have disease beyond the mediastinum and these tumors are not radiosensitive, chemotherapy is the initial treatment of choice. The most effective regimens all used *cis*-platinum at levels used to treat metastatic lesions, and one-third of all patients treated showed long-term survival (Table 5-6).

Treatment

Surgical therapy plays a significant role in the optimal treatment of nonseminomatous mediastinal germ cell tumors, as it does in the treatment of metastatic testicular neoplasms. Initial surgical treatment consisting of debulking of large mediastinal lesions was found to have little usefulness.[35] However, in patients who respond to chemotherapy, particularly those with normalization of their markers, resection of the remaining mediastinal disease is important. Seventy percent of these patients will have either a nonviable tumor or a benign teratoma and on evidence of active malignancy. The importance of resecting this residual disease has recently been recognized because some of these benign lesions will continue to grow and subsequently undergo malignant degeneration.

If viable tumor is found in the resected mediastinal tumors, a salvage chemotherapy regimen should be used because survival in these patients is unusual.[42,43] Salvage regimens currently used include that reported by Hainsworth et al., which consists of VP-16 with cisplatin.[46]

NEOPLASMS OF THE POSTERIOR MEDIASTINUM

Neurogenic tumors make up 75 percent of all posterior mediastinal lesions; they are derived from embryonal neural crest cells. These cells are located at the dorsal border of the closing neural tube and migate to their final destination. Neural crest cells in the thorax give rise to peripheral nerves including the sympathetic and parasympathetic ganglia and the Schwann cells.

BENIGN NEUROGENIC TUMORS

NEUROFIBROMAS

Neurofibromas contain both nerve elements and nerve sheath elements. The thoracic lesions usually arise in intercostal nerves, but can arise from any nerve in the thorax, including the spinal nerve roots, autonomic nerve, and vagus nerve.

There are two pathologic types of these lesions, the solitary type and the plexiform type. The latter is found only in patients with Von Recklinghausen's disease. Treatment of these lesions is exclusively by surgical resection (Table 5-7; Fig. 5-9).

GANGLIONEUROMAS

Ganglioneuromas are tumors arising from the sympathetic ganglion and occur most often in young children. Harjula et al.[45] report that the average age of the patients in their series was 15 years with a 5:2 female-to-male ratio. These tumors are occasionally hormonally active (Table 5-7).

MALIGNANT NEUROGENIC TUMORS

NEUROBLASTOMAS

Neuroblastomas are the most common of the neurogenic tumors arising in children. Although the most common site of origin of these tumors is the retroperitoneum, 15 to 20 percent of them are primary in the mediastinum.

Table 5-7. Major Characteristics of Neurogenic Tumors

Tumor	Mean Age (yr)	Male/Female Ratio	Treatment	Malignant Potential	Associated Diseases
Neurofibroma	35	1:2	Surgical excision	Yes	Von Recklinghausen's disease
Ganglioneuroma	15	2:5	Surgical excision	No	None
Neurolemmoma	40	1:2	Surgical excision	Yes	Von Recklinghausen's disease

Symptoms caused by these tumors can be related to extradural spinal cord compression secondary to extension of the tumor via a spinal nerve route[46] or as a result of the bioactivity of these tumors. Nonepisodic systolic or diastolic hypertension secondary to catecholamine production, the watery diarrhea syndrome due to vasoactive intestinal polypeptide, and opsomyoclonus and nystagmus have been reported to occur with the mediastinal neuroblastomas.[47,48] Involvement of the sympathetic ganglion can produce a Horner's syndrome.

Two staging systems are currently used in the management of patients with neuroblastoma. The Evans system, introduced in 1971,[49] stages the patients on the basis of tumor size and the presence or absence of metastasis. In this system the staging of metastatic disease is subdivided to include a group of patients whose disease is metastatic exclusively to liver, skin, or bone marrow. This latter form of the disease is seen almost exclusively in infants 6 months and younger, and the massive tumor involvement in the abdomen will spontaneously regress in 85 percent of patients within 6 to 15 months without treatment (Table 5-8).

A second staging system proposed by Hayes et al., St. Jude's Hospital, may have greater applicability to thoracic neuroblastoma because of their frequent midline origin (Table 5-9).[50]

A histologic classification of neuroblastomas has been developed by Shimada et al.[51] This grading system is based on the maturation of the tumor toward ganglioneuroma formation and the division of the tumors into stroma-rich and -poor groups.

In addition to these staging criteria, other factors have been recently identified to be associated with prognosis. The presence of a hyperdiploid chromosome number in patients with neuroblastoma predicted responses to chemotherapy. Nonresectable tumors in children less than 1 year of

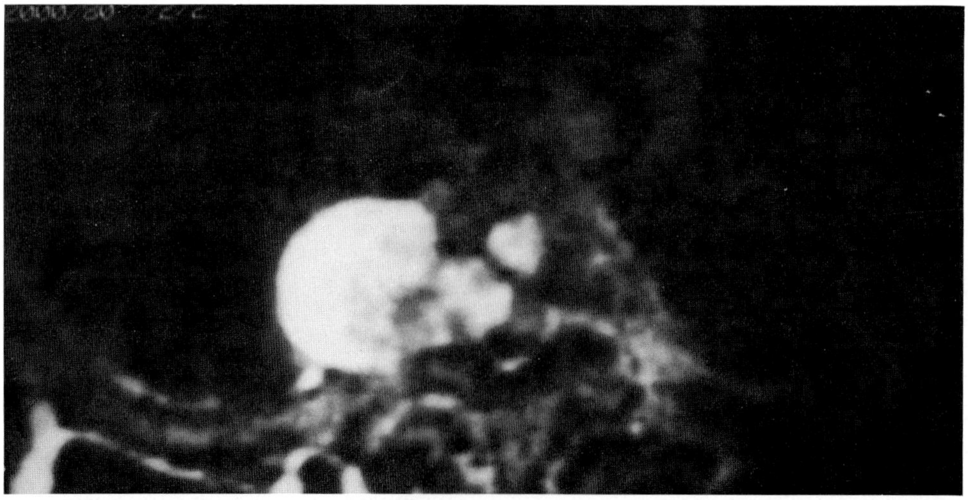

Fig. 5-9. CT scan demonstrating a benign neurofibroma arising in the posterior mediastinum.

Table 5-8. Evans Staging System for Neuroblastoma

Stage	Description
I	Tumor confined to the organ or structure of origin
II	Tumor extending in continuity beyond the organ or structure of origin but not crossing the midline; regional lymph nodes on the ipsilateral side may be involved
III	Tumor extending in continuity beyond the midline; regional lymph nodes may be involved bilaterally
IV	Remote disease involving skeleton, organs, soft tissues, or distant nodal groups
IV-S	Same as I or II, but with remote disease confined to one or more of the liver, skin, or bone marrow

age were analyzed by flow cytometry for cellular DNA content.[52] Of 17 tumors containing hyperdiploid amounts of DNA, 15 had complete responses to chemotherapy compared with none with a diploid content. Patients with Evans IV-S disease were found to have hyperdiploidy as well.

Tumors from patients with Evans stages I to IV and IV-S disease were analyzed as well for N-*myc* DNA amplification using the Southern blot technique.[53] This also correlated with the development of metastasis in stage II patients.

The mainstay of therapy for the treatment of mediastinal neuroblastomas has been surgery. Complete resection for stage I disease is associated with 100 percent survival, and adjuvant therapies are not employed.

For stage II disease, the role of adjuvant therapies has not been clearly defined. Conflicting reports appears in the literature regarding the efficacy of adjunctive radiotherapy,[54] and because there are significant effects on symmetric growth, it is not widely used. A study of the role of adjuvant therapy in stage II disease, showed no benefit of cyclophosphamide.[55]

Table 5-9. St. Jude's Childrens Hospital Staging System for Neuroblastoma

Stage	Description
I	Localized tumor completely resected without local invasion
IIA	Localized tumor resected with residual microscopic disease
IIB	Localized tumor partially or not resected
IIIA	Regional or systemic spread of disease without bone or bone marrow involvement
IIIB	Same as IIIA but with evidence of a single localized destructive lesion of bone without marrow involvement
IIIC	Generalized tumor in bone and marrow or in marrow only

For stage III and IV disease, chemotherapy has been used as the mainstay of therapy, with surgery and radiotherapy relegated to adjunctive treatments. The role of the chemotherapy is to reduce tumor size and either prevent dissemination (stage III) or control disseminated disease (stage IV).

The most commonly used regimens employ some combination of vincristine, doxorubicin, cyclophosphamide, VM-26, *cis*-platinum, and DTIC.[56,57] Rosen et al. report an 82 percent 3-year disease-free survival in stage III patients who were older than 1 year.[58] For stage IV disease, 1-year survival approaches 67 percent.[59] The 5-year survival rate is below 10 percent.[60]

For salvage therapy in patients with advanced disease, high-dose chemotherapy, whole-body radiation, and bone marrow transplantation are in use.[61]

NEUROLEMMOMAS

Neurolemmomas (schwannomas), which can be either benign or malignant, arise from Schwann cells, the cells that sheathe the peripheral nerves from the point at which they penetrate the pia mater to the point at which they terminate at the periphery. These tumors are usually benign and slow growing and are most often found in the costovertebral sulcus of the upper posterior mediastinum. They arise most frequently in the third to fifth decades and appear as a well-circumscribed homogeneous density on chest x-rays.

These tumors arise on the right side in about 70 percent of cases and are associated with Von Recklinghausen's disease and the Noonan syndrome in up to 40 percent of cases. They grow into the intervertebral foramina in up to 20 percent of cases, even though clinical evidence of extension into the spinal column is absent. Surgical excision offers an excellent prognosis (Table 5-7; Fig. 5-10).

Malignant schwannomas can arise from malignant degeneration of a neurofibroma in patients with Von Recklinghausen's disease or can arise de novo from Schwann cells of the peripheral nerve sheaths. They arise only rarely from the malignant degeneration of a benign schwannoma. From 4 to 29 percent of patients with Von Recklinghausen's

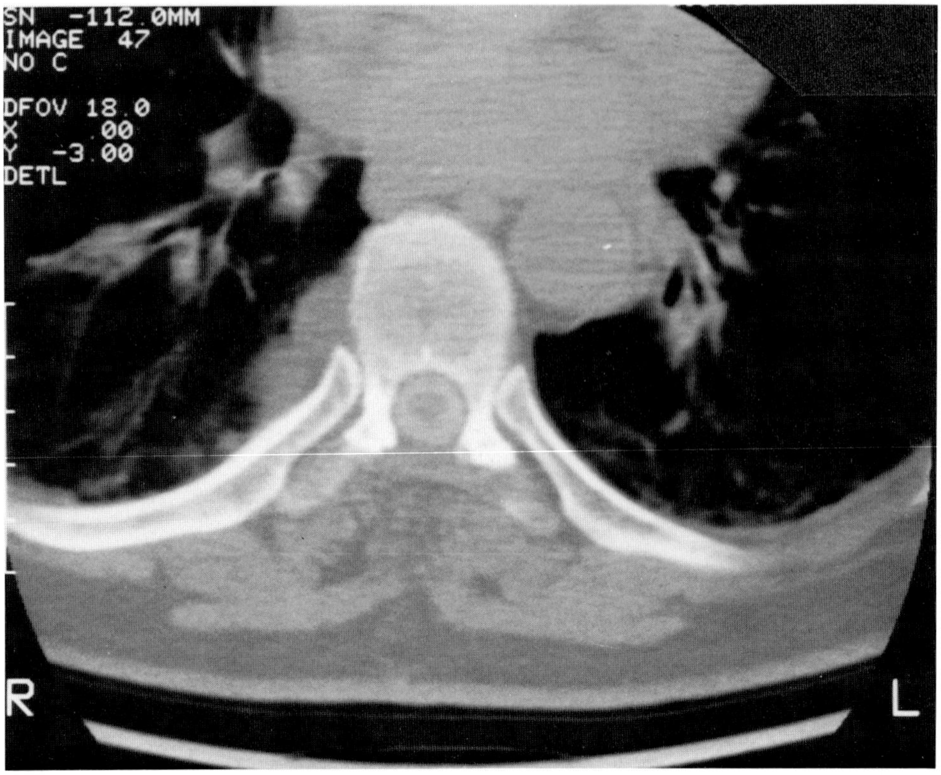

Fig. 5-10. CT scan demonstrating a neurolemmoma with erosion of the thoracic vertebral body.

disease may develop malignant schwannomas during their lifetime.[62,63]

These tumors are usually discovered as a mass detected on chest x-ray in patients complaining of pain, weight loss, and malaise. Metastatic sites, in order of frequency, are lung, liver, skin, bone, peritoneum, and pleura.[64]

The prognosis of these tumors directly correlated with successful surgical extirpation of the tumor and the histologic grade of the lesion. Patients with complete surgical excision have shown cure rates as high as 60 percent.[65] Long-term survivals are reported as well for the low-grade lesions, based on mitosis, cellularity, and necrosis, versus 37 percent in patients with high-grade lesions.[66] There has been no clearly defined role for irradiation or chemotherapy in this disease.

Recently there has been a reported association of an amplification of the N-*myc* gene in malignant schwannomas, much as in neuroblastomas. This preliminary data suggest that the N-*myc* protein may play a role in the oncogenesis of malignant schwannomas.[67]

NEUROEPITHELIOMAS (ASKIN'S TUMOR)

Neuroepitheliomas histologically are indistinguishable from neuroblastomas. In addition to being located in the mediastinum, they frequently present as primary chest well lesions.

Recent studies have shown that these tumors have a specific chromosomal translocation, rcp(11;22) (q24;q12).[68] Ewing sarcoma is also characterized by this translocation but has a different immunocytochemical profile.

This lesion was first described by Askin and colleagues in 20 children and adolescents (average age, 14 years). There is a 3 : 1 female predominance. Patients with this disease have an extremely short life expectancy (8 months) and have been unresponsive to any conventional therapy.

THYMOMAS

Although they are usually anterior mediastinal tumors, thymomas may arise primarily from thymic rests localized in the parietal pericardium. These tumors are considered primary if there is no anterior mediastinal involvement. Five patients are reported in the literature, four females and one male.[69] As with most pericardial lesions, congestive heart failure is the presenting symptom. All patients have a mediastinal or pericardial mass detected by chest x-ray. There is no evidence of myasthenia gravis in these patients.

REFERENCES

1. Silverman NA, Sabiston DC Jr: Mediastinal mass. Surg Clin N Am 60:757, 1980
2. Wychulis AR, Payne WS, Clagett OT et al: Surgical treatment of mediastinal tumors. J Thorac Cardiovasc Surg 62:379, 1971
3. Davis RD, Oldham HN, Sabiston DC Jr: Primary cyst and neoplasms of the mediastinum: recent changes in clinical presentation, methods of diagnosis, management and results. Ann Thorac Surg 44:229, 1987
4. Oldham HN, Sabiston DC Jr: Primary tumors and cysts of the mediastinum: lesions presenting as cardiovascular abnormalities. Arch Surg 9:71, 1968
5. Fontenelle LJ, Armstrong RG, Stanford W et al: The asymptomatic mediastinal tumors. Arch Surg 102:98, 1971
6. Ross JS, O'Donovan PB, Novoa R et al: Magnetic resonance of the chest: initial experience with imaging and in vivo T1 and T2 calculations. J Radiol 152:95, 1984
7. Souadjian JV, Enriquews P, Silvestein MN et al: The spectrum of diseases associated with thymoma. Arch Intern Med 134:374, 1974
8. Le Golvan DP, Abell MR: Thymomas. Cancer 39:2142, 1977
9. Wilkens EW, Castleman B: Thymoma: a continuing survey at the Massachusetts General Hospital. Ann Thorac Surg 28:252, 1979
10. Tanabe T, Kubo Y, Hashimoto M: Patch angioplasty of the superior venal caval obstruction: case reports with long term follow up. Ann Thorac Surg 19:371, 1975
11. Verley JM, Hollmann KH: Thymoma: a comparative study of clinical stages, histologic features and survival in 200 cases. Cancer 55:1074, 1985
12. Gerein AN, Srivastave SP, Burgess J: Thymoma: a ten year review. Am J Surg 138:49, 1978
13. Penn CH, Hope-Stone HF: The role of radiotherapy in the management of malignant thymoma. Br J Surg 59:533, 1972
14. Skeggs DBL: Complication associated with the radiotherapy of thymic tumors. Proc R Soc Med 66:155, 1972
15. Marks RD, Wallace KM, Petit HS: Radiation therapy control of 9 patients with malignant thymoma. Cancer 41:117, 1978
16. Batata MA, Martini N, Huvos AG et al: Thymoma: clinicopathologic features, therapy and prognosis. Cancer 34:389, 1974
17. Shetty MR, Arora RK: Invasive thymoma treated with cis platinum. Cancer Treat Rep 65:531, 1981
18. Boston B: Chemotherapy of invasive thymoma. Cancer 38:49, 1976
19. Daugaard G, Hansen HH, Roth M: Combination chemotherapy for malignant thymoma: role of COPP. Ann Intern Med 99:189, 1983
20. Chaninian AP, Bhardroj S, Nyer M et al: Treatment of invasive or metastatic thymoma: report of eleven cases. Cancer 47:1752, 1981
21. Chahinian AP, Holland JF, Bardwag S: Chemotherapy for malignant thymoma. Ann Intern Med 99:736, 1983
22. Campbell MG, Pollard R, Al-Sarraf M: A complete response to metastatic malignant thymoma to Cisplatinum, doxorubicin and cyclophosphamide. Cancer 48:1315, 1981
23. Fornasiero A, Daniele O, Sperandio P et al: Chemotherapy of invasive or metastatic thymoma: report of five cases. Cancer Treat Rep 68:1205, 1984
24. Giaccone G, Musella R, Bertetto O et al: Cisplatin containing chemotherapy in the treatment of invasive thymoma: report of five cases. Cancer Treat Rep 69:695, 1985
25. Umsawasd T, Chiuten DF, Holoye P et al: Cytoxan + adriamycin + cisplatin + prednisone in the treatment of malignant thymic tumors. Proc Am Soc Clin Oncol 4:149, 1985
26. Nefzger MD, Mostofi FK: Survival after surgery for germinal malignancies of the tests: rates of survival in tumor groups. Cancer 30:1225, 1972
27. Luna MA, Johnson DE: Postmortem findings in testicular tumors. p. 667. In Johnson EG (ed): Testicular Tumors. Medical Examination Publishing Co, New York, 1978
28. Lynch MJG, Blewiott, GL: Choriocarcinoma arising in the male mediastinum. Thorax 8:157, 1953
29. Lewis BD, Hurst RD, Payne WS et al: Benign teratomas of the mediastinum. J Thorac Cardiovasc Surg 86:727, 1974
30. Adeborojo SA, Nicola ML: Teratoid tumors of the mediastinum. Am Surg 42:361, 1976
31. Schlumberger HG: Teratoma of the anterior mediastinum in a group of military age: study of 16 cases and review of theories of genesis. Arch Pathol 41:398, 1946
32. Curry WA, McKay CE, Richardson RL et al: Klinefelter's syndrome and mediastinal germ cell neoplasms. J Urol 125:127, 1981
33. Nichol CR, Hoffman R, Einhorn LH et al: Hematologic malignancies associated with primary germ cell tumors. Ann Intern Med 102:603, 1985
34. Jain KK, Bosl GJ, Bains MS: The treatment of extragonadal seminoma. J Clin Oncol 2:820, 1984
35. Martini N, Golby B, Haidu SI et al: Primary mediastinal germ cell tumors. Cancer 33:763, 1974
36. Raghavan D, Burrett A: Mediastinal seminoma. Cancer 46:1187, 1980
37. Bush SE, Martinez A, Bagshaw M: Primary mediastinal seminoma. Cancer 48:1877, 1981
38. Hainsworth JD, Einhorn H, Williams SD et al: Extragonadal germ cell tumors: successful treatment with combination chemotherapy. Ann Intern Med 97:7, 1982
39. Daugaard G, Roth M, Hansen HH: Therapy of extra-

gonadal germ cell tumors. Eur J Clin Oncol 19:895, 1983
40. Israel A, Bosl GJ, Golby RB et al: The results of chemotherapy for extragonadal germ cell tumors in the cisplatin era: the Memorial Sloan-Kettering Cancer Center experience (1975–1982). J Clin Oncol 3:1073, 1985
41. Levitt RG, Husband JE, Glazer HJ: CT of primary germ cell tumors of the mediastinum. Am J Roentgenol 142:73, 1984
42. Fune HC, Mendez M, Alonso E et al: Mediastinal germ cell tumors treated with cisplatin, bleomycin and vinblastine (PVB). Proc Am Assoc Cancer Res 22:474, 1981
43. Vogelzanj NJ, Raghaven D, Anderson RW et al: Mediastinal nonseminomatous germ cell tumors: the role of combined modality therapy. Ann Thorac Surg 33:333, 1982
44. Hainsworth JD, Williams SD, Einhorn LH et al: Successful treatment of resistant germinal neoplasms with VP 16 and cisplatin: results of a South Eastern Cancer Study Group trial. J Clin Oncol 3:666, 1985
45. Harjula A, Mattila S, Luosto R et al: Mediastinal neurogenic tumors: early and late results of surgical treatment. Scand J Thor Cardiovas Surg 20:115, 1986
46. Holgerson LO, Santulli TV, Schullinger JN et al: Neuroblastoma with intraspinal dumbbell extension. J Pediatr Surg 18:406, 1982
47. Kudo K, Kitajima S, Muindakata H et al: WDHA syndrome caused by VIP producing neuroblastoma. J Pediatr Surg 17:476, 1982
48. Altman A, Baehner RL: Favorable prognosis for survival in children with coincident opsomyoclonus and neuroblastoma. Cancer 37:846, 1978
49. Evans AE, D'Angio GJ, Rasndolph J: A proposed staging system for children with neuroblastoma. Cancer 27:374, 1971
50. Hayes FA, Green A, Hustu HO et al: Surgicopathologic staging of neuroblastoma: prognostic significance of regional lymph node metastasis. J Pediatr 102:59, 1983
51. Shimda H, Chatten J, Newton WA et al: Histopathologic prognostic factors in neuroblastic tumors: definition of subtypes of ganglioneuroblastoma as an age-linked classification of neuroblastomas. JNCI 73:405, 1984
52. Look AJ, Hayes FA, Nitschke R et al: Cellular DNA content as a predictor of response to chemotherapy in infants with unresectable neuroblastoma. N Engl J Med 311:231, 1984
53. Saegur RC, Brodeur GM, Sather H et al: Association of multiple copies of the N-myc oncogene with rapid progression of neuroblastoma. N Engl J Med 313:1111, 1985
54. McGuire WA, Simmons DL, Gorsfeld JL et al: Should stage II neuroblastoma receive irradiation? Proc Am Soc Clin Oncol 3:80, 1984
55. Evan AE Abo V, D'Angio GJ et al: Cytophophamide treatment of patients with localized and regional neuroblastoma: a randomized study. Cancer 36:655, 1976
56. Schusater B, Land VJ, Nitschke R et al: Phase II study of four drug chemotherapy for metastatic neuroblastoma: a pediatric Oncology Group study. Cancer Treat Rep 67:187, 1983
57. Gasparini M, Bellani FF, Musumeci R et al: Response and survival of patients with metastatic neuroblastoma after combination chemotherapy with adriamycin, cyclophosphamide and vincristine. Cancer Chemother Rep 58:365, 1974
58. Rosen EM, Cansady JR, Frantz CN et al: Stage IV-N: a favorable subset of children with metastatic neuroblastoma. Med Pediatr Oncol 13:194, 1985
59. Carl M, Pastore G, Perlongo G: The role of chemotherapy in neuroblastoma. p. 765. In Raybaund C (ed): Pediatric Oncology. Excerpte Medicine, New York, 1982
60. Finkelstein JZ, Klemperer MR, Evans AE et al: Multiagent chemotherapy for children with metastatic neuroblastoma: a report from the Childrens Cancer Study Group. Med Pediatr Oncol 6:179, 1974
61. D'Angelo GJ, August C, Elkins W et al: Metastatic neuroblastoma managed by supra lethal therapy and bone marrow reconstitution: results of a four institution Children's Cancer Study Group pilot study. Prog Clin Biol Res 175:557, 1985
62. Rosenberg JC: Neoplasms of the mediastinum. p. 852. In DeVita VT (ed): Principles and Practice of Oncology. 2nd ed. JP Lippincott, Philadelphia, 1985
63. Brasfield RD, Das Gupta TK: Von Recklinghausen's disease: a clinicopathological study. Ann Surg 175:86, 1972
64. Sordillo PP, Helson L, Hajdu SI et al: Malignant schwanoma—clinical characteristics and response to therapy. Cancer 47:2503, 1981
65. Nombison RN, Ruo N, Moore R et al: Malignant soft tissue tumors of nerve sheath origin. J Surg Oncol 25:268, 1984
66. Bojsen-Moller M, Myhre-Jensen O: A consecutive series of 30 malignant schwannomas. Survival in relation to clinicopathologic parameters and treatment. Acta Pathol Microbiol Scand 92:147, 1984
67. Schwenn MR, Billing PC, Little JB: N-myc amplification and expression in a malignant schwannoma from a patient with neurofibromatosis. Proc Am Assoc Clin Res 26:65, 1985
68. Whang-Peng J, Triche TJ, Knutsen T et al: Chromosomal translocation in peripheral neuroepithelioma. N Engl J Med 311:584, 1984
69. Masaoka A, Monden B, Nakahura K et al: Followup study of thymomas with special reference to their clinical stages. Cancer 48:2485, 1981

6

Chest Wall, Pleura, and Sternum

Primary tumors of the chest wall are uncommon. Of 4,277 primary bone tumors in the Mayo Clinic series, there were 35 benign and 234 malignant lesions (6.29 percent) arising in either the ribs or the sternum.[1] In a similar series of 750 primary bone tumors reported at the Barnes Hospital, 61 (8 percent) occurred in the chest wall. Of these 61 lesions, 58 occurred in the ribs.[2]

Because of the rarity of these lesions, the establishment of an accurate diagnosis is often elusive. Pain and the presence of a mass have been the two most common complaints of patients with chest wall tumors, and many patients experience both. Patients often notice a mass several months before seeking a physician's advice, and frequently some local trauma focuses attention on the lesion.

The sex distribution of these lesions is 2 : 1 males to females, and the age of the patient may be suggestive of the type of benign or malignant lesion. The average age for benign tumors is 26, with eosinophilic granulomas, aneurysmal bone cysts, and osteochondromas occurring in the younger population and fibrous dysplasias and bone islands in older individuals. The average age for primary malignant lesions is approximately 40. Ewing's sarcoma is most common in adolescence, with osteogenic sarcoma, lymphoma, chondrosarcoma, and plasmacytoma occurring more frequently in adults. Metastatic lesions to the thoracic skeleton are the most common of all lesions, and the aveage age of these patients is the fifth and sixth decades (Table 6-1).

Laboratory examinations are usually of little help, with certain exceptions. The erythrocyte sedimentation ratio (ESR) may be elevated in some instances of Ewing's sarcoma, and the alkaline phosphatase level is often elevated in osteogenic sarcomas. Electrophoresis of serum proteins may uncover proteins specific for myelomas, although the Bence Jones protein has only been rarely identified in solitary plasmacytomas.

Radiographic evaluation of the chest wall is helpful in diagnosis and in determining the extent of disease. A local abnormality is almost always visible, and most rib lesions, although visualized on posterior and lateral chest x-rays, are better defined in oblique views. Tomography, both standard and computerized, will better delineate the tumor and the extent of its local involvement. Sharp delineation and intact cortical margins, as seen in radiographs, are characteristic of benign tumors, whereas malignant tumors are usually poorly defined and cortical disruption is common. Occasionally, old rib fractures, calcified prominent costal cartilages, myositis ossificans, prominent or bifid xyphoids, and osteomyelitis of bony structures in the chest can give misleading pictures that may suggest tumors. Because of this, an accurate histologic diagnosis is essential for the treatment of chest wall tumors. In general, needle biopsy is not recommended unless there is a strong suspicion of myeloma or metastatic disease. Small tumors (2 cm) should be excised, a procedure that in most cases will be curative. For larger tumors a carefully planned open biopsy should be undertaken to obtain adequate tissue; this should be performed so as not to compromise the incision for a future definitive resection.

TUMORS OF THE RIBS

The reported distribution of tumors in several large series is summarized in Table 6-2. The most common benign lesions, in order of frequency, are

Table 6-1. Average Age for Benign and Malignant Chest Wall Tumors

Tumor	Age (yr)
Benign	
Eosinophilic granuloma	10
Osteochondroma	15
Chondroma	25
Fibrous dysplasia	40
Malignant	
Ewing's sarcoma	10
Osteogenic sarcoma	15
Chondrosarcoma	30
Plasmacytoma	50

Table 6-2. Histologic Classification of Benign Chest Wall Lesions Reported in the Literature[1,2,3,4]

Type of Tumor	No. of Patients	Percent of Total
Fibrous dysplasia	28	34
Osteochondroma	18	23
Enchondroma	11	14
Eosinophilic granuloma	5	7
Osteoblastoma	3	4
Bone islands	3	4
Aneurysmal bone cyst	2	2
Hemangioma	2	2
Xanthoma	2	2
Fibroma	2	2
Fibroxanthoma	1	1
Giant cell tumor	1	1
Lipoma	1	1
Osteoid osteoma	1	1
Angiomatosis	1	1
Chondroblastoma	1	1
Total	82	100

Table 6-3. Histologic Classification of Malignant Chest Wall Tumors Reported in the Literature[1,2,3,4]

Type of Tumor	No. of Patients	Percent of Total
Chondrosarcoma	29	34
Myeloma	29	34
Ewing's sarcoma	11	13
Osteogenic sarcoma	10	12
Lymphoma	7	7
Total	86	100

fibrous dysplasias (34 percent), osteochondromas (22 percent), and eosinophilic granulomas (6 percent). The most common malignant lesions are chondrosarcomas, plasmacytomas, Ewing's sarcoma, and osteogenic sarcomas (Table 6-3).[1–4]

BENIGN RIB TUMORS

FIBROUS DYSPLASIAS

The lesions of fibrous dysplasia are generally completely asymptomatic and are usually discovered on routine radiographic examination of the chest. The characteristic lesion has a homogeneous gray or ground-glass appearance and a sharply defined edge. There is usually a very thin sclerotic rim due to a narrow zone of deposition of reactive bone around the fibrous tissue.

Pathologically the major feature is a proliferation of fibroblasts that produce a dense collagenous matrix. The fibrous element typically contains trabeculae of osteoid and bone which are too small to be resolved radiographically but can be delineated on computed tomography (CT) with attenuated values of 20 to 40H (Fig. 6-1).

Fibrous dysplasia typically exhibits extremely intense uptake on bone scans, presumably as a result of the diffuse microscopic ossification (Table 6-4).

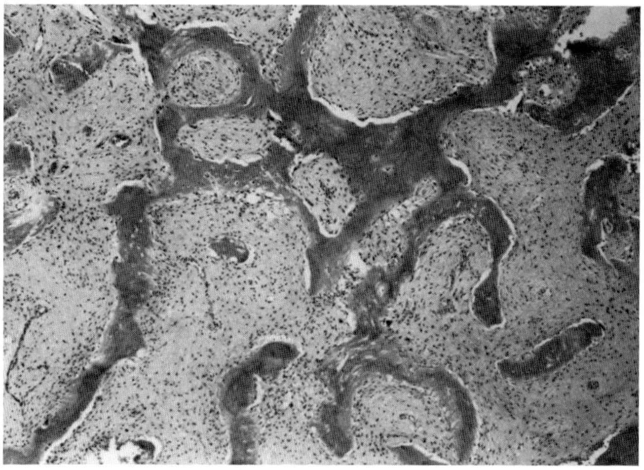

Fig. 6-1. Fibrous dyplasia. Curved randomly interconnecting trabeculae of immature bone in a moderately fibrous stoma. (× 50.)

ENCHONDROMAS

Enchondromas are typically located at the costochondral junctions and occur most often in patients in the second and third decades of life. This tumor usually presents as a painless mass on the anterior chest wall.

Table 6-4. Major Characteristics of Rib Tumors

Tumor	Median Age (yr)	Male/Female Ratio	Location	Treatment	Markers
Benign					
Fibrous dysplasia	40	1 : 1		Surgical excision	
Chondroma	25	1 : 1		Surgical excision	
Osteochondroma	15	1 : 1	First four ribs	Surgical excision	
Eosinophilic granuloma	10	3 : 2		Observation	
Malignant					
Chondrosarcoma	30	2 : 1		Surgical resection	None
Plasmacytoma	57	3 : 1		Radiotherapy	Bence Jones proteins, serum electrophoresis
Ewing's sarcoma	10	2 : 1		Surgical resection, chemotherapy	None
Osteogenic sarcoma	20	2 : 1		Surgery, chemotherapy	Alkaline phosphatase

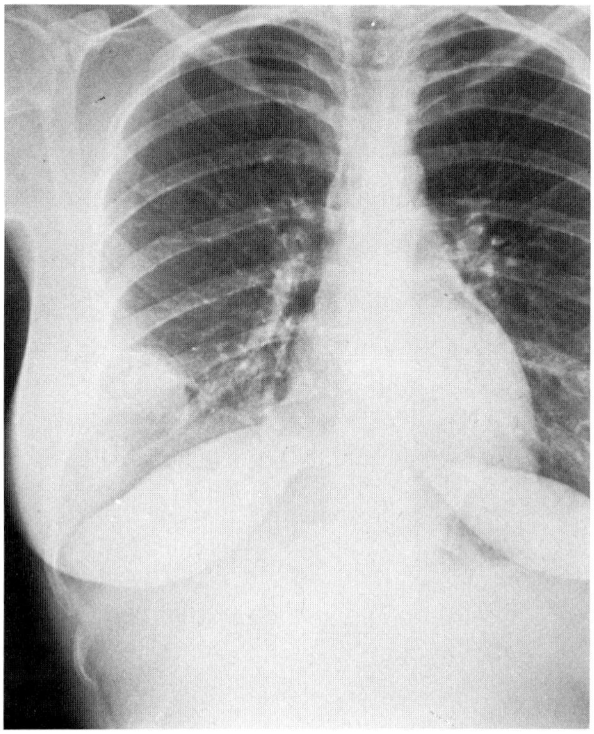

A

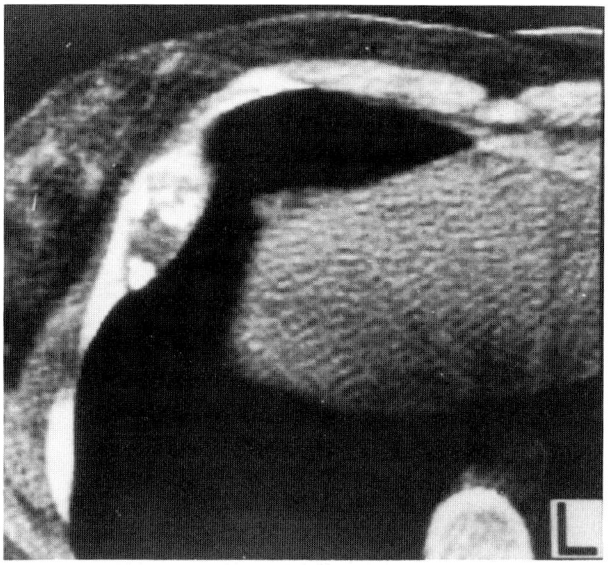

B

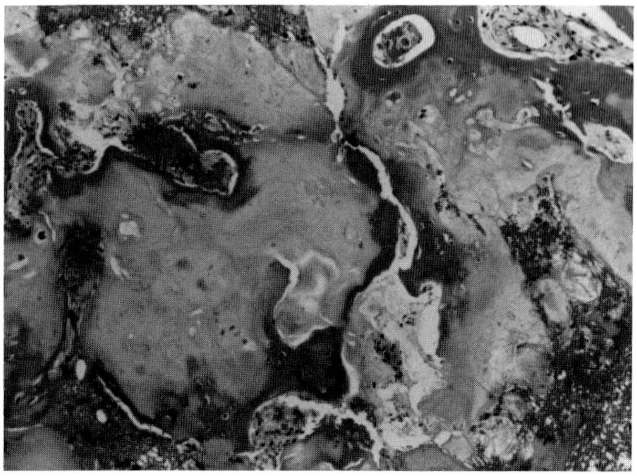

C

Fig. 6-2. **(A)** Plain PA chest x-ray revealing two enchondromas in an asymptomatic 17-year-old patient. **(B)** CT scan revealing the thin cortex and matted calcification within the tumor. **(C)** Enchondroma. Sparsely cellular hyaline cartilage nodules showing "picture framing" by endochondrally ossified bone at the periphery. (× 100.)

On radiography this lesion appears as a medullary mass that may thin the overlying cortex, often in an eccentric manner, but does not disrupt it. Slight to very prominent stippled or matted calcifications of the tumor are frequently seen (Fig. 6-2).

On gross section the characteristic chondroma is composed of confluent masses of bluish semitranslucent hyaline cartilage with a distinctly lobular arrangement. The chondrocytes that make up the cellular component of a chondroma are small cells that lie in lacunar spaces and have a round, regular nucleus. The degree of cellularity varies remarkably in chondromas; hence, cellularity affords little help in differentiating chondroma from chondrosarcoma.

Left untreated, these tumors can grow to a very large size, sometimes exceeding 4 cm, which some pathologists believe is the upper limit for benign tumors.[5] Excision of the involved costal cartilage along with a short segment of the accompanying rib is curative (Table 6-4).

OSTEOCHONDROMAS

Osteochondromas generally are identified in the first and second decades of life, and there is no sex predilection. It is interesting that the majority of the lesions that arise in the ribs are located on the first four ribs.

A palpable mass is ordinarily the only finding. The characteristic appearance on radiography is that of a projection composed of a cortex continuous with underlying bone and spongiosa. The cap is initially cartilagenous, but irregular calcifications may be present.

The gross pathologic features confirm the radiographic pattern. The tumor cortex and its periosteal covering are continuous with those of the underlying bone, with which it often merges. Microscopic studies confirm the gross appearance of regular cortical and underlying medullary bone with its fatty or hematopoietic components (Fig. 6-3).

The presence of an osteochondroma in itself is insufficient reason for surgical extirpation, since malignant transformation is rare. Surgical excision is indicated if the tumor is causing pain, has radiographic features suggestive of malignancy, or shows an abnormal increase in size. Removal of the tumor flush with the bone of origin is the treatment. The entire cartilagenous cap must be removed to avoid recurrence. If the tumor is located on a rib, en bloc excision is often necessary (Table 6-4).

EOSINOPHILIC GRANULOMAS

Eosinophilic granulomas of bone make up 60 to 80 percent of all cases of histiocytoma X and can be solitary or multifocal. Most patients are in the first three decades of life, and the peak incidence is between 5 and 10 years of age. Male patients predominate 3 : 2 over females.

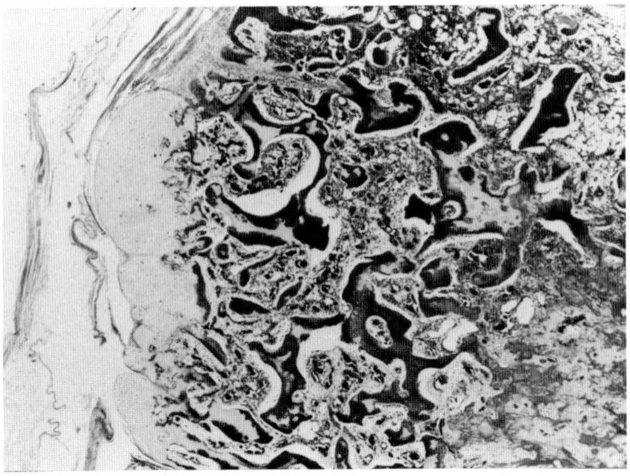

Fig. 6-3. Osteochondroma. Hyaline cartilage cap with overlying fibrous tissue transforming into bone and hematopoietic marrow by endochondral ossification. (× 20.)

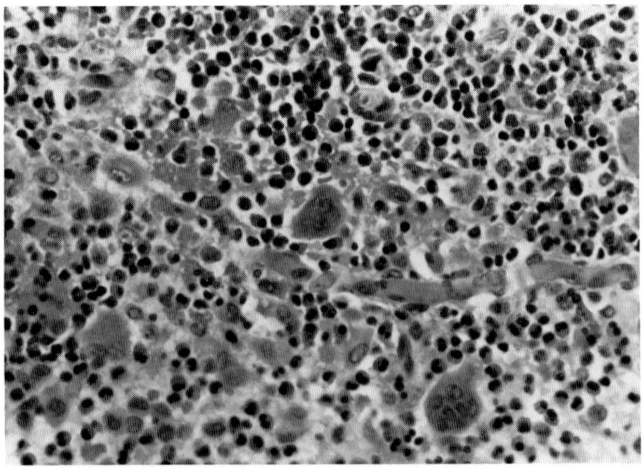

Fig. 6-4. Eosinophilic granuloma. The lesion is composed of two cell populations. Histiocytes are the larger mononuclear cells, which form several multinuclear giant cells in this field. Eosinophils are the numerous smaller background cells with occasional bilobed nuclei. (× 400.)

These are geographic lytic lesions and can be associated with a reactive sclerotic rim or have sharp punched-out areas with no sclerosis. CT often shows the extent of bone destruction much more clearly than does radiography.

Grossly the lesions contain soft grayish-yellow or brownish tissue often with necrotic areas, cysts, and hemorrhage. Microscopically they are characterized by proliferating histiocytes that are large and ovoid (Fig. 6-4).

Many of the bone lesions heal spontaneously, but symptomatic lesions may be healed by resection, curettage, steroid injection, or radiotherapy in low doses (Table 6-4).[6]

MALIGNANT RIB TUMORS

CHONDROSARCOMAS

Chondrosarcomas are the most common of the primary malignant tumors of the chest wall. As with its benign counterpart (chondroma), the costochondral junction is its most frequent location. However, the tumor may occur anywhere along the course of the ribs (Table 6-4).

Pathologic grading of the tumor is most important. Signs of malignancy may be subtle and found only in limited areas of a tumor (Fig. 6-5).

The classic histologic features include the presence of many cells with plump nuclei, cells with two plump nuclei, and giant cartilage cells with large single and multiple nuclei or clumps of chromatin. Grading of chondrosarcomas emphasizing the mitotic rate and cellularity was performed by Evans et al.,[7] and a similar grading system was used by Marcove and Huvos[8] and Gitelis et al.[9] In correlating the grade with distant metastasis and survival in several large series, the following was observed: Grade I chondrosarcoma has 5 percent metastasis, 92 percent 5-year survival, and 85 percent 10-year survival; grade II has 20 percent metastasis, 70 percent 5-year survival, and 50 percent 10-year survival; grade III has 55 percent metastasis, 44 percent 5-year survival, and 28 percent 10-year survival.[10] Because the majority of rib lesions are grade I and II, definitive surgical resection is the treatment of choice, and the extent of resection should not be compromised because of an inability to close the chest wall defect.

Opinions differ about what constitutes a wide resection. King,[11] reporting the Mayo Clinic experience, advocates a minimum 2-cm margin of resection, with wider margins of resection (4 cm) indicated for the higher-grade lesions. For rib cage

A B C

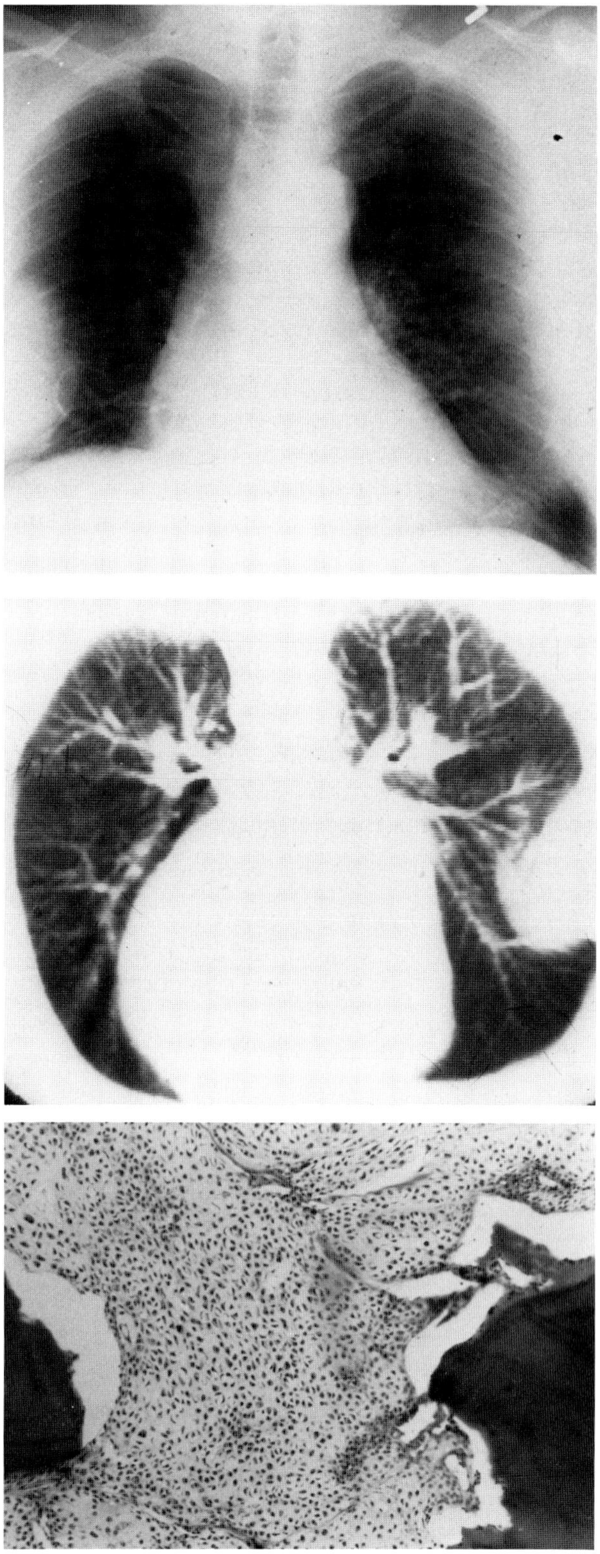

Fig. 6-5. **(A)** Plain PA chest x-ray revealing a large homogeneous mass in the right rib cage. **(B)** CT scan of the same lesion. **(C)** Chondrosarcoma. Intertrabecular spaces of cancellous bone are infiltrated by a moderately cellular cartilage tumor. (× 80.)

resection this includes removal of the involved ribs in toto and several partial ribs above and below the neoplasm. Reconstruction of these defects requires stabilization of the bony thorax and, in rare situations, coverage of any soft tissue defect. For anterior thoracic defects less than 10 cm in diameter no reconstruction is usually necessary.

Because these are generally slow-growing malignant tumors with a high cure rate following adequate surgical resection, high survival rates follow resection. The results following surgical resection in various series reveal that five-year survival rates of 85 to 90 percent are common, with 10-year survival, in most series, approaching 70 percent.[1,2,3,4]

At present radiotherapy and chemotherapy have no proven efficacy in the management of these tumors.

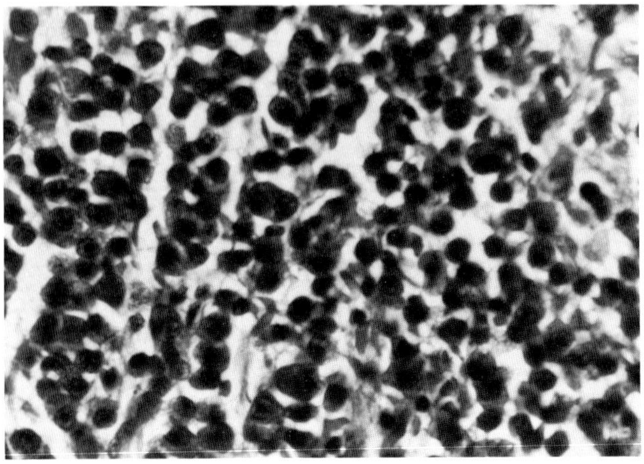

Fig. 6-6. Plasma cell myeloma. A sheet of atypical plasma cells with occasional double nuclei and prominent nucleoli. (× 500.)

PLASMACYTOMAS

Solitary plasmacytomas arising in bone are uncommon, occurring in 3 to 7 percent[12,13] of patients with plasma cell myeloma. Patients with the disease often develop multiple myelomas, but the time to dissemination is variable and may be longer than 20 years.

Approximately 25 to 30 percent of all primary malignant tumors in the chest wall are plasmacytomas. Myeloma, which is familiar as multiple punched-out lytic lesions in the skull, is not as readily recognized when it takes the form of a solitary similar-appearing lesion in the ribs or sternum.[14]

The average age of patients presenting with solitary plasmacytomas is 57 years, and males predominate 3 : 1 over females. The ribs are the third most common site of presentation after the spine and pelvis. Approximately 25 percent of all patients will have elevated levels of paraprotein in serum or urine. The presence of paraproteins is not predictive of subsequent disease progression (Table 6-4).

If examination of the entire skeleton radiographically and by bone scans reveals no additional lesions, tissue should be obtained by needle biopsy initially. If the location of the tumor precludes a safe approach for needle biopsy, open surgical biopsy can be accomplished.

Grossly myeloma tissue is soft, reddish-gray, and friable. Microscopically it is composed of sheets of clearly packed plasma cells, varying in maturity. Each cell contains abundant basophilic cytoplasm and a round or oval eccentric cytoplasm, often with two or three nucleoli (Fig. 6-6).

Local control of a solitary plasmacytoma can be achieved with a high success rate by radiotherapy.[15] More radical surgical resection should be reserved for patients who failed radiotherapy treatment and have symptomatic localized disease.

Overall, patients with plasmacytomas have an indolent course of disease. A review of several reported series[16–20] showed that 55 percent of patients progressed to systemic disease in the first 5 years following diagnosis. An additional 23 percent manifested systemic myeloma at later time. At 15 years, however, 23 percent of all patients had no evidence of disease (NED).

With progression of disease, patients died of disseminated disease. There is a median survival time of 47 months and a 5-year survival of 32 percent after progression. Overall, survival of patients with solitary plasmacytomas is 75 percent at 5 years, 52 percent at 10 years, and 37 percent at 20 years.

Systemic chemotherapy should probably be reserved for patients who manifest disease progression.

EWING'S SARCOMA

Ewing's sarcoma is one of the most common primary bone malignancies and is especially common in young patients. It makes up 6 to 7 percent of all primary bone malignancies and approximately 13 percent of all rib lesions. The peak age incidence is 10 to 20 years of age, and most patients are between 5 and 30 years old. Male patients are affected more commonly than females in ratios from 1.4 : 1 to 2 : 1 (Table 6-4).[21]

Patients usually present with pain that gradually increases in severity over several months. Other common signs and symptoms include a mass, tenderness, and local erythema. Some patients have systemic manifestations including malaise, low-grade fever, anemia, leukocytosis, and an elevated ESR.

The typical appearance on plain radiography is that of permeative bone destruction and laminated periosteal reaction. There is frequently an associated extraosseous soft tissue mass. Incisional biopsy to establish the diagnosis is the initial step in the management of these patients. Ewing's sarcomas are grossly soft or fibrous and sometimes gelatinous. There are often areas of hemorrhage, necrosis, and cyst formation (Fig. 6-7).

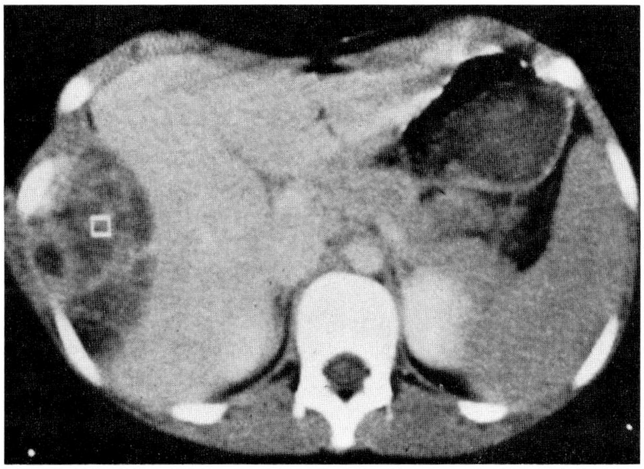

A

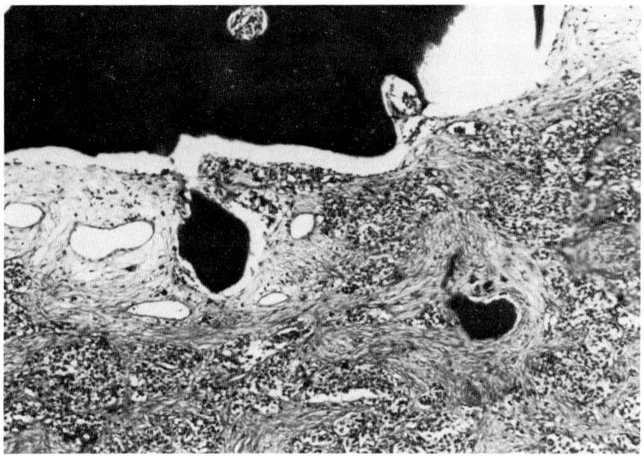

B

Fig. 6-7. **(A)** CT scan revealing a Ewing's sarcoma arising from the tenth rib with compression of the underlying hepatic parenchyma. **(B)** Ewing's sarcoma. A section through the corticomedullary junction revealing sheets of small round nuclei in endosteal marrow and in one haversian canal at the top left of center. (× 70.)

The microscopic appearance is that of monotonous fields of small, round cells that lie together and are often arranged in clusters or cords. The average cell is two or three times the size of a lymphocyte and contains a well-defined, moderately basophilic, oval or round nucleus with few nucleoli. Traditional survival rates for Ewing's sarcomas have been approximately 10 percent. Significant improvement has occurred with the advent of the combined-modality approach.

The role of chemotherapy in Ewing's sarcoma has evolved over the past decade. In the earliest trials the most effective agents were cyclophosphamide, vincristine, actinomycin D, and adriamycin. These single agents were able to induce responses, but long-term survival advantages could not be demonstrated. When multiagent regimens were initially used in single institutional trials,[22–24] at least one series reported a survival of 52 percent at 5 years.[24] The intergroup Ewing's sarcoma group studied four drugs (vincristine, cyclophosphamide, actinomycin D, and adriamycin) versus three drugs (vincristine, actinomycin D, and cyclophosphamide). In addition, the role of prophylactic lung radiation was evaluated in each arm.[25]

The four-drug regimen proved to be more efficacious than the three-drug regimen and marginally more effective than the regimen involving three drugs and prophylactic lung radiation. Also, when the courses of drugs were shortened from 6 weeks to 3 weeks, more patients had a longer disease-free survival. These results have been similarly noted in other studies involving aggressive chemotherapy.[26–29]

OSTEOGENIC SARCOMAS

Osteogenic sarcomas are the second most common tumors of bony origin after myelomas. In the ribs, however, they are the fourth most common and are responsible for only 10 percent of the tumors reported in a collected series.[6] In a Mayo Clinic series, rib osteosarcomas accounted for 1 percent of all lesions.[1]

There is a male predilection for these tumors, and the peak incidence is in the second decade (Table 6-4).

Clinically the tumor may present as a painful, rapidly expanding mass. The duration of symptoms prior to definitive therapy may vary from a few weeks to several months.

About one-half of osteosarcomas exhibit a radiographic appearance typical enough to permit confident diagnosis. The classic "sunburst" pattern secondary to reactive periosteal new bone is often present (Fig. 6-8).

Similar to the current treatment of Ewing's sarcomas, pre- and postoperative multidrug chemotherapy with en bloc resection has become the standard therapy. Single agents in osteosarcoma have yielded response rates approaching 40 percent. The agents considered to yield the highest response rates have been *cis*-platinum, adriamycin, and high-dose methotrexate.[30] Multidrug regimens are currently used in a neoadjuvant setting after biopsy. Chemotherapy is administered prior to surgery to shrink the tumor in preparation for an en bloc resection, as well as to evaluate the regimen chosen.

Rosen et al.[31] reported on the use of preoperative chemotherapy with high-dose methotrexate with Leucovorin rescue, adriamycin, and a combination of bleomycin, cyclophosphamide, and actinomycin D administered 4 to 16 weeks prior to surgery. A second regimen eliminated adriamycin preoperatively, and patients with a good histologic response were treated for only a total of two or more cycles and had their therapy stopped at the end of 15 weeks. Patients with a poor response had adriamycin and *cis*-platinum added to their regimen and high-dose methotrexate and bleomy-

A

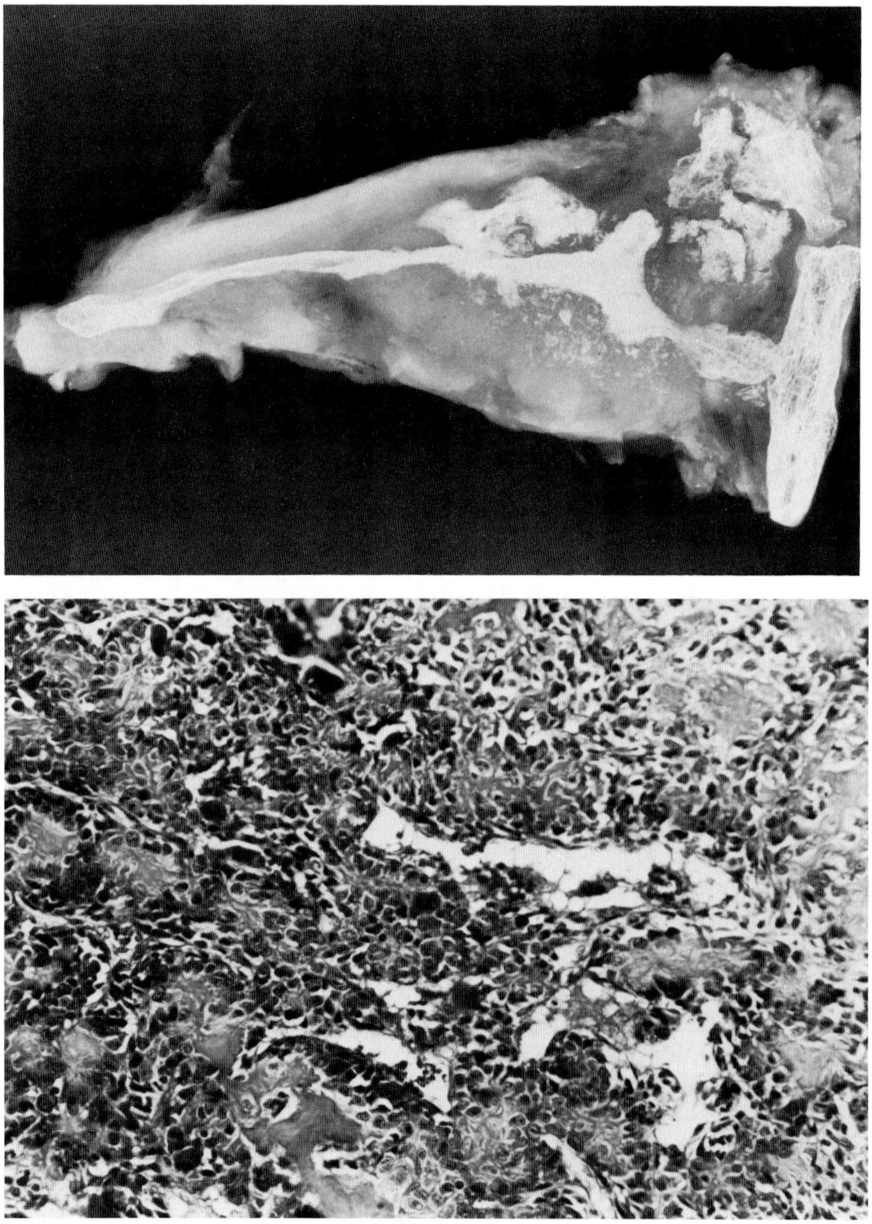

B

Fig. 6-8. **(A)** Specimen radiograph of a primary osteogenic sarcoma revealing the classic sunburst pattern and a markedly destructive lesion. **(B)** Osteosarcoma. Pleomorphic sarcoma cells producing immature bone trabeculae. (× 157.)

cin deleted. Approximately 45 percent of patients demonstrated at least 90 percent necrosis of their tumors preoperatively and were continued on their original regimen. The overall disease-free survival for this regimen was approximately 80 percent.

Similar studies by the Children's Cancer Study Group[32] and the cooperative German-Austrian osteosarcoma study group[33–35] revealed that only 30 percent of their patients had at least 95 percent necrosis of their tumors, with a 2-year disease-free survival of 91 percent. Twenty-nine percent of patients were intermediate responders (50 to 95 percent necrosis). Their 2-year disease-free survival was 83 percent. Forty-one percent of patients were poor responders (less than 50 percent necrosis), and these patients had a 2-year disease-free survival of only 4 percent despite the crossover to adriamycin and *cis*-platinum therapy.

Additional regimens have involved intra-arterial therapy preoperatively. Jaffe et al.[36] reported the results of four cycles of preoperative intra-arterial *cis*-platinum, with an overall disease-free survival of more than 80 percent in patients with complete or partial response (60 to 100 percent necrosis) versus 34 percent in patients who had no response.

SOFT TISSUE SARCOMAS

The majority of malignant soft tissue sarcomas that arise in the thoracic skeleton are categorized as fibrous in origin and are predominantly malignant fibrous hystiocytomas. In addition, dermatofibrosarcoma protuberans, liposarcomas, fibrosarcomas, angiosarcomas, and primitive neuroectodermal tumors have been reported. The last of these is a rare, highly malignant small cell neoplasm that most often arises from the chest wall or paravertebral region. Askin[37] originally described this lesion in 20 children and adolescents whose tumor arose in the soft tissues of the chest wall and in whom aggressive therapy yielded a median survival of only 8 months.

Predisposing factors to the development of sarcomas of the chest wall include a history of irradiation[38] or the finding of one of the various hereditary syndromes such as Von Recklinghausen's neurofibromatosis, Werner syndrome, or Gardner syndrome.[39] Adequate wide excision is accepted as the mainstay of therapy. The most significant prognostic factors for these patients is the histologic grade. Overall, the 5-year survival is 55 percent for fibrosarcomas.[40] Other sarcomas with a similar prognosis include dermatofibrosarcomas and liposarcomas.[41] Patients with angiosarcomas and neuroectodermal tumors have the worst prognosis.[42]

CHEST WALL RECONSTRUCTION

With larger resections, reconstruction may be considered necessary to obtain sufficient chest wall fixation in an area for vital respiratory effort or to achieve additional chest wall fixation for more adequate respiratory function.

Marlex mesh alone[43] has been used to stabilize the bony thorax. Crucial to the use of this material is that it must be placed under tension when sewn into place to the ribs of the chest wall defect. Prolene sutures are placed through muscle and fascia and around and through the ribs. When secured taut, its initial high tensile strength ensures a stable thoracic wall early. However, there may be a loss of support with time (Fig. 6-9).

Another polypropylene mesh, Prolene, has also been used for chest wall reconstruction. Prolene is a double-stitch knit, whereas Marlex is only a single-stitch knit.[44] Prolene is therefore considered rigid in all directions, whereas Marlex is rigid in only one direction.

GoreTex soft tissue patch has recently been advocated for chest wall reconstruction because it is impermeable to the flow of both air and water across the chest wall.[45]

To enhance rigidity, methyl methacrylate has been used. This was originally described by LeRoux in 1956 and promoted by McCormack et al.[46] They used a Marlex sandwich that consists of methyl methacrylate and steel mesh embedded between two layers of Marlex mesh. In this procedure a piece of stainless steel slightly smaller than the defect to be repaired is used. An excess arm of Marlex mesh surrounding the sandwich is available for securing the prosthesis to the chest wall. An advantage of methyl methacrylate is that as it is setting it can be bent and curved into the appropriate shape (Fig. 6-10).

A modification of this technique has been described by Pass et al.[47] Marlex is first sutured lightly to the edges of the defect, and the lung is deflated. The methyl methacrylate is then spread on the Marlex, and the steel mesh is placed on the hardening and warming methacrylate. A final layer is then placed over the mesh.

Other materials used to repair defects include periosteum, rib grafts, titanium mesh, and fiberglass. These materials have not gained wide acceptance.

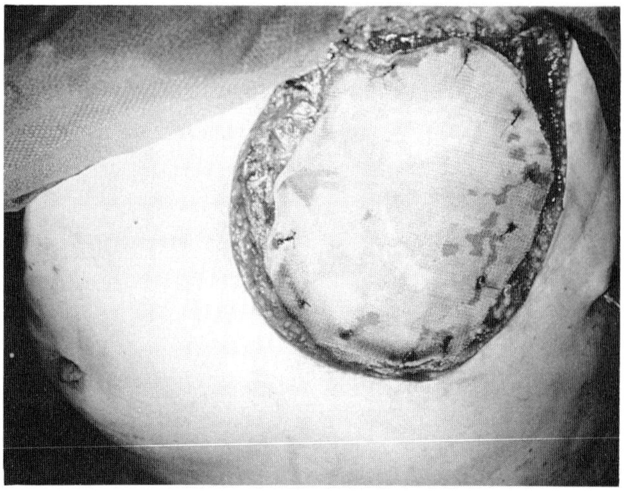

Fig. 6-9. Marlex mesh reconstruction of the chest wall secured with prolene sutures.

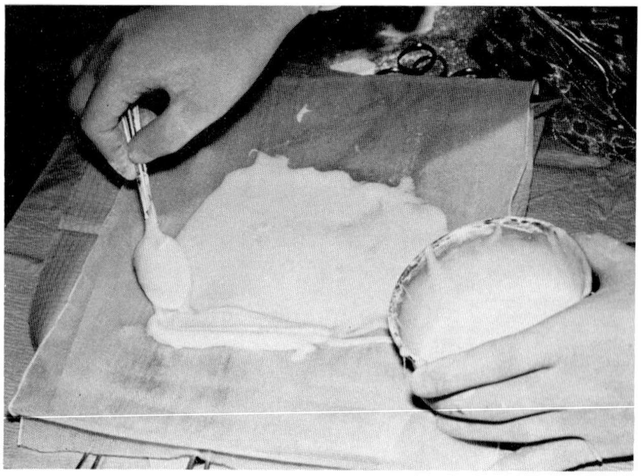

Fig. 6-10. Marlex mesh–methyl methacrylate sandwich being constructed.

A

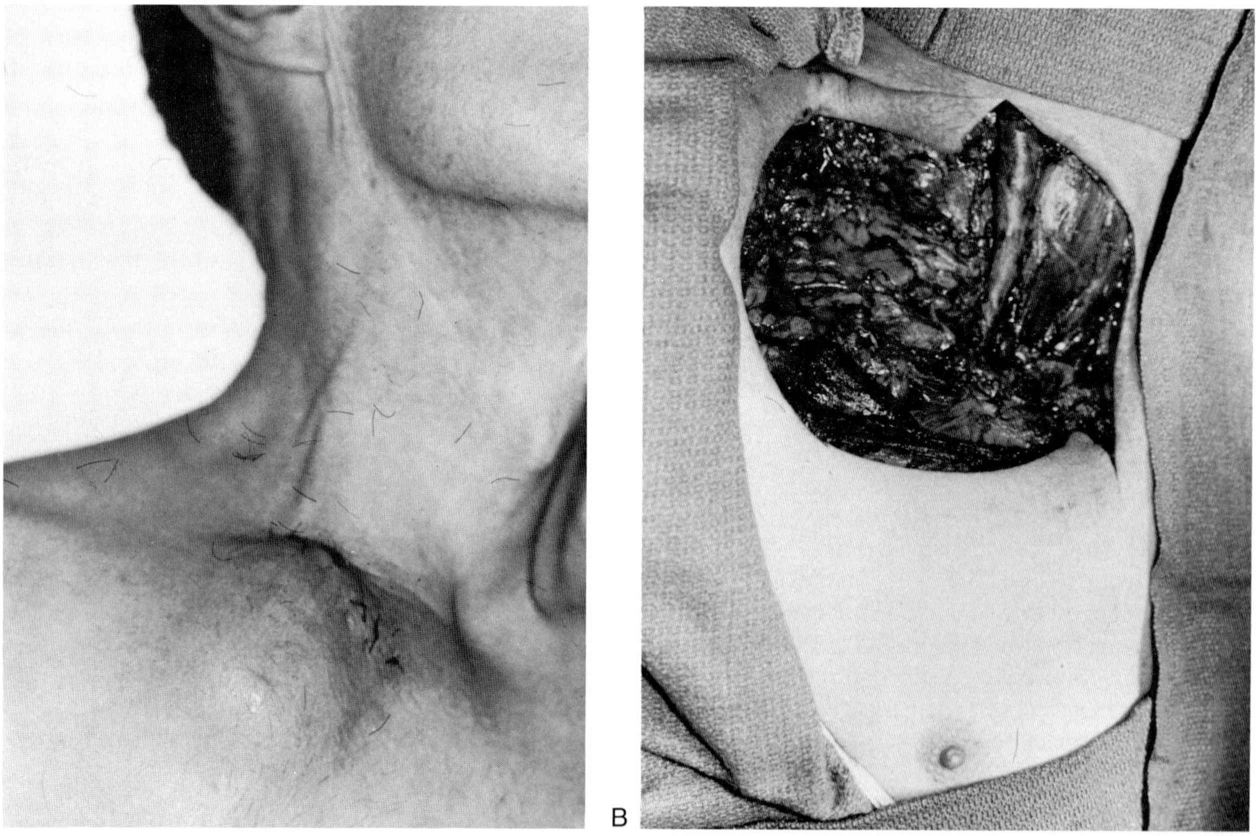

B

Fig. 6-11. **(A)** Radiation-induced osteogenic sarcoma. **(B)** The resultant defect following resection of the clavicle and the first two ribs. (*Figure continues.*)

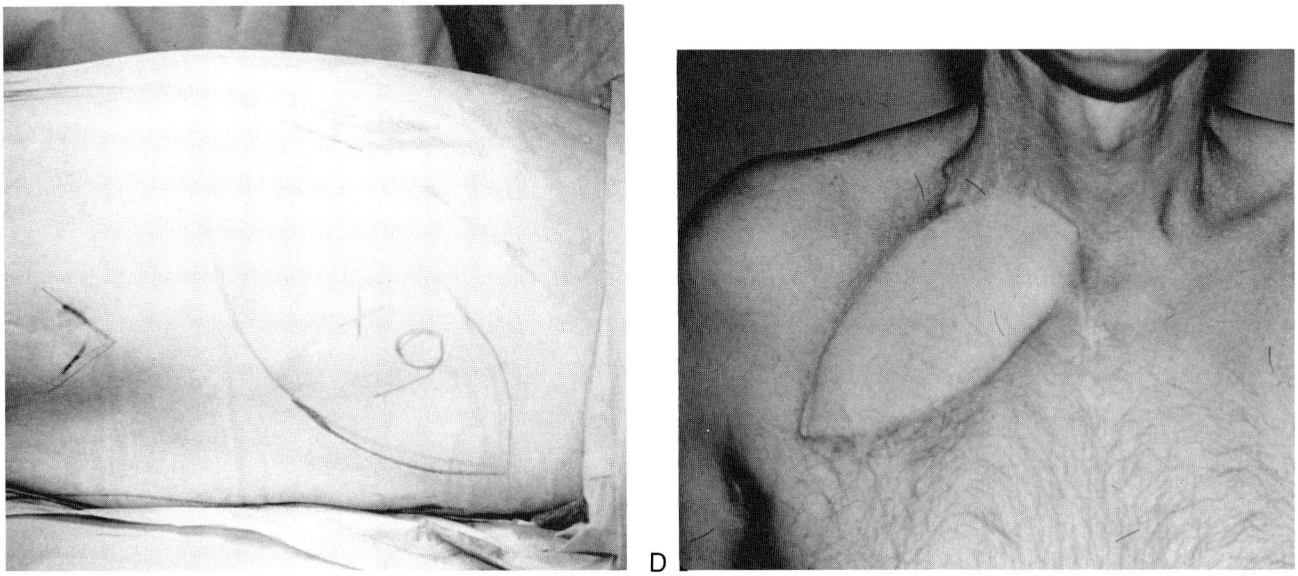

C D

Fig. 6-11 (*Continued*). **(C)** A latissimus dorsi myocutaneous flap designed to cover the chest wall defect. **(D)** The flap in position 1 month postoperatively.

In situations in which a soft tissue defect in addition to bony defects must be closed, various myocutaneous flaps have been used. Campbell[48] first reported the use of a latissimus dorsi muscle flap in 1950. This muscle has an axial blood supply, which permits elevation and rotation of this muscle for a substantial distance (Fig. 6-11). The TRAM flap described by Rablins in 1979 for breast reconstruction is useful for large defects of the chest wall as well.[49] The vascular supply to the muscle and skin is supplied by both the superior and inferior epigastric arteries coursing on the posterior surface of the muscle. The flap is usually based superiorly on the internal mammary artery and can easily cover an entire hemithorax (Fig. 6-12).

In addition to the myocutaneous flaps, large chest wall defects can be closed by utilizing the greater omentum and skin grafting[50–54] and also, most recently, with microvascular free flaps. The latter technique is particularly useful if local flaps have failed or if the local tissues have previously undergone radiation (Fig. 6-13). A tensor fascia lata myocutaneous flap based on the lateral circumflex femoral vessels has been reported for an area that received heavy irradiation.[55]

STERNUM

Tumors of the sternum are uncommon, and the vast majority are malignant. They are most likely to be metastatic and to originate from the breast, kidney, or thyroid.[56] Testicular, lung, stomach, and colon cancers also frequently metastasize to the sternum.

Primary tumors of the sternum are always malignant. The most common lesion is the chondrosarcoma.[57–59] Slow growth and a tendency to local recurrence after limited excision are characteristic of this tumor. Adequate radiographic investigation is necessary to assess the true extent of the lesion correctly. The presenting mass is often part of a much larger tumor invading the sternum. These tumors are radioresistant, and surgery is the mainstay of therapy.

The second most common group of tumors are those of reticuloendothelial origin. This includes Ewing sarcomas, myelomas, and lymphomas. In the majority of these cases the tumors are systemic but occasionally are localized to the sternum. In such cases the role of surgery is to establish the diagnosis.

Plasmacytomas are treated with melphalan and prednisone, with radiation therapy for the localized lesion.[15,16] En bloc resection of Ewing sarcoma may be indicated in some instances, but the tumor is so radiosensitive that a course of radiation therapy between treatments with vincristine and actinomycin D is most effective.[29]

Occasionally lesions such as angiosarcomas, neurosarcomas, and liposarcomas have been reported.[60,61]

Benign lesions arising in the sternum include

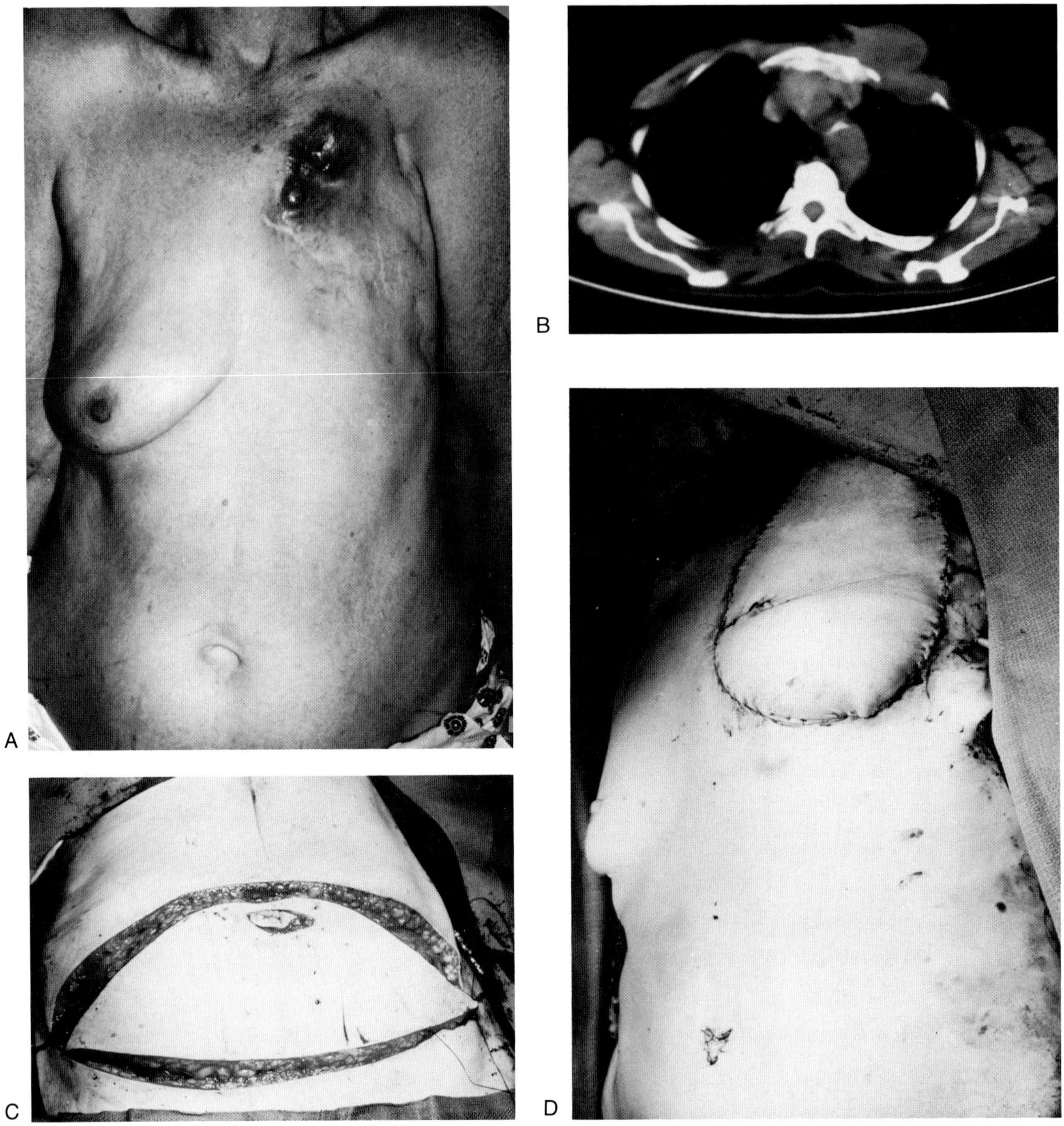

Fig. 6-12. **(A)** Radiation-induced sarcoma 10 years after a mastectomy and postoperative radiation therapy to the chest wall. **(B)** CT scan delineating the full AP extent of the lesion. **(C)** A TRAM flap being elevated to cover the defect. **(D)** The flap rotated and secured into position. The patient's umbilicus has been relocated.

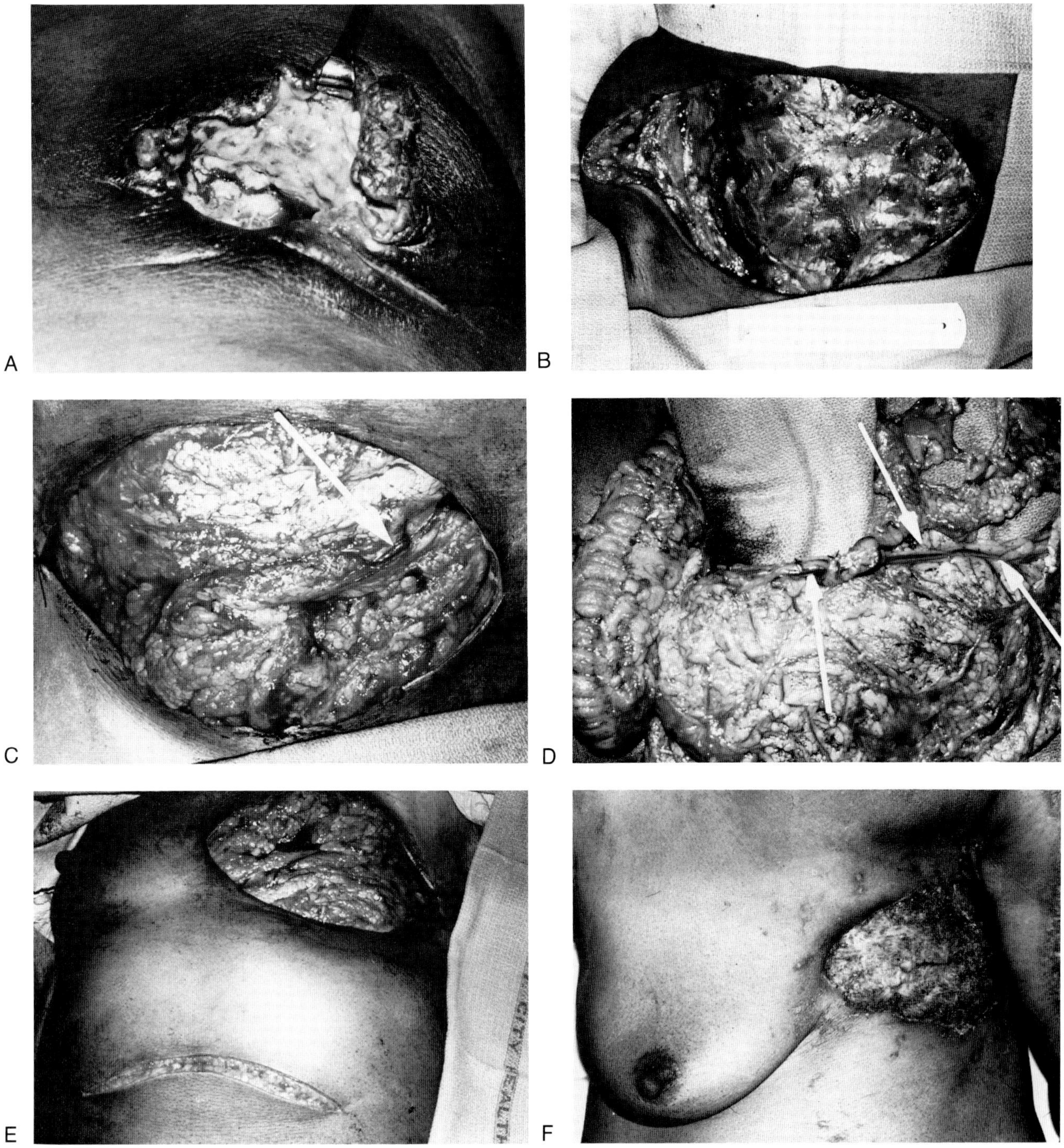

Fig. 6-13. **(A)** An ulcerated lesion of the chest wall secondary to a recurrent breast cancer. **(B)** The defect to be repaired following resection. **(C)** The abdomen is opened, and the omentum and its vascular pedicle (arrows) are identified. **(D)** The omentum is fully mobilized on its vascular pedicle. **(E)** A tunnel is created, the omentum is brought up to the defect, and the abdomen is closed. **(F)** The healed skin graft placed on the transposed omentum.

chondromas, giant cell tumors, and inflammatory and parasitic masses.

For tumors in which resection of the sternum is indicated, the incision is carried down to the rigid chest wall, leaving any involved skin, subcutaneous tissue, or muscle adherent to the tumor wall. The deep aspect of the tumor is evaluated by entering a normal intercostal space. Adherent pleura or pericardium is resected with the tumor mass. If the manubrium is resected, the medial portion of the clavicles should be excised with a 4-cm margin of normal sternum and costal cartilage. If a portion of the sternum is preserved, the sternal defect can usually be repaired by using Marlex mesh under moderate tension. When a total sternectomy is performed, a Marlex–methyl methacrylate sandwich will give secure fixation and rigidity to the anterior chest wall. This is essential to preserve the 360-degree circumferential integrity of the thorax without significant paradoxical motion. It is important that the prosthesis be the exact size of the part excised. There is a tendency of the defect to widen after the tumor is excised. If too large a prosthesis is used, a wider chest results, with a smaller anteroposterior diameter. This also can constrict the major vascular inflow to the heart. Secure skin closure over the area of repair can be accomplished primarily or if necessary with bipedical advancement flaps or with myocutaneous flaps (Figs. 6-14 to 6-18).

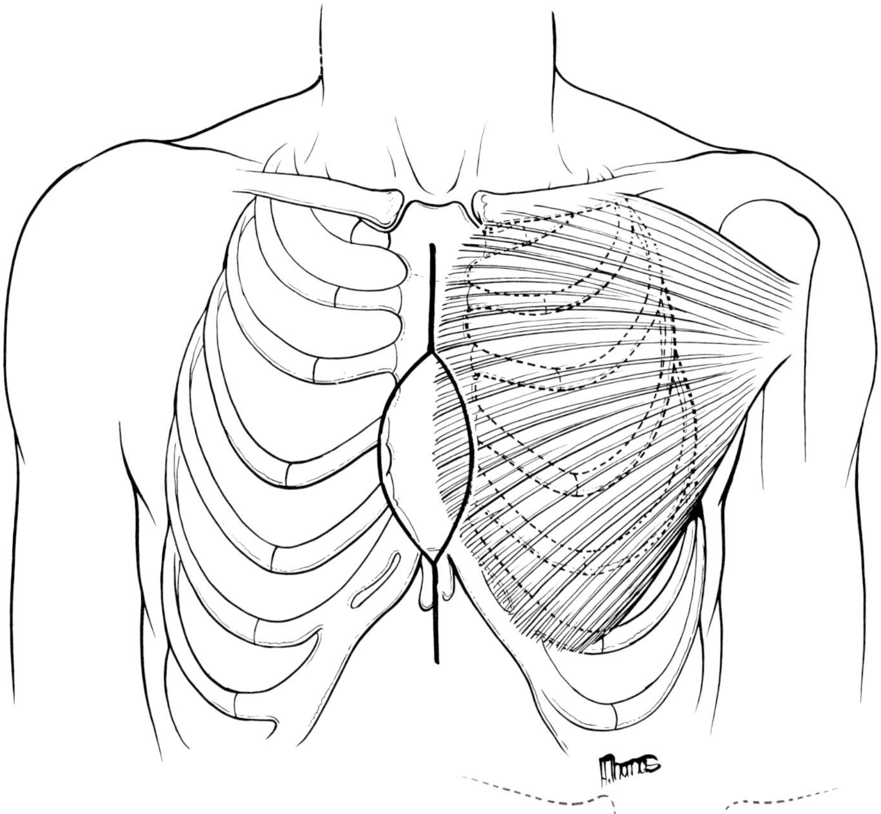

Fig. 6-14. Drawing indicating incision for resection of a primary chondrosarcoma of the lower sternum.

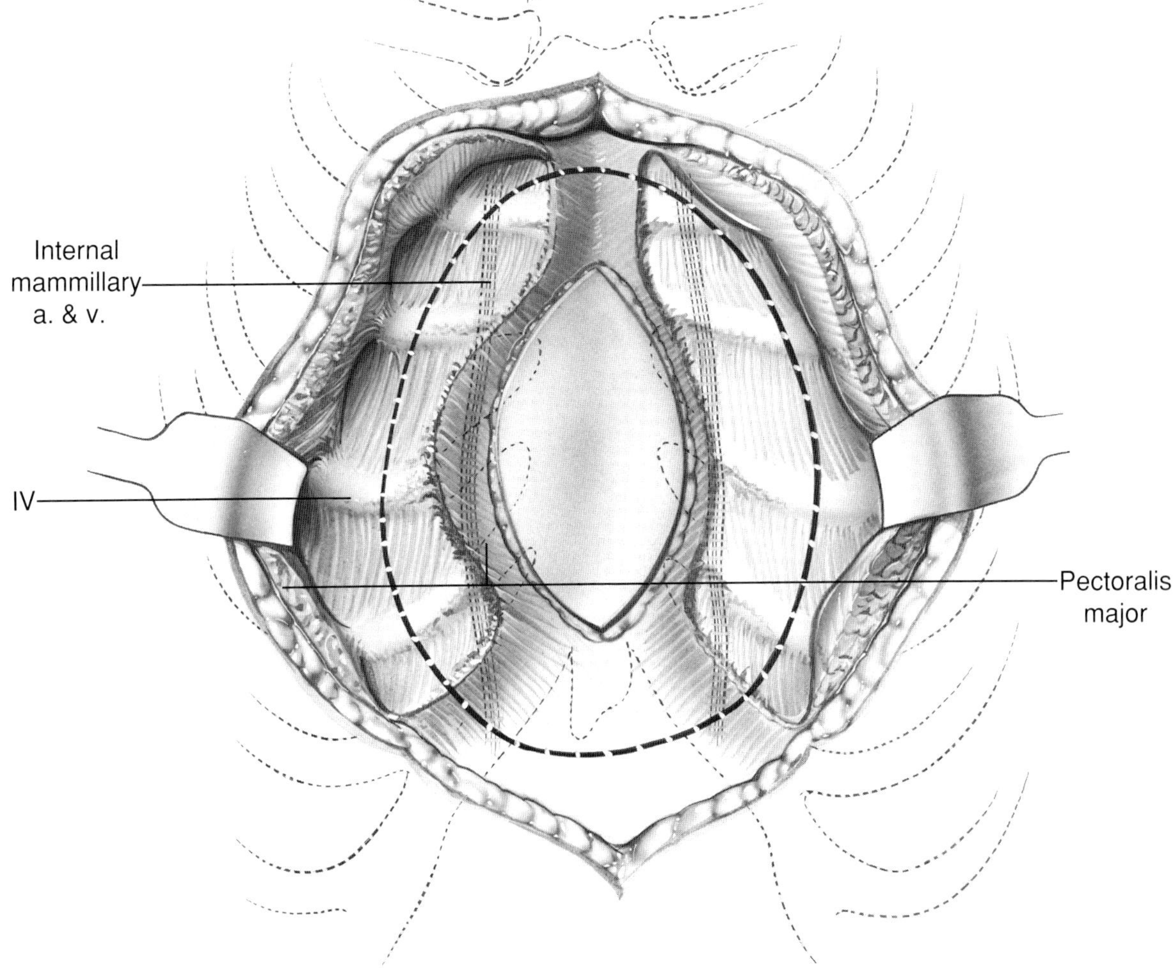

Fig. 6-15. Skin and muscle excision to be incorporated with the sternal resection.

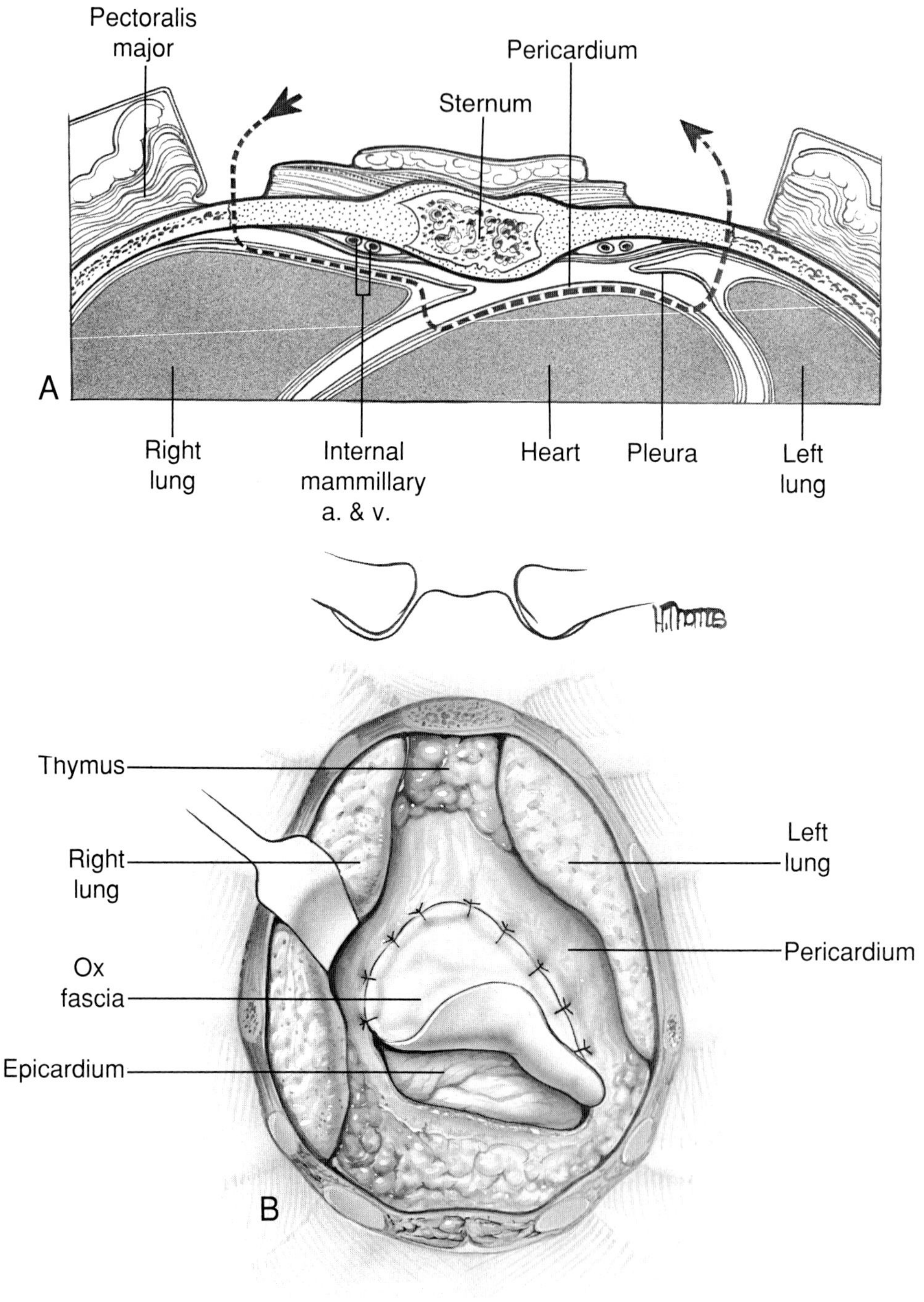

Fig. 6-16. **(A)** Cross-sectional view showing removal of tumor, with a portion of the pericardium. **(B)** Repair of pericardial defect with Martex mesh.

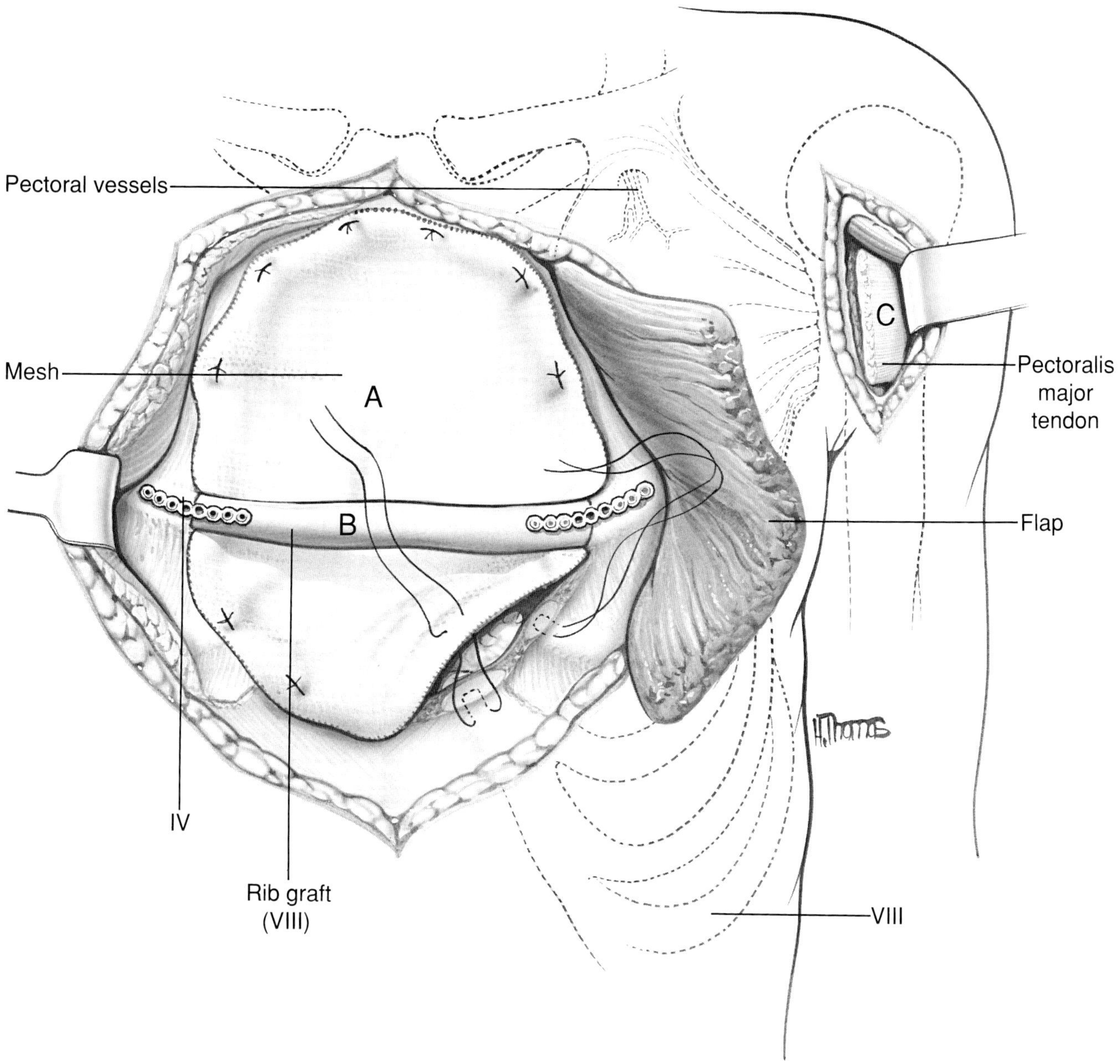

Fig. 6-17. **(A)** Martex mesh is used to reconstruct the sternal defect; attachment is to the cut sternum superiorly and the ribs laterally. **(B)** An autologous rib graft is made to the fourth rib for added support and is secured with a plate. **(C)** Incision of the pectoralis major insertion to allow advancement of the pecoralis muscle to cover the Martex and autologous rib reconstruction. (From Sherman et al.,[62] with permission.)

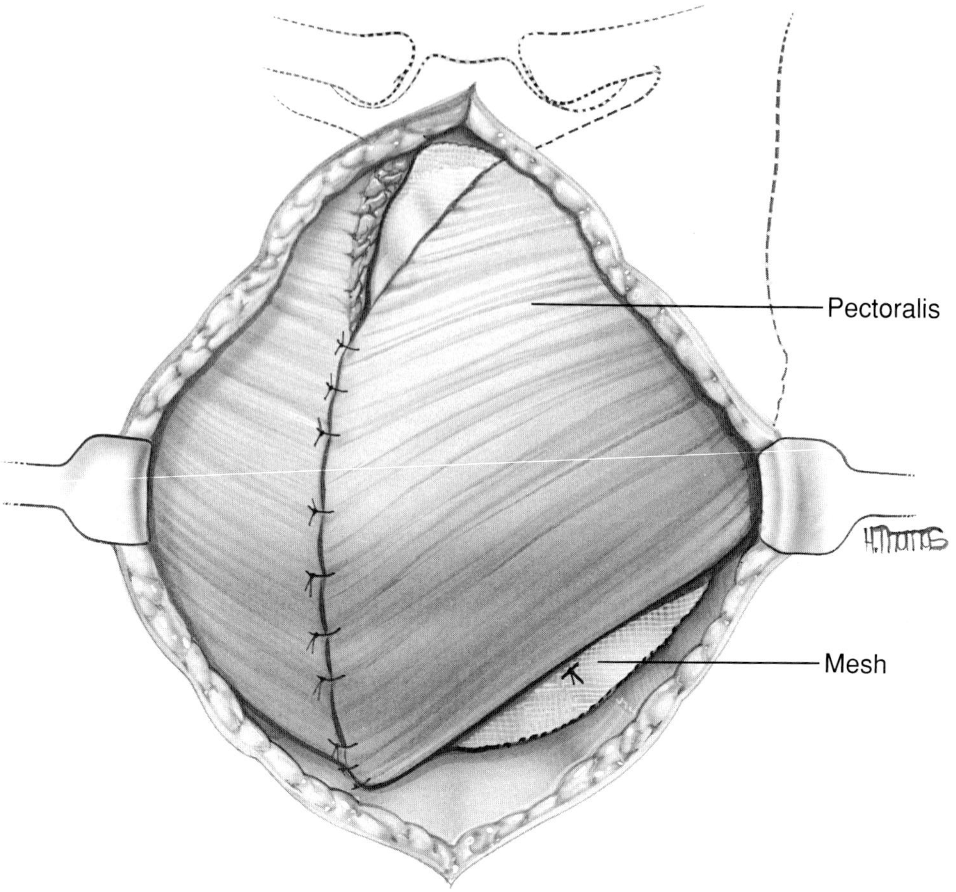

Fig. 6-18. Completion of the bipectoral advancements prior to skin closure.

PLEURA

MALIGNANT MESOTHELIOMA

In 1932 Klemperer and Rabin proposed the name "mesothelioma" for primary malignant tumors of the pleura.[63] In 1960 Wagner et al. demonstrated the association between the diffuse malignant mesothelioma and asbestos exposure.[64] It has been proved that the zerosolized fibers of asbestos cause the health hazard, but the threshold level of exposure below which the risk is negligible has not been determined.[65] The dose and duration of exposure are important factors in calculating threshold levels, but the length of time since the first exposure is more crucial in determining risk. Once the fibers are inhaled and trapped in the pulmonary parenchyma, in situ exposure continues for life.[65]

Asbestos is not the only factor that leads to the development of mesothelioma. Only half of all patients with malignant mesothelioma are able to document a history of asbestos exposure. The vast majority of all exposed workers will never develop mesotheliomas in their lifetimes.

CLINICAL PRESENTATION

The majority of the signs and symptoms of mesothelioma are related to the presence of a unilateral pleural effusion. The average age at the time of presentation is between the fifth and eighth decades of life. The majority of patients complain of progressive shortness of breath or a vague nonpleuritic chest pain that can radiate to the shoulder or the abdomen. Pericardial involvement can lead to effusions, arrhythmias, congestive heart failure, or tamponade.

Chest x-rays will reveal a unilateral pleural effusion or contracture of the hemithorax. The CT scan defines the anatomic extent of the tumor and effusion, extension to the chest wall, the status of the contralateral lung, and the presence of disease below the diaphragm.

The diagnosis of malignant pleural mesothelioma is difficult to establish by pleural fluid aspiration or a closed pleural biopsy. An open pleural biopsy is usually necessary to obtain sufficient tissue to make a definitive diagnosis.[67]

This procedure could compromise any later attempt at surgical resection because of the interruption of the extrapleural plane when the biopsy specimen is taken from the parietal pleura. In addition, there is a propensity for the tumor to extend through the intercostal incision and invade the chest wall. Therefore, the open biopsy should be performed at a center at which definitive care will be given and an accurate frozen-section diagnosis can be made.

STAGING

The Butchart staging system is simple and correlates statistically with survival.[68] To stage the patients accurately, CT scanning is the most effective modality to define the extent of local disease and involvement of the opposite thorax, abdomen, or lymph nodes outside the chest[69] (Table 6-5).

Mesotheliomas may be classified as benign or malignant, and the latter may be subclassified as localized or diffuse. Benign mesotheliomas are solitary, rounded lesions arising from either the visceral or parietal pleura. They enter into the differential diagnosis of solitary rounded peripheral opacities on chest x-ray.[70,71]

Localized malignant mesotheliomas have fibrosarcomatous elements microscopically and show little or no tendency to spread around the pleural cavity. Their local involvement of the chest wall may be extensive, but they are amenable to surgical resection with inclusion of a chest wall resection.[72]

TREATMENT

The diffuse malignant mesotheliomas show little tendency to invade the chest wall in the early stages and therefore may benefit from radical surgery for cure.

Pleuropneumonectomy was first performed by Mason in 1949, but it was not until the mid-1970s that several large series appeared in the literature. Pleuropneumonectomy refers to the excision of the total parietal pleura, hemidiaphragm, pleuropericardium, and lung. Worn[73] and Massen et al.[74] reported on their results after performing this operation in 87 patients in the Ruhr area of Germany. The 5-year survival in these two series was approximately 15 percent, and there was a 20 percent hospital mortality rate.

Table 6-5. Staging of Malignant Mesothelioma

Stage	Description
I	Tumor confined to ipsilateral pleura and lung
II	Tumor involving the chest wall, mediastinum, pericardium, or contralateral pleura
III	Tumor involving both thorax and abdomen or lymph nodes outside the chest
IV	Distant metastasis

De Lara et al.[75] reported on 11 cases from the Rush Presbyterian Hospital Center with no hospital mortality. Butchart et al.[68] reported on 29 cases analyzed by the stage of tumor. There were only two long-term survivors, who were both stage I and had epithelial-type tumors.

In analyzing these and other results, Butchart et al. concluded that the selection of patients for this operation should be limited to patients with presumptive stage I disease and who were less than 60 years of age with no evidence of significant cardiac or respiratory disease other than the mesothelioma itself.[76]

Palliative surgery has a wider role in the management of mesothelioma. The aims of palliative surgery are the prevention of recurrent effusions and amelioration of the discomfort and respiratory embarassment produced by tumor bulk. The most favorable results for pleurectomy and decortication combined with radiation were reported by Hilaris et al.[77] A variety of radiation techniques were used, including brachytherapy with iodine 125 (10 percent), irridium (27 percent), or phosphorus 32 (17 percent) combined with external radiation therapy. The latter was used alone in 46 percent of cases. A 49 percent 2-year survival was reported.

At present the only prospective trial to evaluate the role of radical surgery for mesotheliomas is being conducted in Great Britain. This will attempt to answer the question of whether radical surgery is beneficial in the stage I patient population. If not, palliative pleurectomy with radiation should be applied to all patients. This is suggested by the results reported by Harvey et al. summarizing their experience in the treatment of 93 patients in the Kaiser Permanente institutions.[78] At present the role of chemotherapy, if any, is not defined.

REFERENCES

1. Pasquini CA, Dahlin DC, Clagett OT: Primary tumors of the ribs and sternum. Surg Gynecol Obstet 104:390, 1957
2. Teitlebaum S: Twenty years experience with intrinsic tumors of the bony thorax at a large institution. J Thorac Cardiovasc Surg 63:776, 1972
3. Graeber GM: Initial and long term results in the management of primary chest wall neoplasms. Ann Thorac Surg 63:664, 1982
4. Theikel JB, Adkins S: Primary chest wall tumors. Ann Thorac Surg 11:450, 1971
5. Jaffe HL: Tumor and Tumorous Conditions of the Bone and Joints. Lea & Febiger, Philadelphia, 1958
6. Lichtenstein L: Bone Tumors. CV Mosby, St. Louis, 1977
7. Evans HL, Ayala AG, Romsdahl MM: Prognostic factors in chondrosarcoma of bone. Cancer 40:818, 1971
8. Marcove R, Huvos A: Cartilaginous tumors of the ribs. Cancer 27:749, 1971
9. Gitelis S, Bertoni F, Picci P et al: Chondrosarcoma of bone. J Bone Jt Surg 63A:1248, 1981
10. McAfee MK: Chondrosarcoma of the chest wall: factors affecting survival. Ann Thorac Surg 40:535, 1985
11. King RM: Primary chest wall tumors: factors affecting survival. Ann Thorac Surg 41:597, 1986
12. Chak L, Coix RS, Bostwick DC et al: Solitary plasmacytoma of bone: treatment progression and survival. J. Clin Oncol 5:811, 1987
13. Knowling MA, Harwood AR, Bergsagel DE: Comparison of extramedullary plasmacytomas with solitary and multiple plasma cell tumors of bone. J Clin Oncol 1:255, 1983
14. Corvin J, Lindber RD: Solitary plasmacytoma of bone vs extramedullary tumors and their relationship to myeloma. Cancer 43:1007, 1979
15. Mill WB, Griffith R: The role of radiation therapy in the management of plasma cell tumors. Cancer 45:647, 1980
16. Bergsagel DE, Baily AS, Lusegly GR: The chemotherapy of plasma cell myeloma and the incidence of acute leukemia. N Engl J Med 301:743, 1979
17. Tong D, Griffin TW, Laramore GE et al: Solitary plasmacytoma of bone and soft tissues. Radiology 135:195, 1980
18. Batkle R, Sany J: Solitary myeloma: clinical and prognostic features of a review of 114 cases. Cancer 48:845, 1981
19. Meyer JE, Schults MD: Solitary myeloma of bone: a review of 112 cases. Cancer 34:438, 1974
20. Woodruff RK, Malpas JS, White FE: Solitary plasmacytoma: solitary plasmacytoma of bone. Cancer 43:2344, 1979
21. Kissane JM, Askin FB, Foulkes M et al: Ewings sarcoma of bone: clinicopathologic aspects of 303 cases from the Intergroup Ewings Sarcoma Study. Hum Pathol 14:773, 1983
22. Fernandez CH, Lindberg RD, Sautow WW et al: Localized Ewings sarcoma: treatment and results. Cancer 34:143, 1974
23. Hustu OH, Pinkel D, Pratt CB: Treatment of clinically localized Ewings sarcoma with radiotherapy and combination chemotherapy. Cancer 30:1522, 1972
24. Pomeray TC, Johnson RE: Combined modality therapy of Ewings sarcoma. Cancer 35:36, 1975
25. Nesbitt ME, Perez CA, Tefft M et al: Multimodality therapy for the management of primary nonmetastatic Ewing sarcoma of bone: an Intergroup study. Natl Cancer Inst Monogr 56:225, 1981
26. Rosen GA, Caparros B, Nirenberg A et al: Ewings sarcoma: ten year experience with adjuvant chemotherapy. Cancer 47:2204, 1981
27. Jurgens H, Exner U, Gadner H et al: Multidisciplinary treatment of primary Ewings sarcoma of bone. Cancer 61:23, 1988
28. Rosen GA, Caparros B, Mosende C et al: Curability of Ewings sarcoma and considerations for future therapeutic trials. Cancer 41:888, 1978
29. Rosen G, Wollnen H, Tan C et al: Disease free survival in children with Ewings sarcoma treated with radiation therapy and adjuvant four drug sequential chemotherapy. Cancer 33:384, 1974
30. Jaffe N, Paed D: Recent advances in the chemotherapy of metastatic osteogenic sarcoma. Cancer 30:1627, 1972
31. Rosen G, Marcove R, Capanos B et al: Primary osteogenic sarcoma. The rationale for preoperative chemotherapy and delayed surgery. Cancer 43:2163, 1979
32. Krailo M, Ertel I, Makley J et al: A randomized study comparing high-dose methotrexate with moderate-dose methotrexate as components of adjuvant chemotherapy in childhood nonmetastatic osteosarcoma: a report from the Children's Cancer Study Group. Med Pediatr Oncol 15:69, 1987
33. Winkler K, Beron G, Kotz R: Neoadjuvant chemotherapy for osteogenic sarcoma: results of a cooperative German/Austrian study. J. Clin Oncol 2:617, 1984
34. Winkler K, Beron G, Kotz R: Adjuvant and neoadjuvant chemotherapy of osteosarcoma: experience of the German-Austrian cooperative osteosarcoma studies (COSS), p. 275. In Van Oosteram AT, Van Unnik JAM (eds): Management of Soft Tissue and Bone Sarcomas. Raven Press, New York, 1986
35. Jaffe N, Prudich J, Knappo J: Treatment of primary osteosarcoma with intraarterial and intravenous high-dose methotrexate. J Clin Oncol 1:428, 1983
36. Jaffe N, Raymond K, Ayala A: Effect of cumulative courses of intraarterial cis-diamminedichloroplatin-II on the primary tumor in osteosarcoma. Cancer 63:63, 1989
37. Askin FB, Rosa J, Siobley RK et al: Malignant small cell tumor of the thoracopulmonary region in childhood. Cancer 43:2438, 1979

38. Mindell ER, Shah NK, Webster JH: Postradiation sarcoma of bone and soft tissue. Orthop Clin N Am 8:821, 1977
39. Lynch HT, Krush AS, Harlan WL et al: Association of soft tissue sarcoma, leukemia and brain tumors in families affected with breast cancer. Am Surg 39:194, 1973
40. Graeger JA, Patel MK, Briele HA et al: Soft tissue sarcomas of the adult thoracic wall. Cancer 59:370, 1987
41. Graeber GM, Snyder RJ, Fleming AW et al: Initial and long term results in the management of primary chest wall neoplasms. Ann Thorac Surg 34:664, 1982
42. Stefanko J, Turnbul AD, Helson LA et al: Primitive neuroectodermal tumors of the chest wall. J Surg Oncol 37:33, 1982
43. Graham J, Usher FC, Perry SL: Marlex mesh as a prosthesis in the repair of thoracic wall defects. Ann Surg 151:469, 1960
44. Arnold PG, Pairolero PC: Chest wall reconstruction. Ann Thorac Surg 31:45, 1981
45. Pairolero PC, Arnold PG: Chest wall tumors. J Thorac Cardiovasc Surg 90:367, 1985
46. McCormack P, Bains M, Beattie EJ et al: New trends in skeletal reconstruction after resection. Ann Thorac Surg 31:45, 1981
47. Arnold PG, Pairolero PC: Use of the pectoralis major muscle flaps to repair defects of the anterior chest wall. Plast Reconst Surg 73:240, 1984
48. Campbell DA: Reconstruction of the anterior thoracic wall. J Thorac Cardiovasc Surg 19:456, 1950
49. Arnold PG, Pairolero PC, Waldorrf JC: The serratus anterior muscle: intrathoracic and extrathoracic utilization. Plast Reconstr Surg 73:240, 1984
50. Carberry DM, Ballantyne LW: Omental pedicle graft in closure of large anterior chest wall defects. NY State J Med 75:1705, 1975
51. Jacobs EW, Hoffman S, Kirschner P et al: Reconstruction of large chest wall defects using greater omentum. Arch Surg 113:886, 1978
52. Jurkiwicz MJ, Arnold PG: The omentum: an account of its use in the reconstruction of the chest wall. Ann Surg 185:548, 1977
53. Arnold PG, Witzke DJ, Frong B et al: Use of omental transposition flaps for soft tissue reconstruction. Ann Plast Surg 11:508, 1983
54. Vetto M, Rubin S, Bernards W: Closure of large thoracic wall defects using an omental pedicle. Am Surg 43:724, 1977
55. Boyd AD, Shaw WW, McCarthy JG: Immediate reconstruction of full thickness chest wall defects. Ann Thorac Surg 32:337, 1981
56. Crile G: Pulsating tumors of the sternum. Ann Surg 199:103, 1936
57. O'Neal LW, Ackerman L: Cartilaginous tumors of ribs and sternum. J Thorac Surg 21:71, 1951
58. Martini N, Huvos A, Smith J et al: Primary malignant tumors of the sternum. SGO 138:391, 1974
59. Peabody CN: Chondrosarcoma of the sternum: report of a six year survival. J Thorac Cardiovasc Surg 61:636, 1971
60. Pollack A: Angiosarcoma of the sternum. Am J Surg 72:522, 1949
61. Hoop RM: Surgical Diseases of the Pleura and Chest Wall. WB Saunders, Philadelphia, 1986
62. Sherman JE, Salzberg A, Raskin NM et al: Chest wall stabilization using plate fixation. Ann Thorac Surg 46:467, 1988
63. Klemperer P, Rabin CB: Primary neoplasms of the pleura. A report of 5 cases. Arch Pathol 11:385, 1932
64. Wagner JC, Sleggs CA, Marchand P: Diffuse pleural mesothelioma and asbestos exposure in the North Western Cape Province. Br J Ind Med 17:260, 1960
65. Selikoff IJ: Cancer risk of asbestos exposure. p. 1764. In: Origins of Human Cancer. Cold Spring Harbor Laboratory, Cold Spring Harbor, NY, 1977
66. Peto J, Seidman H, Selikoff IJ: Mesothelioma mortality in asbestos workers: implications for models of carcinogenesis and risk assessment. Br J Cancer 44:1, 1981
67. Antman KH: Clinical presentation and natural history of benign and malignant mesothelioma. Semin Oncol 8:313, 1981
68. Butchart FG, Ashcroft T, Barnsley WC et al: Pleuropneumonectomy in the management of diffuse malignant mesothelioma of the pleura: experience with 29 patients. Thorax 31:15, 1976
69. Cohen BA, Efemidis A, Chahinian AP et al: Computed tomography of the chest in diffuse malignant pleural mesotheliomas. Am Rev Respir Dis 123:131, 1981
70. Hutchinson WB, Friedenber MJ: Intrathoracic mesothelioma. Radiology 80:937, 1963
71. Briselli M, Mark EJ, Dickerson GR: Solitary fibrous tumors of the pleura: eight new cases and a review
72. McCormack PM, Nagasaki F. Hilaris BS: Surgical treatment of pleural mesothelioma. J Thorac Cardiovasc Surg 84:834, 1982
73. Worn H: Maglichketten und ergebnisse der churugischen Behanlung des malignent Pleuramesotheliomas. Thoracchirurgie 22:391, 1974
74. Maasen W, Kappes R, Petro W et al: Surgical therapy of pleural diseases. Arch Monaldsi 37:255, 1982
75. De Lara GA, Jensik R, Faber LP: Surgical management of malignant mesothelioma. Ann Thorac Surg 26:375, 1978
76. Butchart EG, Adams M, Wilkins MF et al: Malignant mesothelioma. p. 566. In Roth J (ed): Thoracic Oncology.
77. Hilaris BS, Nori D, Kwong E et al: Pleurectomy and intraoperative brachytherapy and postoperative radiation in the treatment of malignant pleural mesothelioma. Int J Radiat Oncol Biol Phys 10:325, 1984.
78. Harvey JC, Fleischman EH, Kagan AR, Streeter OE: Malignant pleural mesothelioma: a survival study. J Surg Oncol 45:40, 1990

7

Trachea

The trachea is a fibromuscular tube 10 to 12 cm in length. It originates at the cricoid cartilage and descends through the anterosuperior mediastinum to bifurcate at the lower border of the fourth thoracic vertebrae. Half of the trachea lies in the neck, and the remaining half is in the thorax. The trachea, varying in diameter from 13 to 22 mm, is supported by approximately 20 U-shaped hyaline cartilages which make up three-quarters of the circumference.

The mucous membrane of the trachea, which consists of ciliated epithelial cells and a few goblet cells, rests on an elastic lamina propria beneath which is the submucosa. An additional fibrous coat containing the hyaline cartilages and smooth muscle of the membranous portion of the trachea. Tumors can arise in any portion of the trachea and from any cell type which contributes to the normal tracheal anatomy.

TUMORS OF THE TRACHEA

In 1953 Gilbert et al.[1] summarized the most common benign lesions reported in the literature. In adults benign lesions made up 50.9 percent of all primary tracheal tumors. The most common benign tumors were the osteochondroma, papilloma, fibroma, angioma, and osteochondroma (Table 7-1). The most frequent site of origin is the upper one-third of the trachea in children and the lower one-third in adults.

BENIGN TUMORS

CHONDROMAS

Chondromas are benign tumors that histologically duplicate the normal cartilage, whether it be the elastic or hyaline type. The chondroma may exhibit an increased cellularity, but the individual cells retain a uniform structure similar to that in normal cartilage. Vascular invasion can be seen with chondromas and thus cannot be used as a criterion of malignancy. There is a male preponderance of roughly 4 : 1, and the age of the patients ranges from 56 days to 81 years.[2]

No definitive cause has been found for these lesions. The higher incidence between the ages of 40 and 60 years has led to speculation that their development may be related to disorders of ossification of the hyaline cartilages or to a metaplasia secondary to chronic inflammation.[3]

Radiologically chondromas usually appear on plain radiographs of the neck as a discrete smooth soft tissue mass, contiguous with one of the cartilages and usually with narrowing of the air column. Coarse macrocalcifications occur in 75 percent of patients and, when present, are pathognomonic for this type of tumor.[4]

Computed tomography (CT) has in recent years been the most valuable radiographic study because of its ability to show the size and extent of the tumor as well as possible invasion of surrounding structures.

PAPILLOMAS

Papillomas account for almost 60 percent of benign tracheal tumors in children and approximately 25 percent in adults. The sex incidence is equal, and these tumors rarely occur in adults older than 30. The recurrence rate of these lesions can be as high as 90 percent.

It is believed that the etiology of these lesions is secondary to a papillomavirus infection. Studies have demonstrated an increased risk of papillomavirus infection in children of mothers who have

Table 7-1. Benign Tracheal Tumors of Adults and Children

	Children	Adults
Tumor Type	No. (%)	No. (%)
Chondroma	1 (3)	76 (51)
Papilloma	23 (59)	42 (29)
Fibroma	9 (23)	30 (20)
Angioma	6 (15)	2 (1)

condyloma acuminatum, and serum complement-fixing antibodies against autologous papillomavirus antigens have been found.

Various treatment modalities have caused regression of these lesions. Local application of estrogenic hormones has produced regressions, and there have been spontaneous remissions in conjunction with pregnancy.[5]

Current management is used only in symptomatic patients and involves frequent and repeated endoscopic removal of papillomas with cup forceps and/or laser surgery.[6] Radiotherapy has been associated with up to 14 percent incidence of malignant transformation, with little added success in controlling this lesion.[7]

Chemotherapeutic regimens and interferon therapy have also been unsuccessful in controlling these lesions.[8] Currently photodynamic therapy with dihematoporphyrin ether and a rhodamine B dye laser has been successful in the treatment of several patients with unremitting disease, as well as in the treatment of foci of carcinoma in situ.[9]

HEMANGIOMAS

Hemangiomas occur in the subglottic areas of the larynx and trachea in infants. Because of the location of these lesions, sudden ventilatory obstruction is the most frequent presentation. The lesions are similar to hemangiomas of the skin in infants, with an increase in size after a month or more of life followed by spontaneous diminution at about the first year.

Tracheotomy may be necessary to allow ventilation, along with repeated small doses of radiation to shrink the tumor in obstructing lesions.

FIBROMAS

The first tracheal fibroma was described in 1767 by Lerutaud. It accounts for approximately 20 percent of all benign lesions in adults. Stridor is the most frequent presenting symptom, and endoscopic excision is the most effective therapy.

MALIGNANT TUMORS

Of 503 primary tracheal tumors in adults reported in the literature 247 (49 percent) were malignant. In children only 7 percent of 40 tumors were malignant and all were sarcomatous in origin. In adults almost 80 percent of malignant lesions were carcinomas. The two most common malignant tumors are squamous cell carcinomas and adenoid cystic carcinomas.[1]

SQUAMOUS CELL CARCINOMAS

Recently Grillo and Mathiesen[10] reported the end results of treatment of 52 patients with squamous cell carcinoma of the trachea. An additional nine patients have been reported by Pearson et al.[11] These lesions occurred exclusively in patients who were smokers. The peak incidence was in the sixth and seventh decades of life.

Of the 61 patients in both series, 50 underwent resection of their primary lesions. There were three operative deaths. Fifteen patients (30 percent) died secondary to tumor recurrence. An additional six patients (12 percent) died of other causes. The remainder were alive from 6 months to 15 years postresection. All patients who were unresectable succumbed to their disease within 6 months.

Sixteen patients who had resections of a squamous cell carcinoma of the trachea had either a history, a concurrent finding, or later occurrence of squamous cell cancers elsewhere. All resected patients had either pre- or postoperative radiation treatment, the preferred treatment being postoperative.

The median survival for patients who failed surgical resection and irradiation was 34 months versus an average survival of 10 months for patients treated by irradiation alone.

ADENOID CYSTIC CARCINOMAS

In the combined series of Grillo and Mathiesen[10] and Pearson et al.,[11] there were 108 patients with adenoid cystic carcinomas of the trachea. These lesions occurred equally in men and women, and there was no association with cigarette smoking. The age distribution was uniform from the third to seventh decades.

Eighty-six patients (80 percent) underwent surgical resection, and there were 13 (15 percent) operative deaths, most of which occurred in patients undergoing carinal resection. Of the 64 patients who had a complete and potentially curative resection, 10 (16 percent) died of their disease. The remainder (84 percent) are alive and well, with a median survival of 8 years.

Nine patients underwent incomplete resection only, and postoperative radiation was unsuccessful in controlling the disease in eight patients. Recurrence were noted from 2 to 9 years after resection. Five of these seven deaths were due to a local recurrence of the tumor; two were due to brain metastasis, and one was due to diffuse pulmonary metastasis.

It is apparent that these tumors are slow growing and relatively radioresistant, with little likelihood of cure without adequate surgical resection. Long-term palliation, however, can be achieved following incomplete resection and radiotherapy.

MISCELLANEOUS TUMORS

A variety of other malignant lesions have occurred in the trachea. The most common of these are the sarcomas. Leiomyosarcomas, spindle cell sarcomas, rhabdomyosarcomas, and chondrosarcomas are among the most frequently reported. Additional tumors include small cell carcinomas and melanomas. As with the other malignancies arising in the trachea, surgical resection followed by radiotherapy is the definitive therapy for the sarcomas. The small cell tumors are best managed with resection and adjunctive chemotherapy.

TRACHEAL RECONSTRUCTION

Circumferential resection and primary reconstruction of the trachea are possible in the majority of patients. Carinal resection with and without an associated pulmonary or sleeve resection is the most difficult of the primary reconstructions. In 1974 Eshapasse[12] reported on 19 cases of carinal resection and reconstruction. Twenty-nine cases were reported in 1980 by Perelman and Koroleva,[13] and 36 cases were reported in 1982 by Grillo.[14] The primary indication for carinal resections includes both primary tracheal lesions extending to the carina and bronchogenic or inflammatory lesions with carinal involvement. Depending on the extent of the trachea to be resected and whether there is more involvement of the right or left mainstem bronchus, a variety of primary reconstructions have been performed (Figs. 7-1 to 7-6).

The surgical approach to the carina has been primarily through a right posterolateral thoracotomy. Perelman and Koroleva[13] and Grillo[14] used this approach in the majority of their cases. Cooper et al.[15] advocated the use of the median sternotomy approach in performing distal trachea and carina reconstruction. After opening the superior pericardium, the carina and main bronchi are near the surface and the construction of the anastomosis is easier. Two additional advantages to this approach are that the patient is in a good position for a laryngeal release if further mobilization of the proximal trachea is necessary and that it permits removal of the left lung if the left main bronchus cannot be advanced far enough to use in a reconstruction. Mobilization of the left mainstem bronchus is inhibited by its adherence to the aorta.

In situations when the left main bronchus could not be attached through a right thoracotomy, Perelman and Koroleva[13] stapled the left mainstem bronchus distal to the tumor. In 10 patients they noted no difficulty with shunting or infection in the left lung. Grillo,[14] using this technique, observed tachycardia and tachypnea due to massive vascular shunting through the nonaerated left lung, and a left pneumonectomy was required in one patient 8 months later. An additional patient underwent a completion pneumonectomy performed through a separate incision after completion of the resection and anastomosis of the trachea to the right mainstem bronchus.

The main disadvantage of the median sternotomy approach is that it is more restrictive than a right thoracotomy if extensive tumor dissection is required beyond the confines of the airway (Fig. 7-7).

TRACHEAL REPLACEMENTS

Because up to one-half of the trachea in adults and one-third in infants can be resected with a primary anastomosis, few primary tracheal tumors require a tracheal replacement. The majority of the cases requiring tracheal replacement are for inflammatory disease, with the majority of malignant cases being adenoid cystic carcinomas in which the diagnosis has been made late or definitive treatment has been delayed by prolonged palliative treatment such as laser therapy. Because of the experimental nature of tracheal reconstruction, Grillo recommends definitive irradiation as palliation for such lesions.[16]

FOREIGN MATERIAL REPLACEMENT OF THE TRACHEA

The ideal foreign materials for tracheal reconstruction must be well accepted by the host, cause minimal inflammatory reaction but still be incorporated by the surrounding tissues, be impervious to fibroblastic and bacterial invasion of the lumen, and permit ingrowth of respiratory epithelium along the lumen. Over the years a variety of prostheses have been used in the laboratory by various investigators. These have included polyethylene,[17] vitallium,[18] stainless steel mesh,[19] homologous tracheal grafts over an acrylic tube,[20] Teflon and Marlex mesh combined,[21] lucite cylinders with external fixation rings,[22] Ivalon sponge,[23] and Marlex mesh cylinders.[24] The results have been varied, as have the attempts to use these materials in humans. Major complications include massive hemorrhage due to innominate artery erosion, dislodgement of the prosthesis, suture line granulomas, and ulceration and strictures.

In 1976 Neville et al.[25] reported on the successful replacement of the trachea utilizing a synthetic polydimethyl siloxane prosthesis in 26 patients. This material had been initially used by Graziano et al.[26] in dogs several years earlier. Late complications involved distal suture line granulomas, which were endoscopically removed, and one distal shift of the prosthesis. Long-term results were excellent.[27] The prosthesis fulfilled all the requirement except for reepithelialization. The smooth lining of the prosthesis, however, allowed for clearing of mucous without the presence of cilia within the graft.

It was thought that wrapping the distal anastomosis with Dacron and pericardium would prevent the fatal complication of innominate artery erosion after prosthetic displacement and that telescoping the prosthesis distally would eliminate the granulomas that were noted only in patients with end-to-end anastomosis.

AUTOGRAFT REPLACEMENT

With the failure of most replacement techniques, as well as homograft replacements, many experiments with autologous grafts have been performed. In 1940 Toffel[28] attempted to repair tracheal and bronchial defects with free fascia grafts. Rush and Clifton[29] and Marshak et al.[30] reported on the experimental reconstruction of the trachea with bladder mucosa and bladder wall. Other attempts at reconstruction included diaphragmatic pedicles,[31] autologous periosteum[32] and perichondrium,[33] and pleuroperiosteal flaps.[33] Recently experimental reconstructions have been attempted with small bowel interposition and microvascular reanastomosis. Letang et al.[34] reported on 20 dogs undergoing replacement of the cervical trachea with a vascularized small bowel segment as a tubular graft. A silicone stent was placed in the lumen of the intestinal fragment and was removed the second week after the operation. Endoscopic and histologic examinations were performed up to 2 months after surgery and revealed no evidence of anastomotic stricture or mucus formation. Microscopically there was substitution of the bowel mucosa by squamous epithelium, as well as development of connective tissue fixing the neck musculature to the small bowel serosa, thus avoiding collapse of the new airway.

Kast et al.[35] reported as well on the interposition of the local esophagus into a tracheal defect. This provided a bed into which a silicone T tube is placed, avoiding the problems of the chronic ulcerated bed that result when a prosthetic material alone is used. The esophagus in humans would then have to be reconstructed via a gastric, colonic, or free jejunal interposition. This would dictate a much more formidable surgical procedure than may be warranted. Nonetheless, these last two studies demonstrate the potential efficacy of autologous intestinal interpositions for tracheal reconstruction.

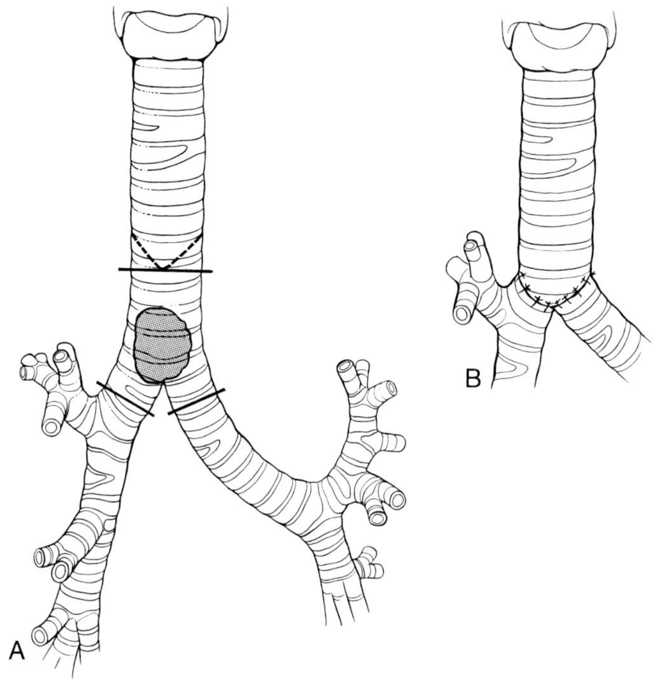

Fig. 7-1. **(A)** Resection of the carina and portions of the right and left mainstem bronchi. **(B)** Primary reconstruction of the right and left mainstem bronchus to the proximal trachea.

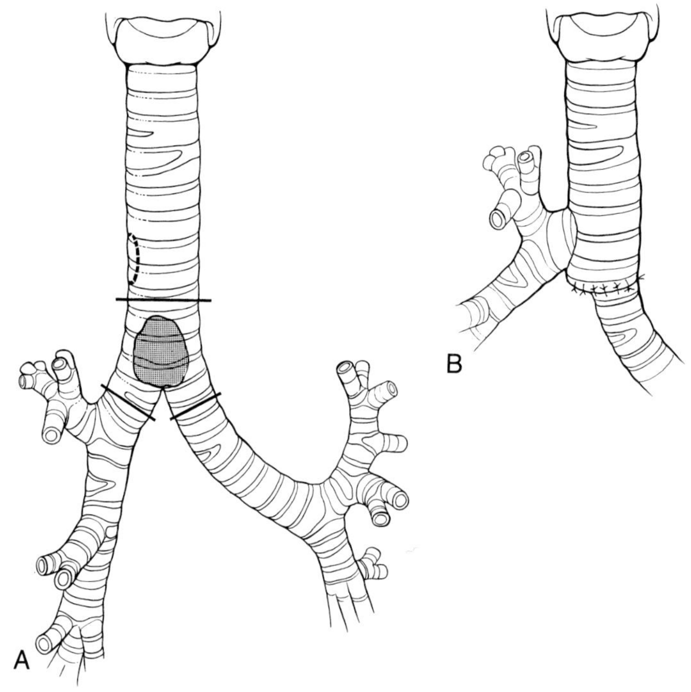

Fig. 7-2. **(A)** Primary resection of the carina and portions of the right and left mainstem bronchi. **(B)** End-to-end anastomosis of the left mainstem bronchus to the proximal trachea. End-to-side anastomosis of the right mainstem bronchus at a level above the anastomosis of the left mainstem bronchus.

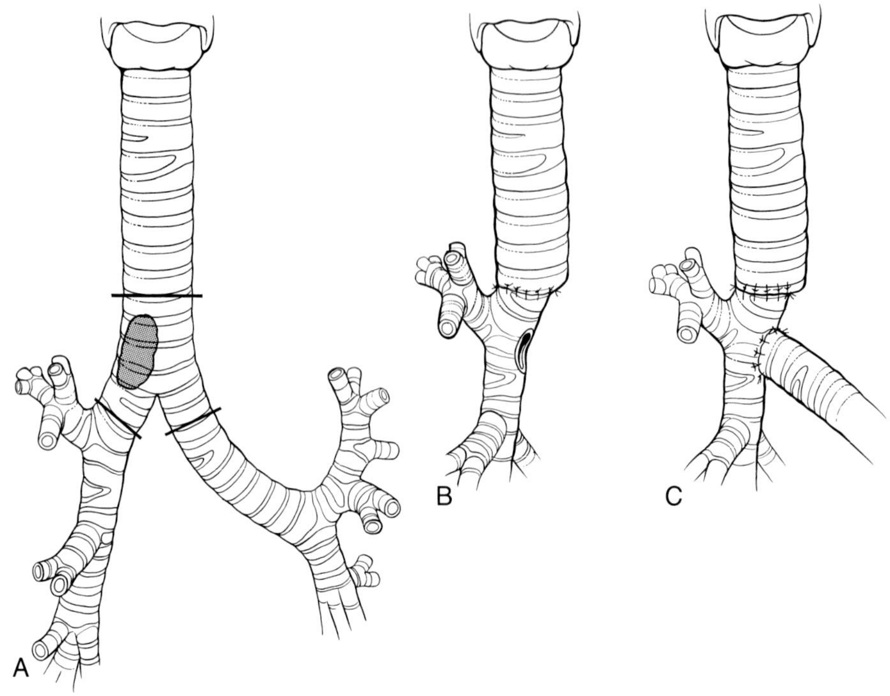

Fig. 7-3. **(A)** A more extensive tracheal resection. **(B)** Advancement of the right mainstem bronchus to the end of the trachea. **(C)** Implantation of the left mainstem bronchus to the bronchus intermedius.

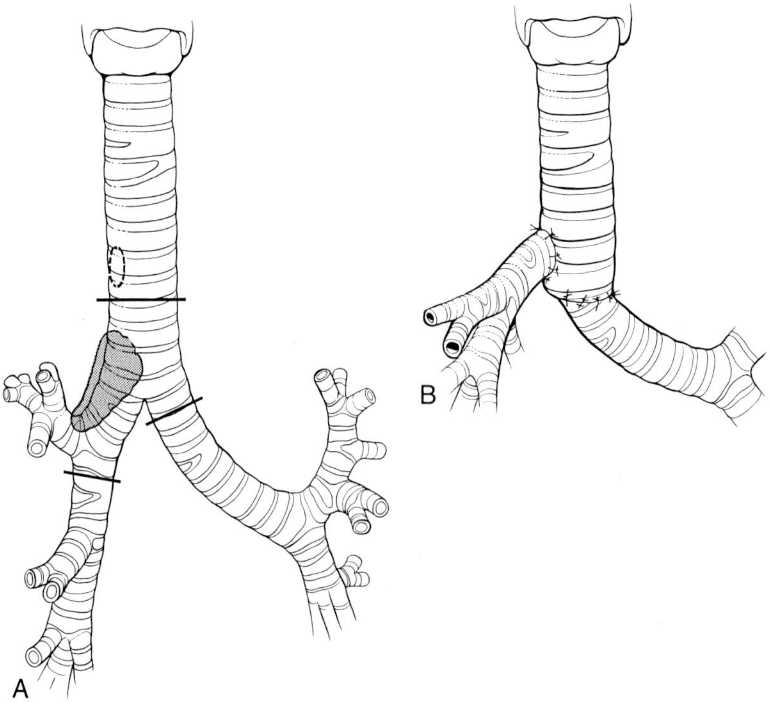

Fig. 7-4. **(A)** Resection of the carina and the right upper lobe. **(B)** Reanastomosis of the left mainstem bronchus end to end with the trachea. The bronchus intermedius is advanced to the side of the trachea above the level of the reanastomosis of the left mainstem bronchus.

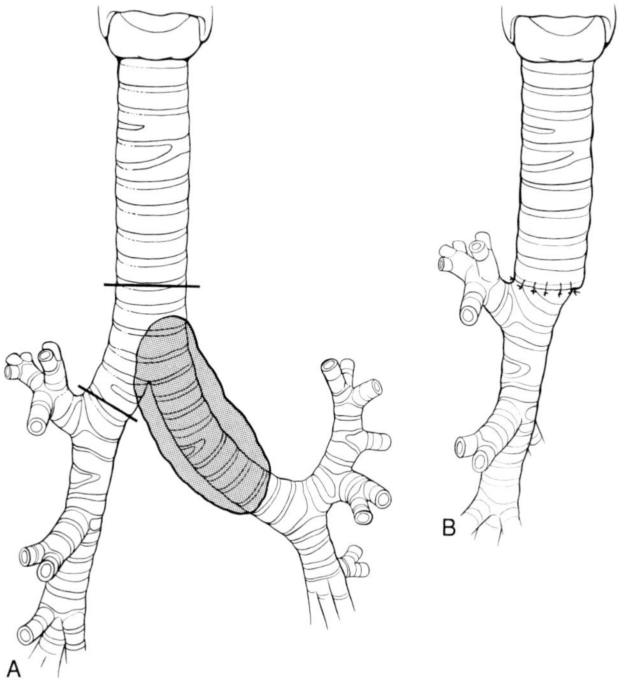

Fig. 7-5. **(A)** Resection of a lesion requiring left pneumonectomy and carinal resection. **(B)** End-to-end reconstruction of the right mainstem bronchus to the trachea.

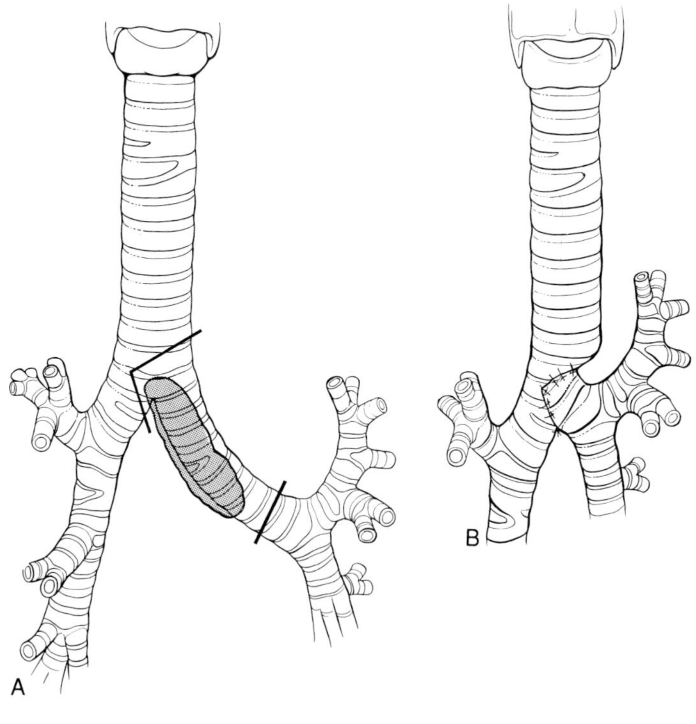

Fig. 7-6. **(A)** Excision of the carina and the left mainstem bronchus with preservation of the takeoff of the right mainstem bronchus. **(B)** End-to-side anastomosis of the left mainstem bronchus to the trachea.

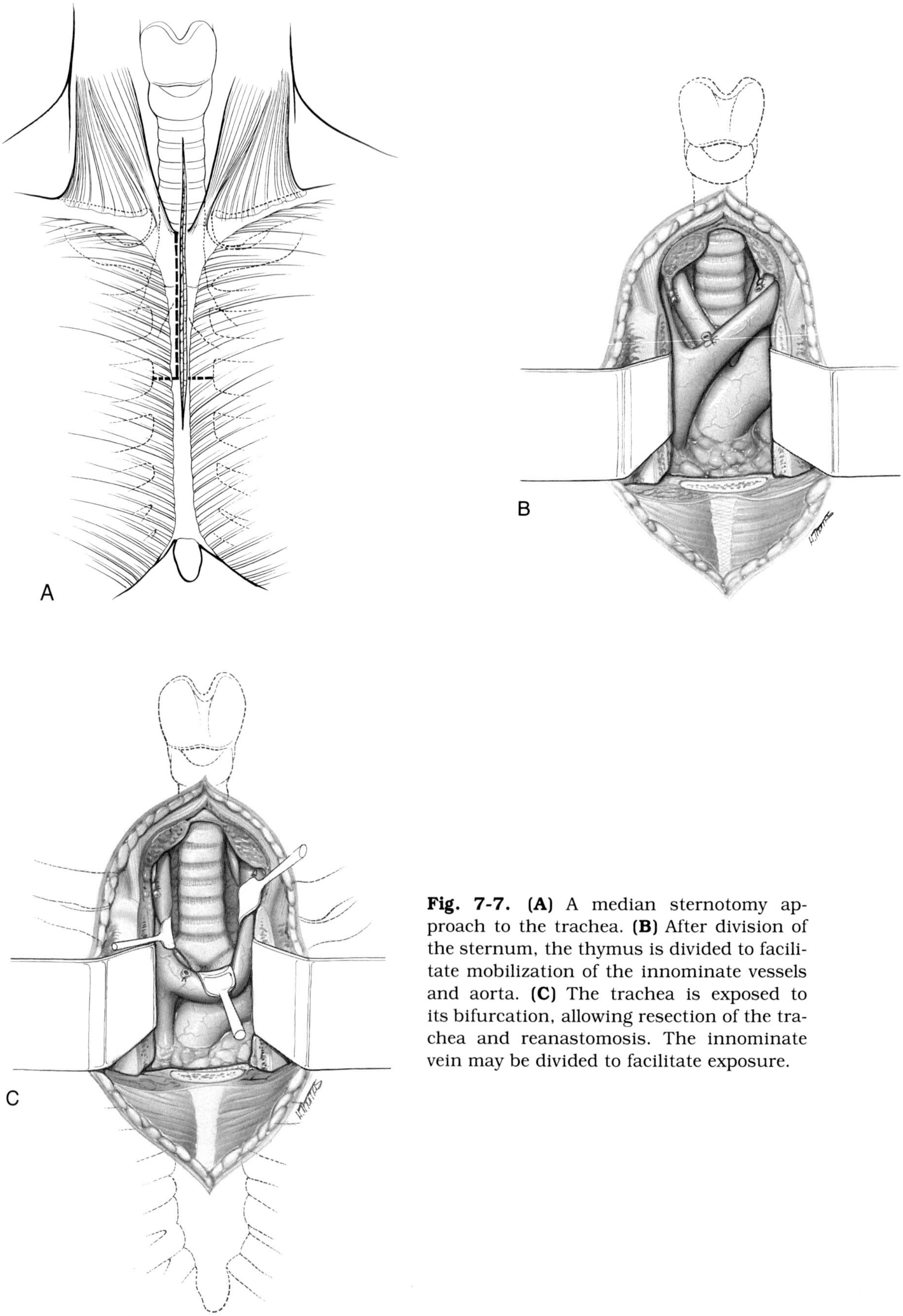

Fig. 7-7. **(A)** A median sternotomy approach to the trachea. **(B)** After division of the sternum, the thymus is divided to facilitate mobilization of the innominate vessels and aorta. **(C)** The trachea is exposed to its bifurcation, allowing resection of the trachea and reanastomosis. The innominate vein may be divided to facilitate exposure.

REFERENCES

1. Gilbert JG, Mazzarella LA, Feit L: Primary tracheal tumors in the infant and adult. Arch Otolaryngol 58:1, 1953
2. Arevalo M, Ordi S, Renado G et al: Chondrosarcoma of the trachea: report of a case. Respiration 49:147, 1986
3. Barsochhini LM, NcCoy G: Cartilaginous tumors of the larynx: a review of the literature and a report of four cases. Ann Otol Rhinol Laryngol 77:146, 1968
4. Zizman J, Noyek AM, Lewis JS: Radiologic diagnosis of chondroma and chondrosarcoma of the larynx. Arch Otolaryngol 101:232, 1971
5. Byrne JC, Tsao MS, Fraser RS et al: PV human papillomavirus 11 DNA in a patient with chronic laryngotracheobronchial papillomatosis and metastatic squamous carcinoma of the lung. N Engl J Med 317:873, 1987
6. Singleton GT, Adkins WY: Cryosurgical treatment of juvenile laryngeal papillomatosis: an eight year experience. Ann Otol Rhinol Laryngol 81:784, 1972
7. Siegel SE, Cohen SR, Isaacs H et al: Malignant transformation of tracheobronchial juvenile papillomatosis without prior radiation therapy. Ann Otol Rhinol Laryngol 80:192, 1979
8. Healy GB, Gelber RD, Trowbvridge AL et al: Treatment of recurrent respiratory papillomatosis with human leukocyte interferon. N Engl J Med 319: 401, 1988
9. Kavura IS, Mehta AC, Eliachar I: Effect of photodynamic therapy and external beam radiation therapy on juvenile laryngotracheobronchial papillomatosis. Am Rev Respir Dis 141:509, 1990
10. Grillo HC, Mathiesen DJ: Primary tracheal tumors: treatments and results. Ann Thorac Surg 49:69, 1990
11. Pearson FG, Todd RJ, Cooper JD: Experience with primary neoplasms of the trachea and carina. J Thorac Cardiovasc Surg 88:511, 1984
12. Eshapasse H: Les tumeurs tracheales primitives. Traitement chirugical. Rev Fr Mal Respir 2:425, 1974
13. Perelman MI, Koroleva N: Surgery of the trachea. World J Surg 18:16, 1974
14. Grillo HC: Carinal reconstruction. Ann Thorac Surg 34:356, 1982
15. Cooper JD, Pearson WG, Patterson GA et al: Use of silicone rubber stents in the management of airway problems. Ann Thorac Surg 47:371, 1989
16. Grillo HC: Tracheal replacement. Ann Thorac Surg 49:864, 1990
17. Clagett OT, Grindlay JH, Moersch HJ: Resection of the trachea: an experimental study and a report of a case. Arch Surg 57:253, 1948
18. Daniel RA: The regeneration of defects of the trachea and bronchi: an experimental study. J Thorac Surg 17:335, 1948
19. Bucher RM, Burnett E, Rosemond GP: Experimental reconstruction of the tracheal and bronchial defects with stainless steel wire mesh. J Thorac Surg 21:572, 1951
20. Davies OG, Edminston JM, McCorkle HJ: The repair of experimental tracheal defects with fresh and preserved homologous tracheal grafts. J Thorac Surg 23:367, 1952
21. Kramish D, Marfit HM: The use of Teflon prosthesis to bridge complete sleeve defects in the human trachea. Am J Surg 106:704, 1963
22. Michelson E, Solomon R, Mann L et al: Experiments in tracheal reconstruction. J Thorac Cardiovasc Surg 41:748, 1961
23. Traber, RE, Tomatis T: Experimental and clinical utilization of prosthesis for replacement of the trachea. Arch Surg 77:576, 1958
24. Beall AC, Harrington B, Usher FC et al: Circumferential replacement of the trachea with maarlex mesh. Surg Forum 11:40, 1960
25. Neville WE, Hamouda F, Anderson J et al: Replacement of the intrathoracic trachea and both stem bronchi with a molded silastic prosthesis. J Thorac Cardiovasc Surg 63:659, 1973
26. Graziano JS, Spinazolla A, Neville WE: Prosthetic replacement of the tracheal carina. Ann Thorac Surg 4:421, 1967
27. Neville WE: Reconstruction of the trachea and stem bronchi with Neville prosthesis. Int Surg 67:229, 1982
28. Taffel M: The repair of tracheal and bronchial defects with free fascia grafts. Surgery 8:56, 1940
29. Bush BF, Clifton EE: Experimental reconstruction of the trachea with bladder mucosa. Surgery 40: 1105, 1956
30. Marshak G, Proter JH, McAdams AJ: Reconstruction of the canine trachea with urinary bladder wall. Laryngoscope 83:1090, 1973
31. Westaby S, Sheperd M, Mohl-Olsen J: The use of diaphragmatic pedicle grafts for reconstructive procedures in the esophagus and tracheobronchial tree. Ann Thorac Surg 33:486, 1976
32. Finholsrud EW, Plested WG, Mulder DG: Tracheobronchial reconstruction with autologous periosteum. J Thorac Cardiovasc Surg 52:666, 1966
33. Kon A, Vamden-Hoff A: Cartilage tube formation by perichondrium: a new concept for tracheal reconstruction. Plast Reconstr Surg 72:791, 1983
34. Letaing E, Sanchez-Floret J, Gimferrer JM et al: Experimental reconstruction of the canine trachea with a free revascularized small bowel graft. Ann Thorac Surg 49:955, 1990
35. Kato R, Onuki AS, Watanabe M et al: Tracheal reconstruction by esophageal interposition: an experimental study. Ann Thorac Surg 49:951, 1990

8

Thoracic Spine

The functions of the spinal column are as follows: it allows coordinated movement, it protects the neural elements, and it supports the weight of the trunk. Interference with any of these functions can produce symptoms. Tumor control or ablation, with restoration of normal function, is the primary goal of treatment of spinal cord tumors.

PRESENTING SYMPTOMS

The most common presenting symptom of a tumor of the spinal column is pain. The pain may be localized or radicular and may be secondary to bony element collapse, tumor itself, or neurologic involvement. Tumor pain characteristically worsens at night and is often persistent. The second most common symptom is a spinal deformity. A history of painful scoliosis is sometimes associated with osteoid osteoma and osteoblastoma.[1] Spinal deformity can also result either from direct bony involvement, from secondary fracture, or as a postsurgical complication. Neurologic dysfunction, sensory and/or motor, is another complaint associated with tumor involvement. The neurologic involvement may be upper motor neuron, if the cord is involved, or lower motor neuron, if the cauda equina or nerve roots are involved. The prognosis for neurologic involvement is directly linked to the rate of onset of motor weakness. A neurologic deficit that insidiously worsens over several months has a far better prognosis than weakness that develops suddenly. Acute neurologic compromise is more commonly seen in patients with thoracic metastasis, in whom the ratio of the canal to the cord is smallest.[2,3]

Multiple myeloma is more common in patients aged 40 to 60. Metastatic disease is more common past the age of 60. Ewing's sarcoma and eosinophilic granuloma are more common in the younger age group, as are osteoid and osteoblastoma.

Finally, a patient with a history of a malignancy and spinal complaints should alert the physician to the possibility of metastases. This is often an emergency situation.

DIAGNOSIS

The spine is carefully examined for direct bony tenderness, deformity, and range of motion. A careful neurologic examination must be performed, including a rectal examination with assessment of perianal and perivaginal sensation. Radicular pain, reflex changes, muscle weakness, and muscle atrophy are recorded. Radicular pain may help localize the level of spinal involvement. A sensory deficit is not as specific as a motor deficit for the level of involvement, because such a deficit can be several segments below a myelographically apparent block.[4]

After a complete history and physical examination, the following laboratory tests are routine: complete blood count with differential, platelet count, coagulation evaluation, erythrocyte sedimentation ratio (ESR), alkaline phosphatase, calcium, and acid phosphatase. Serum and urine electrophoresis should also be ordered in patients over the age of 40 years to rule out multiple myeloma.

Radiographic evaluation of the spine should include anterior, posterior, lateral, and oblique views. Technetium 99 (Tc-99) scanning is necessary when primary or metastatic bony involvement is suspected. Since a minimum of 50 percent decalcification of bone is necessary to produce detectable radiographic changes in the vertebral column, a bone scan is an excellent skeletal survey for metastatic lesions and is helpful in determining very small lesions, such as an osteoid osteoma (Fig. 8-1). Because bone scanning reflects bone turnover in the presence of vascularity, it may not detect the primarily destructive lesions without reactive bone, such as multiple myeloma. It may also fail to demonstrate lesions less than 3 mm in diameter.

Single photon emission computed tomography (SPECT) bone scanning may provide an accurate assessment of smaller lesions. Computed tomography (CT), combined with the use of contrast media, demonstrates the direction and extent of bone and soft tissue involvement around the spinal canal. CT particularly allows for a good visualization of the anterior and middle columns (Fig. 8-2). It must be used in association with myelography to evaluate a patient's neurologic involvement, and there may be more than one level of vertebral involvement. If there is a complete block on the myelogram, CT may demonstrate the length of the lesion, with some contrast slipping by (Fig. 8-3). If not, dye should be introduced above or below the block for proper demonstration. The cerebrospinal fluid should be analyzed for protein content and for malignant cells after the myelogram.

Magnetic resonance imaging (MRI) is sensitive to paraspinal involvement by tumor, as well as to the effects of irradiation on the vertebral elements. It is particularly good for demonstrating cord involvement. Spinal lesions exhibit prolongation of T_1 and T_2 relaxation times, with decreased signal intensity in T_1-weighted studies, and increased

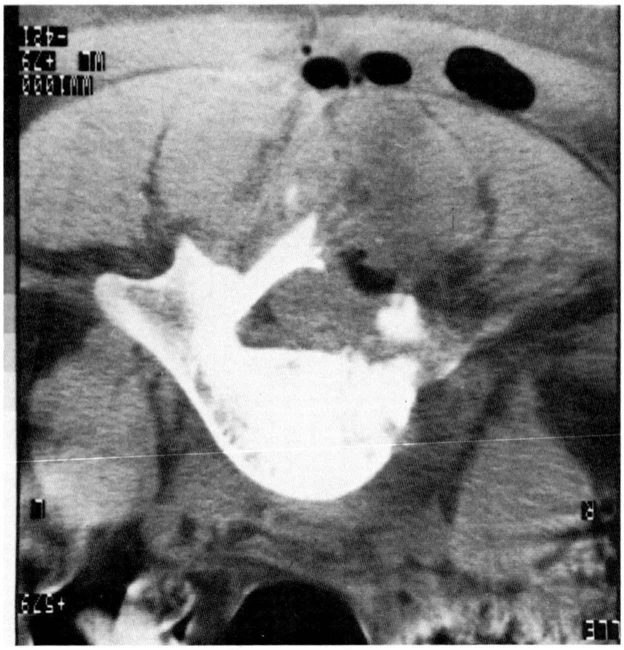

Fig. 8-2. Large destructive lesion with destruction of the middle column and significant spinal cord compression.

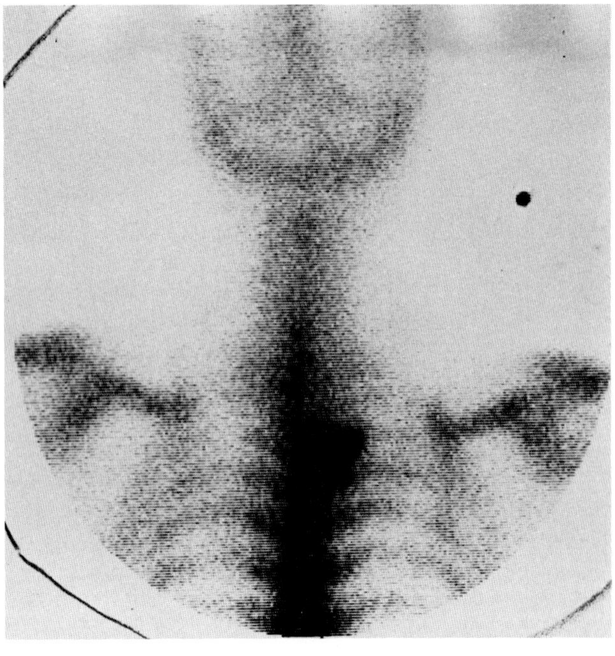

Fig. 8-1. Positive bone scan depicting an active lesion in the upper thoracic vertebra consistent with osteoid osteoma.

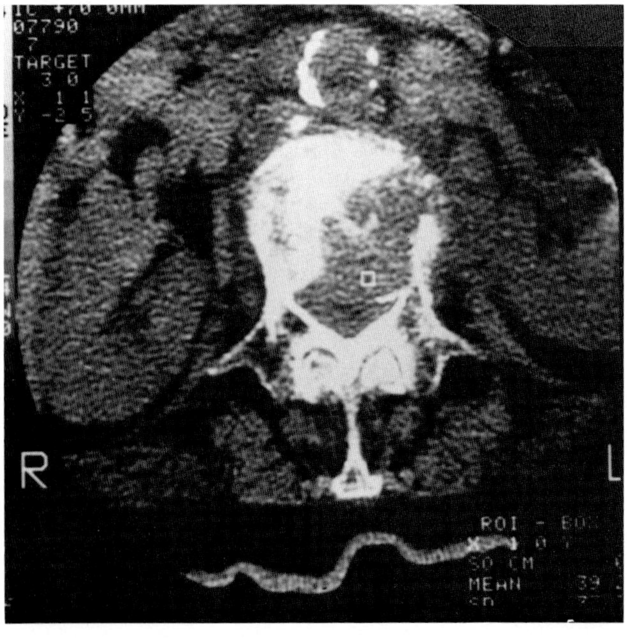

Fig. 8-3. CT with myelography indicating a complete block.

signal intensity in T_2-weighted images. Modic has shown that hemangiomas are an exception to the pattern, with short to intermediate T_1 and long T_2 times. MRI is superior to CT without contrast media, and at least equal to CT with contrast media, in demonstrating anatomic relationships of tumors.[5,6] As MRI develops, it will probably become the procedure of choice for demonstrating neurologic involvement. Currently, however, CT is better than MRI in demonstrating the amount of bony involvement.

Angiography may additionally aid the surgeon in outlining the borders of a particularly vascular tumor, such as hemangioma or metastatic renal cell carcinoma, that has a high risk of hemorrhage (Fig. 8-4). It may also be used for preoperative em-

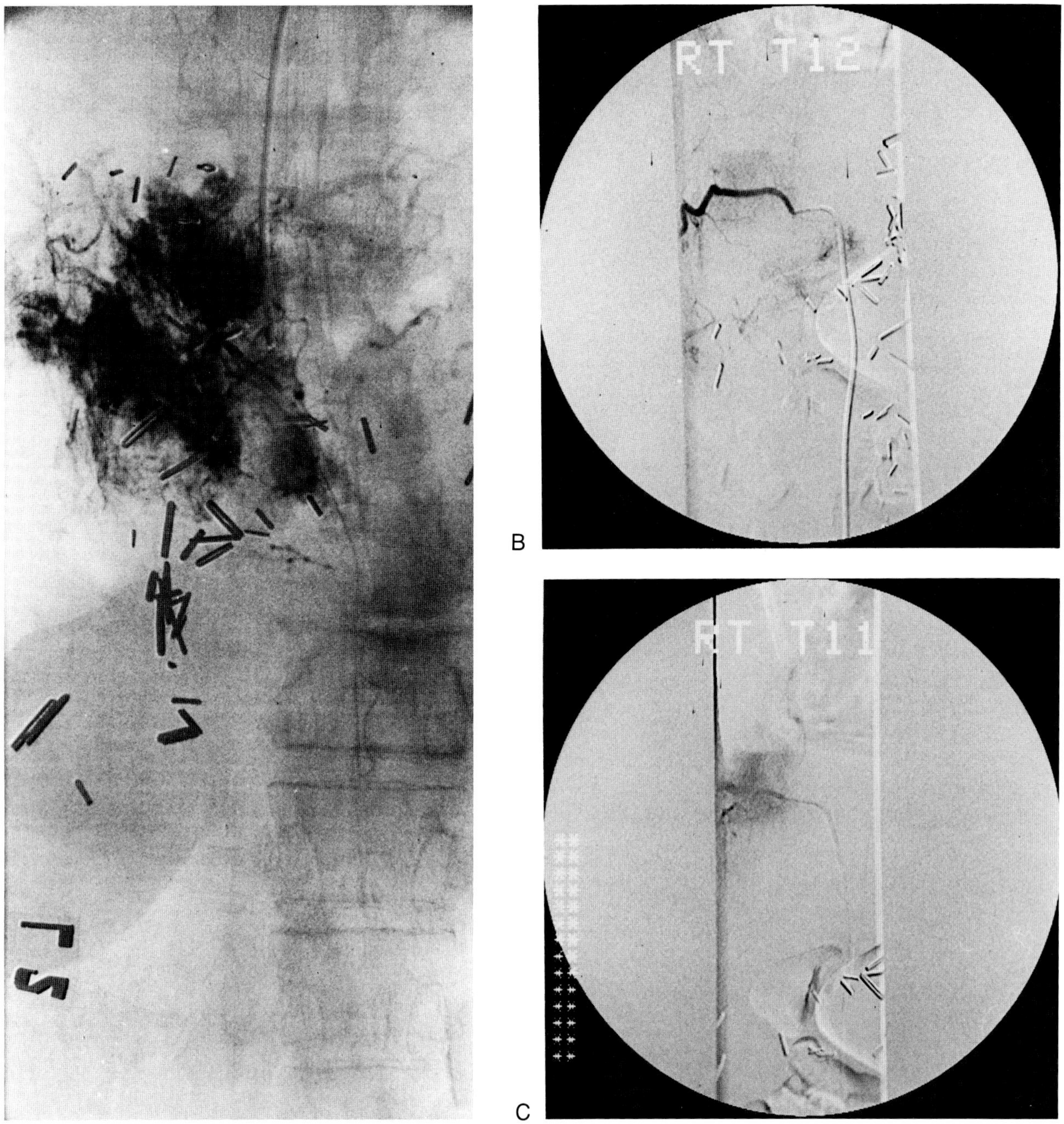

Fig. 8-4. **(A)** Angiograph demonstrating a highly vascular metastatic renal cell cancer to the thoracic spine. **(B)** Selective angiograph of the segmental vessel feeding the metastatic lesion. **(C)** Postembolization angiograph showing obliteration of the segmental vessel.

bolization. It is also essential in delineating the spinal cord blood supply prior to radical spine operations.

DIFFERENTIAL DIAGNOSIS

The differential diagnosis is derived from the history, physical examination, laboratory work-up, and radiographic evaluation. Clinically, localized pain is often seen in vertebral osteomyelitis.[7] Low back pain and associated radiculopathy are nonspecific for herniated disc and/or spinal stenosis.[8] Patients with herniated discs often obtain relief with bed rest, whereas individuals with spinal tumors often have nocturnal pain with increased pain in the supine position. Syringomyelia, which may be idiopathic or post-traumatic, may also have symptoms similar to those of a neoplastic lesion.[9] Some of the vertebral tumors are similar radiographically. Osteogenic sarcoma, for example, which is either mixed or lytic, can be confused with other lytic lesions, including osteoblastoma, hemangioma, plasmacytoma, lymphoma, and metastatic disease. Multiple myeloma, with its lytic appearance, must also be differentiated from osteoporosis. Pathologic fractures of myeloma must be differentiated from pathologic fractures secondary to senile osteoporosis.

Once a differential diagnosis is established, the next step is often biopsy. The final diagnosis is based on the pathologist's evaluation of a tissue sample. Prognosis and further medical and/or surgical treatment often depend on the pathologist's diagnosis. A biopsy, open or closed, is therefore critical. Although the thoracic spine can be approached closed from the posterolateral approach, open biopsy is often preferred in lesions of the thoracic spine. However, a CT-guided needle biopsy can be used occasionally, but may not provide sufficient tissue for diagnosis. Anterior lesions in the vertebral body can be biopsied posteriorly through the pedicle or via a costotransversectomy. An intrathoracic approach is best when benign lesions are suspected and excisional curettage is planned as treatment. An intrathoracic approach is also necessary when an anterior decompression is intended, so that an appropriate vertebrectomy can be performed. Occasionally, lesions of the thoracolumbar junction or extensive lesions can be approached with a thoracoabdominal approach. This is often necessary for anterior spinal reconstruction (Table 8-1).

Table 8-1. Typical Location of Spinal Tumors in the Spinal Column

Anterior Elements	Posterior Elements
Aneurysmal bone cysts	Aneurysmal bone cysts
Giant cell tumors	Giant cell tumors
Hemangiomas	Osteoid osteomas
Eosinophilic granulomas	Osteoblastomas
Ewing's sarcomas	Osteosarcomas
Lymphomas	
Chondrosarcomas	
Osteosarcomas	
Metastatic carcinomas	

PRIMARY BONE TUMORS

BENIGN TUMORS

OSTEOID OSTEOMAS AND OSTEOBLASTOMAS

Osteoid osteomas and osteoblastomas, characteristically involve the posterior elements of the spine. Both lesions have a central lytic area with surrounding reactive bone. Osteoblastomas can, however, appear more aggressive and can be confused with osteosarcomas. Characteristically, osteoid osteomas and osteoblastomas are differentiated by the size of their central lytic defects, with osteoid osteomas being less than 1.5 cm in diameter. Osteoblastomas can be less sclerotic and more expansile than osteoid osteomas. The two tumors are usually seen in patients less than 25 years old.

Characteristically, osteoid osteomas produce pain, often nocturnal, which is relieved by aspirin. Because of the small size of the nidus, radiographic demonstration of these lesions can be difficult. The lesion, by definition, is less than 2.0 cm in diameter and is easily obscured by the overlapping shadows of the vertebral column. CT demonstrates the lesion well, but the most sensitive method of locating an osteoid osteoma is by bone scan. The technetium bone scan provides accurate localization of the lesion, permitting an early diagnosis and prompt treatment. Grossly the lesion is grainy, soft, and wine-red, and microscopically there is a mixture of thin and twisted osteoid trabeculae that in the center are more compact, highly calcified, and with fewer cells, corresponding to the nidus of the lesion (Fig. 8-5; Table 8-2).

Osteoblastomas differ from the osteoid osteomas primarily in size and greater local aggressiveness. The tumor often develops outside the bone and spreads into the surrounding soft tissues without infiltrating them. The majority of these patients who have a lesion at the thoraco-

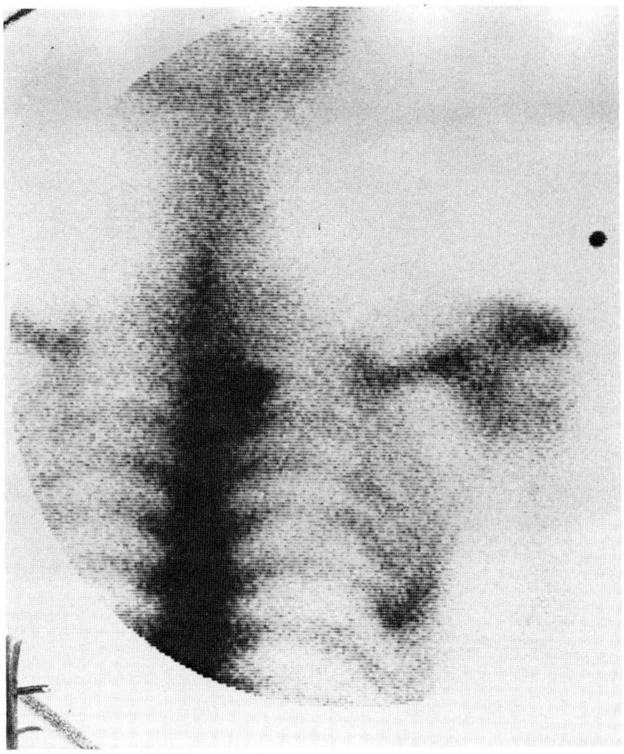

A

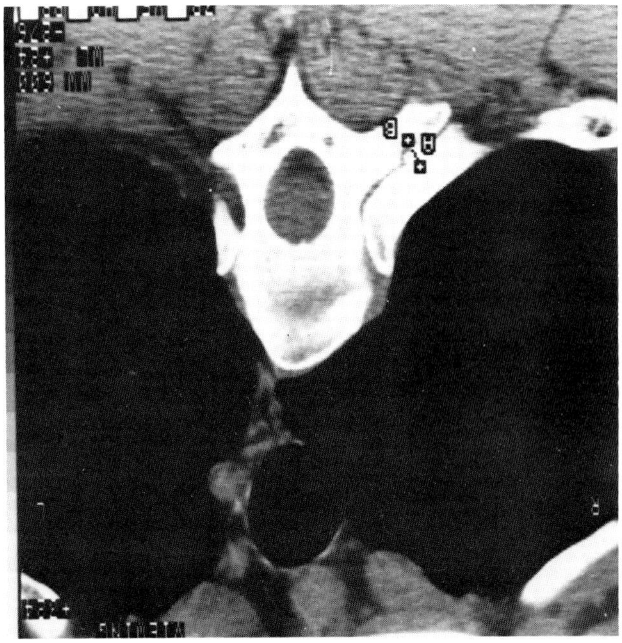

B

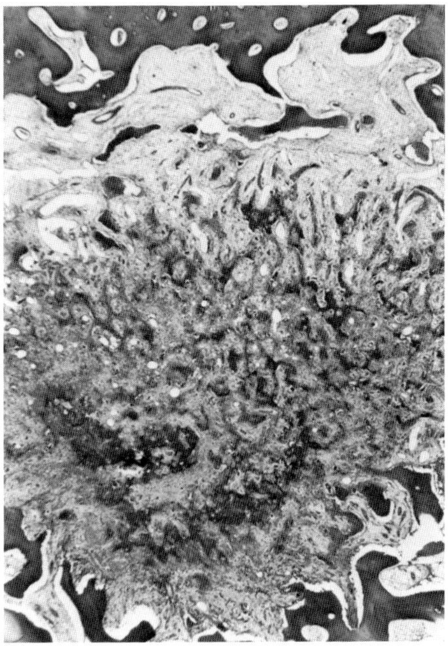

C

Fig. 8-5. **(A)** Bone scan indicating activity suggestive of an osteoid osteoma in the thoracic vertebrae. **(B)** CT scan demonstrating an osteoid osteoma in the pedicle of a midthoracic vertebra. **(C)** Osteoid osteoma. Circumscribed nidus of fibrovascular tissue containing immature osseous trabeculae subjacent to the cortex. (× 16.)

lumbar junction will present with an accompanying scoliosis measuring between 10 and 30 degrees. Histologically this tumor is characterized by a group of mesenchymal cells that have a tendency toward osteoblastic differentiation and by the presence of a rich capillary and sinusoidal vascularization (Fig. 8-6; Table 8-2). Treatment involves surgical excision, but may be supplemented by low-dose radiotherapy in patients in whom an incomplete excision is performed.

Osteoid osteoma and osteoblastoma are the most common causes of a painful scoliosis in the thoracolumbar spine.[1] It is rare for spinal fusion to be necessary after the excision of these lesions,

Table 8-2. Major Characteristics of Primary Spinal Tumors

Tumor	Median Age (yr)	Male/Female Ratio	Size (cm)	Location	Treatment	Associated Diseases	Markers
Benign							
Osteoid osteoma	25	1.5 : 1	<2.0	Posterior elements	Surgical excision		
Osteoblastoma	25	2 : 1	>2.0	Posterior elements	Surgical excision plus low-dose radiotherapy		
Osteochondroma	40	2 : 1		Cervical spine, upper thoracic vertebrae	Surgical excision (symptomatic patients only)		
Aneurysmal bone cyst	15	1 : 2		Posterior elements (rare in thoracic spine)	Surgical curettage plus grafting		
Giant cell tumor	35	2 : 1		Anterior elements	Surgical resection or radiotherapy and stabilization		
Eosinophilic granuloma	10	2 : 1		Vertebral body	Observation or radiotherapy	Hand-Schüller-Christian syndrome, Letterer-Siwe disease	
Malignant							
Solitary, plasmacytoma	55	2 : 1		Vertebral body	Radiotherapy		Bence Jones proteins, serum electrophoresis
Ewing's sarcoma	15	2 : 1		Vertebral body	Radiotherapy plus chemotherapy		Erythrocyte sedimentation ratio
Osteogenic sarcoma	20	1 : 1		Anterior elements	Surgical resection plus chemotherapy		Alkaline phosphatase
Chondrosarcoma	35	1 : 1		Anterior and posterior elements	Surgery		None

but it is more commonly necessary after the excision of an osteoblastoma, which is inherently a larger and more aggressive lesion.

The preoperative use of tetracycline and intraoperative evaluation of the specimen with a Wood's lamp may help in identifying the tumor at the time of surgery, particularly in osteoid osteoma.

OSTEOCHRONDROMAS

Osteochondromas are the most common benign tumors of bone. In the vertebral column they are

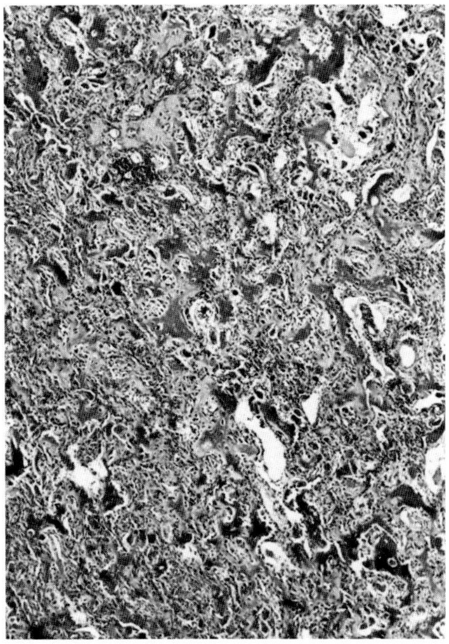

Fig. 8-6. Osteoblastoma. Numerous microtrabeculae of bone in a vascularized fibrous stroma are rimmed by osteoblasts and occasional osteoclasts. (× 50.)

rare, and they occur most often in association with hereditary multiple exostoses. Approximately 7 percent of patients with osteochrondromatosis will have lesions in the vertebral column. Of the symptomatic lesions 60 percent arise in the cervical spine, with an additional 20 percent in the thoracic spine above the T6 level.[10–12]

Solitary occurrences are unusual, but there are cases of solitary osteochondroma presenting with neurologic dysfunction. The plain radiograph often will not reveal the characteristic osteochondroma, a radiolucent cartilaginous cap on a stalk. The intraluminal extension of the radiolucent component is obscured on the plain radiographs and is best visualized on the MR scan. Because of the very slow progression of these compressive cord lesions, excision of the tumor en bloc or piecemeal provides excellent recovery of neurologic function with little likelihood of recurrence. It should be performed only in symptomatic patients[13,14] (Fig. 8-7; Table 8-2).

ANEURYSMAL BONE CYSTS

Aneurysmal bone cysts are found in children and adolescents and are found most commonly within the vertebral body, although at times they occur in the posterior elements. They consist of an expansile mass surrounded by a thin rim of reactive bone. They may be quite aggressive on presentation and can be confused with malignant lesions. Clinical symptoms manifest themselves in a short time, indicating the rapid evolution of the pathologic process. Pain in the spine is often accompanied by radicular symptoms fairly quickly, and often fairly progressive myeloradiculopathy or sudden paraparesis occurs.

Radiographs of the spine reveal a destructive radiolucent lesion with a thin sclerotic capsule. The CT scan with myelogram will reveal the full extent of the intraluminal extension of this lesion. The gross appearance of this lesion is a thin, fibrous capsule with a bluish color reflective of the hemorrhagic cystic mass inside. Histologically the lesion contains histiofibroblasts with many fine capillaries and scattered thin osteoid trabeculae. Because these lesions are very vascular, the surgical treatment, which consists of curettage and bone grafting may be associated with an excessive blood loss. Many surgeons prefer preoperative embolization of these lesions to reduce intraoperative blood losses, but if one is approaching these lesions anteriorly the feeding segmental vessel can be easily identified and ligated before the lesion is curetted. Low-dose radiation should be considered if the tumor has recurred locally, but is associated with malignant transformation years later (Fig. 8-8; Table 8-2).

GIANT CELL TUMORS

Giant cell tumors are often found in the anterior elements of the thoracic spine and are slow-growing but locally aggressive lesions. Their peak incidence is in the third and fourth decades, and the plain radiographs demonstrate an area of focal rarefaction and marginal sclerosis. A CT scan is especially important in the evaluation of these tumors because complete excision is vital for the eradication of these lesions. CT scanning is also important in the early identification of a local recurrence. Histologically these lesions contain multinucleated giant cells uniformly and randomly distributed with mononuclear cells (Fig. 8-9; Table 8-2).

Because of their locally invasive nature, giant cell tumors have been reported to have a particularly poor prognosis.[15] Prolonged disease-free survival has been reported following resection or curettage with radiotherapy. With more aggressive surgical resection, good disease-free survival has been obtained without radiotherapy as well. Unlike with most of the other benign lesions, aggres-

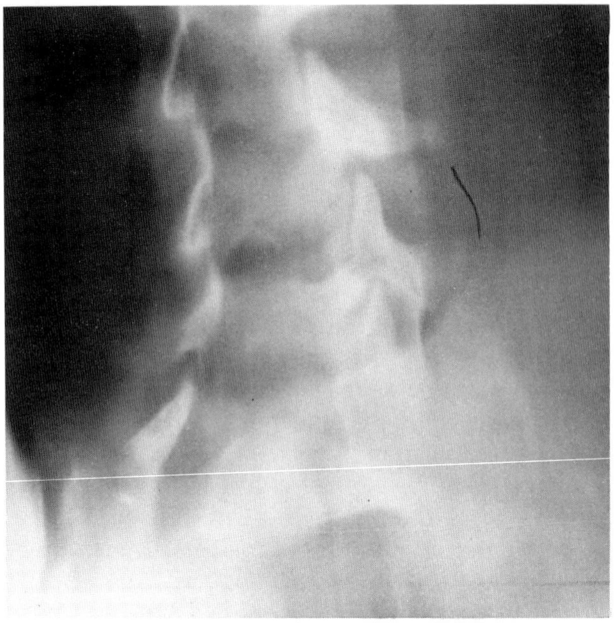

A

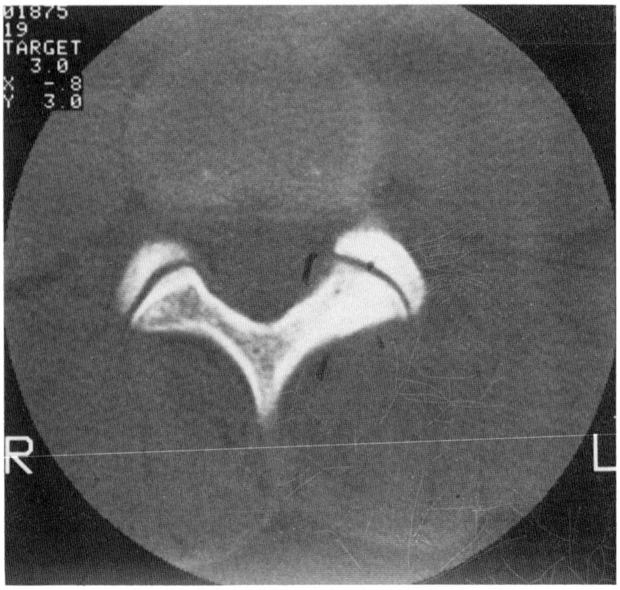

B

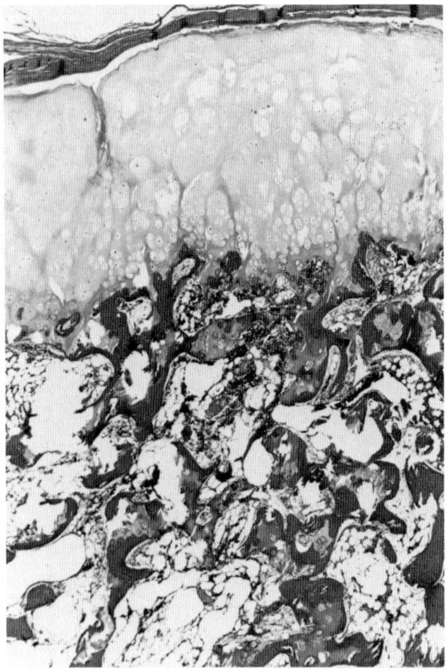

C

Fig. 8-7. **(A)** Tomograph demonstrating an osteochondroma arising in the middle column. **(B)** CT scan, further delineating the lesion. **(C)** Osteochondroma. The lesion consists of a cartilage cap covered by fibrous tissue undergoing endochondral ossification and forming bone and marrow. (× 20.)

sive surgical resection for these lesions may require some form of spinal stabilization.[4,16,17]

EOSINOPHILIC GRANULOMAS

Eosinophilic granulomas are found most often in the vertebral body of children and adolescents. The tumor consists of eosinophils and histiocytes and may result in complete destruction and flattening of the vertebral body, causing vertebra plana. The majority of the lesions are self-limiting, however, and the treatment, in general, is observation and support while the lesion is going through a painful stage. These lesions are associated with Hand-Schüller-Christian syndrome and Letterer-Siwe disease, a granulomalike reticuloendotheliosis with a probable viral etiology. The long-term prognosis is good, and therefore low-dose radiotherapy (1,000 rads) should be used only in cases that do not respond to spinal support and appear

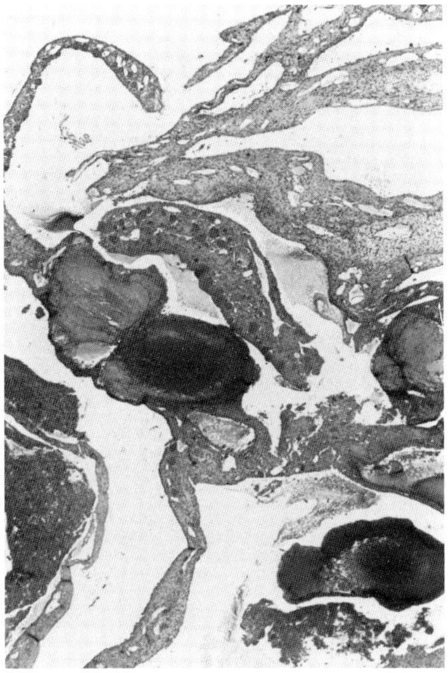

Fig. 8-8. Aneurysmal bone cyst. There are numerous honeycombed sinusoidal spaces lined with vascularized fibroconnective tissue containing multinucleated giant cells. (× 20.)

to be more aggressive than usual. Histologically the eosinophilic component predominates but may be associated with lymphomonocytic cells as well (Fig. 8-10; Table 8-2).

HEMANGIOMAS

Hemangiomas are the most common benign tumors of the spine and involve the vertebral body, with its characteristic vertical striped radiographic appearance. The lesion may occur at any age, but has a peak incidence from ages 40 to 50. Most of these tumors are asymptomatic and require no treatment. Tumors that become symptomatic may be treated with low-dose radiation therapy. Occasionally, they may present with a painless but progressive paralysis secondary to epidural tumor extension. They may also cause a pathologic fracture with neurologic involvement secondary to bony compression of the spinal cord. Treatment is surgical excision with preoperative embolization to control intraoperative bleeding.[18] The histology of these lesions is characterized by the presence of newly formed and anomalous vascular spaces. During childhood, when the form is in its developmental stage, the appearance is that of a capillary hemangioma (Fig. 8-11).

MALIGNANT TUMORS

MULTIPLE MYELOMAS

Multiple myelomas affect primarily the vertebral bodies, and the median age is 55 years. A solitary plasmacytoma will occur in approximately 3 percent of cases, and these lesions have a more indolent course. Whereas three-quarters of patients with multiple myeloma involving the spinal column are dead within 1 year of their diagnosis and all are dead within 4 years, the 5-year survival rate for solitary plasmacytomas is approximately 60 percent, with survival periods as long as 20 years reported.[19,20] Plasma cells proliferate, replacing the normal bone marrow, and produce a lytic lesion on plain radiography. In the systemic form of the disease, multiple levels of the disease may be evident. This may be confirmed by an abnormal immunoglobulin band, anemia, and ESR. Bence Jones proteins may be found in the urine. These markers, however, may be absent completely in the solitary plasmacytomas, and the diagnosis has to be made via a Craig needle biopsy. This reveals the characteristic sheets of plasma cells, which are the hallmark of this disease. Treatment usually includes irradiation and chemotherapy. Rarely, if the disease is localized or if there has been a failure of previous treatment, surgical decompression and stabilization are necessary[21] (Fig. 8-12; Table 8-2).

EWING'S SARCOMA

Ewing's sarcoma is a highly aggressive tumor that occurs primarily in early adolescence and childhood. The spine is an uncommon site of origin for this disease (only 3 percent of cases originate in the spine).[22] Kornberg et al.[23] reported only 78 cases of spine involvement in a series of 217 Ewing's sarcomas. Pilepich et al.[24] reported on 22 patients with primary vertebral Ewing's sarcoma and noted that 14 of the patients had neurologic deficits at the time of diagnosis. Other patients have presented with slight pain lasting from several months to up to 1 year. The radiographic appearance is of a permeative lytic lesion of the body, usually with an associated soft tissue mass as well. The diagnosis can be made by a Craig needle biopsy. The histologic appearance of uniform small cells with globelike nuclei is characteristic of this disease (Fig. 8-13). The treatment of choice for Ewing's sarcoma involves multiagent chemotherapy for two cycles initially followed by high-dose

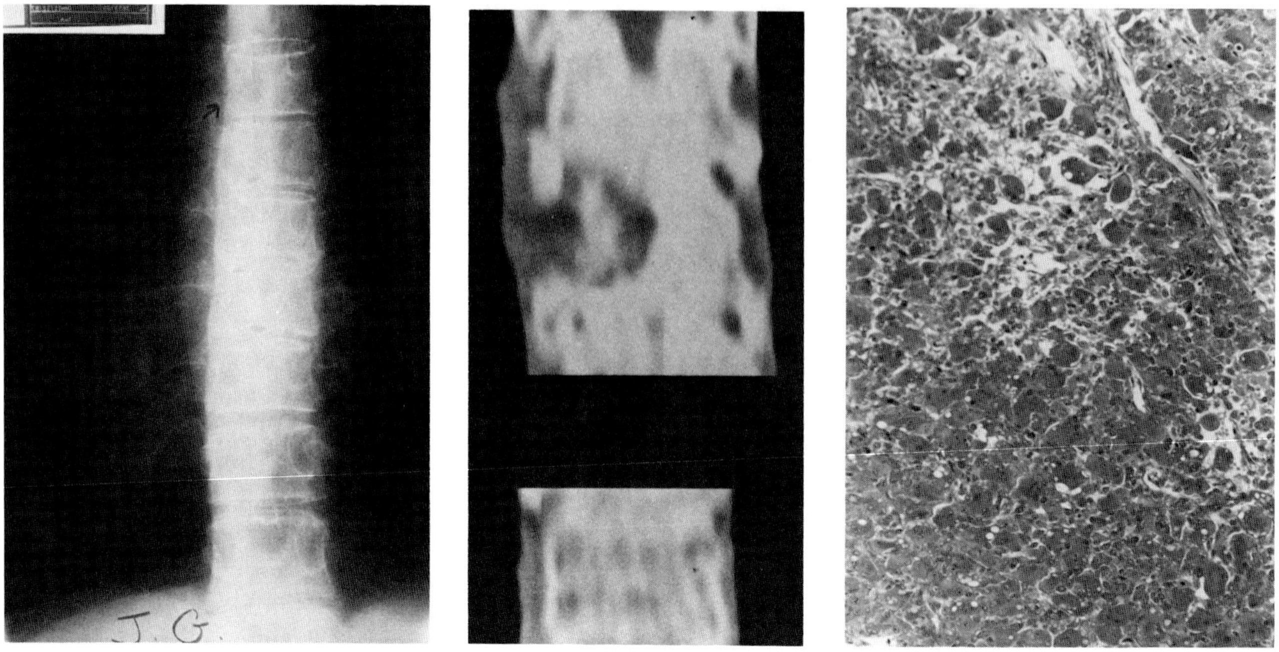

A B C

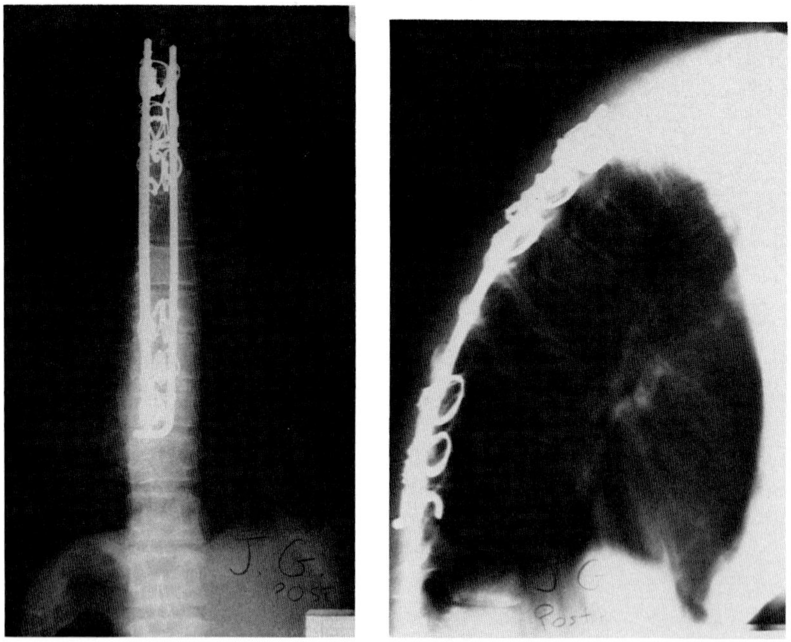

D E

Fig. 8-9. **(A)** Plain radiograph showing some scalloping of the T7 thoracic vertebra. **(B)** Coronal MR scan showing a destructive lesion of the T7 vertebra. **(C)** Giant cell tumor. The tumor consists of a syncytial sheet of mononuclear cells in which multinucleated giant cells are uniformly and randomly distributed. (× 125.) **(D)** Postoperative radiograph showing partial vertebral resection and stabilization with Harrington rods and sublaminar wires. **(E)** Lateral postoperative chest x-ray.

radiotherapy and then consolidation chemotherapy for up to 18 months. Local control and encouraging disease-free survival rates are achieved with this regimen. Surgical treatment is reserved for individuals who have failed primary therapy and then present with neurologic deficits (Table 8-2).

LYMPHOMAS

Lymphomas involve the vertebral body and radiographically appear lytic. Occasionally they have an ivory or sclerotic appearance. Biopsy is necessary to differentiate them from Ewing's sarcoma or

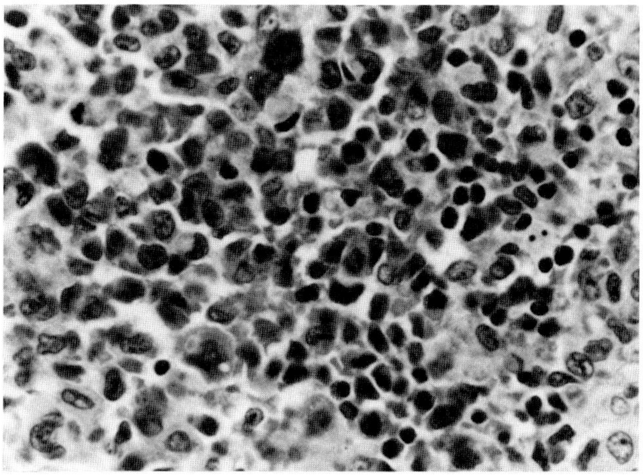

Fig. 8-10. Eosinophilic granuloma. The lesion is composed of two cell populations. Histiocytes are the larger mononuclear cells, which form several multinuclear giant cells in this field. Eosinophils are the numerous smaller background cells with occasional bilobate nuclei. (× 400.)

metastatic disease. Treatment is by radiotherapy, but occasionally chemotherapy is indicated if there is widespread disease. If the spine becomes unstable secondary to bony destruction, surgical stabilization may be indicated (Fig. 8-14).

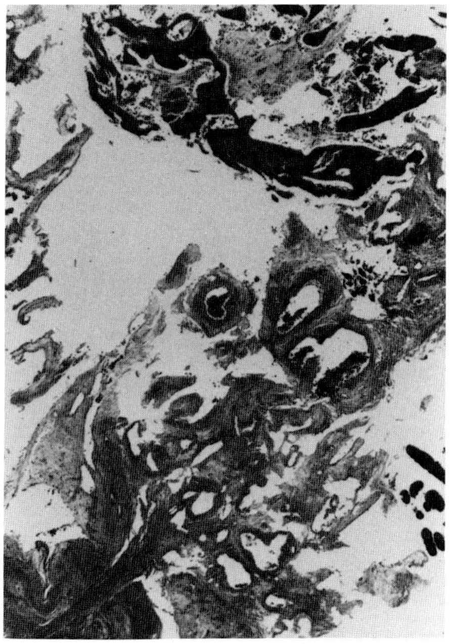

Fig. 8-11. Hemangioma. Multiple interconnecting cavernous spaces are lined with flattened endothelial cells within a bony trabecula. (× 25.)

OSTEOSARCOMAS

Osteosarcomas are more commonly seen as metastatic lesions than as primary lesions of the spine. When they are seen in the spine, the patient may have developed a tumor secondary to Paget's disease, irradiation, or malignant transformation of a benign tumor such as an osteochondroma. Approximately 2 percent of all primary osteogenic sarcomas arise in the spine. This aggressive neoplasm is also seen in adolescents. Radiographically, the lesion may be lytic, sclerotic, or mixed.[25] The typical radiographic findings include cortical destruction, soft tissue calcification, and, in advanced cases, collapse. In 95 percent of cases the lesion arises from the anterior elements of the vertebral column. CT demonstrates intraspinal and paraspinal soft tissue masses more clearly, allowing for a more accurate preoperative plan. Treatment must be individualized, but wide resection is usually important. Perioperative chemotherapy is often necessary.[13] Sundaresan et al. reported on seven patients undergoing wide resection or vertebral body resection combined with radiotherapy.[26] With this regimen four patients were alive and free of disease with a median survival of 52 months. The other three patients succumbed to their disease during the 11-month interval that has been traditionally reported. The histologic appearance of the typical osteogenic sarcoma reveals pleomorphic sarcomatous cells (Fig. 8-15; Table 8-2).

CHONDROSARCOMAS

Approximately 10 percent of chondrosarcomas arise in the spinal column. They may involve either anterior or posterior elements and are usually slow-growing lesions. They are seen in adults and are radiographically lytic. An associated soft tissue mass and soft tissue calcifications may be evident as well. As with the other malignant lesions, CT scans will better demonstrate the full extent of the lesion and any cord compression. The tumor is radioresistant, and treatment requires en bloc excision. Repeated debulking procedures may be necessary for recurrences. Long-term survivals have been reported with intralesional excisions, but an en bloc resection, although rarely possible, is preferable. Histologically these lesions show infiltration of the intratrabecular spaces of cancellous bone by a cellular cartilage tumor (Table 8-2).

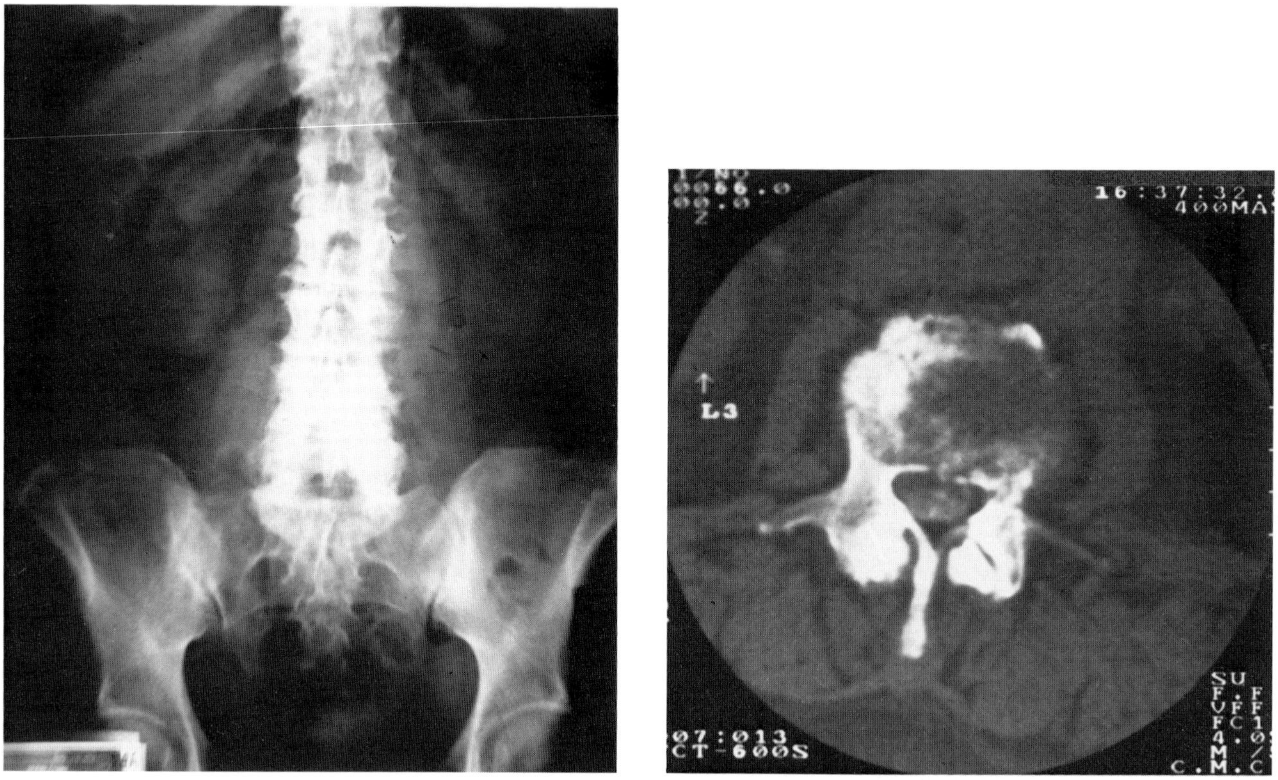

A B

Fig. 8-12. **(A)** Solitary plasmacytoma arising in the lumbar vertebra. **(B)** CT scan revealing a destructive lesion at L3 with extension into the spinal canal. **(C)** Postoperative radiograph following decompression and stabilization with methyl methacrylate and CD rods. **(D)** Several years later a second lesion is noted in the L1 vertebral body. **(E)** Sagittal MRI scan showing involvement of multiple vertebral bodies.

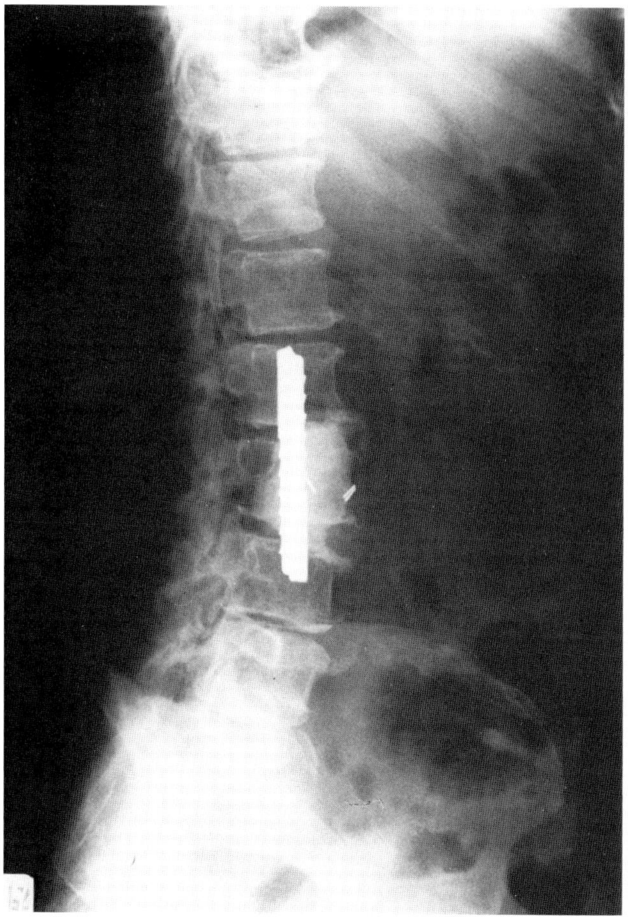

C

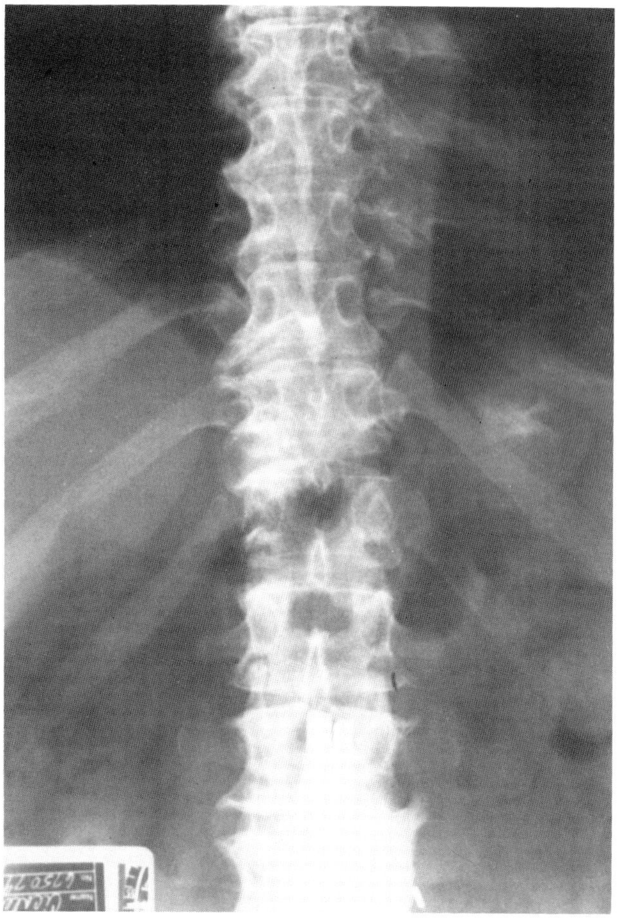

D

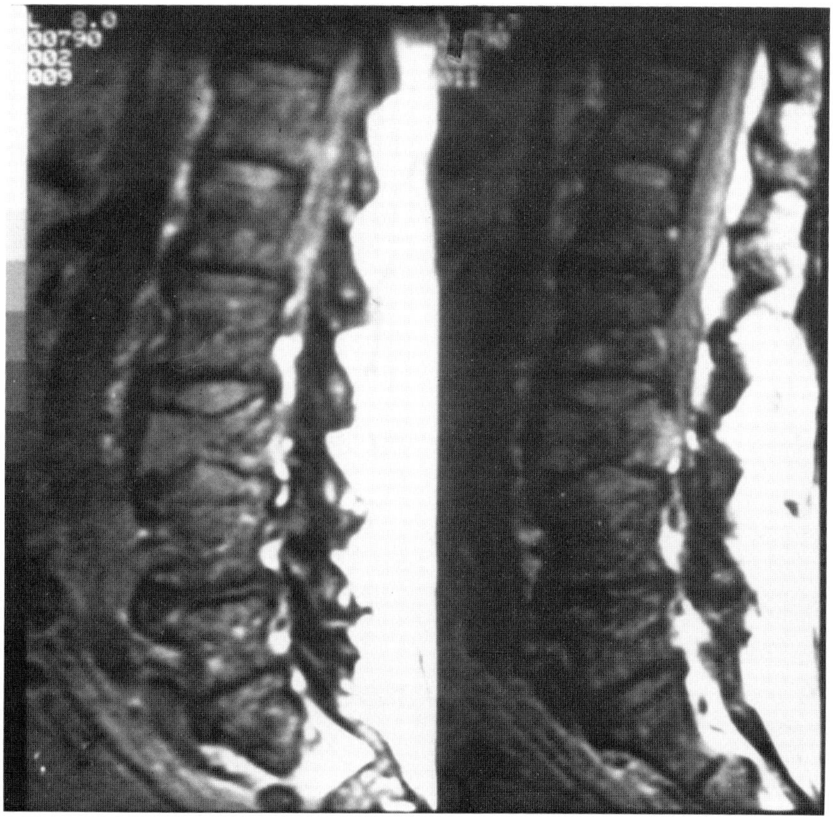

E

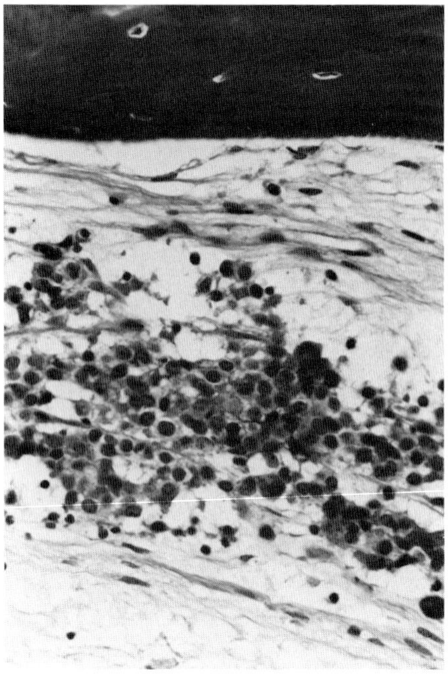

Fig. 8-13. Ewing's sarcoma. A uniform sheet of small, round cells with scant cytoplasm is shown. The uniform, hyperchromatic nuclei are almost devoid of nucleoli, and no mitotic activity is noted. (× 320.)

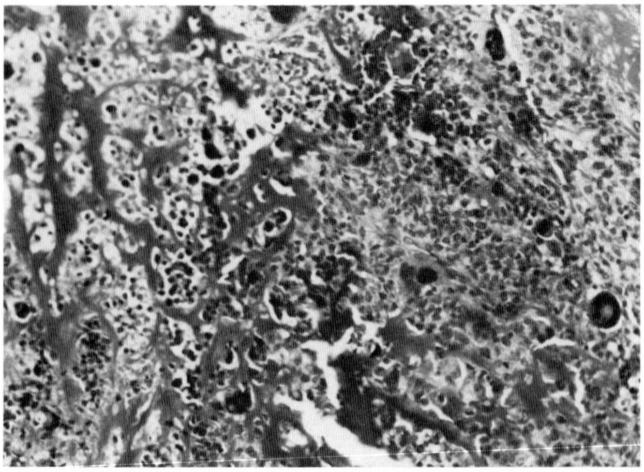

Fig. 8-15. Osteosarcoma. Pleomorphic sarcomatous cells produce wisps of delicately interconnected osteoid and bone. (× 125.)

METASTATIC BONE TUMORS

Metastases to the vertebral column most commonly affect the lumbar vertebrae. However, the thoracic spine, with its smaller canal diameter and more tenuous blood supply, has greater potential for neurologic compromise. Lung cancer, breast cancer, prostate cancer, and lymphoma are the leading primary tumors that metastasize to the spine. Others that metastasize frequently include kidney, gastrointestinal, and thyroid tumors. The metastases generally seed hematogenously to the vertebral body containing active red marrow. At times the tumor can metastasize by direct extension. Batson's venous plexus, which lies within the epidural space, is a conduit for tumor spread. While in contact with the intercostal and lumbar veins, this valveless system allows metastases from the heart and prostate through the azygos and pelvic venous systems, respectively.[27,28] Five percent of patients with metastatic disease are said to develop spinal cord compression[29] (Fig. 8-16). Neurologic compromise may result from direct extension of the tumor, pathologic fracture (with resulting compression), or intradural metastases. The primary cancer may well go on to seed the spine silently, without symptoms, and plain radiographs may be the first indication of metastatic disease. Biopsy of lytic lesions has shown a much higher incidence of definitive histologic diagnosis than has biopsy of blastic lesions. Debate continues about the necessity of open biopsy of metastatic lesions. Harrington believes that open biopsy is rarely indicated, except at the time of surgical stabilization and/or decompression.[2,3]

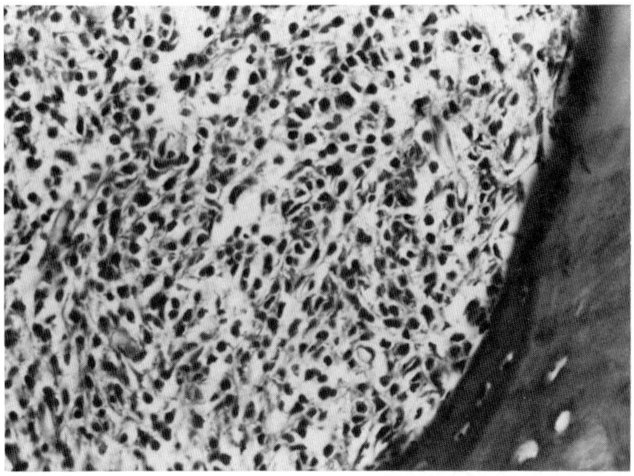

Fig. 8-14. Lymphoma. Intertrabecular spaces are infiltrated by monomorphic round tumor cells. (× 80.)

PRINCIPLES OF TREATMENT

In treating both benign and malignant lesions of the spine, the general principle is excision of the tumor, if possible, with or without adjuvant therapy. The goal of this should be control of pain, prevention and correction of spinal instability and

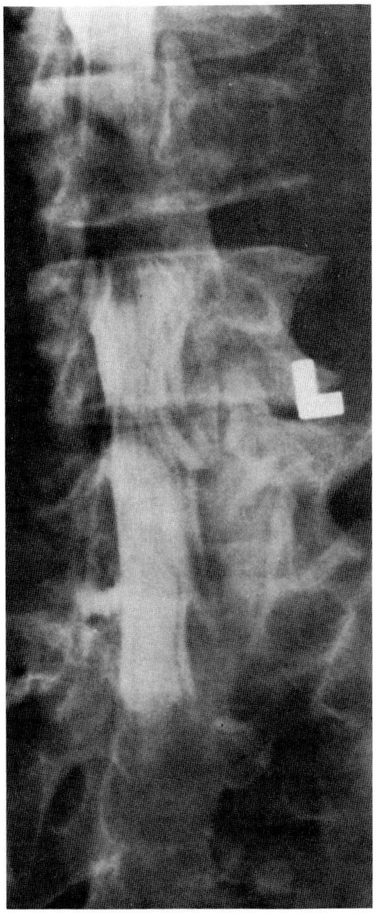

Fig. 8-16. Myelogram demonstrating a complete block due to metastatic cancer.

deformity, and reversal, if possible, of neurologic compromise. The spine is a weight-bearing structure.[30,31] Vertebral collapse leads to progressive spinal deformity and progressive cord compromise. Therefore, the spine must be treated like any weight-bearing long bone and prophylactically stabilized if there is impending fracture and collapse. Benign lesions require thorough excision. Bone graft may or may not be necessary, depending on the size and location of the lesion. With lesions that involve the posterior elements, complete excision is often possible. Anterior involvement may allow only partial removal, but current advanced surgical techniques can permit vertebral replacement. Low-dose irradiation is recommended as an alternative therapy or additive approach for lesions that commonly involve the vertebral body, such as hemangiomas, giant cell tumors, aneurysmal bone cysts, and eosinophilic granulomas. Caution must be emphasized in using adjuvant radiation in young patients because of the risk of secondary malignant transformation.[32] However, most studies that report malignant transformation were done with much higher doses of radiation than would currently be used for such lesions. With benign lesions that are highly aggressive, such as giant cell tumor and osteoblastoma, a more aggressive resection may be necessary. If spinal stability has been compromised by either the lesion or surgery, stabilization with fusion may be required. Pettine and Klassaen reported that localized spinal fusion was needed after facet resection with osteoid osteoma or osteoblastoma.[1] Usually, however, resection of one facet unilaterally is not an indication for fusion.

Historically, metastatic lesions and aggressive primary malignant lesions were treated by radiation alone, posterior laminectomy alone, or laminectomy with adjuvant radiation or chemotherapy. However, since many malignant metastatic lesions present primarily anteriorly in the vertebral bodies, a posterior approach may be inadequate to resect the tumor or decompress the spinal canal.[33–35] Malignant lesions, with cord compression, must be decompressed anteriorly with the subsequent placement of segmental spinal stabilization. Decompressive laminectomy may, in fact, sacrifice any remaining stability provided by an intact posterior column and is therefore generally contraindicated except when the lesion is in the epidural space and spinal stabilization will not be compromised. If a posterior approach is chosen and the spine is destabilized as a result of surgery, immediate stabilization should be added.

Unremitting pain that cannot be controlled by medical treatment, the presence or imminent probability of neurologic dysfunction, spinal instability, and what DeWald et al. term "loss of structural support" are all indications for surgical treatment.[36] For metastatic tumors, the indications have become more clearly defined. DeWald et al. have outlined five distinct classes of spinal malignant tumors and treatment. Class 1 patients present without deformity but with moderate pain. With less than 50 percent destruction of the vertebral body, only radiotherapy and chemotherapy are necessary. With 50 percent or greater destruction of the anterior elements or with significant pedicle involvement, surgical stabilization is recommended. For Class 2 patients, who present with moderate deformity and collapse and are immunocompetent, surgical reconstruction is recommended. Class 3 patients, who have moderate deformity and collapse but are immunocompromised, should have surgical decompression and/or stabilization after medical management in an attempt to control the immunocompromised status. Class 4 patients, who have marked deformity and paralysis, should have immediate surgical decompression and stabilization. Class 5 patients, who have marked deformity and paralysis and are immunocompromised, have an extremely poor prognosis, and therefore the oncologist and the spine surgeon together should decide whether treatment is indeed a viable option for these patients.[36]

Harrington has divided patients with metastatic disease into five classes, a classification that also emphasizes the degree of neurologic involvement and bony destruction. Class 1 patients, without significant neurologic involvement, and Class 2 patients, with involvement of bone without instability, are initially offered either chemotherapy, hormonal therapy, or local irradiation. Class 3 patients, with major neurologic dysfunction and without significant involvement of bone, should be treated with irradiation. Radiotherapy alone has been shown to be as effective as a decompressive laminectomy.[37] If the disease was acute in onset, steroids should be administered. Class 4 patients, who have vertebral collapse and pain but are neurologically stable, and Class 5 patients, who have collapse and instability with neurologic involvement, both require surgical decompression and stabilization.[2,3] Harrington has further defined his indications for surgical intervention. Patients with a progressive painful kyphotic deformity with an intact posterior column require anterior decompression and stabilization. Patients with a progressive kyphotic deformity, with all three columns affected, require anterior and posterior decompression and stabilization. Class 4 and 5 individuals require decompression on the side of the involvement. Other patients who should be considered for surgery include those with radioresistant tumors and those who failed radiotherapy.[29]

A determination of stability is the basis for the spinal surgeon's eventual choice of the approach to stabilization. If the anterior spine is involved, these patients are best approached anteriorly or anterolaterally. If the posterior spine is involved, a posterior approach is required. With extensive involvement, a combined anterior and posterior approach is indicated.

The rib cage provides additional stability in the thoracic spine. Because the anterior elements are small at T1 and T2, anterior access is restricted and a posterior approach is usually preferred. Although an anterior approach to the upper thoracic vertebrae has been described by Sundarasen et al., the surgery must be individualized and may be performed in one or two stages.[38]

Upon anterior decompression, the segmental vessels should be ligated around the vertebral level of the lesion. Stabilization can then be carried out in several fashions. Methyl methacrylate has been used alone successfully by several surgeons after corpectomy for one or more vertebral levels (Fig. 8-17).[29,39] Radiotherapy can then be carried out postoperatively, because methyl methacrylate has been shown to have no weakening effect from radiation, nor does it interfere with local radiotherapy.[40] Harrington has in some cases reinforced methyl methacrylate with Harrington distraction rods anteriorly, and this is preferred when technically possible because it makes for a more stable construct.[20] The vertebral endplates are removed to ensure better cement fixation. Rush rods or Kirschner wires, or just the serrated portion of the Harrington rod, can be used. Traditionally, autologous iliac, fibular, and rib bone grafts have been used to enhance stability. These strut grafts in neoplastic disease usually require additional ex-

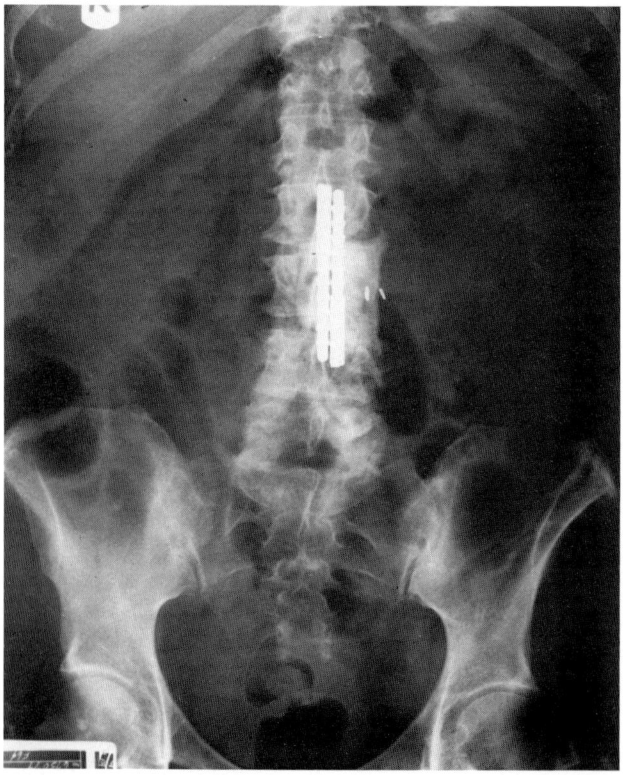

Fig. 8-17. Decompression and stabilization of a metastatic lesion with methyl methacrylate and Cotrell-Dubusset rods.

ternal fixation. Fusion may not be achieved in the face of postoperative irradiation. Radiotherapy has to be limited to a subtherapeutic dosage (1,500 to 2,000 rads, compared with a therapeutic dosage of 4,000 to 5,000 rads). In certain cases, stabilization alone, without fusion, is performed when it is unclear how long patients will live. Brachytherapy is also useful.

Fusion can always be added if longevity is assured. Stener has performed spondylectomies and reconstructed the absent vertebral body space with corticocancellous blocks fixed with screws posteriorly.[41] Metallic fixation is added above and below the inserted grafts. Besides cement and bone for spinal stabilization, stabilizations can be performed with metallic devices. The Chinese have used a stainless steel prosthetic vertebral body that incorporates bone graft inside and around the prosthesis.[42] Posterior segmental spinal stabilization is the best choice and has been used by Roy-Camille, DeWald, Fidler, Harrington, and Flatley[3,36,43–45] (Fig. 8-18). If life expectancy is greater

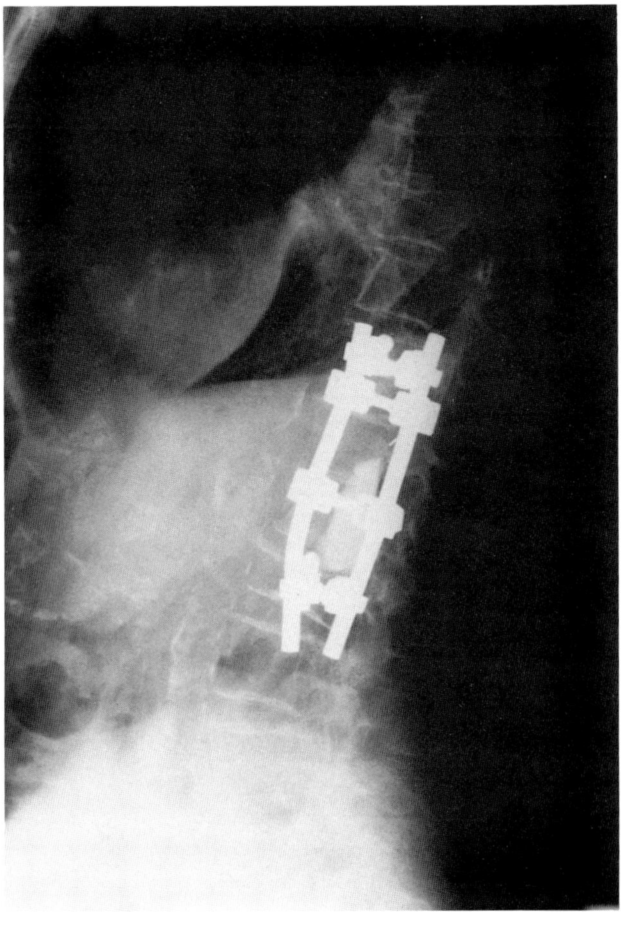

Fig. 8-18. Posterior segmental stabilization following anterior decompression.

than 1 year and stabilization alone has been performed, fusion can be performed later. The choice of segmental fixation is dependent upon the specifics of the individual case. Sublaminar wires with a Harrington-Lugue or Lugue system can be used. Pedicle screws with rods or plates can be used, and Cotrel Dubousset instrumentation as well. The key, however, in all of these cases is segmental fixation to prevent failure of fixation and to distribute the forces to the entire length of the spine that is being surgically treated.

SURGICAL APPROACH

The thoracic and/or lumbar spine can be approached through one of three operative procedures depending on the level required.[46–50] For lesions between C7 and T3, a standard left or right thoracotomy incision can be used. The scapula can be lifted off the chest wall and the third rib excised. To improve exposure to a higher level, the second rib can also be excised. Because the scapula covers the defect, no reconstruction is required for multiple rib resections above the fifth rib (Fig. 8-19). For lesions between T4 and T11, a standard posterolateral thoracotomy can be used with resection of any single rib that will gain direct access to the lesion to be resected (Fig. 8-20). In young children, unless a rib is required for a graft, a rib resection is not necessary for exposure. For exposure of the T12 to L2 vertebral bodies, the following approach has provided the best exposure with very acceptable cosmetic results.

The skin incision is placed directly over the 10th rib and extends through the costal arch onto the anterior abdominal wall (Fig. 8-21). The incision on the abdominal wall is a pararectus incision and can be extended as low as necessary, approximately 3 cm medial to the iliac crest. This incision allows access to the iliac crest if a bone graft is required, and it is much more cosmetic than the traditional paramedian or midline extensions.

The external oblique fascia is opened, and the muscle is split in the direction of the fibers. The internal oblique and transversus abdominus muscles are divided (Fig. 8-22), and the retroperitoneal space is entered. The peritoneal envelope is easily mobilized off the iliacus muscle and reflected medially off the psoas. The attachments of the peritoneum to the undersurface of the diaphragm can then be easily mobilized (Fig. 8-23).

After the thoracic incision has been completed by dividing the latissimus and resecting the 10th

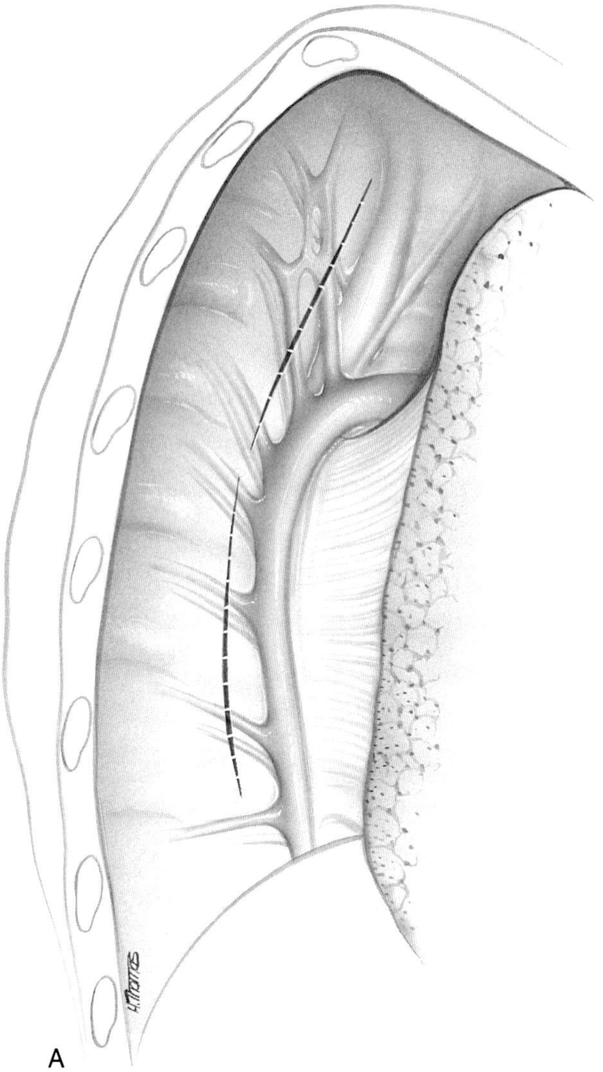

A

Fig. 8-19. (A) Following a right posterolateral thoracotomy the parietal pleura is incised along the line indicated to expose the thoracic segmental vessels. (B) For a high-level lesion the segments overlying T2 to T5 are divided. The discs and vertebral bodies at this level are exposed.

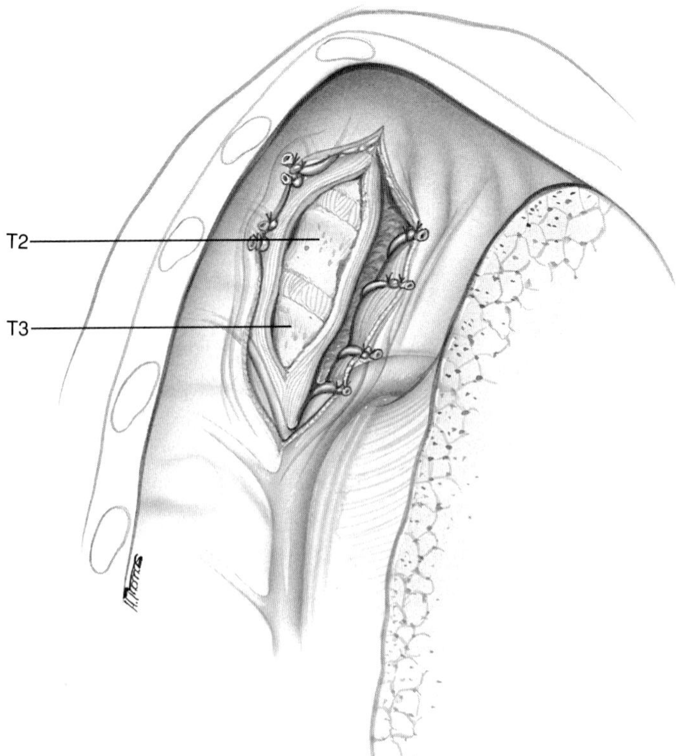

B

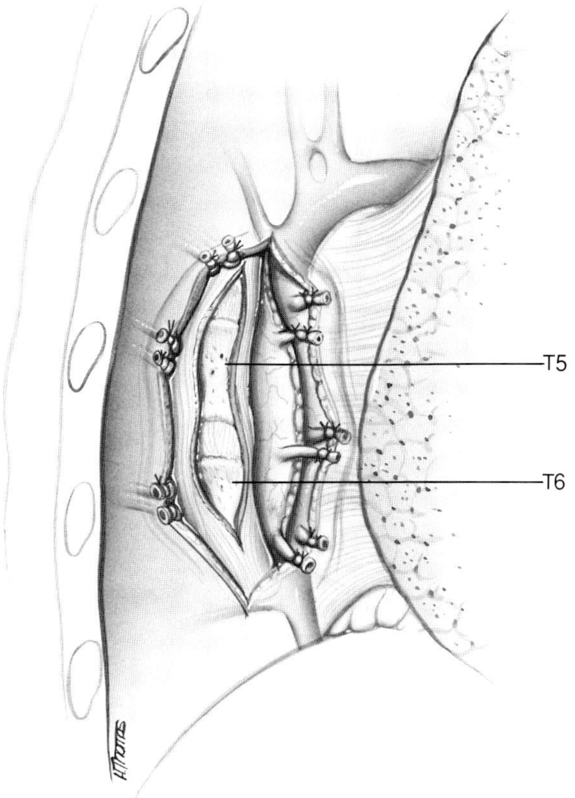

Fig. 8-20. Exposure of the midthoracic vertebrae in a similar fashion to that in Fig. 8-19.

rib, the thoracic cavity can be entered. The costal arch is divided, and the diaphragmatic insertion on the undersurface of the 10th rib is detached. The diaphragm can then be incised, leaving a 2-mm cuff for repair (Fig. 8-24). The major vessels are mobilized off the front of the spine by dividing the segmental vessels off the levels to be exposed (Fig. 8-25 and 8-26). Following completion of the spinal portion of the operation, the diaphragm is closed with 2-silk vertical mattress sutures. A chest tube is placed through the resected bed of the 10th rib. The ribs are reapproximated by placing percostal sutures around the upper border of the ninth rib and through holes drilled through the 11th rib. This prevents entrapment of the 11th rib intercostal nerve and a subsequent neuroma.

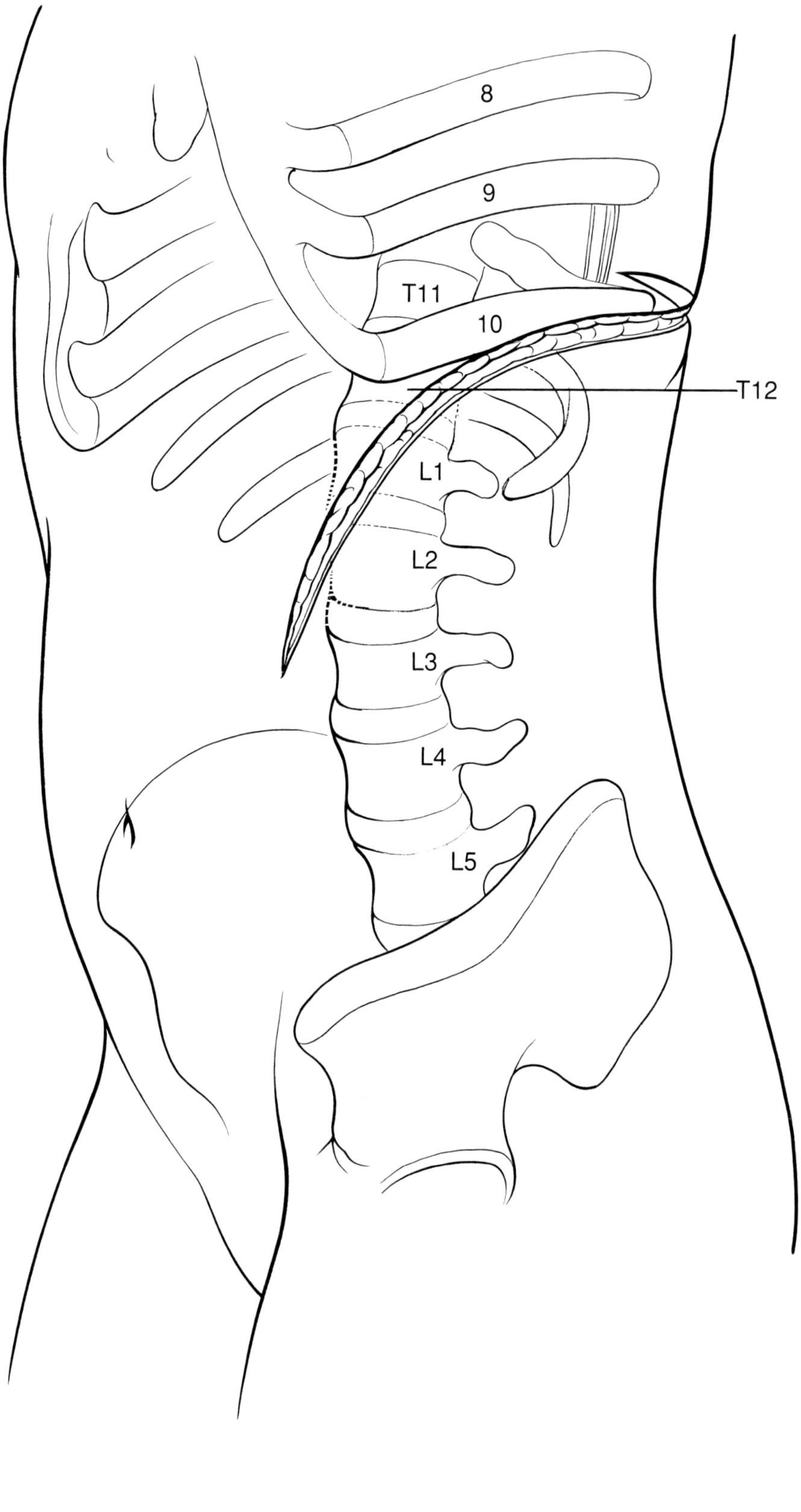

Fig. 8-21. The skin incision used for a 10th-rib thoracolumbar approach.

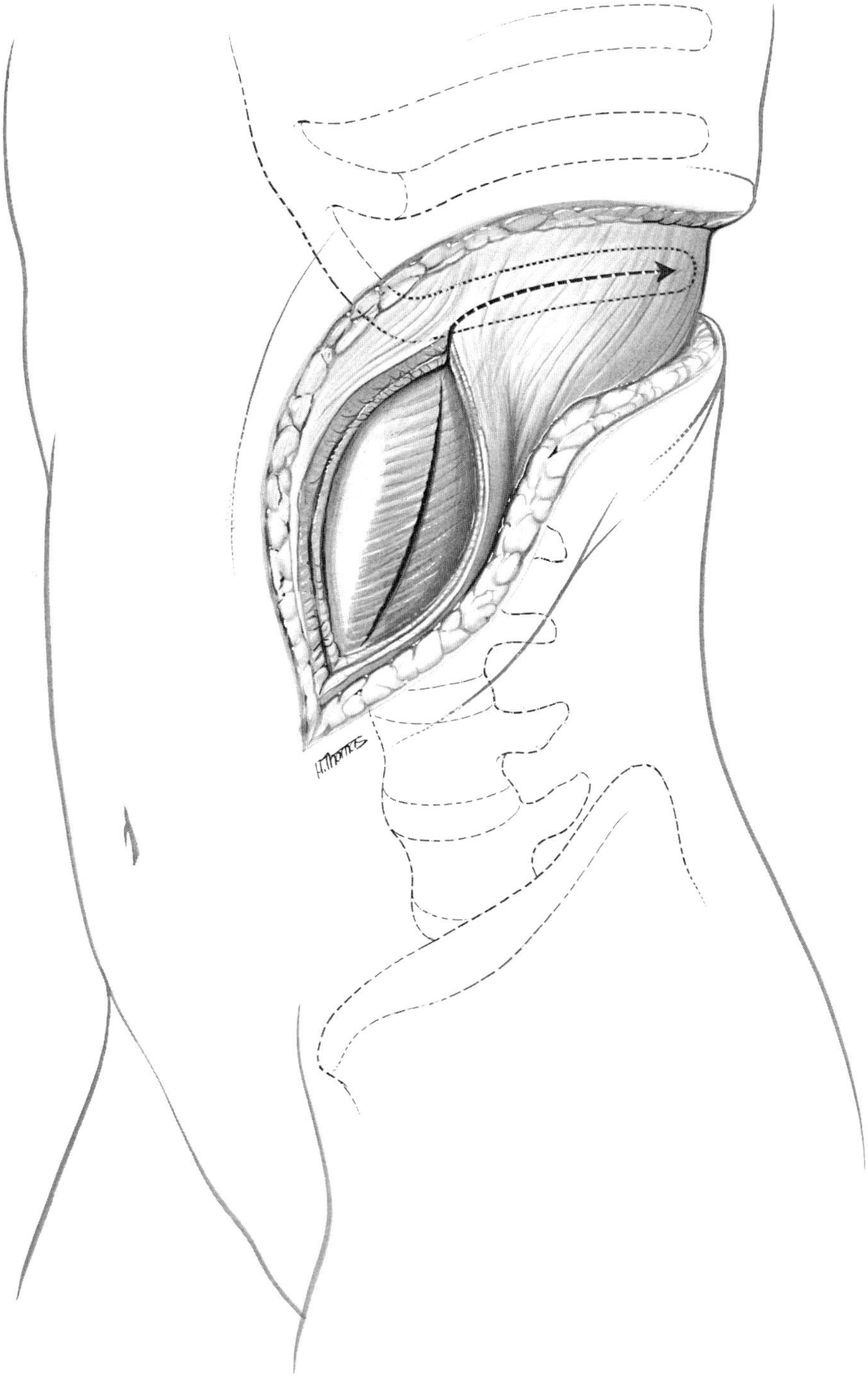

Fig. 8-22. The abdominal portion of the incision in Fig. 8-21 is completed initially by dividing the external oblique muscle in the direction of its fibers and incising the internal oblique and transversus abdominus musculature to gain entry into the retroperitoneal space.

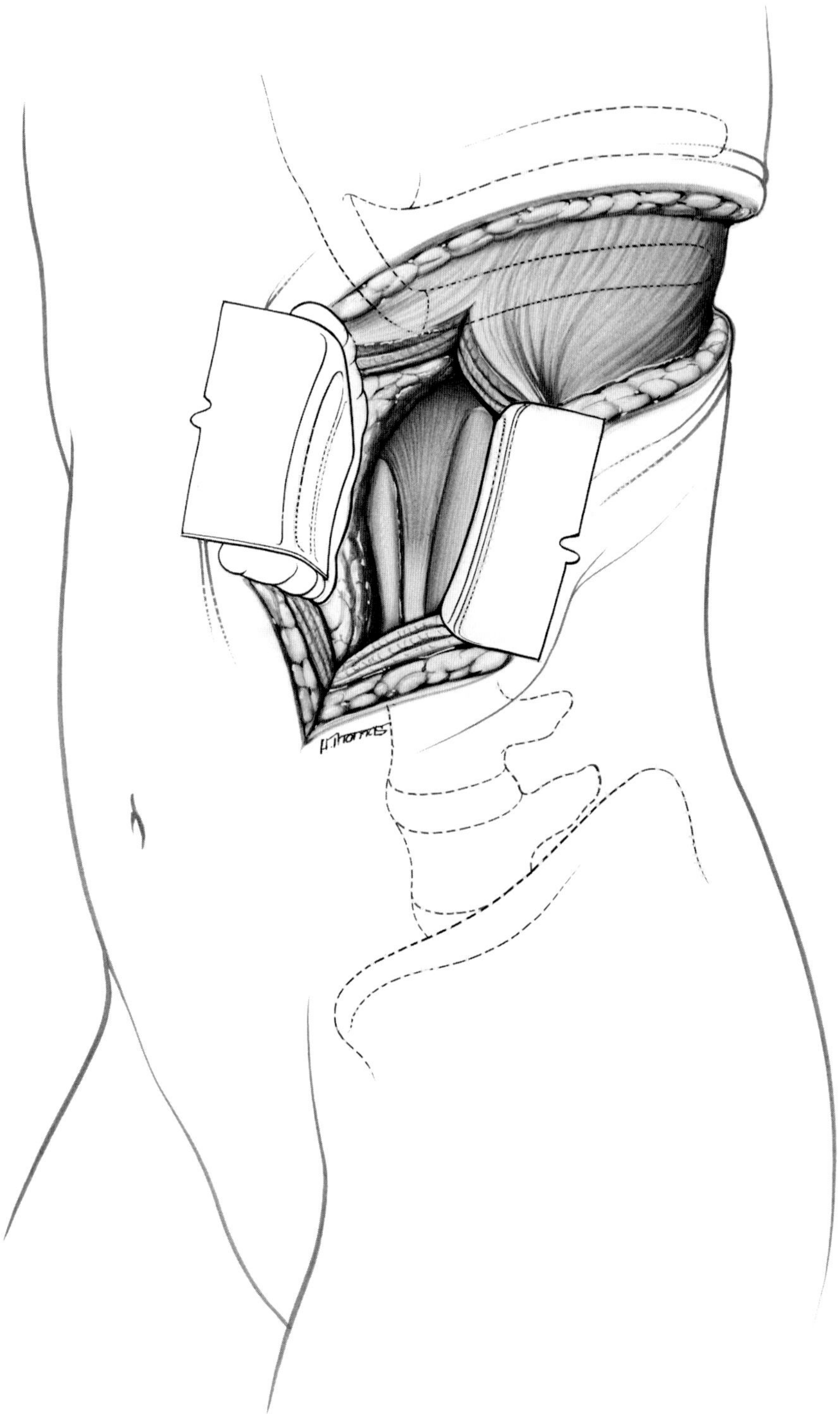

Fig. 8-23. The peritoneal envelope is dissected off the iliacus and psoas, exposing the major vasculature and segmental vessels overlying the upper lumbar vertebrae.

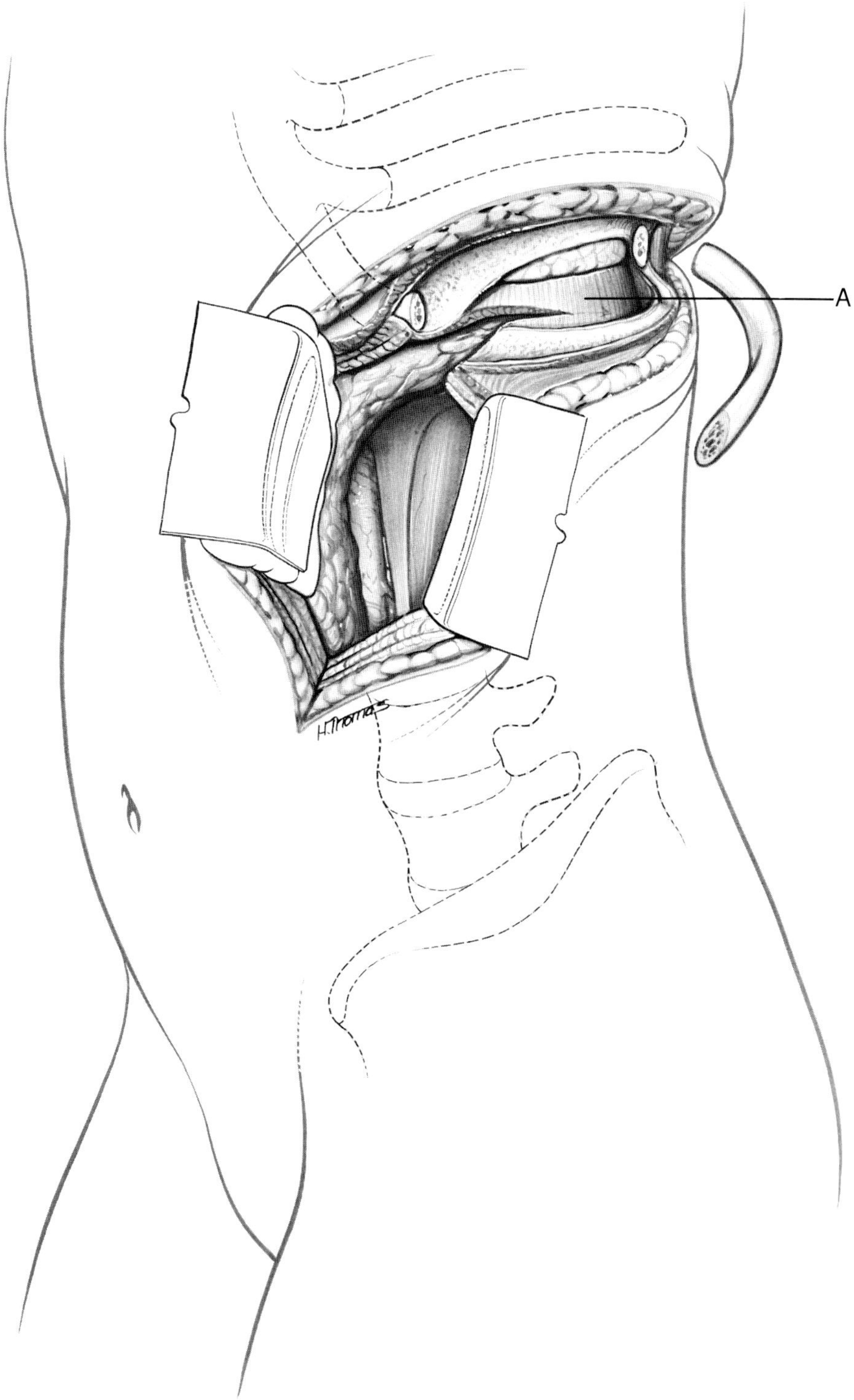

Fig. 8-24. The 10th rib is incised, and the chest cavity is entered. The diaphragm is incised **(A),** leaving a cuff for repair after the spinal portion of the operation is completed.

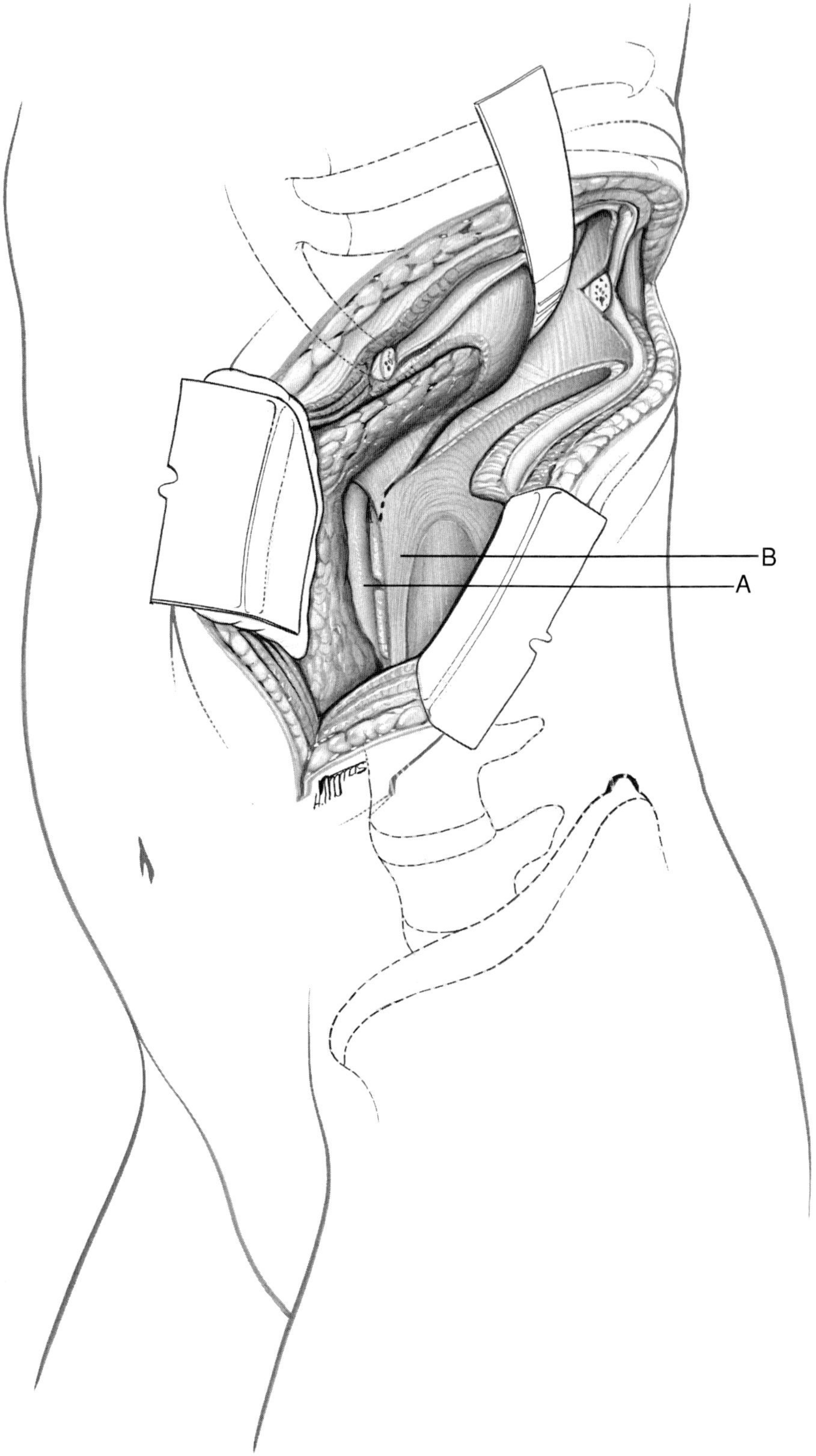

Fig. 8-25. Following complete incision of the diaphragm, the segmental vessel of the thoracolumbar junction **(A)** can be divided, as well as the crux of the diaphragm on that side **(B).**

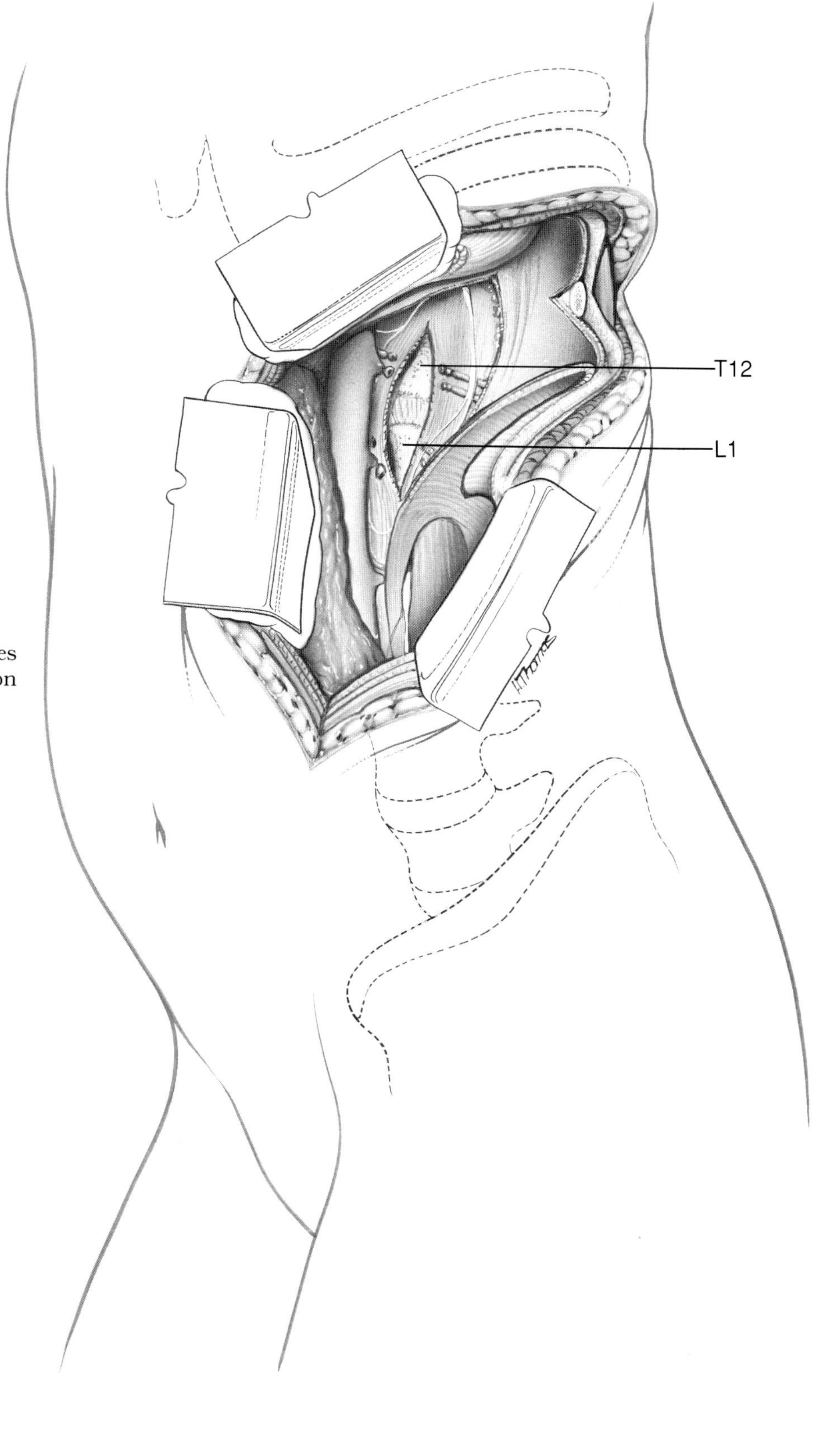

Fig. 8-26. The vertebral bodies at the thoracolumbar junction are exposed.

COMPLICATIONS

Complications may relate to the disease process itself or to the choice of treatment, such as radiotherapy, chemotherapy, and/or surgery; they may also be secondary to unrelated medical or postsurgical complications. Sundaresan et al. have written about postradiation sarcoma.[51] The latent period for this is usually 5 to 20 years. Irradiation of the spine increases blood loss during surgery and certainly impairs the quality of tissue and bone healing.

There are also increased skin problems following radiation and chemotherapy, with a higher incidence of wound diastasis and postoperative infection. Because bone stock is often poor, instrumentation may loosen and dislodge in the spine. MacAfee et al. document complications after the use of methyl methacrylate in stabilization of the vertebral spine secondary to trauma or metastatic disease.[52] Most of the complications, however, were in the cervical spine. Therefore, the listed complications of loss of fixation, neural deficit, and infection may be more of a problem specific to the cervical spine than the thoracic spine in general. It is important to remember that methyl methacrylate works only in compression and is of no value to resist torsion or tension.

Late complications, beside postradiation sarcoma, include additional sites of spinal cord compression and late collapse secondary to extensive tumor involvement.

REFERENCES

1. Pettine KA, Klassaen RA: Osteoid osteomas and osteoblastoma of the spine. J Bone Jt Surg 68A:354, 1986
2. Harrington KD: Current concepts review: metastatic disease of the spine. J Bone Jt Surg 68A: 1110, 1986
3. Harrington KD: Orthopedic Management of Metastatic Bone Disease. CV Mosby, St. Louis, 1988
4. Friedlander GE, Southwick WO: Tumors of the spine. p. 1022. In Rothman RH, Simeone FA (eds): The Spine. WB Saunders, New York, 1982
5. Bale JF, Bell WE, Dunn V et al: Magnetic resonance imaging of the spine in children. Arch Neurol 43: 1253, 1986
6. Beltran J, Noto AM, Chakeres DW et al: Tumors of the osseous spine: staging with MR imaging versus CT. Radiology 162:565, 1987
7. Eismont FJ, Green BA, Brown MD et al: Coexistent infection and tumor of the spine. J Bone Jt Surg 69:452, 1987
8. Sim FH, Dahlin DC, Stauffer RN et al: Primary bone tumors simulating lumbar disc syndrome. Spine 2: 65, 1977
9. Booth RE: Pathogenesis of signs and symptoms of spinal disorders. Instr Course Lect 34:37, 1985
10. Kak VS, Prabhaver S, Khosla VK et al: Solitary osteochrondroma of the spine causing spinal cord compression. Clin Neurol Neurosurg 867:135, 1985
11. Malat J, Virapongse C, Levine A: Solitary osteochrondroma of the spine. Spine 11:625, 1986
12. Slepian A, Hamby WB: Neurologic complications associated with hereditary deforming chondrodysplasia. J Neurosurg 8:529, 1951
13. Enneking WF: Musculoskeletal Tumor Surgery. Churchill Livingstone, New York, 1983
14. Marchand EP, Villemure JG, Rubin J et al: Solitary osteochondroma of the thoracic spine presenting as spinal cord compression. Spine 11:1033, 1986
15. Weinstein JN, McLaine RF: Primary tumors of the spine. Spine 12:843, 1987
16. Dahlin DC: Giant cell tumors of the vertebrae above the sacrum. Cancer 39:1350, 1977
17. Savini R, Gherlinzoni F, Morandi M et al: Surgical treatment of giant cell tumors of the spine. J Bone Jt Surg 65:1283, 1983
18. Dilorenzo N, Nardi P, Ciappetta P et al: Benign tumors and tumorlike conditions of the spine: radiologic features, treatment and results. Surg Neurol 25:449. 1969
19. McLain RF, Weinstein JN: Solitary plasmacytomas of the spine: a review of 84 cases. J Spinal Disorders 2:69, 1989
20. Valderrama JA, Bullough PG: Solitary myeloma of the spine. J Bone Jt Surg 50:82, 1988
21. Torma T: Malignant tumors of the spine and spinal extradural space. Acta Chir Scand 225:1, 1957
22. Russin LA, Robinson MJ, Engle HA et al: Ewing's sarcoma of the lumbar spine: a case report of long term survival. Clin Orthop 164:126, 1982
23. Kornberg M: Primary Ewing's sarcoma of the spine. Spine 11:54, 1986
24. Pilepich MV, Vietti TJ, Nesbit ME et al: Ewing's sarcoma of the vertebral column. Int J Radiat Oncol Biol Phys 7:27, 1981
25. Jeanmart L: Radiology of the Spine: Tumors. Springer-Verlag, New York, 1986
26. Sundaresan N, Rosen G, Huvos AG et al: Combined treatment of osteosarcoma of the spine. Neurosurgery 23:714, 1988
27. Boland PJ, Lane JM, Sundaresan N: Metastatic disease of the spine. Clin Orthop 169:95, 1982
28. Emseelem HA: Metastatic disease of the spine: diagnosis and management. South Med J 79:1405, 1986
29. Siegal T, Tiqva P, Siegal T: Vertebral body resection for epidural compression by malignant tumors. J Bone Jt Surg 67:375, 1985
30. Denis F: The three column spine and its significance in the classification of acute thoracolumbar spinal injuries. Spine 8:917, 1983

31. White AA, Panjabi MM: Clinical Biomechanics of the Spine. JB Lippincott, Philadelphia, 1978
32. Lorx CF, Herndon JH: Spinal cord compression secondary to kyphosis associated with radiation therapy for metastatic disease. Clin Orthop 210: 120, 1986
33. Lee CK, Rosa R, Fernand R: Surgical treatment of tumors of the spine. Spine 11:201, 1986
34. Martin NS, Williamson J: The role of surgery in the treatment of malignant tumors of the spine. J Bone Jt Surg 52:227, 1970
35. Onimus M, Scraub S, Bertin D et al: Surgical treatment of vertebral metastasis. Spine 11:883, 1986
36. DeWald R, Bridwell K, Prodromas C et al: Reconstructive spinal surgery as palliation for metastatic malignancies of the spine. Spine 10:21, 1985
37. Gilbert RN, Kim JM, Posner JB: Epidural spinal cord compression from metastatic tumor: diagnosis and treatment. Ann Neurol 3:40, 1978
38. Sundaresan N, Shah J, Foley KM et al: An anterior surgical approach to the upper thoracic vertebrae. J Neurosurg 61:686, 1984
39. Harrington KD: The use of methyl methacrylate for vertebral body replacement and anterior stabilization of pathological fracture dislocations of the spine due to metastatic malignant disease. J Bone Jt Surg 63:36, 1981
40. Murray JA, Bruels MC, Lindber RD: Irradiation of polymethylmethacrylate: in vitro gamma radiation effect. J Bone Jt Surg 56:311, 1974
41. Stener B: Musculoskeletal tumor surgery. Clin Orthop 191:8, 1984
42. Ma YZ, Tang HF, Chai BF et al: The treatment of primary vertebral tumors by radical resection and prosthetic vertebral replacement. Clin Orthop 215: 78, 1987
43. Fidler MW: Anterior decompression and stabilization of metastatic spinal features. J Bone Jt Surg 66:47, 1984
44. Flately TJ, Anderson MH, Anast GT: Spinal instability due to malignant disease. J Bone Jt Surg 66: 47, 1984
45. Roy-Camille R, Saillant G, Mazel C: Internal fixation of the lumbar spine with pedicle screw plating. Clin Orthop 303:7, 1986
46. Burrington JO, Brown C, Wayne ER et al: Anterior approach to the thoracolumbar spine: technical considerations. Arch Surg 111:456, 1976
47. Dwyer AF, Newton MC, Sherwood AA: An anterior approach to scoliosis. Clin Orthop 62:192, 1969
48. Southwick WO, Robinson A: Surgical approaches to the vertebral bodies in the cervical and lumbar regions. J Bone Jt Surg 39:631, 1957
49. Hodgson AR, Yau AC: Anterior surgical approaches to the spinal column. p. 289. In Apley AG (ed): Recent Advances in Orthopaedics. Williams & Wilkins, Baltimore, 1969
50. Watkins RG: Surgical Approaches to the Spine. Springer-Verlag, New York, 1986
51. Sundaresan N, Huvos AG, Krol G et al: Postradiation sarcoma involving the spine. Neurosurgery 18: 721, 1986
52. McAfee PC, Bohlman HH, Drucker T et al: Failure of stabilization of the spine with methylmethacrylate. J Bone Jt Surg 68:1145, 1986

9

Heart, Diaphragm, and Great Vessels

TUMORS OF THE HEART

Primary tumors of the heart are rare; they are found on autopsy in only 0.0017 percent of all cases.[1] It is found 20 times less frequently than cardiac involvement by metastasis or direct extension on autopsy. Approximately 75 percent of all cardiac tumors are benign, and two-thirds of these tumors are atrial myxomas. Although benign, pathologically these lesions can have a malignant clinical behavior (Table 9-1).

BENIGN CARDIAC TUMORS

MYXOMAS

In 1952 Goldberg et al. reported the first clinical diagnosis of atrial myxoma.[2] The first successful surgical excision involving cardiopulmonary bypass was performed by Craaford in 1954.[3]

The most common constitutional symptoms and laboratory findings associated with these lesions are prolonged fever, weight loss, myalgia or arthritis, elevated erythrocyte sedimentation rate (ESR), anemia, and leukocytosis. They can obstruct either the pulmonary or systemic venous drainage or both and interfere with valve function. Obstruction to valve flow is often related to posture and may lead to shortness of breath, syncope, or sudden death.

The myxomas frequently cause recurrent strokes, peripheral embolization, and, when right-sided, pulmonary embolization. The emboli may be tumorous or due to mural thrombi. Myomas may manifest a malignant behavior by infiltrating and destroying the arterial wall, giving rise to myxomatous pseudoaneurysm.[4] The diagnosis is readily made by two-dimensional echocardiography and can be confirmed by cardiac angiography.

The majority of the myxomas occur in the left atrium (80 percent); 15 percent occur in the right atrium, and the remaining 5 percent are bilateral or ventricular in origin.[5,6]

The operative mortality in several series varies from 0 to 3 percent.[5–7] Intracardiac recurrence of myxoma has been reported at a rate of 5 to 14 percent. Recurrences have been documented at the site of the original tumor, at other single or multiple intracardiac sites, and at extracardiac sites.[8] Tumors not arising from the atrial septum are thought most likely to recur. These recurrences are most often sessile and multiple and exhibit faster growth and more infiltration than the original tumor.[9] The proposed mechanisms of recurrence are inadequate resection, tumor implantation from the original tumors, unrecognized multicentric origin, and the growth of pretumor reserve cells.

RHABDOMYOMAS

Benign rhabdomyomas are the most common cardiac tumors in both infants and children. These are considered to be hamartomas, and there is a strong association between cardiac rhabdomyoma and tuberous sclerosis. Early operation under 1 year of age, as reported by Reece et al.,[10] leads to successful long-term survival.[11] Frequently these

Table 9-1. Malignant Tumors of the Heart

Angiosarcoma
Rhabdomyosarcoma
Fibrosarcoma
Malignant lymphoma
Extraskeletal osteosarcoma
Neurogenic sarcoma
Malignant teratoma
Leiomyosarcoma
Liposarcoma
Synovial sarcoma

lesions present with ventricular tachycardia, which is corrected after surgical excision. Additional benign lesions have been reported in both children and adults. Benign fibromas are common in the former group, and lipomas and hemangiomas are frequent in the latter.

MALIGNANT CARDIAC TUMORS

ANGIOSARCOMAS

Angiosarcoma was first described by Menny in 1888[12] and is the most frequent primary malignant tumor, accounting for 15 percent of the cardiac sarcomas. McCallister[13] studied 39 patients, who were adults ranging in age from 15 to 76 years with 70 percent between the ages of 20 and 50. There was a male predominance, and 77 percent of the patients presented with clinical findings of right heart failure, with the right atrium being the most common site.

Microscopically these tumors are composed of malignant cells forming vascular channels, and there is considerable histologic variation within the same tumor. Most contain foci of solid areas and spindle cells.

The combined role of surgery and chemotherapy has been associated with prolonged survival in some patients,[14] although 88 percent of all patients reported in the literature have died within 9 months.[15] Hollingsworth and Strugill[16] suggest a possible benefit of radiotherapy in inadequately excised tumors.

RHABDOMYOSARCOMAS

Rhabdomyosarcomas are the second most common primary sarcomas of the heart. These neoplasms are composed of malignant cells with features of striated muscles and have been found in patients from 3 months to 80 years of age, but is primarily a tumor of adults. There is slight male predominance.

In the AFIP series[13] the majority of patients demonstrated cardiomegaly on chest x-ray and nonspecific electrocardiogram (ECG) changes including S-T segment and T wave abnormalities, low voltage, and various degrees of bundle branch block. These tumors occurred with equal frequency in the right and left sides of the heart, and the majority of the patient died within 1 year. Various combinations of local excision, radiation, and chemotherapy have extended survival up to 3 years.

MALIGNANT FIBROUS HISTIOCYTOMAS

Malignant fibrous histiocytomas generally arise in the left atrium of the heart and often involve the mitral valve.[17] They have been described as fibrosarcomas, myxosarcomas, and, most commonly now, malignant fibrous histiocytomas. Microscopically they consist of spindle-shaped cells with elongated and blunt-ended nuclei. Although mitoses are common, pleomorphism and anaplasia are minimal.

In most reported cases, excision is not possible and the majority of patients die postoperatively. Radiation and chemotherapy have been tried with minimal success.[18,19]

In addition to these more common lesions, the following primary malignant tumors of the heart have been reported: lymphoma, nerve sheath tumor, teratoma, leiomyosarcoma, liposarcoma, synovial sarcoma, and extraosseous osteogenic sarcoma.

SURGICAL TREATMENT

Poole et al.[20] reviewed the surgical results in 28 patients cases who underwent surgery for primary sarcomas of the heart, predominantly angiosarcomas, rhabdomyosarcomas, and malignant fibrous histiocytomas. Of the 28 patients, 26 required cardiopulmonary bypass. There was one postoperative death, and survival ranged from 2 to 55 months (mean, 14 months). Death was caused by peripheral metastasis in 11 patients and by local recurrence with blood flow obstruction in 6 patients. Two patients died of other causes. Patients who received postoperative irradiation survived more than twice as long (22 versus 9 months). The average radiation dose administered was 5,000 rads over 30 days. Eight patients received adjunctive chemotherapy, with no benefit observed.

More recently Cooley et al.[21] used autotransplantation of the heart for a paranganglioma of the left atrium, and Jamieson et al.[22] used cardiac transplantation of the heart for an unresectable left ventricular lesion. The latter technique probably offers an optional therapy for the sarcomatous lesions confined to the heart on presentation.

PRIMARY TUMORS OF THE PERICARDIUM

Mesotheliomas are the most common malignant tumors of the pericardium and are dervived from the mesothelial cells of either the visceral or the parietal pericardium. The most common clinical finding is dyspnea secondary to the associated pericardial effusion, and chest x-rays reveal significant cardiomegaly.

Approximately 120 cases of primary pericardial mesothelioma have been reported. In the AFIP series there were 19 cases of mesothelioma in patients ranging in age from 17 to 83 years. The male-to-female ratio is 2 : 1, and there is no evidence linking pericardial mesothelioma to asbestosis.

Most pericardial mesotheliomas diffusely cover the pericardium and encase the heart. They invade the heart only superficially and can be readily differentiated from primary cardiac sarcomas, which are invariably intracavitary. These lesions spread to the adjacent pleura and mediastinum and may also invade the mediastinal lymph nodes. Distant metastases are uncommon.[23]

Benign lesions that can mimic the symptoms of pericardial mesothelioma are pericardial cysts, bronchogenic cysts, and mesothelial hyperplasia as a complication of radiotherapy in patients with carcinoma.

There is no specific treatment for pericardial mesothelioma. Surgical excision is usually not possible, and chemotherapy and radiotherapy have been reported to produce temporary improvement,[24] but there is no well-established correlation between this treatment and the course of the disease. Prognosis is generally poor, and as many as 60 percent of patients diagnosed with the disease die within 6 months, although occasional long-term survivals of 5 years have been reported.[25]

PRIMARY TUMORS OF THE DIAPHRAGM

The first report of a primary tumor of the diaphragm was by Groncher in 1868.[26] This tumor was discovered at autopsy and was diagnosed as a fibroma. Wiener and Chau[27] reviewed the world literature from 1868 to 1963 and reported on 71 cases. Of these 71 cases, 43 were benign, the most common tumors being bronchial, mesothelial, or teratoid cysts, and 28 were malignant, the most common tumors being fibrosarcomas (Table 9-2). An additional 14 cases were reported by Olafsson et al.[28] in 1971 (Table 9-3). Seven additional cases have been reported through 1989.[29–31]

In these two collective reviews, cases not believed to be primary, as well as cases in which no pathologicoanatomic diagnosis had been established, were eliminated. Most of the patients were in the fourth decade, but all ages were represented. The youngest patient was a 26-day-old infant with hemangioendothelioma, and the oldest was an 80-year-old woman with mesothelioma.

Table 9-2. Primary Tumors of the Diaphragm (1868–1963)

Tumor	No. of Cases	Tumor	No. of Cases
Angiofibroma	3	Fibroangioendothelioma	1
Chondroma	1	Fibromyosarcoma	2
Cyst	12	Fibrosarcoma	8
Fibroma	3	Hemangioendothelioma	1
Fibrolymphangioma	1	Hemangiopericytoma	1
Fibromyoma	1	Leimyosarcoma	1
Hamartoma	1	Myosarcoma	2
Lymphangioma	1	Neurofibrosarcoma	2
Leiomyoma	2	Rhadbomyosarcoma	2
Lipoma	9	Sarcoma	2
Mesothelioma	2	Sarcoma—vascular	2
Neurolemmoma	2	Sarcoma—mixed	2
Neurofibroma	4	Sarcoma—undifferentiated	1
Rhabdomyofibroma	1	Synovial cell sarcoma	1

(Data from Wiener and Chau.[27])

Table 9-3. Primary Tumors of the Diaphragm (1963–1969)

Tumor	No. of Cases
Benign	
Angiofibroma	1
Cyst	6
Fibroma	1
Hamartoma	1
Malignant	
Fibrosarcoma	1
Hemangioendothelioma	1
Sarcoma	2
Mesenchymoma	1

(Data from Olafsson et al.[28])

The male-to-female ratio was 1 : 1, as was right- or left-sided location. The ratio of benign to malignant lesions was 2 : 1.

The diagnosis is difficult to establish because of the rarity of these lesions as well as the nonspecific nature of the majority of the presenting symptoms. The most common symptoms are pains in the epigastrium or in the lower part of the chest, cough, dyspnea, and gastrointestinal discomfort. Twenty percent of patients are asymptomatic. The tumor is detected in asymptomatic patients routinely on chest x-rays.

PRIMARY TUMORS OF THE GREAT VESSELS

Primary tumors of the aorta are rare. Since they were first described by Brodowski in 1873,[32] fewer than 25 such tumors have been reported. They were of various histologic types and characteristically presented with diverse clinical manifestations that precluded accurate preoperative or antemortem diagnosis. The underlying common denominators were major vascular obstruction and tumor embolization.

Table 9-4. Histologic Types of Primary Aortic Tumors

Tumor	No. of Cases
Benign	
Myxoma	1
Fibromyxoma	3
Malignant	
Fibrosarcoma	2
Fibromyxosarcoma	3
Medullary sarcoma	1
Spindle cell sarcoma	1
Giant cell sarcoma	2
Endothelioma	2
Leiomyosarcoma	2
Undifferentiated sarcoma	2
Angiosarcoma	1
Malignant fibroushystiocytoma	2

Table 9-5. Location of Primary Aortic Tumors

Anatomic Site	No. of Cases
Ascending aorta and arch	1
Thoracic aorta	7
Thoracoabdominal aorta	5
Abdominal aorta	9

In the 22 cases reported in the literature (Tables 9-4 and 9-5), 16 occurred in males and 6 in females. The ages ranged from 3.5 months to 70 years. Nonspecific symptoms such as headache, weakness, anorexia, and poorly localized chest and or abdominal pain were reported.[33–40]

Aortic tumors metastasize frequently and widely, with the primary route via arterial tumor embolization. Metastatic lesions to skin, bone, pleura, liver, spleen, pancreas, kidneys, adrenal gland, and intestinal mucosa have been reported. In most cases the primary aortic tumor did not invade locally but remained confined to the aortic walls and lumen.

The best radiographic techniques available include aortography and computed tomography (CT). On aortography, irregular filling defects project in the lumen of the aorta and reflect the gross morphology of the tumor. The remaining aorta is relatively smooth and of normal caliber, and it demonstrates a normal arterial wall. The CT scan confirms the intra-aortic origin and excludes extra-aortic abnormalities. These tests do not differentiate intraluminal tumor from thrombus.

The prognosis for patients with primary malignant aortic neoplasms is poor. The majority of patients are dead within 3 to 6 months as a result of cachexia, tumor embolism, and widespread metastasis.

There have been six attempts at surgical treatment of aortic neoplasms.[41] Two long-term survivals were reported in patients with benign lesions.[1] In patients with malignant neoplasms, primary excisions, endarterectomies, and exclusion techniques have been used, but survival has not exceeded 1 month.[42]

REFERENCES

1. Straus R, Merlis R: Primary tumors of the heart. Arch Pathol Lab Med 39:74, 1945

2. Goldberg HP, Glenn F, Dotter CT et al: Myxoma of the left atrium: diagnosis made during life with operative and post-mortem findings. Circulation 6:762, 1952
3. Craaford C: Discussion on late results of mitral commissurotomy. p. 202. In Lam CR (ed): International Symposium on Cardiovascular Surgery. WB Saunders, Philadelphia, 1955
4. Semh BKH: Surgical considerations in the treatment of cardiac myxoma. J Thorac Cardiovasc Surg 87:251, 1984
5. Hanson EC, Gill CC, Razavi M et al: The surgical treatment of myxomas: clinical experience and late results in 33 patients. J Thorac Cardiovasc Surg 89:298, 1985
6. Larssons B, Le Pore V, Kennergreen C: Atrial myxomas: results of 25 years experience and review of the literature. Surgery 105:695, 1989
7. Richardson JV, Brandt B, Doty JB et al: Surgical treatment of atrial myxomas: early and late results of 11 operations and review of the literature. Ann Thorac Surg 28:354, 1979
8. Markel LM, Waller B, Armstrong W: Cardiac myxoma: a review. Medicine 66:114, 1987
9. Read RC, White HJ, Murphy ML et al: Malignant potentiality of left atrial myxoma. J Thorac Cardiovasc Surg 68:857, 1974
10. Reece IJ, Codely PA, Fracier OH et al: Cardiac tumors: clinical spectrum and prognosis of lesions other than classical benign myxoma in 20 patients. J Thorac Cardiovasc Surg 88:430, 1984
11. Engle MA, Ebert PA, Redo SF: Recurrent ventricular tachycardia due to resectable cardiac tumor: report of two cases. Circulation 50:1052, 1977
12. Hudson REB: Cardiovascular Pathology. Williams & Wilkins, Baltimore, 1970
13. McAllister HA, Fenoglio JJ: Tumors of the cardiovascular system. In Atlas of Tumor Pathology, 2nd series, Fascicle 15. Armed Forces Institute of Pathology, Washington, D.C., 1978
14. Coqveran J: Primary heart sarcomas: two operated cases. Ann Chir Thorac Cardiovasc 11:57, 1972
15. Glancy DL, Morales JB, Roberts WC: Angiosarcoma of the heart. Am J Cardiol 21:413, 1968
16. Hollingsworth JH, Strugill BC: Treatment of primary angiosarcoma of the heart. Am Heart J 78:254, 1971
17. Caley F, Bijapur HI: Fibrosarcoma of the left atrium. Br Med J 1:1134, 1963
18. Baldell P, DeAngeli D, Polara A et al: Primary fibrosarcoma of the heart. Chest 62:234, 1968
19. Eckstein R, Gossner W, Reinmuller R: Primary malignant fibrous histiocytoma of the left atrium. Surgical and chemotherapeutic management. Br Heart J 52:354, 1984
20. Poole GV, Meredith JW, Beyer RH: Surgical implications in malignant cardiac disease. Ann Thorac Surg 36:484, 1983
21. Cooley DA, Reardon MJ, Frazier OH: Human cardiac explantation and autotransplantation: application in a patient with a large cardiac pheochromocytoma. Tex Heart Inst J 12:171, 1986
22. Jamieson SW, Gaudiani VA, Reits BA: Operative treatment of an unresectable tumor of the left ventricle. J Thorac Cardiovasc Surg 81:797, 1981
23. Chun PKC, Leeburg WT, Coggin ST: Primary pericardial malignant epitheloid mesothelioma causing acute myocardial infarction. Chest 77:559, 1980
24. Sytman AL, MacAlpin RN: Primary pericardial mesothelioma: report of two cases and a review of the literature. Am Heart J 81:760, 1971
25. McAllister HA: Primary tumors and cysts of the heart and pericardium. Curr Probl Cardiol 4:1, 1979
26. Groncher M: Tumor vegelant du centre phrenique du diaphragme. Bull Soc Anat Paris 43:385, 1868
27. Weiner MF, Chou WH: Primary tumors of the diaphragm. Arch Surg 90:143, 1965
28. Olafsson G, Raussing AS, Holen O: Primary tumors of the diaphragm. Chest 59:568, 1971
29. Porker MC: Leiomyosarcoma of the diaphragm: a case report. Eur J Surg Oncol 11:171, 1985
30. McClenathan JH, Opkada F: Primary neurilemmoma of the diaphragm. Ann Thorac Surg 48:126, 1989
31. Sarot IA, Schwimmer D, Schecter DC: Primary neurilemmoma of the diaphragm. NY State J Med 69:837, 1969
32. Brodowski W: Primäres sarkom der aorta thoracica mit verbreitung des neugebildes in der unteren körperhälfte. Uber Leist Fortschr Ges Med 8:243, 1873
33. Kattus AA, Longmire WB, Camon JA et al: Primary intraluminar tumor of the aorta producing malignant hypertension. N Engl J Med 262:694, 1960
34. Smeloff EA, Reece JM, Master JH: Primary intraluminal malignant tumor of the aorta. Am J Cardiol 15:107, 1965
35. Stevenson J, Burkhend H, Trueheart RE et al: Primary malignant tumor of the aorta. Am J Med 51:553, 1971
36. Salm R: Primary fibrosarcoma of the aorta. Cancer 29:73, 1972
37. Silverman JF, Wexler L: Primary intraluminal tumor of the aorta. Radiology 102:581, 1972
38. Bowles LT, Ring EM, Hill WT et al: Hemangiopericytoma in a resected thoracic aortic aneurysm. Ann Thorac Surg 1:746, 1965
39. Blenkinsopp WK, Hobbs JT: Pedunculated hemangiopericytoma attached to the thoracic aorta. Thorax 21:193, 1962
40. Mason MS, Wheeler JR, Gregory RT et al: Primary tumors of the aorta: report of a case and review of the literature. Oncology 39:167, 1982
41. Guttentag A, Lazar H, Franklin P et al: Malignant fibous histiocytoma obstructing the thoracic aorta. Ann Thorac Surg 47:775, 1989
42. Chen KTK: Primary malignant fibrous hystiocytoma of the aorta. Cancer 47:540, 1981

10

Illustrative Cases

The following 29 cases are not all to be interpreted as representative. Rather, they are examples of what can be achieved through thoracic surgery. More than 50 percent of these patients either had no sign of disease when lost to follow-up or died of other ailments. In all instances, life was prolonged by surgical intervention; in one case (B.W.) the patient lived for 23 years after diagnosis. Such cases serve to encourage the continued efforts to advance the science and treatment of thoracic oncology, with the hope that in the future these exceptional cases shall be the norm.

LUNG

Patient: J.P.K. (Fig. 10-1)

Sex: Female

Age: 59

Diagnosis: Adenocarcinoma of the lung

Stage: T2, N0, M0, stage I

Complaint: Left lower lobe lesion on routine chest x-ray

History and Examination: The examination was entirely negative. The CT scan of the chest failed to show any lymph node involvement. A percutaneous needle biopsy was performed, and adenocarcinoma was found.

Treatment: On 11/26/85 a left lower lobe lobectomy was carried out. The tumor measured 3.3 cm with puckered visceral pleura. It was staged as T2. All lymph nodes were negative. The patient had an uneventful convalescence.

Follow-up: The patient has no evidence of disease (NED) at 5.5 years postsurgery.

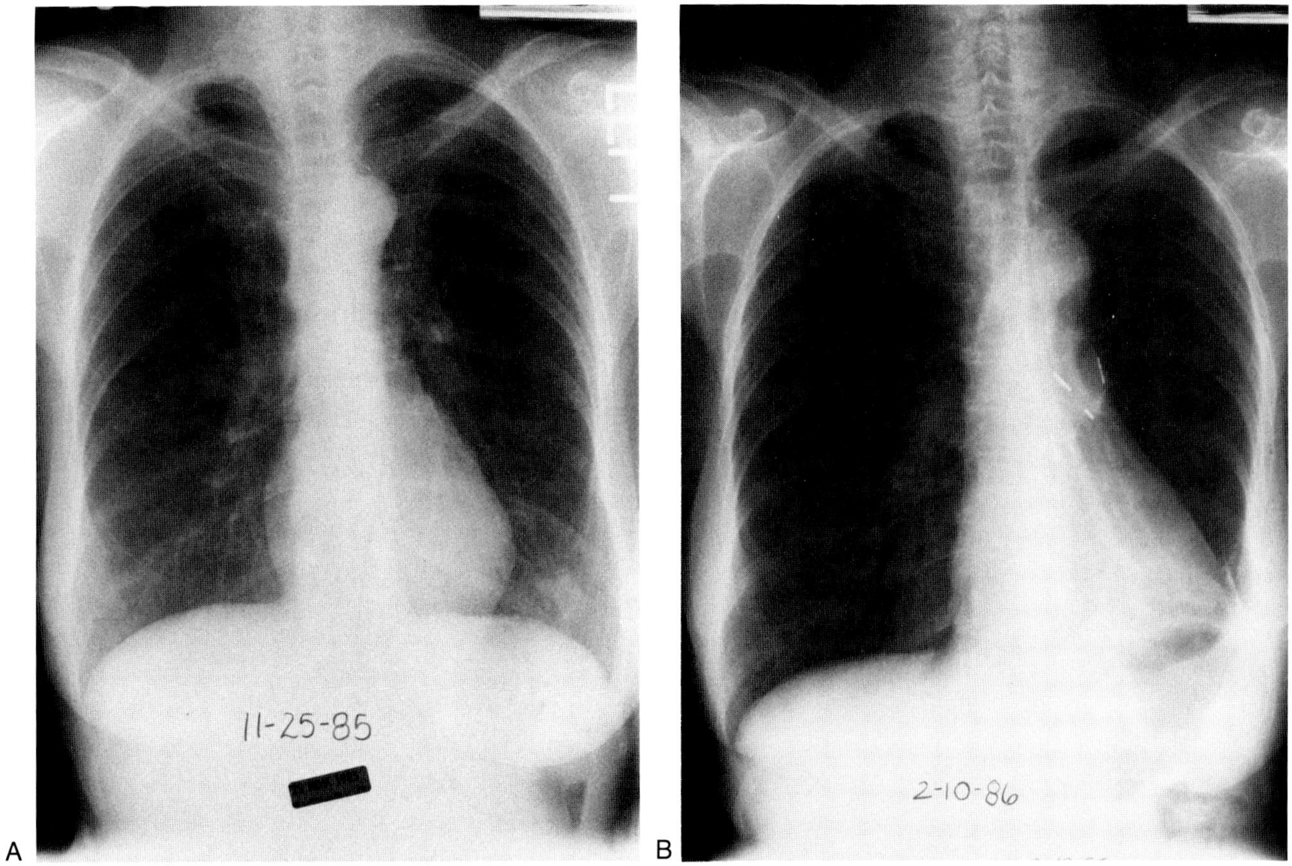

Fig. 10-1. **(A)** PA chest x-ray taken on 11/25/85. A mass can be seen in the left lower lung field. **(B)** PA chest x-ray taken on 2/10/86 after a left lower lobe lobectomy with mediastinal lymph node excision.

Patient: M.D. (Fig. 10-2)

Sex: Female

Age: 69

Diagnosis: Adenocarcinoma of left lower lobe

Stage: T2, N1, M0, and T2, N0, M0 double primary or? T2, N1, M1 (metastasis to upper lobe)

Complaint: Lesion behind the heart on routine chest x-ray

History and Examination: The patient was a nonsmoker with no chest complaints. She had had a dilatation and curettage (D and C) 3 months earlier. A bronchoscopy was negative. Percutaneous needle biopsy was nondiagnostic. Exploratory thoracotomy was advised.

Treatment: Left thoracotomy was performed on 1/7/86. A mass (2.5 × 2.0 × 2.0 cm) was found in the left posterior basal segment involving the basal pleura. A left lower lobectomy was performed. Lymph node 12 in the left lower lobe contained metastatic carcinoma. A separate 2-mm nodule was excised from the lingula. This contained adenocarcinoma involving visceral pleura.

Follow-up: The patient is NED after 5.5 years. ? changes in pleura by chest x-ray.

Fig. 10-2. **(A)** PA chest x-ray taken on 1/6/86. Barely visible behind the heart is a mass in the left lung. **(B)** Lateral chest x-ray taken on 1/6/86. A mass is visible over the inferior portion of the aorta. **(C)** PA chest x-ray taken on 2/13/91. There are changes consistent with the left lower lobe lobectomy and the wedge excision of the lingula with mediastinal lymph node dissection. There are some pleural changes at left base.

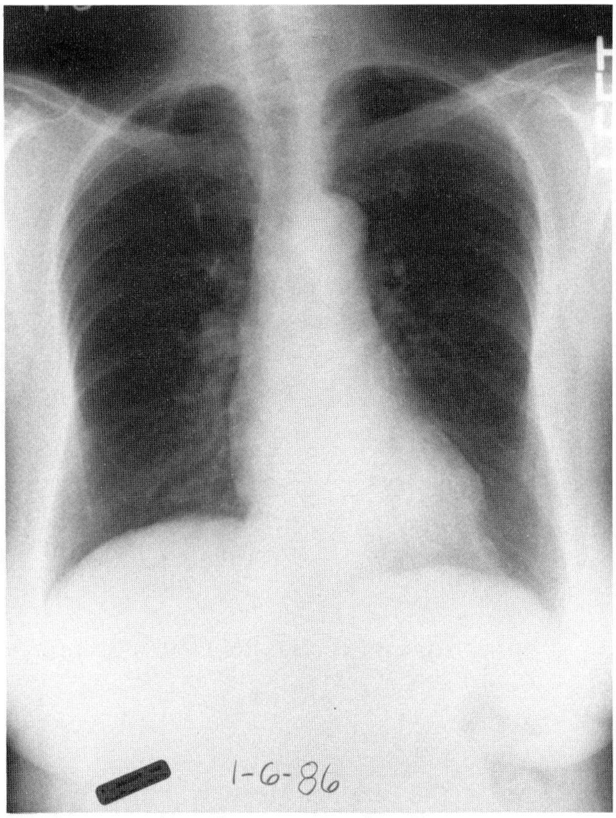

A

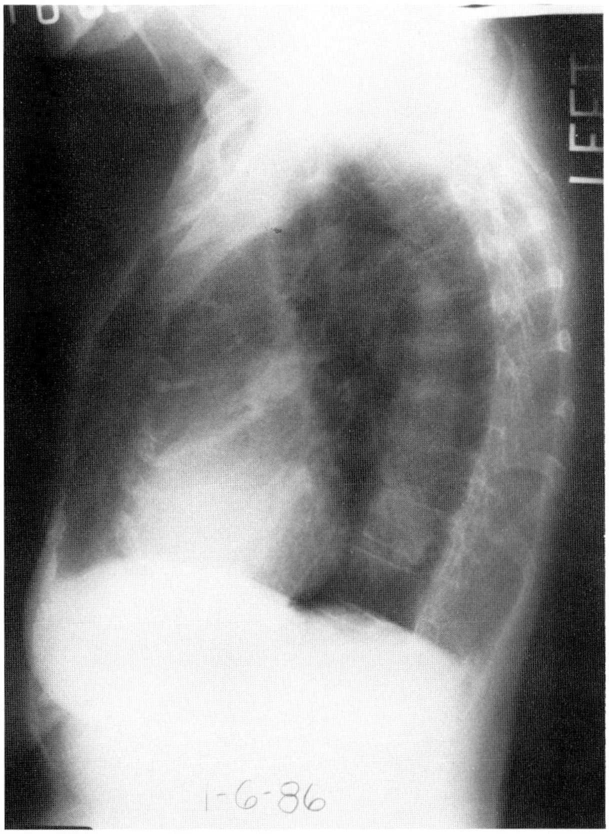

B

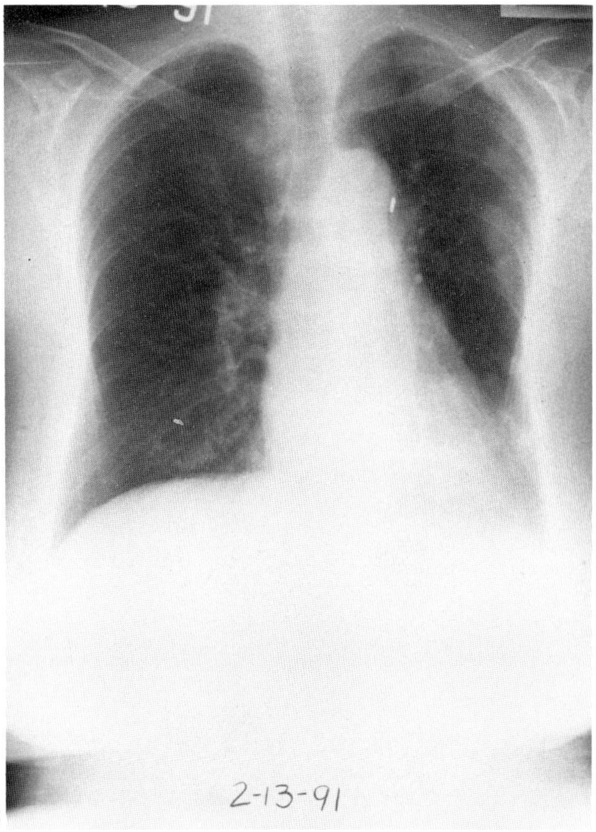

C

Patient: M.S. (Fig. 10-3)

Sex: Female

Age: 30

Diagnosis: Adenocarcinoma, right upper lobe, with mediastinal lymph node metastases

Stage: T1, N2, M0 (IIIA)

Complaint: Abnormal chest x-ray

History and Examination: This 30-year-old woman had a chest x-ray taken elsewhere, which showed a mass in the right upper lobe associated with hilar and mediastinal increased density. She had a direct mediastinotomy performed elsewhere, and adenocarcinoma was biopsied from the mediastinum. This was declared nonresectable and not treatable for cure. Radiotherapy was begun, and she received 4,500 rads, which was discontinued at our request. Approximately 1 month later (2/15/77) we carried out a right thoracotomy. A right upper lobe lobectomy was performed. Iodine 125 (I-125) seeds were implanted in the mediastinum tumor, and afterloading catheters were placed across the superior mediastinum for additional mediastinal radiotherapy. The catheters were brought out parasternally. This was our second patient in whom afterloading catheters were placed in the mediastinum. Since a right upper lobe lobectomy had just been carried out, we placed a patch of silastic to protect and keep the direct radiation effect from the hilum.

Follow-up: She got along well postoperatively and was maintained on low-dose chemotherapy. She became quite ill elsewhere, and almost 1 year later, after a stormy session that required a right pneumonectomy, she continued to do well. This infection may have been related to the silastic prosthesis that we placed. She continues to do relatively well 14 years later.

Fig. 10-3. **(A)** PA chest x-ray taken on 2/13/77. This chest x-ray was taken after 4,500 rads of radiotherapy to the right upper lobe and mediastinum. A lesion is barely visible in the right upper lobe where the anterior first rib, clavicle, and third rib cross. There is also some mild fullness of the right hilum. **(B)** PA chest x-ray taken on 3/3/77 following a right upper lobe lobectomy. The mediastinum has been implanted with I-125 seeds, and after afterloading catheters had been placed along the superior mediastinum. **(C)** PA chest x-ray taken on 9/15/80. A right pneumonectomy has been done. With careful scrutiny one can see small I-125 seeds in the mid-mediastinal region. The clips along the mediastinum and in the upper portion of the chest mark the areas where afterloading catheters had been placed to deliver temporary internal radiotherapy.

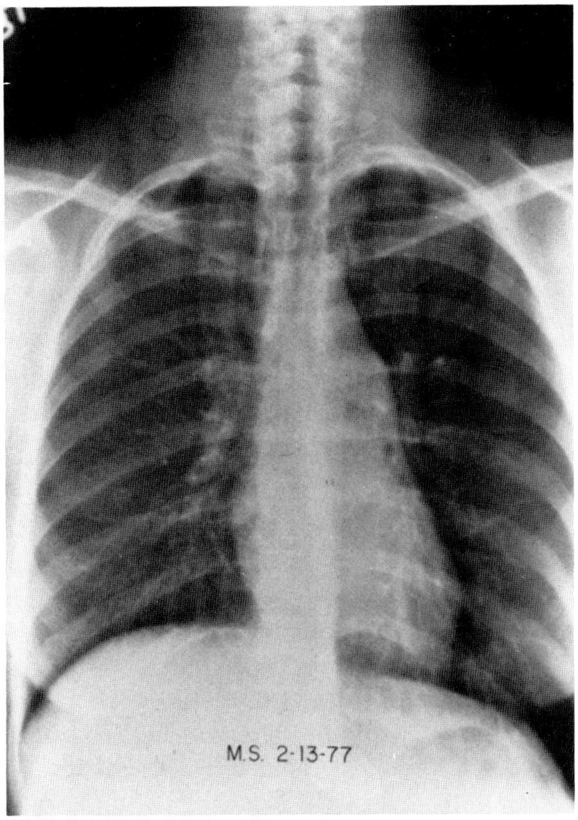

A

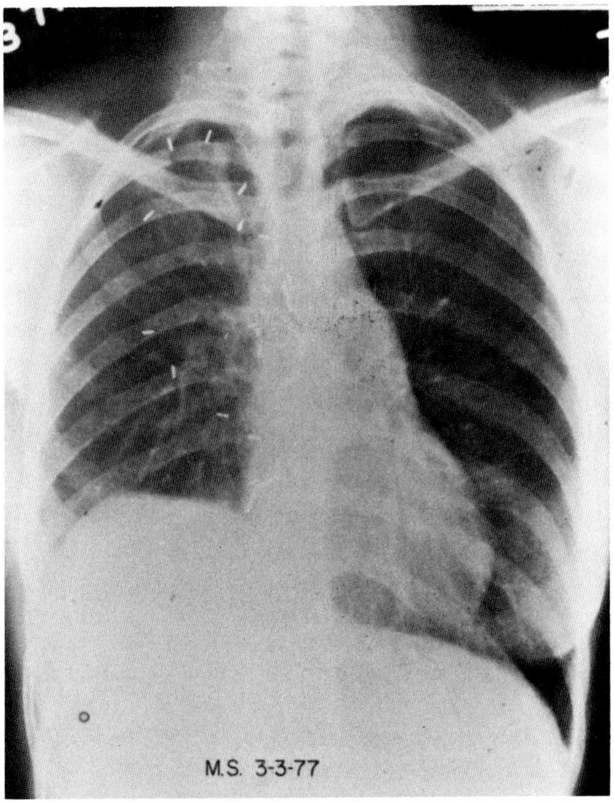

B

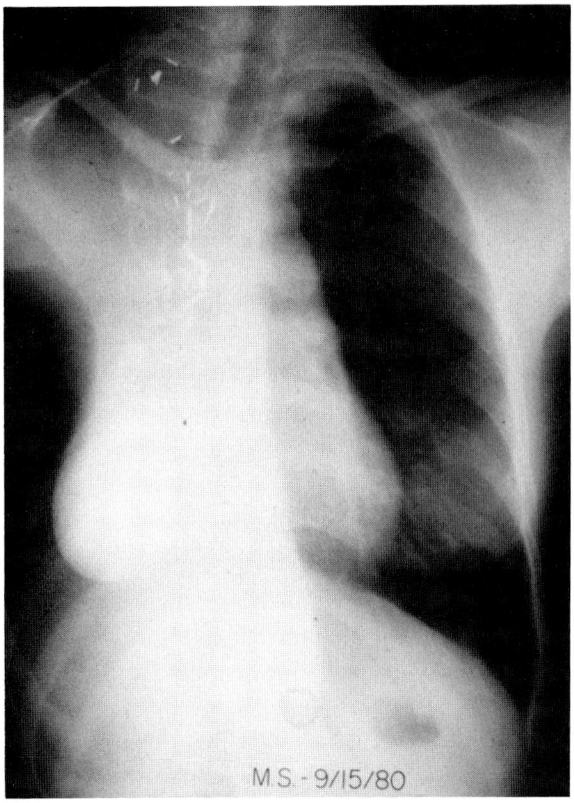

C

Patient: G.M. (Fig. 10-4)

Sex: male

Age: 49

Diagnosis: Poorly differentiated adenocarcinoma of the left lung

Stage: T3, N2, M0, stage IIIA

Complaint: Pain in left chest, fever, hemoptysis

History and Examination: This patient has smoked three packs of cigarettes per day for 30 years. A chest x-ray showed two areas of increased density in the left upper lobe with enlarged mediastinal lymph nodes. The bone scan, brain scan, and liver scan were negative. The tumor was declared nonresectable and not treatable for cure.

Treatment: A left thoracotomy was performed on 5/13/80. There were two lesions in the left upper lobe, each approximately 1.5 × 3.0 × 5.0 cm. There were enlarged, not completely removable lymph nodes in the mediastinum. Thirty-four I-125 seeds were implanted into the two lung tumors. The activity was 0.501 mCi, with a total activity of 17.03 mCi. In the left superior mediastinum a 1.5-cm lymph node was implanted with 12 I-125 seeds, with a total activity of 6.01 mCi. In addition, seven afterloading catheters, approximately 1.0 cm apart, were placed across the left superior mediastinum and brought out anteriorly. The area covered was 4.0 × 9.0 cm^2. Subsequently these catheters were used to deliver 3,000 rads of Iridium-192 (Ir-192). Postoperatively from 6/24/80 to 7/23/80 the patient received an additional 3,776 rads to the tumor areas in 19 treatment sessions.

Follow-up: Immediately postoperatively the patient had to be rebronchoscoped and intubated. He was kept on a respirator for several days but ultimately was discharged home in good condition. He is now alive and well with no evidence of disease more than 11 years postimplant. The tumor was biopsied at operation, and this final tissue diagnosis was confirmed. The official pathology diagnosis was anaplastic small cell adenocarcinoma.

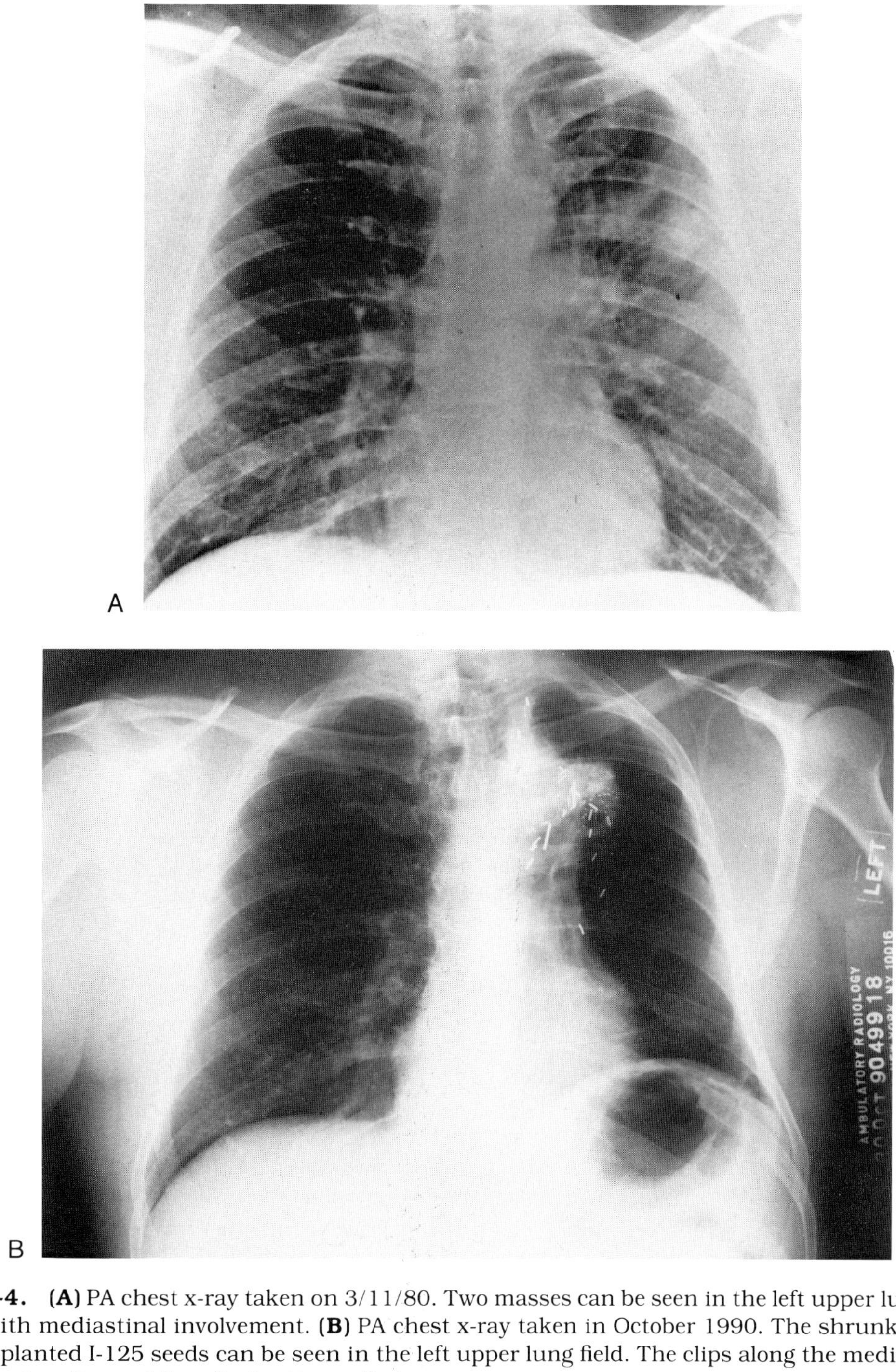

Fig. 10-4. **(A)** PA chest x-ray taken on 3/11/80. Two masses can be seen in the left upper lung field, along with mediastinal involvement. **(B)** PA chest x-ray taken in October 1990. The shrunken mass with implanted I-125 seeds can be seen in the left upper lung field. The clips along the mediastinum mark the locations of the afterloading catheters.

Patient: F.D. (Fig. 10-5)

Sex: Female

Age: 38

Diagnosis: Adenocarcinoma

Stage: T3, N2, M0, stage IIIA

Complaint: Abnormal chest x-ray

History and Examination: This patient was 38 years of age in June 1977 when she was found to have an adenocarcinoma in the right lung with metastases in the mediastinum. She received 5,000 rads of radiotherapy. This tumor was believed not to be resectable, and she received radiotherapy elsewhere. She came to see us in July 1977. We carried out a right thoracotomy on 7/21/77. We excised the superior segment of the right lower lobe and implanted the right middle lobe with I-125 seeds. Temporary afterloading catheters were placed across the mediastinum for the use of Ir-192. Postoperatively she ultimately received methyl-CCNU and Leukeran for 2 years and immunotherapy consisting of *Corynebacterium parvum* for 1 year. During this time she developed pain in her right shoulder, which responded to a nerve block by our pain service. She continued to do well until the summer of 1983, when a small new lesion was found in her left lung. A left thoractomy was done, and a tumor wedge was excised that was believed to be a new lung cancer.

In January 1984 she developed right flank pain. The carcinoembryonic antigen (CEA) level, which had been elevated prior to the removal of the tumor in the left lung, persisted at a range of 16 to 17. The CEA rose to 40. The right adrenal gland was suspicious for metastasis, and in April 1984 a percutaneous needle biopsy was done and carcinoma found. She was restarted on chemotherapy consisting of mitomycin C plus Velban, and at one point the CEA level returned to normal. It subsequently rose to a range of 16 to 17, where it remained. A bone scan was negative. The CT scan of the abdomen performed on 10/15/85 showed only enlargement of the right adrenal gland. Her physical examination at that time was remarkable only for a blood pressure (BP) of 188/98. Her chest x-ray was believed to be stable. She was surgically explored through the right flank on 12/5/85. The right adrenal gland contained a tumor that had invaded the liver and the superior pole of the right kidney, and also involved lymph nodes behind the inferior vena cava. At this point we favored discontinuing the operation and obtaining appropriate angiograms. They had not been obtained preoperatively because of her history of sensitivity to the contrast material. The angiogram showed no significant abnormalities to contraindicate the surgery. On 12/16/85 she was reexplored. The lesion could not be removed without first removing the right kidney. The kidney was mobilized and removed, leaving the tumor attached to the liver and to lymph nodes behind the vena cava. A wedge excision of the inferior portion of the right lobe of the liver was carried out, leaving the metastatic tumor attached to the adrenal gland. As the tumor was mobilized, we found involved lymph node along the spine. The tumor did not seem to extend to the left of the vena cava. It was possible to remove this chain of lymph nodes without disrupting the vena cava itself. Our radiation oncology consultant placed 50 I-125 seeds along the anterior spine from the body of T12 to the body of L3.

In the immediate postoperative period the patient did well. However, 4 days later while sitting up in the surgical intensive care unit and apparently in good health, she had a sudden feeling of apprehension accompanied by a fall in blood pressure. She was returned to bed and was promptly found to be pulseless. Resuscitative efforts failed.

At postmortem examination no tumor was found in the lungs, and limited examination revealed only microthromboemboli in the lungs. We concluded that she had died of cardiac arrhythmia probably secondary to microemboli to the lungs.

She had survived 8 years following the diagnosis of her stage IIIA lung cancer but had succumbed to the effects of metastasis to the right adrenal gland.

A

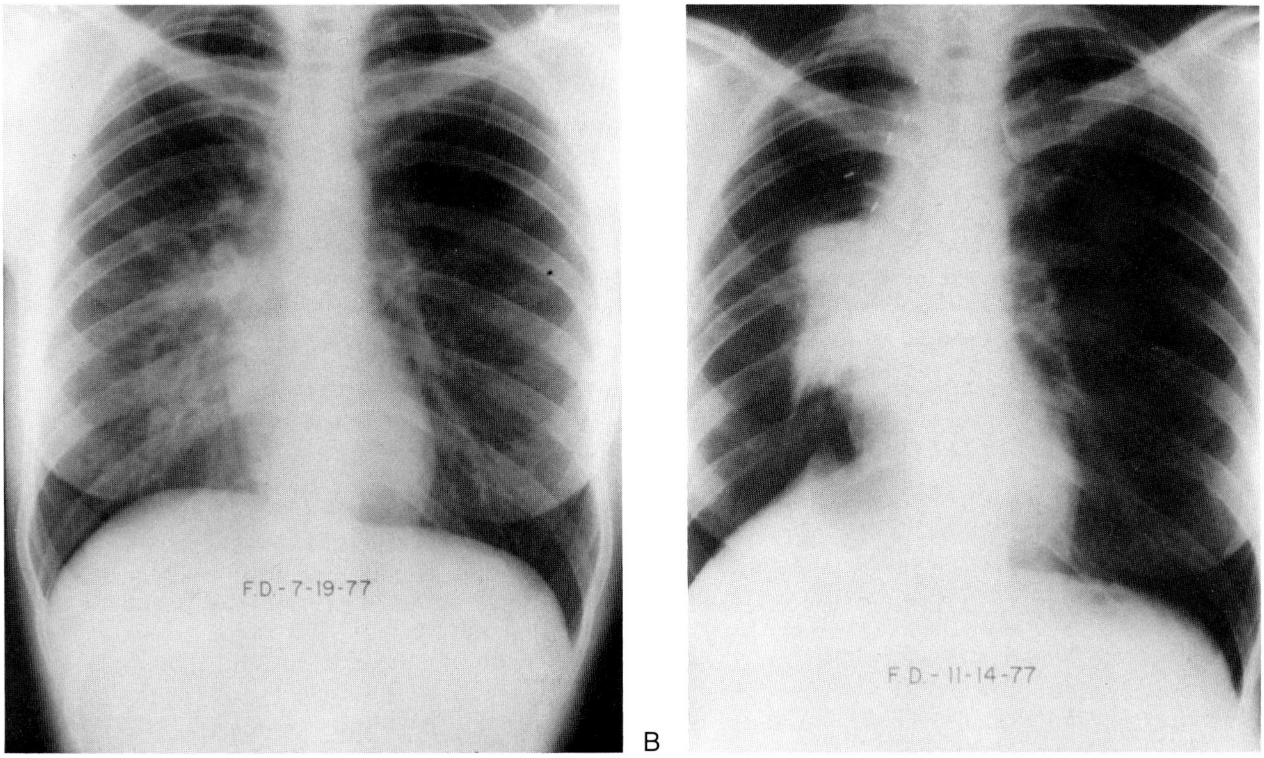

B

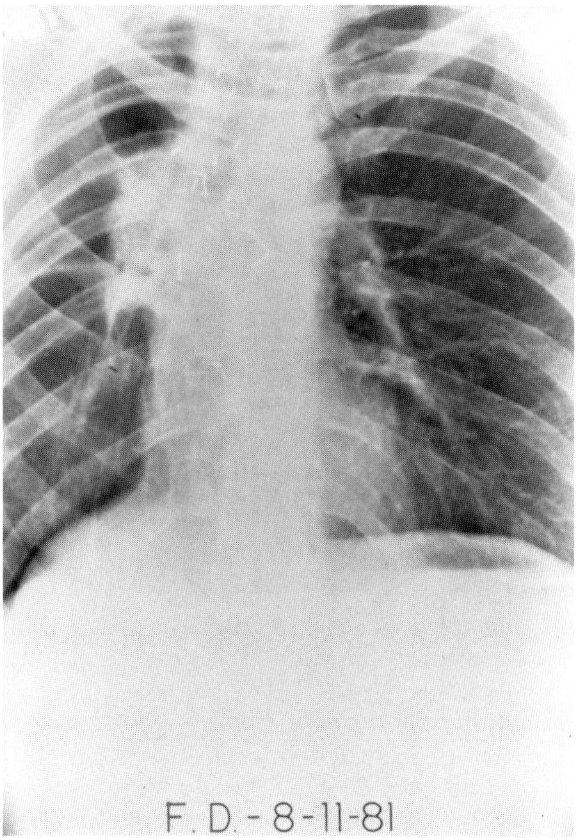

C

Fig. 10-5. **(A)** PA chest x-ray taken shortly after external radiotherapy but just prior to surgery on 7/21/77. **(B)** PA chest x-ray taken on 11/14/77, 4 months after surgery in which internal radiotherapy was used. **(C)** PA chest x-ray taken 4 years after external radiotherapy and surgery for internal radiotherapy. Patient was relatively well at this time.

Patient: V.T. (Fig. 10-6)

Sex: Male

Age: 70

Diagnosis: Squamous cell carcinoma of the lung

Stage: T4, N1, M1

Complaint: Cough of several months' duration

History and Examination: There was dullness at the right lung base along with a recent thoracotomy incision. The chest x-ray showed a large mass occupying most of the right lower lob.

Treatment: The patient had been explored elsewhere, and it was found at that time that the tumor in the right lower lobe had grown inside the left atrium. This was declared to be a nonresectable tumor, and the patient was closed. He was reexplored by us on 6/9/70 with cardiopulmonary bypass available. At exploration an 8.0-cm mass was found in the right lower lobe. The tumor had grown through the inferior pulmonary vein, and as the pericardium was opened, we could palpate a 3.0-cm mass inside the right side of the left atrium. It was possible to proceed with a pneumonectomy. The pulmonary artery was dissected free, suture ligated, and divided. The bronchus was divided and sutured. Since the pericardium was already widely opened, it was possible to place two vascular clamps such that the right half of the left atrium could be resected from the right chest. The specimen and lung were removed. The atrium was closed with two layers of continuous 4-0 silk. There was only lymph node containing tumor in the hilum, which we believed was probably N1.

Follow-up: The patient made an uneventful postoperative recovery and was discharged home approximately 12 days after surgery. He did well for many years. The patient died in 1979, and at postmortem it was found that he had developed a new small cell lung cancer in the left lung with metastases. His T4 right lung cancer was apparently cured, and he had remained free of disease for 9 years.

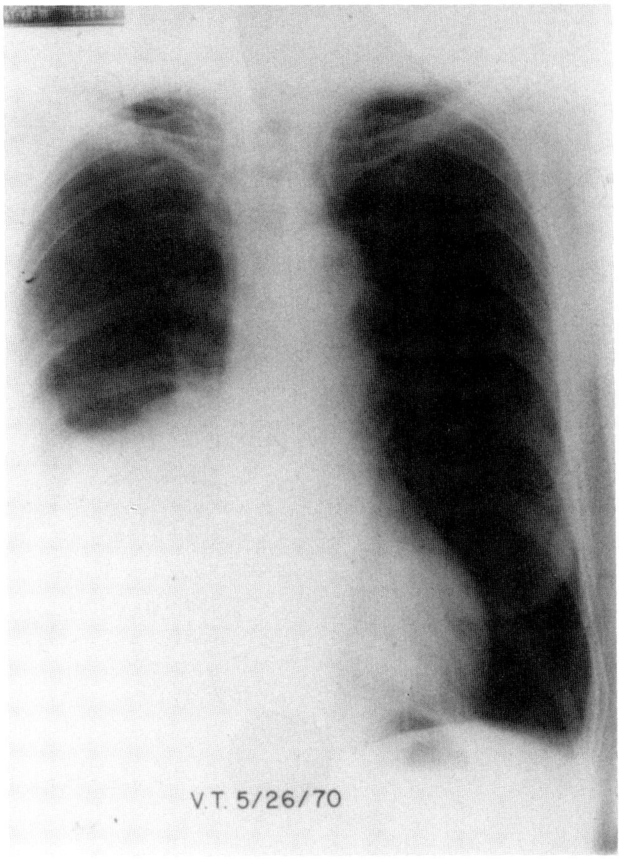

A

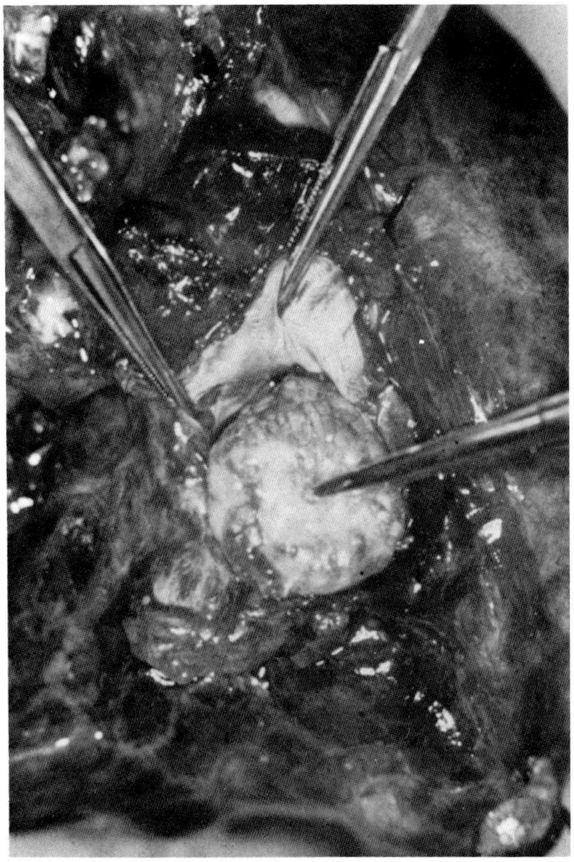

B

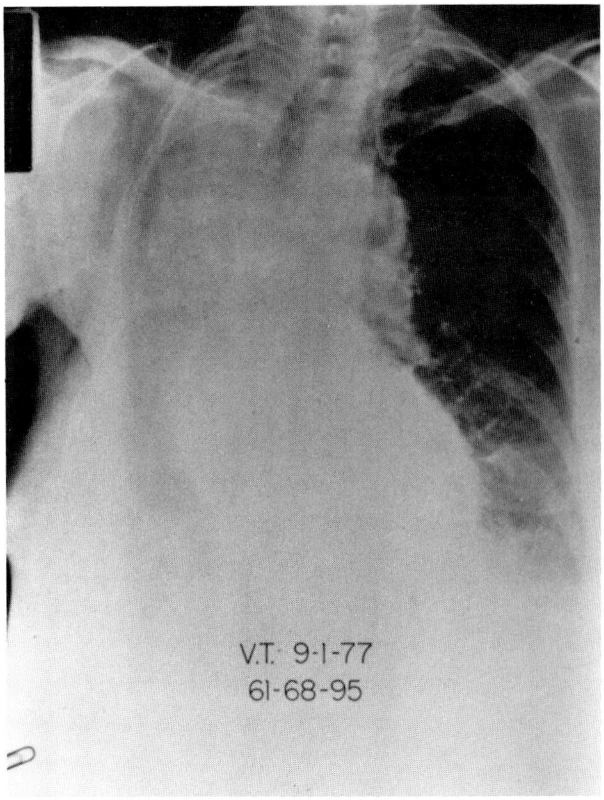

C

Fig. 10-6. **(A)** PA chest x-ray taken on 5/26/70. A large tumor mass fills the right half of the right chest. There is missing rib as a result of the previous thoracotomy. **(B)** Pneumonectomy specimen. Two of the instruments are picking up the cuff of left atrial wall, which in fact circles all the way around this tumor. The third instrument is indicating the center of the tumor, which had grown into the left atrium. **(C)** PA chest x-ray of the patient 7 years after his pneumonectomy. At this time he was continuing to do well.

Patient: J.B. (Fig. 10-7)

Sex: Male

Age: 64

Diagnosis: Non-small cell lung carcinoma of the right upper lobe involving the chest wall; lymph nodes negative.

Stage: T3, N0, M0; chest wall involved

Complaint: Right chest pain for 1 month

History and Examination: The patient suffered from cardiac arrhythmias and emphysema. He was an asbestos worker and a cigarette smoker.

Treatment: Surgery was performed on 2/15/90. A 6.0-cm tumor was found in the right upper lobe, invading the chest wall and ribs 1 to 3. There was a pathologic fracture of rib 1. A wedge excision of right ribs 1 to 3 with wedge excision of the posterior portion of the right upper lobe was carried out. Seventy I-125 seed sutures were placed in the Marlex used for repair.

Follow-up: The chest wall remained negative. The patient developed mediastinal adenopathy.

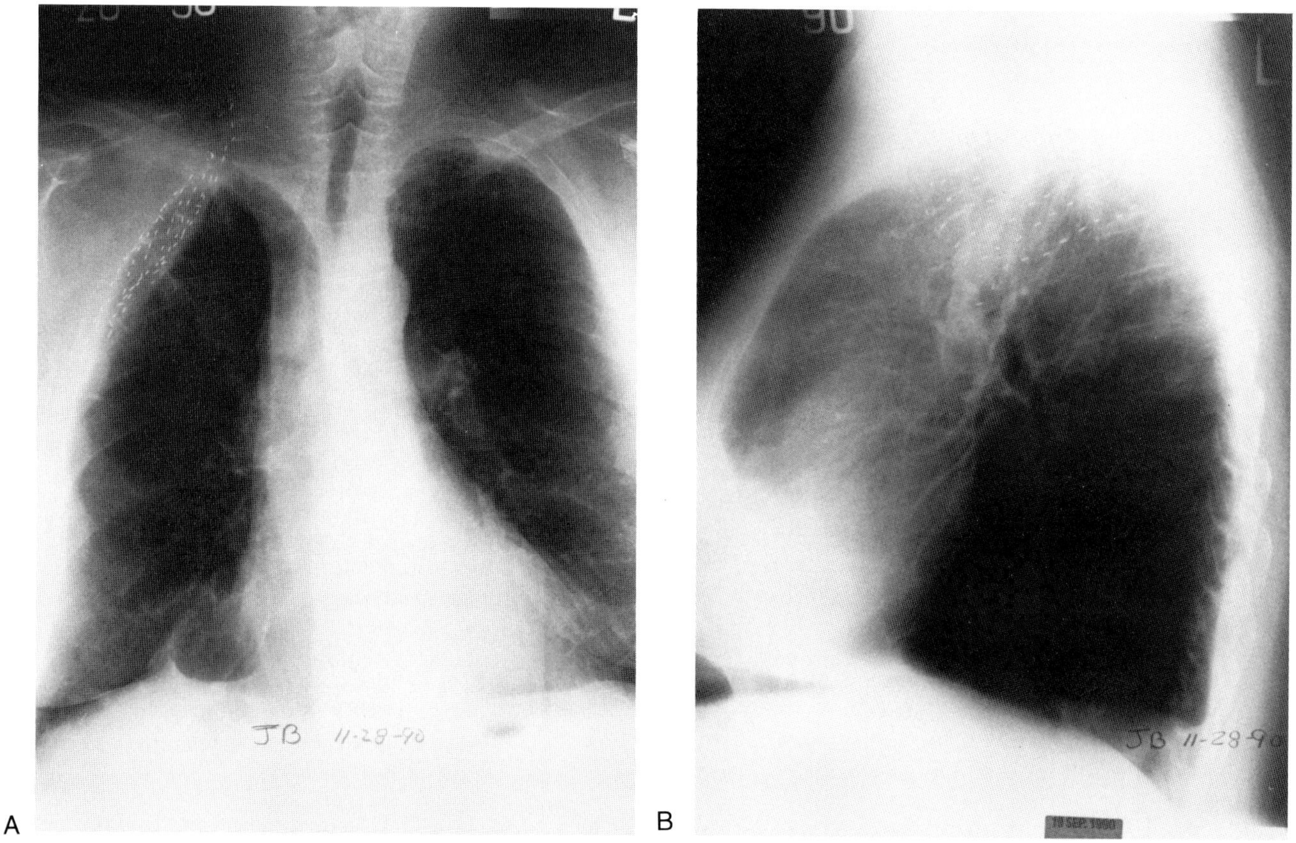

Fig. 10-7. **(A)** PA chest x-ray taken 11/28/90, shows that the right upper ribs are missing. The linear I-125 seed sutures can be seen. **(B)** Lateral chest x-ray, taken on 11/28/90, shows more clearly the location of the I-125 seed sutures.

Patient: P.T. (Fig. 10-8)

Sex: Female

Age: 67

Diagnosis: Adenocarcinoma of the lung with skull metastasis

Stage: Cured stage I lung carcinoma; T1, N0, M1, stage IV, second primary

Complaint: Mass on skull for 1 month

History and Examination: This patient had a left upper lobectomy in 1980 for a primary stage I lung cancer. It was thought that she was cured of this cancer.

In 1988 she discovered a mass on the skull and sought medical attention. A repeat chest x-ray showed the left lung to be clear, but there was a small coin lesion in the right upper lobe. A radiograph of the skull revealed a defect. A CT scan of the head revealed that there was swelling around the left occiput and a defect in the bone but no intracranial lesions. On physical examination there was a soft tissue swelling several centimeters in diameter in the left occipital area. Otherwise the examination was negative.

Treatment: She was started on two cycles of chemotherapy consisting of high-dose *cis*-platinum, VP-16, 5-fluorouracil (5-FU), and mitomycin C. There was an excellent response to treatment, and the swelling on the skull disappeared. The chest x-ray was unchanged. On 8/18/88 she was operated upon by our neurosurgeon consultant and the segment of skull bone involved was excised. The defect in the bone was noted grossly. However, no microscopic carcinoma was found in the specimen. As far as the skull lesion was concerned, this response was complete.

On 10/11/88 a right thoracotomy was carried out, and because of her previous lobectomy and emphysematous changes, a local wedge excision of the tumor was done. This was found to be adenocarcinoma and measured some 1.5 cm in diameter. There was no involvement of lymph nodes.

She received more chemotherapy and clinically did well until she developed a headache. A CT scan of the brain demonstrated a presumed metastasis in the carebellum posterior to the brain stem. This was surgically excised on 1/8/91. Unfortunately the patient developed *Staphylococcus* meningitis postoperatively, and she succumbed on 2/15/91.

Follow-up: This was an 11-year follow-up with the patient NED from left upper lobe lung cancer. She died of infection 2.5 years after the diagnosis of a second lung cancer (Stage IV) with a skull metastasis as the chief complaint.

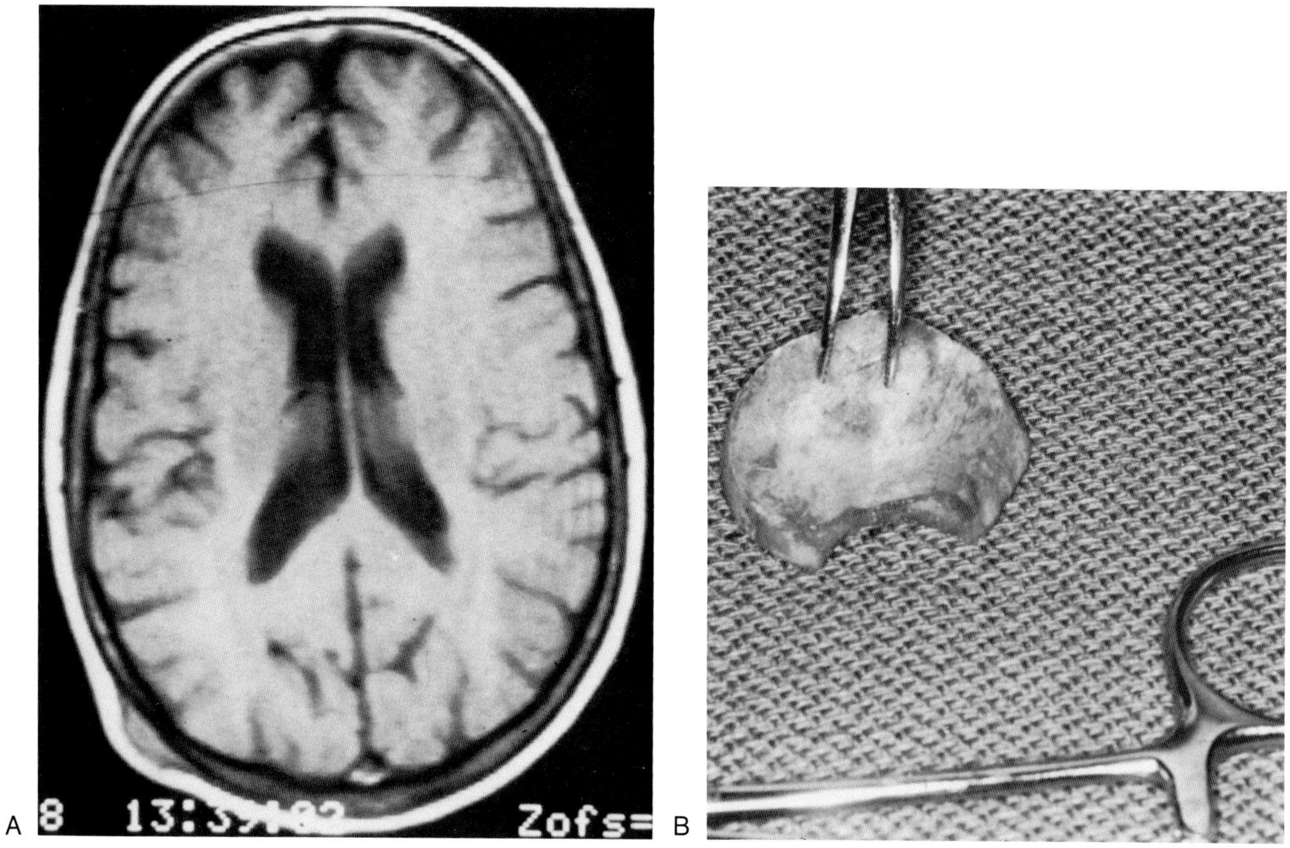

Fig. 10-8. **(A)** Section of a CT scan of the head. A soft tissue mass is visible in the left occipital region. **(B)** Photograph taken in the operating room of the piece of occipital bone excised on 8/18/88. The defect is seen centrally in the bone. (*Figure continues.*)

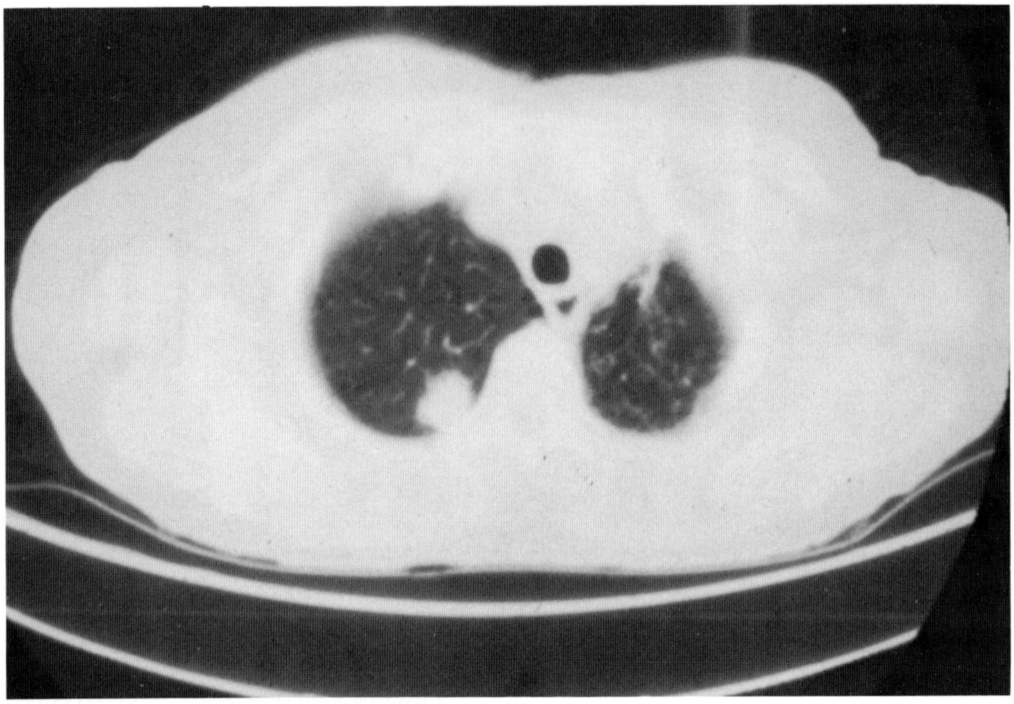

C

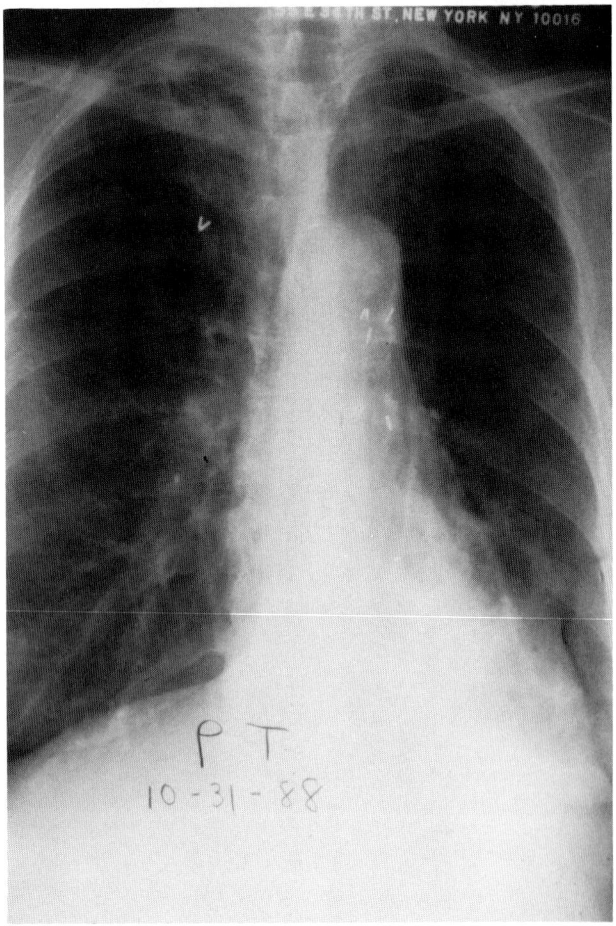

D

Fig. 10-8 (*Continued*). **(C)** CT scan of the chest. It is taken in the upper portion. There is a scar anteriorly in the left lung consistent with the previous left upper lobe lobectomy. Visible in the right chest posterior and spinally is the coin lesion, which was believed to be the primary tumor that produced the skull metastasis in 1988. **(D)** PA chest x-ray taken on 10/31/88. The clips seen in the left chest are from the left upper lobe lobectomy performed in 1980. On 10/11/88 a right thoracotomy was performed and the tumor in the upper lobe was wedge excised. A surgical clip is visible in the right upper lung field. (*Figure continues.*)

E

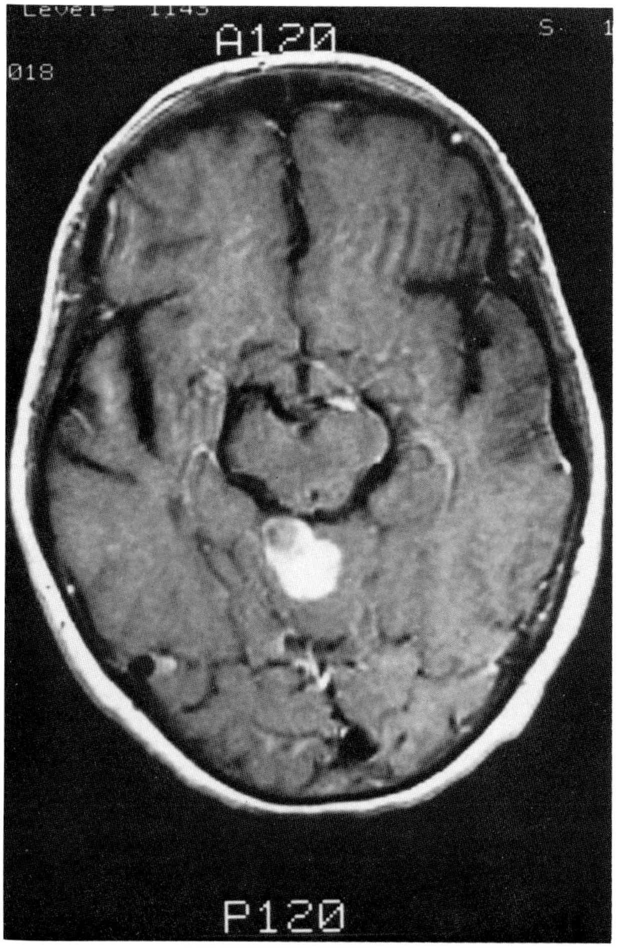

F

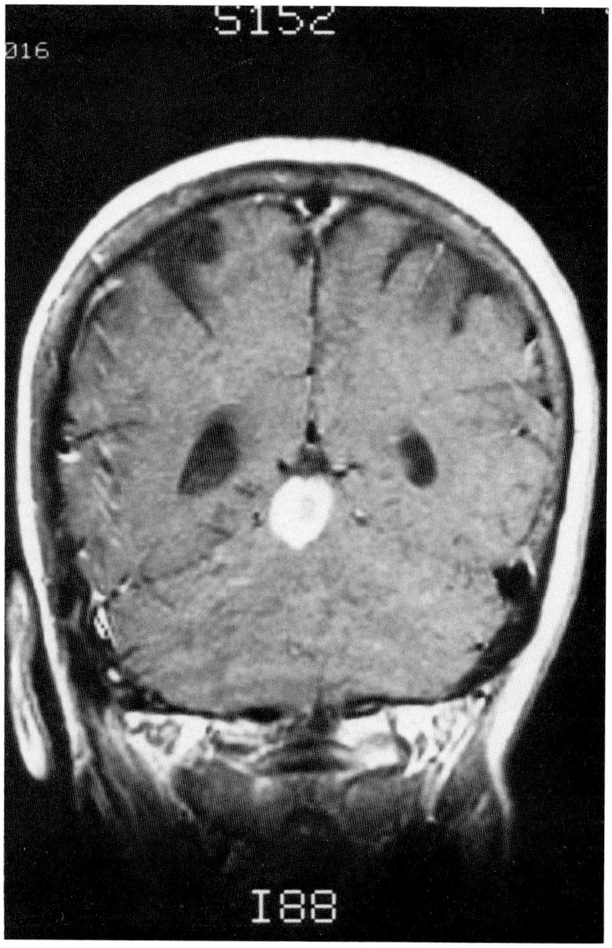

Fig. 10-8 (*Continued*). **(E)** Brain scan taken on 12/3/90. A metastasis in the cerebellum, close to the brain stem, can be seen. **(F)** Front brain scan taken on 12/3/90, also showing the metastasis.

Patient: L.N. (Fig. 10-9)

Sex: Male

Age: 63

Diagnosis: Recurrent squamous cell carcinoma in the bronchial stump after right pneumonectomy

Stage: T3, N0, M0, recurrent

Complaint: Hemoptysis for 2 days

History and Examination: This 63-year old man had had a cough for 3 months when he was first seen on 11/25/51. Squamous cell carcinoma was found protruding from the right upper lobe orifice, and a right pneumonectomy was performed on 11/28/51. The surgical margins were clear, and all lymph nodes were negative.

He was well for the next 18 months, when he developed hemoptysis of bright red blood for 2 days and returned to the hospital. Bronchoscopy at that time found a 2-mm papillary squamous cell carcinoma on the medial carinal wall of the short residual right bronchial stump.

On 6/10/53 the right chest was reoperated upon. It was necessary to resect ribs 2 to 5 en bloc. The scar tissue in the chest was excised down to the clear superior mediastinum, which was entered. It was then possible to redissect free the bronchial stump of the right main bronchus. No extraluminal tumor was found. A segment of bronchial stump trachea and carina some 5.0 cm long in the cephalic-caudal direction by 2.5 cm in the anteroposterior direction encompassing almost 180 degrees in circumference was removed. This left a defect of 5 × 2.5 cm, which was repaired with a double layer of stainless steel mesh, covered, and made airtight with an autologous fascia lata graft. The patient recovered uneventfully and was discharged home 21 days postoperatively.

He maintained a good airway for the rest of his life, although the stainless steel mesh did fragment and at repeat bronchoscopies at intervals some wire fibers were removed. He died at home more than 6 years after the operation, which, from the history we obtained at that time, indicated that he had had a cerebrovascular accident or heart failure at age 71.

Follow-up: He was cancer free 7.5 years after the primary pneumonectomy and 6 years after the reoperation for recurrent lung cancer.

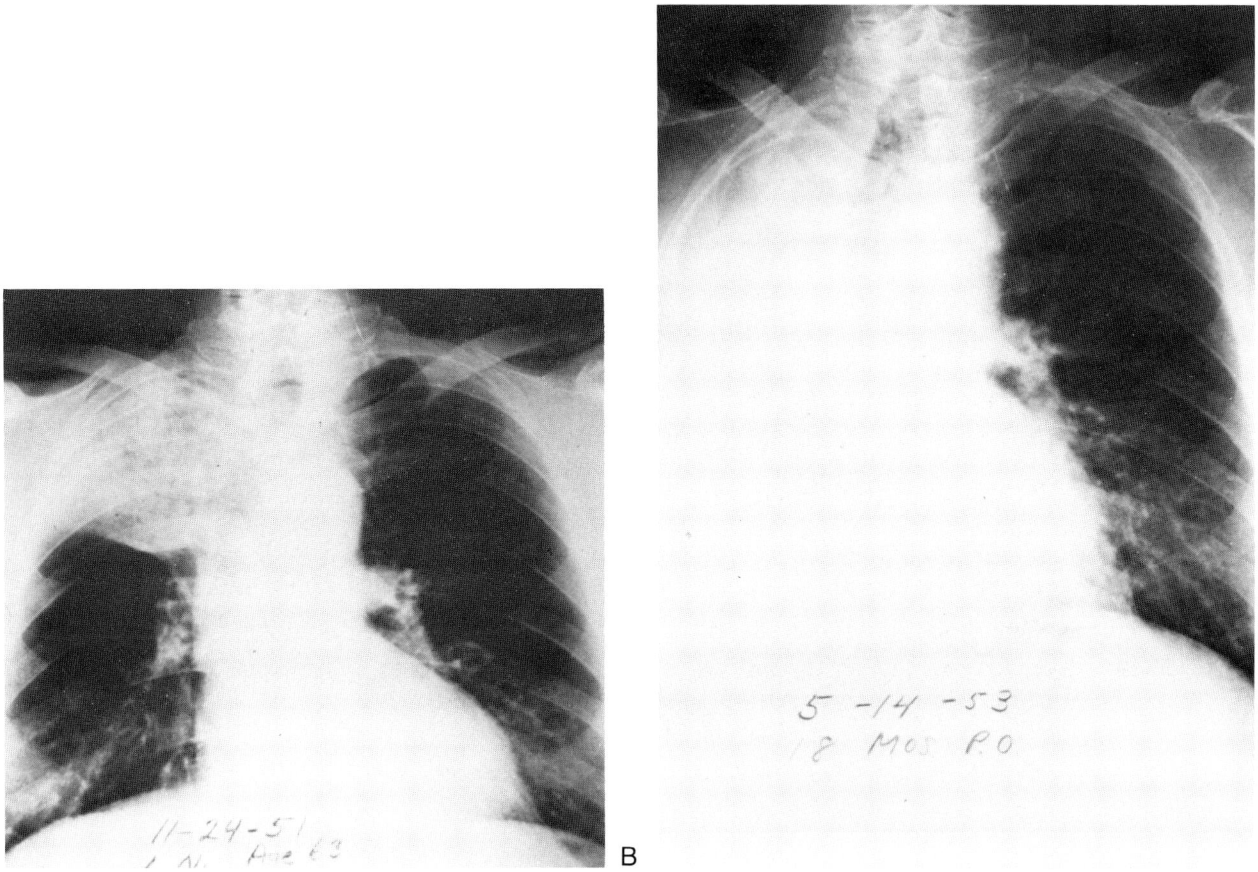

A B

Fig. 10-9. **(A)** PA chest x-ray taken on 11/24/51. It shows consolidation of the right upper lobe secondary to a carcinoma in the right upper lobe orifice. **(B)** PA chest x-ray taken on 5/14/53, 18 months following the right pneumonectomy. (*Figure continues.*)

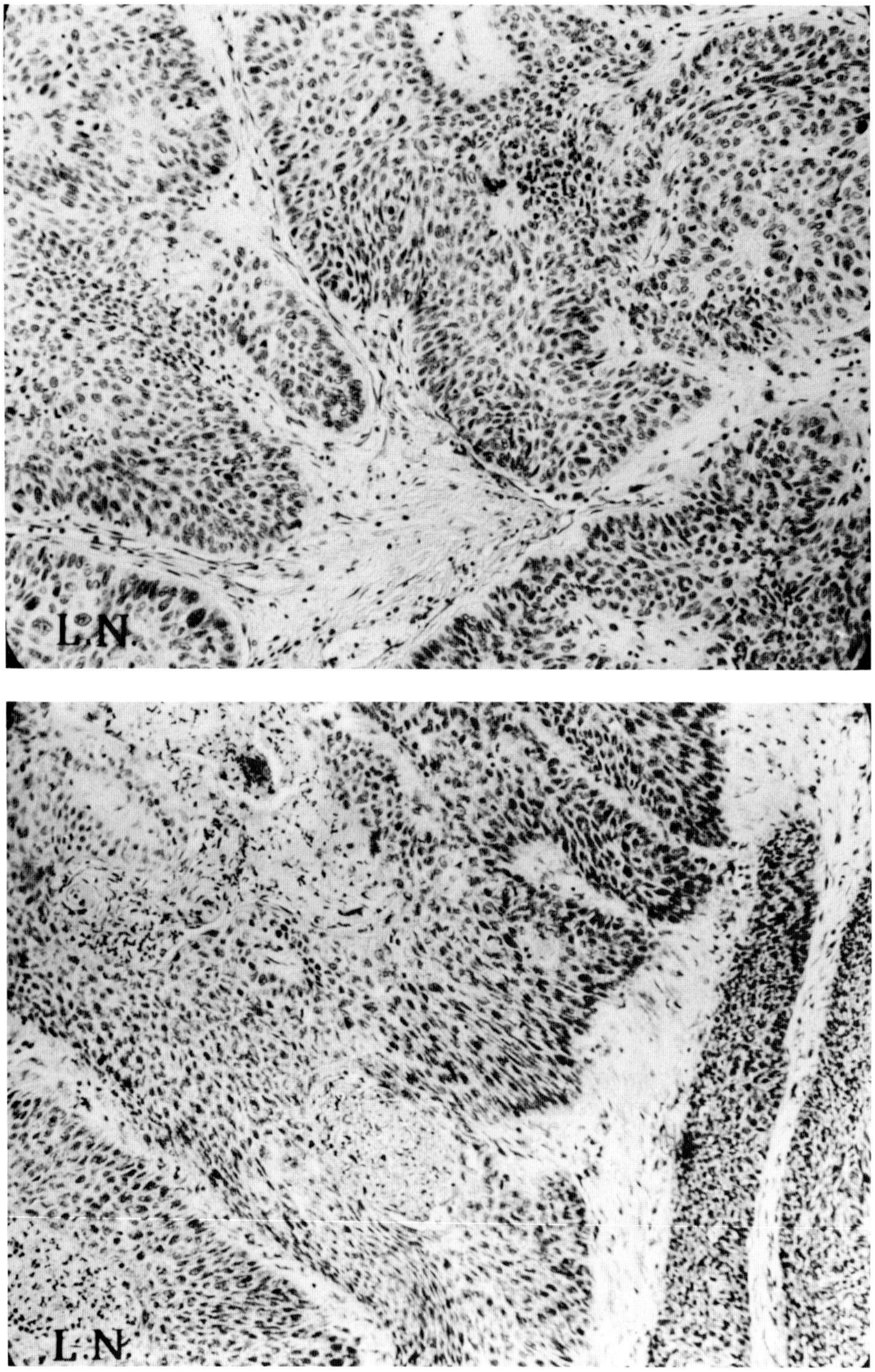

C

D

Fig. 10-9 (*Continued*). Photomicrographs of **(C)** the original tumor removed on 11/28/51 and **(D)** the tumor found on biopsy 18 months later in the bronchial stump. The tumors are believed to be similar epidermoid carcinomas. (*Figure continues.*)

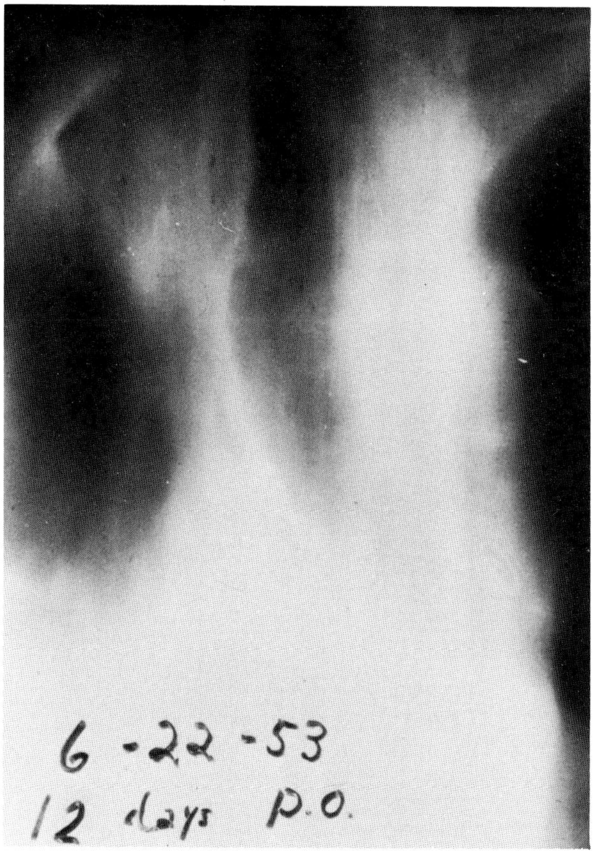

E

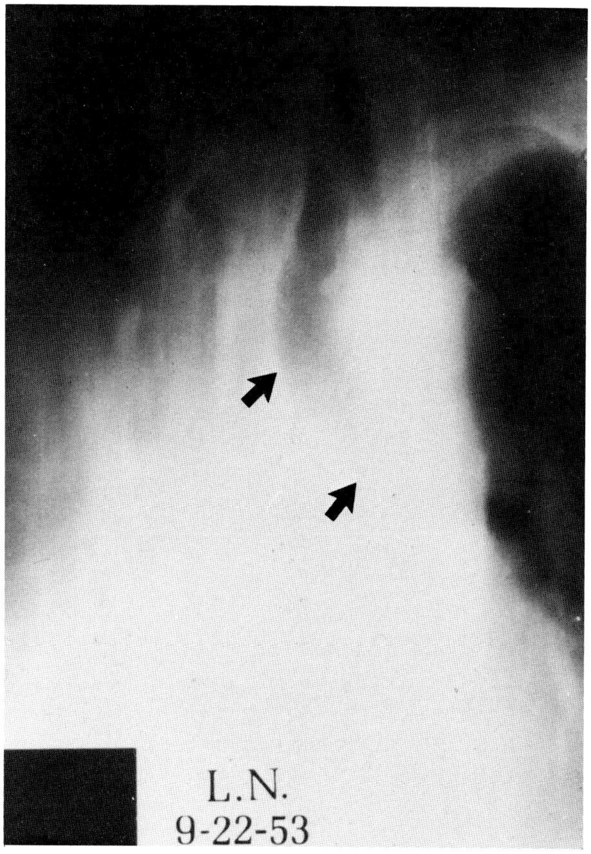

F

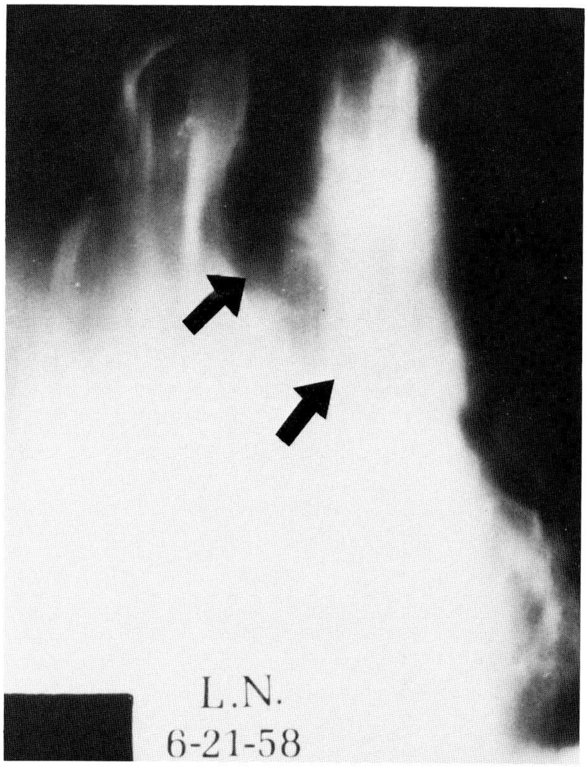

G

Fig. 10-9 (*Continued*). **(E)** PA tomogram taken on 6/22/53, 12 days after the resection of the recurrent tumor in the bronchial stump. A defect has been created in the scarred right thorax to gain access to this region. A patent airway can be seen in the region of the reconstructive surgery. **(F)** PA tomogram of the same region of the chest taken on 9/22/53, 3 months after the operation. The reconstructed area lies between the two arrows. There is a good lumen through this area. **(G)** PA tomogram taken on 6/21/58, 5 years after the reconstruction of the airway following resection of the recurrent cancer. The area between the arrows represents the surgical defect. The lumen through this region is adequate by both radiography and bronchoscopy. (From Beattie EJ, Jr, O'Kane C, Davis CB, Jr, Friedberg SA: Surgical intervention in recurrent bronchogenic carcinoma. JAMA 155:835, 1954, with permission.)

Patient: J.S.P. (Fig. 10-10)

Sex: Female

Age: 52

Diagnosis: Small cell lung cancer of the right upper lobe

Stage: Limited disease (LD)

Complaint: In June 1987 the patient developed fatigue and pain under her right shoulder blade associated with myasthenia.

History and Examination: The patient was unremarkable on physical examination. The chest x-ray showed a hard-to-see density in the right upper lung, and a CT scan of the chest showed a lesion in the right upper lobe associated with widening of the mediastinum. She had a mediastinoscopy elsewhere, and a small cell lung cancer was found in the mediastinal lymph nodes.

Treatment: She received four cycles of *cis*-platinum, adriamycin, vincristine (CAV) elsewhere. The mediastinum was markedly improved. However, the lesion in the lung had not changed. The brain, bone, and liver scans were within normal limits.

On 2/4/88 a right upper lobe lobectomy was carried out. The pathologic examination revealed no residual small cell lung cancer in the lobe, but there was a focal multiloculated abscess containing fungal colonies of aspergillosis in the lung lesion. She did well postoperatively and had two further cycles of chemotherapy postoperatively. Prophylactic radiotherapy to the mediastinum, neck, and brain was given, which was completed on 4/29/88. A third cycle of postoperative chemotherapy was completed on 5/25/88.

Follow-up: The patient is now NED 4 years after diagnosis of her SCLC.

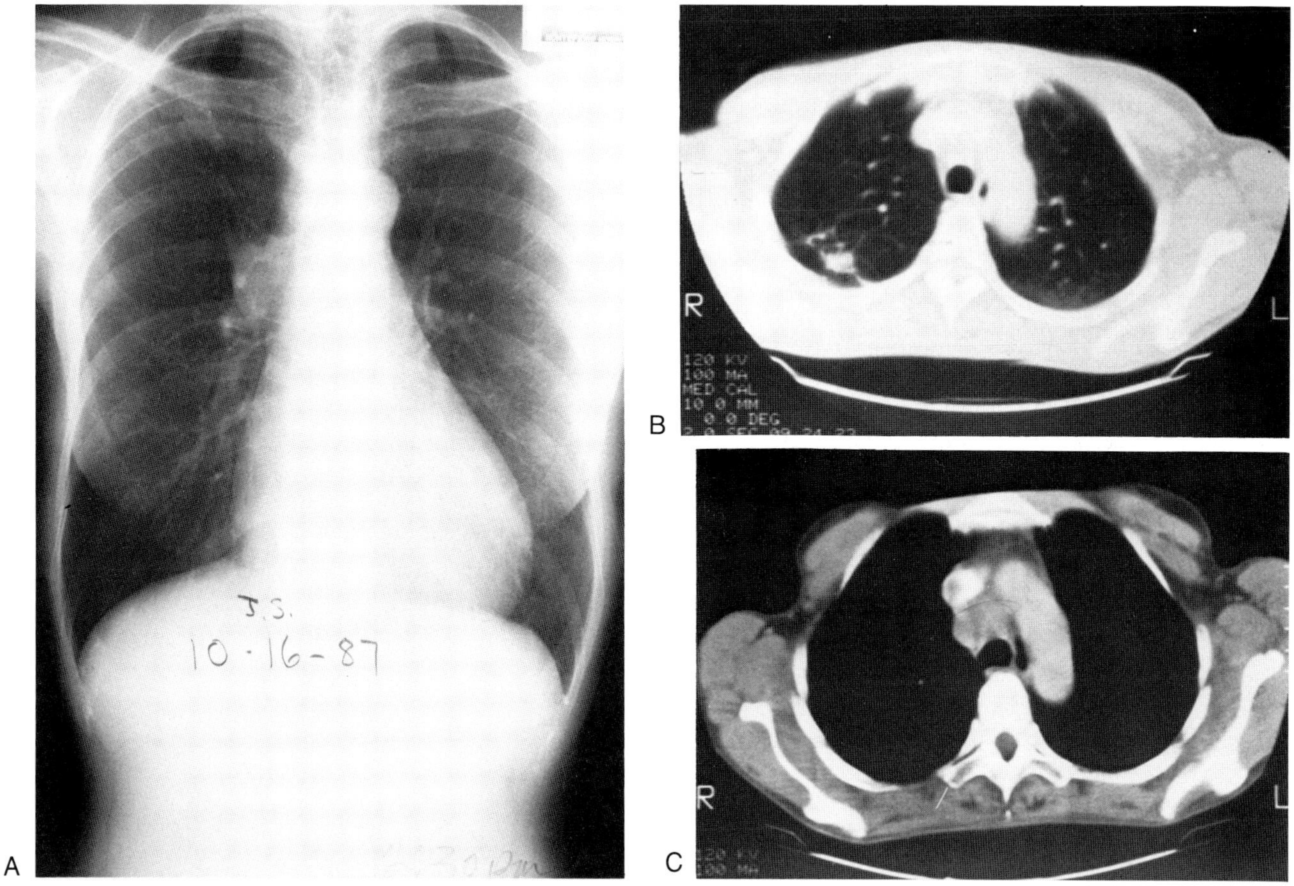

Fig. 10-10. **(A)** PA chest x-ray taken on 10/16/87. There is a mass in the right upper lung field that is difficult to see, and there is also a prominence in the right hilar region. **(B)** CT scan of the chest showing lung windows. There is a mass posteriorly in the right upper lobe. **(C)** CT scan of the chest showing mediastinal windows. There is a lymph node tumor mass anterior to the trachea, posterior to the superior vena cava, and with the aortic arch seen to the left.

Patient: B.G. (Fig. 10-11)

Sex: Male

Age: 52

Diagnosis: Metastasis of osteosarcoma to the left lung and to the right chest wall subcutaneous region

Stage: Metastatic

Complaint: Abnormal chest x-ray

History and Examination: This 52-year-old man had been diagnosed with a giant cell tumor of his left lower tibia in December 1942. This was treated by radiotherapy. In December 1961 he had an ulceration of the leg associated with arterial insufficiency. A lumbar sympathectomy was done, with no relief of pain. A biopsy of the ulcer elsewhere was found to contain osteosarcoma. A mid-thigh amputation was done at an outside hospital for this apparently radiotherapy-induced osteosarcoma. Following this, he did relatively well until May 1966, when he noticed a subcutaneous nodule in his right chest posterior axillary line. This was excised at another outside hospital and found to be metastatic osteosarcoma. A chest x-ray taken at that time demonstrated two lesions in the left upper lobe, and for this reason he came to us.

Treatment: After extensive study and much debate, since this seemed to be an osteosarcoma that had spread both into the lungs and systemically, he had a left upper lobe lobectomy performed on 7/14/66. There were no other signs of osteosarcoma found.

His chest x-ray remained clear after that time, but in October 1966 it was noticed that there was a regrowth of the subcutaneous nodule on the right chest. There was a palpable 1.5-cm mass. On 10/17/66 under local anesthesia a wide excision was made, leaving a defect of 10 by 5 cm. This was closed per primum.

Follow-up: He had no further trouble from the osteosarcoma. He was in good condition when examined on 10/1/88 and has remained relatively well since.

Fig. 10-11. **(A)** Radiograph of the right lower extremity taken in 1962. The abnormal area in the distal tibia can be seen; this ultimately was found to contain osteosarcoma. **(B)** PA chest x-ray dated 5/26/66, showing two areas of increased density in his left upper lobe. They were ultimately removed and were found to be metastatic osteosarcoma. **(C)** PA chest x-ray dated 11/26/73, 7 years after the left upper lobe lobectomy. The patient has remained well.

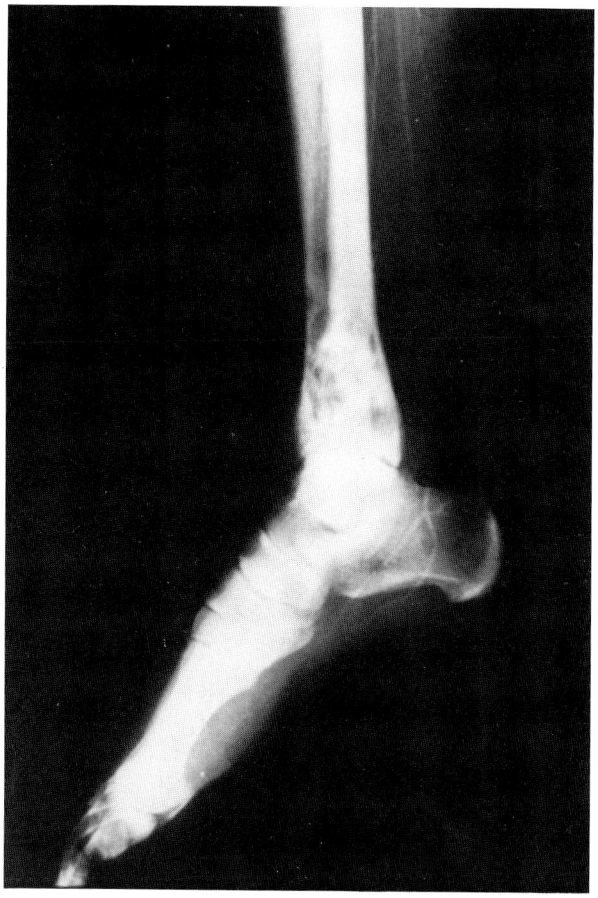

A

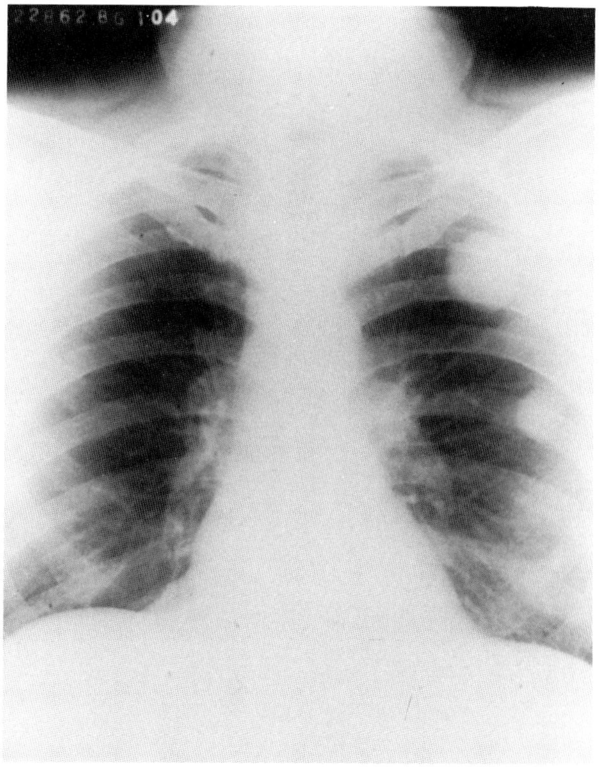

B

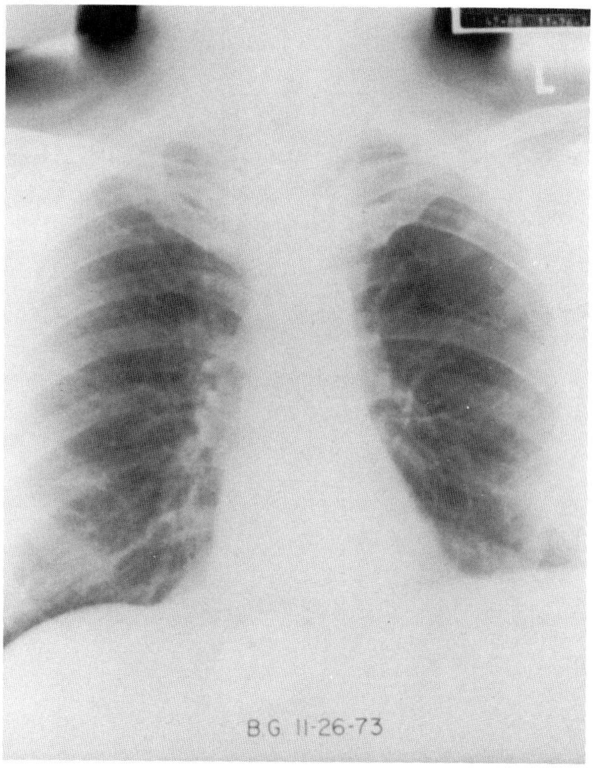

C

Patient: B.W. (Fig. 10-12)

Sex: Female

Age: 16

Diagnosis: Osteosarcoma in the left hip

Stage: Metastatic

Complaint: Pain in the left hip

History, Examination, and Treatment: This 16-year-old girl developed a tumor in the left hip. It was biopsied and found to be osteosarcoma. A left hemipelvectomy was performed at that time. Her chest x-ray was normal at the time of surgery. However, in the summer of 1967 a routine chest x-ray showed metastases in both lungs, and right and left thoracotomies were carried out. Five metastases were wedge excised from the right lung, and four metastases were wedge excised from the left lung.

Six months later, early in 1968, a second left thoracotomy was done and a 3- to 4-cm metastasis was resected from the lower lung field. She did well until early 1969, when a new lesion was visible in the left upper lobe adherent to the chest wall. A third left thoracotomy was carried out, and a small segment of chest wall involving two ribs plus the lesion were wedge excised. Thus, 11 metastases were resected in four thoracotomies.

Follow-up: She continued to do well from then on and for the next 23 years had no further difficulty with osteosarcoma.

One daughter was born in 1982, and a second daughter was born in 1985. B.W. felt that her right breast was enlarging, and in June 1988 a mass was found in the right breast along with enlarged with lymph nodes in the right axilla. In spite of chemotherapy, mastectomy, radiotherapy, and additional chemotherapy, metastases of the breast cancer developed. She died of breast cancer in 1990, 23 years after her hemipelvectomy and 2.5 years after developing the right breast carcinoma.

A

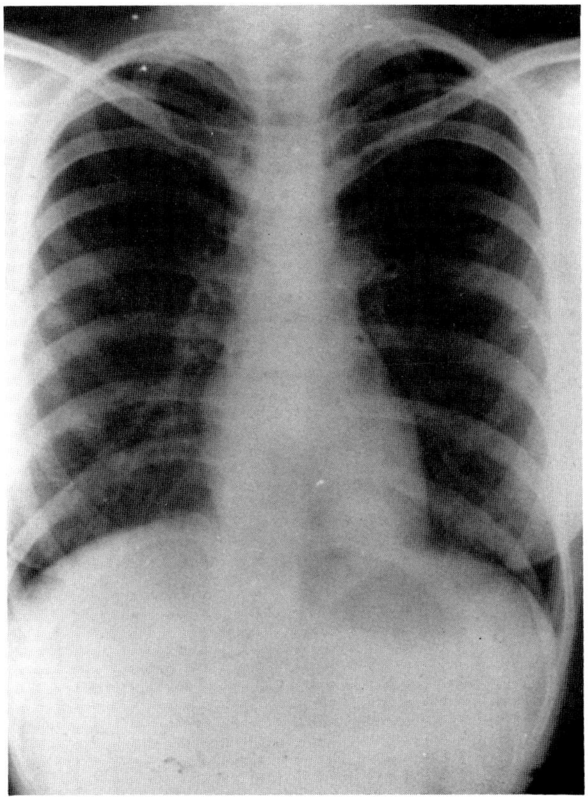

B

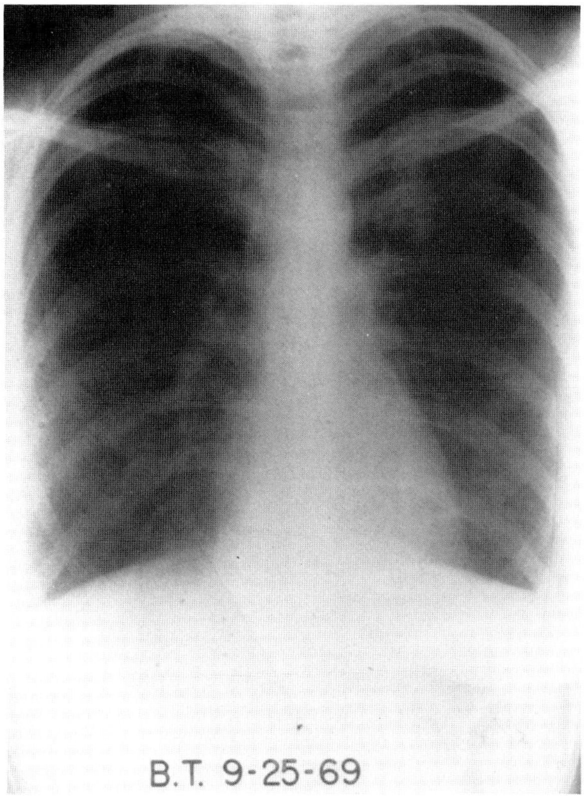

Fig. 10-12. **(A)** PA chest x-ray taken on 8/18/67. There are five metastases in the right lung and four in the left lung. A mass is visible behind the heart. Another smaller mass on the left side is below the seventh rib posteriorly. On the right side one can see a mass posteriorly below the seventh rib and one posteriorly below the ninth rib. The other lesions readily found at operation are difficult to see in this radiograph. **(B)** Chest x-ray taken on 9/25/69 showing the lesion located in the left upper lobe posteriorly adherent to the fifth rib posteriorly. **(C)** Chest x-ray taken on 2/3/88 following one right thoracotomy and three left thoracotomies with total excision of 11 metastases. The lungs are clear at this time.

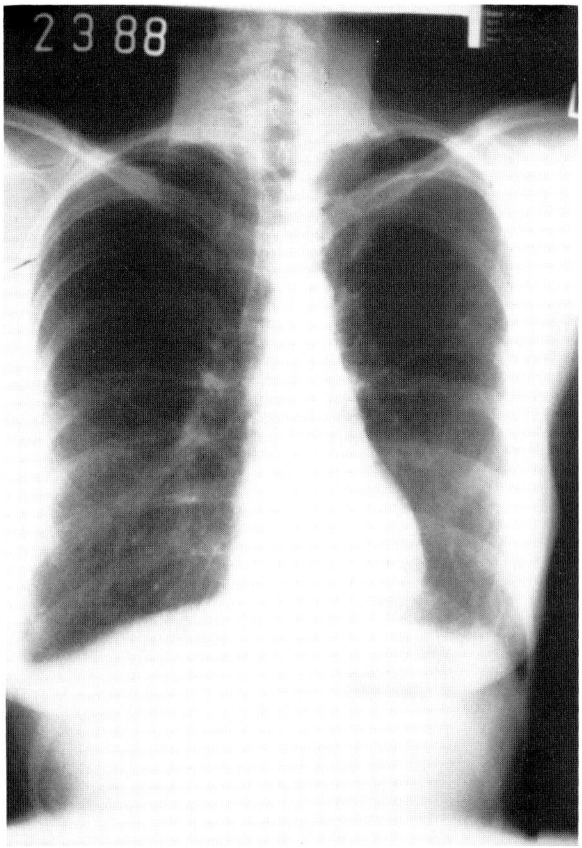

C

Patient: J.S. (Fig. 10-13)

Sex: Female

Age: 10

Diagnosis: Osteosarcoma of the left hip

Stage: Recurrent metastases to lungs, bilateral

Complaint: Pain in the left hip

History and Examination: Examination of this 10-year-old girl showed some limitation of the left hip. Radiography confirmed the probable diagnosis of osteosarcoma, and it was proven by biopsy.

Treatment: On 5/16/68 a left hemipelvectomy was carried out. In the fall of 1969, bilateral pulmonary metastases were seen, and the first and second (left and right) thoractomies were carried out on 9/26/69. Between then and July 1972 a total of two left and four right thoracotomies were carried out, with removal of more than 30 pulmonary metastases. She received a course of high-dose methotrexate, adriamycin, chlorambucil, and cytoxan for 10 months.

She was well until 1986, when a density recurred in the right chest. This was drained by thoracotomy elsewhere on 3/16/86. A cavity refilled with blood clot, and tumor grew in the right upper lobe. On 9/16/86 a right upper lobectomy was performed with removal of all tumor seen. Osteosarcoma was found in the specimen. She received four cycles of chemotherapy consisting of adriamycin and high-dose *cis*-platinum. However, metastases developed. On 1/14/88 a ninth thoracotomy consisting of anterior mediastinotomy was done. Extensive osteosarcoma was found. She died of disease on 2/19/88, 19 years after her hemipelvectomy and after having had nine thoracotomies.

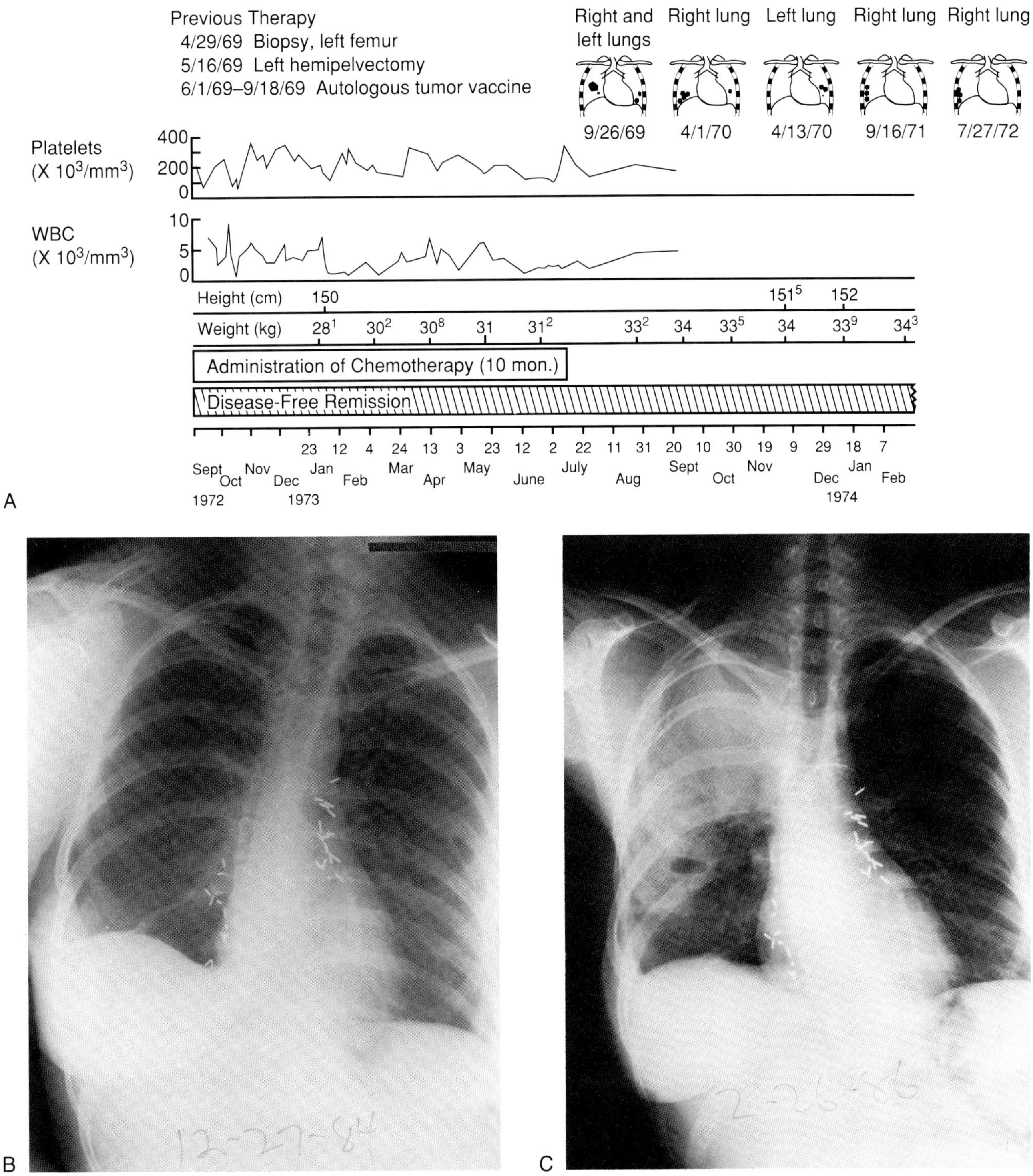

Fig. 10-13. **(A)** Summary of six thoracotomies performed from September 1969 through July 1972 and the chemotherapy course through July 1973. WBC, white blood cell. (Redrawn from Beattie EJ, Jr, Martini N, Rosen G: The treatment of pulmonary metastases in children with osteogenic sarcoma with surgical resection combined with chemotherapy. Cancer 35:618, 1975, with permission.) **(B)** PA chest x-ray taken on 12/27/84, 16 years after hemipelvectomy and 12 years after six thoracotomies for multiple bilateral pulmonary metastases of osteosarcoma. **(C)** PA chest x-ray taken on 2/26/86. A new density is visible in the right upper lung field. (*Figure continues.*)

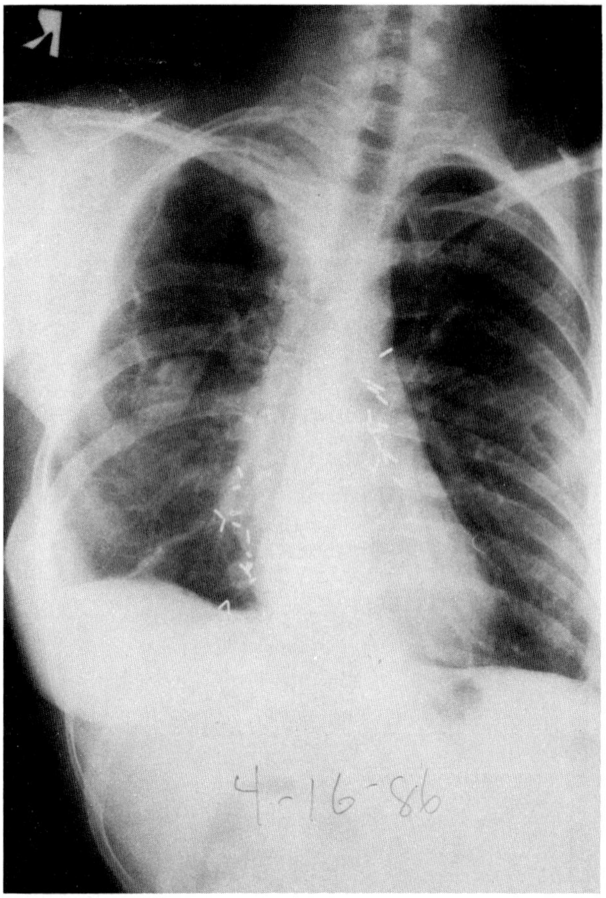

D

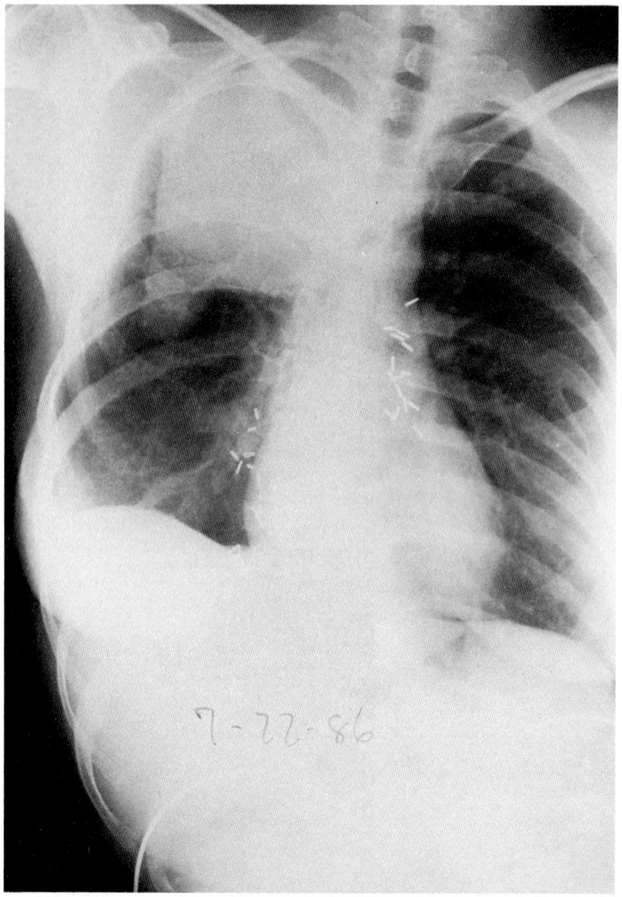

E

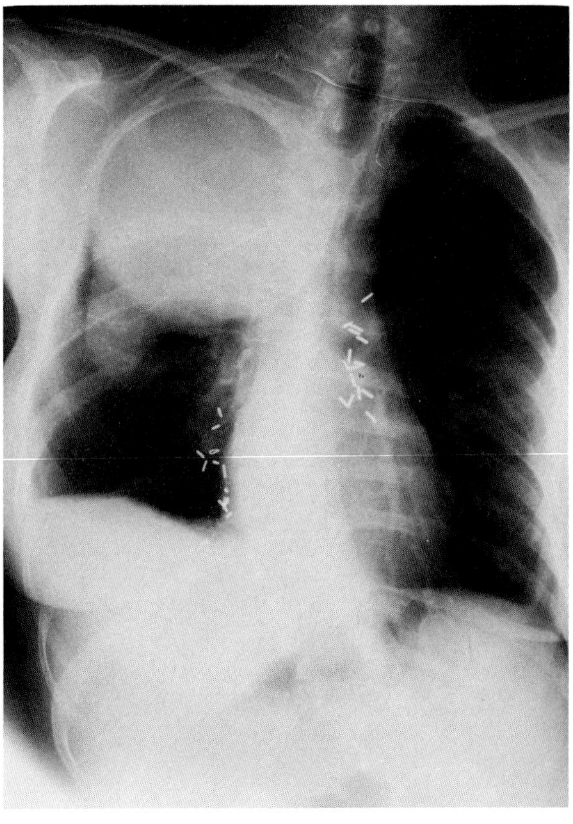

F

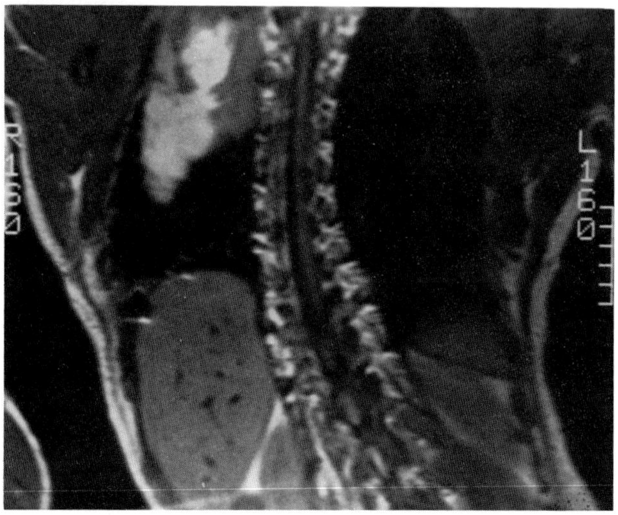

G

Fig. 10-13 (*Continued*). **(D)** PA chest x-ray taken on 4/16/86. A hematoma was drained elsewhere. A cavity can be seen. **(E)** PA chest x-ray taken on 7/22/86. A cavity in the right upper lung field has filled with a larger area of increased density. **(F)** PA chest x-ray taken on 9/16/86. The area of increased density in the right upper lung field has rounded and increased in size and has caused some respiratory difficulty. **(G)** MRI view taken on 9/16/86. This is interpreted as showing blood in the lesion with tumor in the apical and medial portion. (*Figure continues.*)

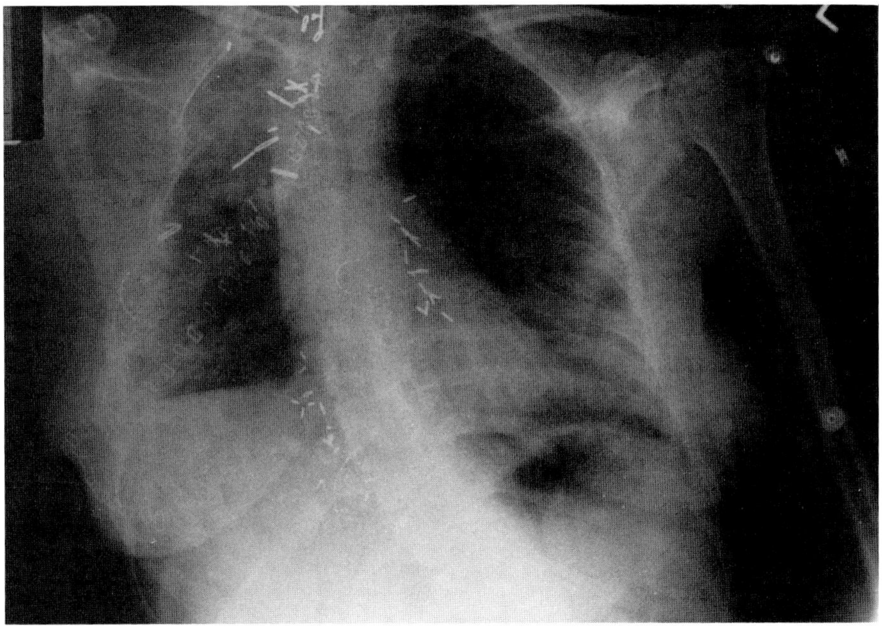

H

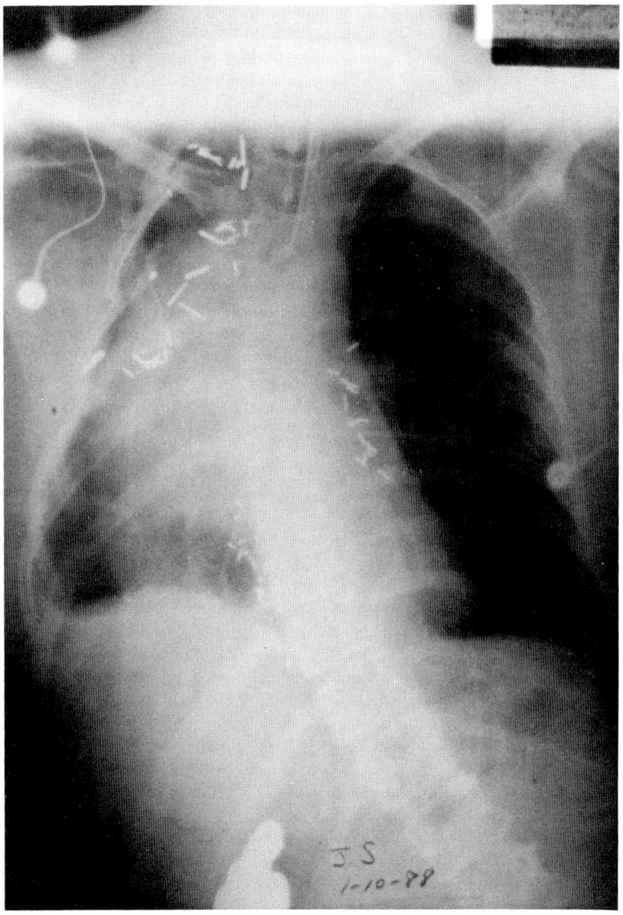

I

Fig. 10-13 (*Continued*). **(H)** PA chest x-ray taken in September 1986 after a right upper lobectomy. I-125 seeds were placed in the superior segment of the right lower lobe when the tumor margin was close. It was thought that lung tissue had to be conserved at this eighth thoracotomy. **(I)** PA chest x-ray taken on 1/1/88, showing recurrent disease in the mediastinum, widened to the right.

Patient: C.M. (Fig. 10-14)

Sex: Female

Age: 55

Diagnosis: Hepatoma metastatic to left lung

Stage: Distant metastases

Complaint: Shortness of breath

History and Examination: In 1979 a left lobe hepatectomy was performed for hepatoma. In 1984 a wedge excision was performed to remove metastasis in the left lower lobe. In 1985 wedge excision was performed to remove multiple metastases from the left lung and to implant I-125 seeds along the left bronchus with involved lymph nodes. In 1988 a wedge excision of the left upper lobe and portion of chest wall was carried out. In October 1990 a thoracotomy found tumor inside the pericardium, metastasis to the left lower lobe, and carcinoma in the left main bronchus. Pneumonectomy was not done. Postoperatively, atelectasis developed in the left lung from tumor obstruction.

Treatment: On 11/20/90 transbronchial afterloading for internal radiotherapy with Ir-192, 1,000 rads, was done.

Follow-up: On 11/27/90 the left lung was reinflated. In July 1991 the left lung was still inflated. Tumor was found metastatic to the left axillary lymph nodes, which were excised and treated with afterloading radiotherapy.

A B

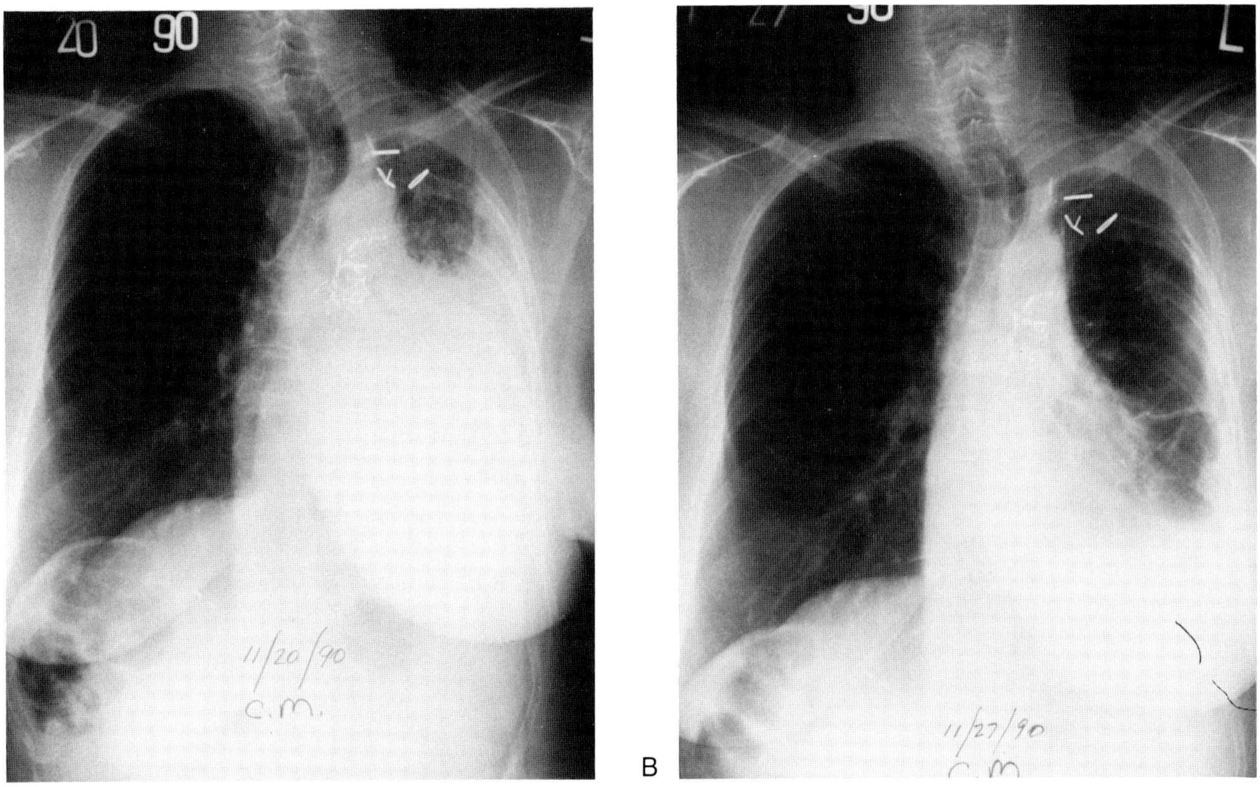

Fig. 10-14. **(A)** PA chest x-ray taken on 11/20/90, shortly after the fourth thoracotomy in October 1990 when a pneumonectomy was not done because of extensive pericardial implants. The left lung has become largely atelectatic. **(B)** PA chest x-ray taken on 11/27/90, 1 week after afterloading I-192 was used in the left mainstem bronchus to treat the tumor. The left lung has largely reinflated. Its smaller size is secondary to the numerous resections of metastases, which had been confined to the left lung.

ESOPHAGUS

Patient: H.R. (Fig. 10-15)

Sex: Female

Age: 65

Diagnosis: Squamous cell carcinoma of the upper esophagus

Stage: T3, NX, M0

Complaint: Dysphagia for several months

History and Examination: This patient was seen early in 1962 with dysphagia. An esophagogram revealed a filling defect and partial obstruction of her esophagus in the upper thorax. Esophagoscopy found squamous cell carcinoma. She received 6,000 rads of radiotherapy. Following this, in one stage she had an essentially total esophagectomy, leaving her with a cervical esophagostomy and gastrostomy. In a later stage the left colon was used in a antiperistaltic fashion with anastomosis of distal colon to the cervical esophagus and of proximal colon to the stomach. A barium enema had been obtained preoperatively to ensure that the colon utilized was free of known disease.

In October 1965, some 3 years later, she again developed dysphagia. A repeat esophagogram at that time showed a filling defect in the distal portion of the transplanted colon a few centimeters above the cologastrostomy. She had a laparotomy in October 1965, and a mass lesion was palpated in the colon near the stomach. The colon was divided at the level of the former cologastrostomy, and a segment of colon was removed without disturbing its blood supply. The colon cephalic to the obstruction was then reapproximated to the stomach in a new cologastrostomy.

Follow-up: The patient did well postoperatively. The lesion in the colon was diagnosed as an adenocarcinoma of the colon and was a distinctly separate new tumor. Approximately 5 years after her second operation she was lost to follow-up when she refused further radiographs. This patient was a 7-year survivor of carcinoma of the upper thoracic esophagus.

A

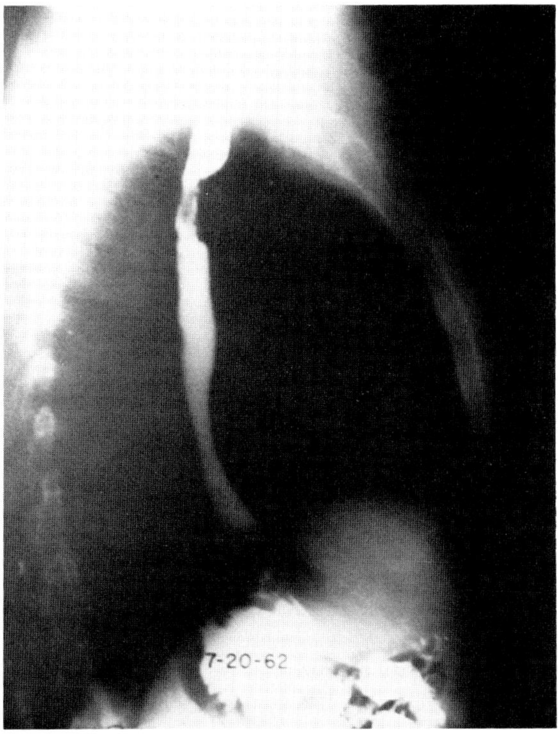

B

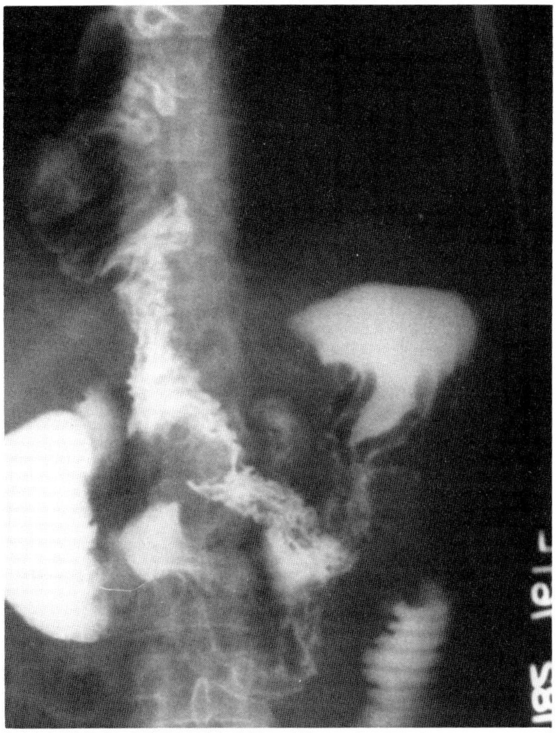

C

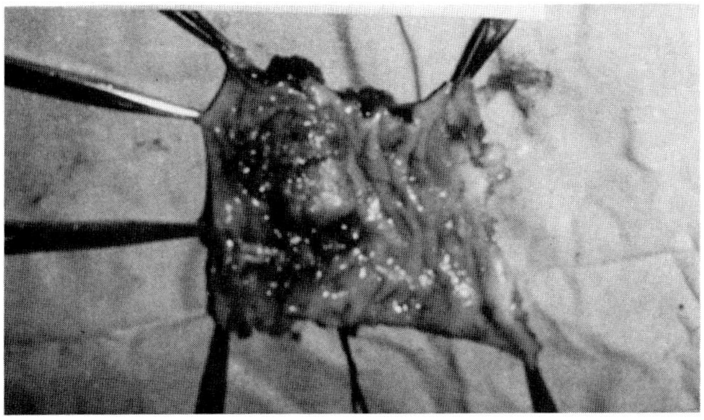

D

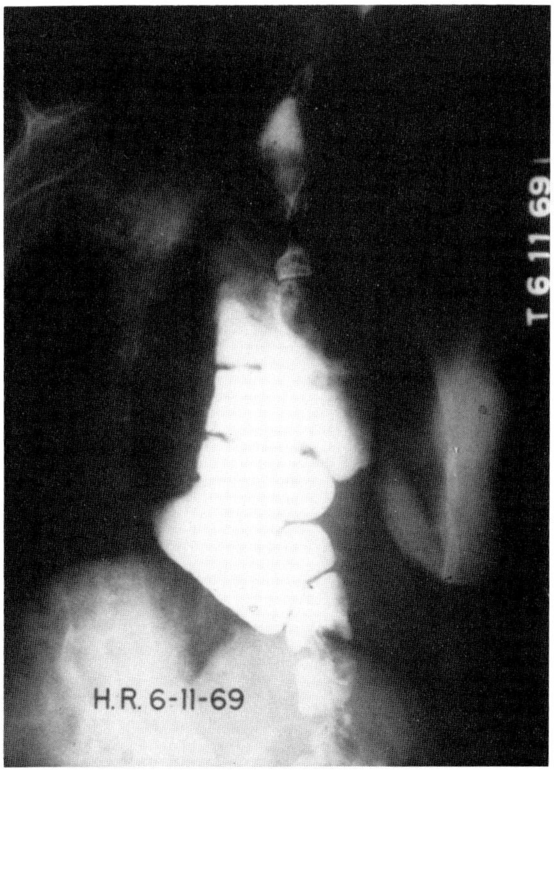

Fig. 10-15. **(A)** Lateral esophagogram taken on 7/20/62. The 3-cm filling defect in the upper esophagus can be seen. **(B)** Frontal view of an esophagogram taken on 10/13/65. The colon, which has been transplanted to connect the cervical esophagus with the stomach, can be seen running down to the stomach. There is a rounded filling defect in the descending portion of this colon a few centimeters above its junction with the stomach. **(C)** Photograph taken in the operating room of the segment of colon resected. To the right is the previous cologastrostomy; to the left is the division of this segment from the colon. In the center of the specimen is a tumor mass, which was found to be an adenocarcinoma of the colon. **(D)** Esophagogram seen in the frontal projection taken on 6/11/69. The residual normal esophagus is seen at the top of the figure. The somewhat dilated colon is seen descending and connecting with the stomach at the bottom of the figure. The patient was asymptomatic at this time and refused any further radiography. Shortly thereafter she was lost to follow-up.

Patient: P.M. (Fig. 10-16)

Sex: Female

Age: 59

Diagnosis: Adenocarcinoma of the esophagus

Stage: Stage II

Complaint: Food sticking on swallowing for approximately 1 month

History and Examination: This 59-year-old woman had been known to have a hiatus hernia for some 13 years. She had had heartburn and frequent belching, but only recently had noted that solid food was sticking in her esophagus. An esophagogram showed a lesion consistent with tumor obstructing the distal esophagus. On esophagoscopy adenocarcinoma was biopsied 32 cm from the incisor teeth.

Treatment: On 7/13/73 a left thoracotomy was carried out and an esophagogastrectomy was performed with pyloroplasty. The anastomosis was created as high as possible just under the aortic arch. The pathologic examination showed that the margins were clear and that no lymph nodes were involved with tumor. The tumor was deep in the wall of the esophagus but had not completely penetrated the wall of the esophagus.

Follow-up: The patient has remained free of tumor and is alive and well 18 years post-surgery.

A

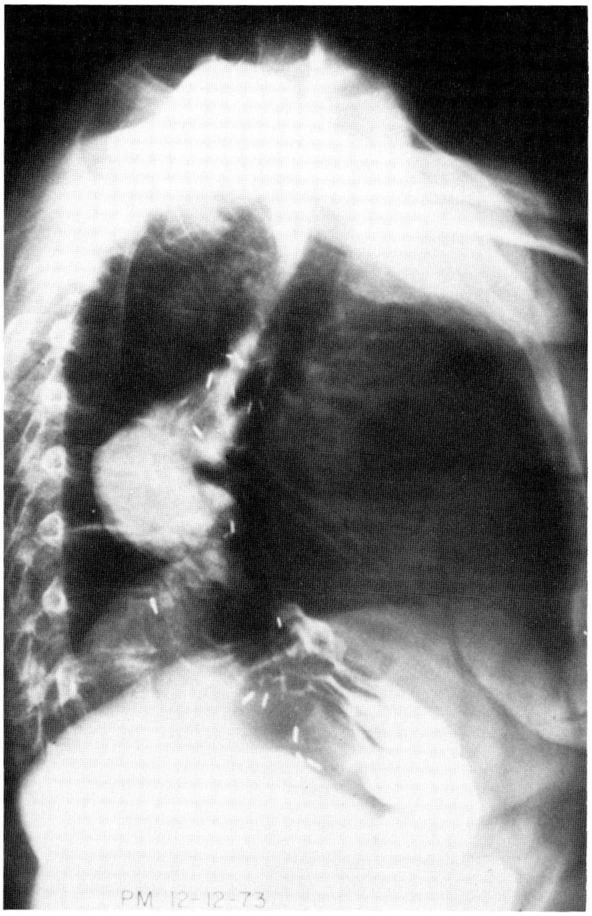

B

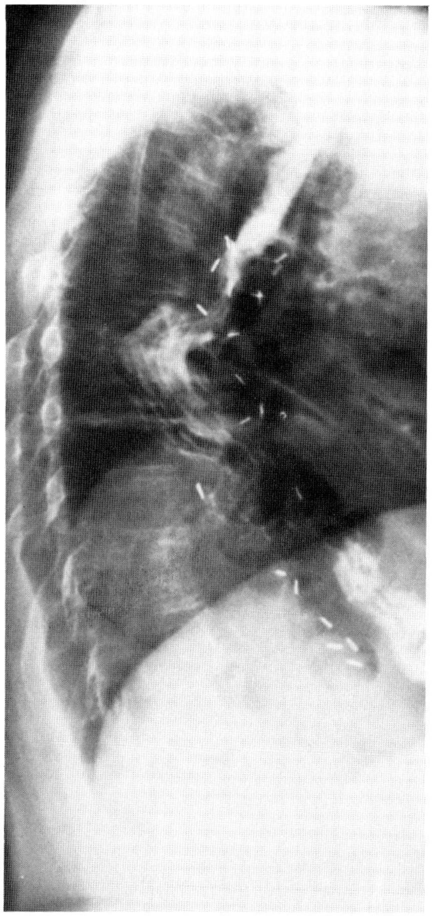

C

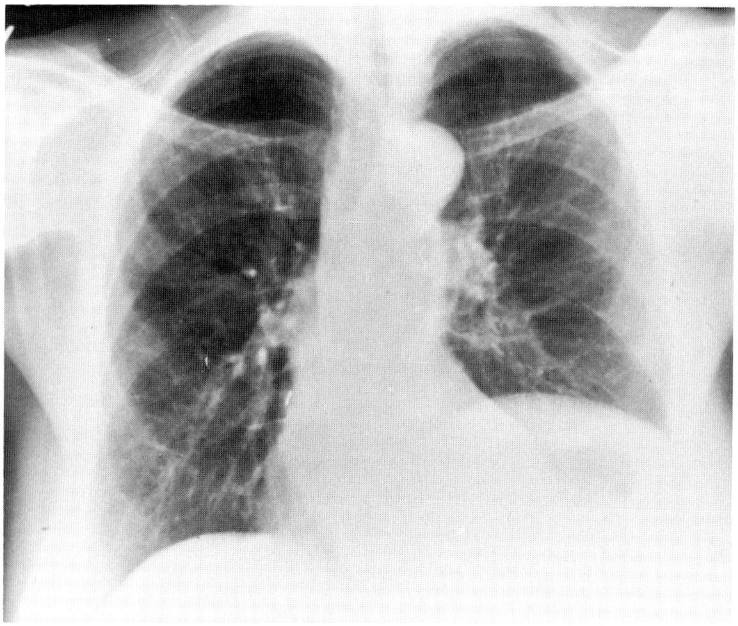

Fig. 10-16. **(A)** Lateral esophagogram taken on 12/12/73 some 5 months after the esophagogastrectomy. The anastomosis is about mid-chest. The slightly enlarged stomach can be seen above the left diaphragm and continuing on through the diaphragm. **(B)** Esophagogram taken on 4/13/81 in the same position as in Fig. A. The esophagogram is essentially unchanged 8 years postoperatively. **(C)** PA chest x-ray taken on 2/23/82 showing the elevated diaphragm resulting from the operation but otherwise clear lung fields. The stomach in the thorax is not visible in this view.

MEDIASTINUM

Patient: M.M. (Fig. 10-17)

Sex: Female

Age: 6

Diagnosis: Ganglioneuroma

Stage: Bilateral chest and abdomen

Complaint: Urinary tract infection

History and Examination: This 6-year-old girl, when aged 6 months, had had a diagnosis of tumor in her left upper quadrant. Surgical exploration and biopsy at that time done elsewhere revealed a neuroblastoma. It was recommended that she have a course of radiotherapy, but she had only a few treatments. She then had a course of Krebiozen.

She did well with no complaints until the age of 6, when she had what appeared to be a urinary tract infection and her pediatrician obtained an intravenous pyelogram (IVP). The IVP showed that there was a large posterior mediastinal mass beginning at about the level of the seventh thoracic vertebra posteriorly and extending paraspinally down below the diaphragm. Nothing else was found on examination, and the patient was otherwise a normal 6-year-old girl.

Treatment: On 2/1/68 a left thoracoabdominal exploration was carried out. There was a large tumor mass that was located in the posterior mediastinum at the level of T7. It lay between the anterior border of the spine and the rest of the thoracic and abdominal viscera. On the left side it extended several centimeters lateral to the costospinal angle. It also extended below the diaphragm posteriorly to about the level of L2. It was densely scarred in the abdominal part, where it seemed to be near the tail of the pancreas. This tumor mass on the left side had nerve attachments to each of the spinal sympathetic ganglia from T7 to L2. After careful dissection and detachment of this tumor from its nerve connections, the tumor was divided with the electrocautery slightly to the right of the midline. This permitted removal of the tumor in the left thorax and left abdomen, with residual tumor remaining on the right.

The pathologic diagnosis was ganglioneuroma. It seemed that the previous neuroblastoma had dedifferentiated into a benign tumor. It was decided to remove the right side of the tumor. On 2/13/68 a right thoracoabdominal approach was made. The right-sided tumor in similar fashion extended from T7 down into the abdomen but stopped at a higher level (about T12). It also was attached to the ganglia and the intercostal nerve roots at each level. The patient made an uneventful postoperative recovery and was discharged home.

She returned in November 1970 complaining of left upper quadrant abdominal pain. Examination revealed a mass deep in the epigastrium. An IVP showed hydronephrosis of the left kidney. She underwent surgery on 11/24/70. There was a large recurrent ganglioneuroma, which seemingly had been centered around the tail of the pancreas. It was necessary to remove the hydroneophrotic left kidney along with a portion of the left adrenal gland. The tumor extended across the abdomen, posterior to the aorta and posterior to the vena cava, to the hilum of the liver. With dissection and mobilization of the inferior vena cava and the aorta, it was possible to remove this lesion intact along with the left kidney.

The patient made an uneventful postoperative recovery. She has done well since and has no complaints at present. She was last seen by us in 1985. It is now 29 years since her neuroblastoma and 23 and 21 years after resection of her ganglioneuroma.

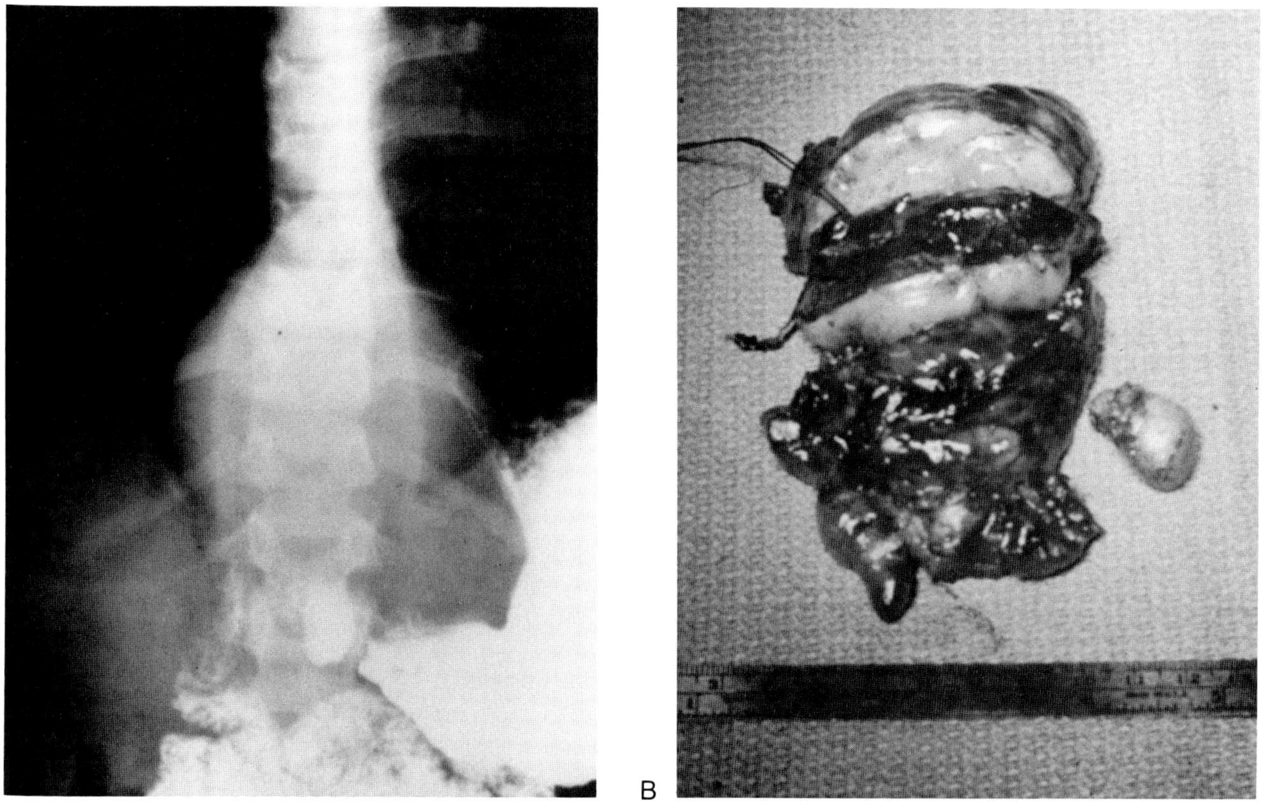

A B

Fig. 10-17. **(A)** Upper gastrointestinal series showing a view of the spine. The paraspinal mass can be seen as a double shadow behind the heart arising from about T7 and descending below the diaphragm. **(B)** Photograph taken in the operating room of the specimen removed from the right chest. The mass extended from the midline of the anterior spine laterally to the right and from approximately T7 to T12. (*Figure continues.*)

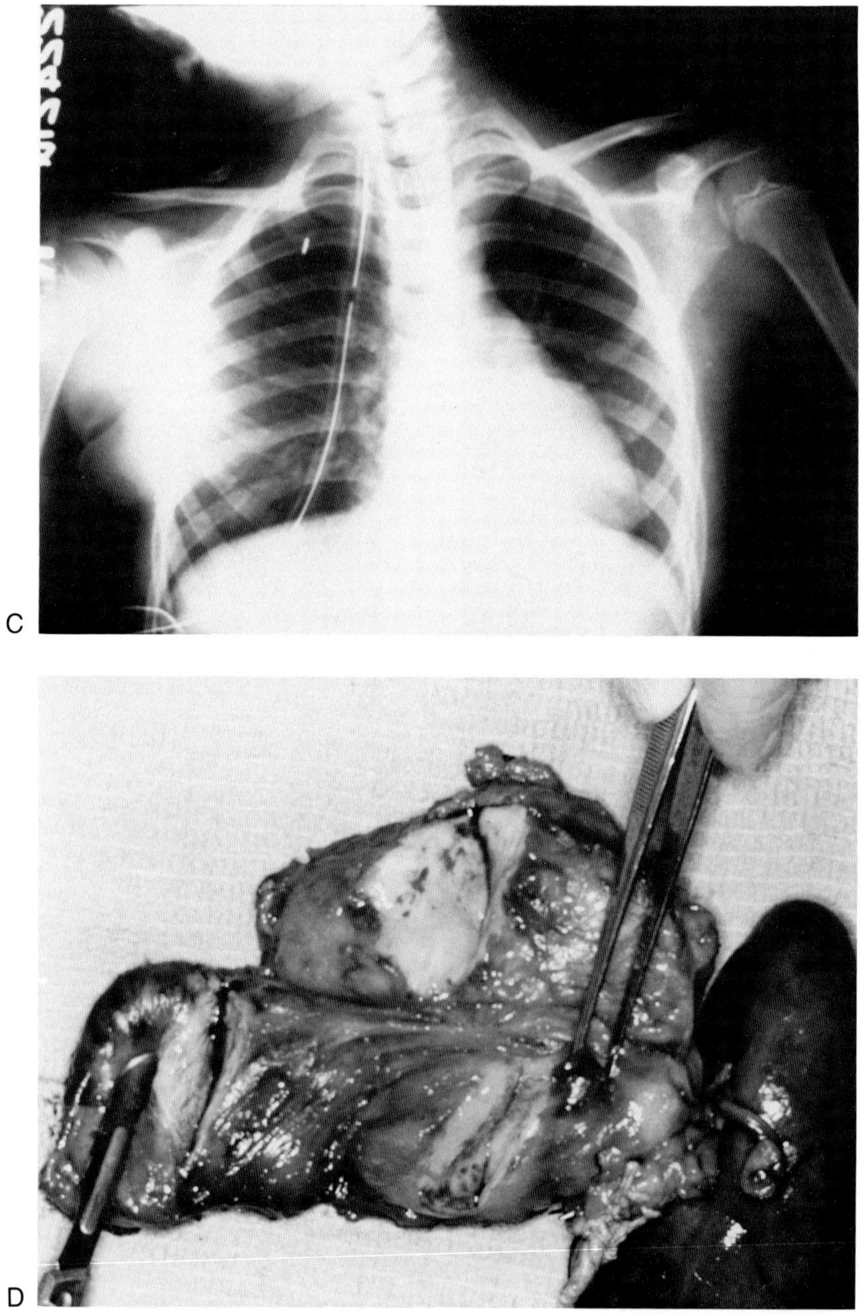

Fig. 10-17 (*Continued*). **(C)** PA portable chest x-ray taken in the postoperative period after the right thoracotomy. The chest is clear, with a chest tube still in place. **(D)** Surgical specimen removed in the operating room on 11/24/70. The left kidney is visible to the right. The tumor mass extended posterior to the aorta and posterior to the vena cava over to the hilum of the liver. The tumor has been incised in several places, showing its nature. It was relatively well encapsulated and had grooves in its anterior border for the aorta and vena cava. (*Figure continues.*)

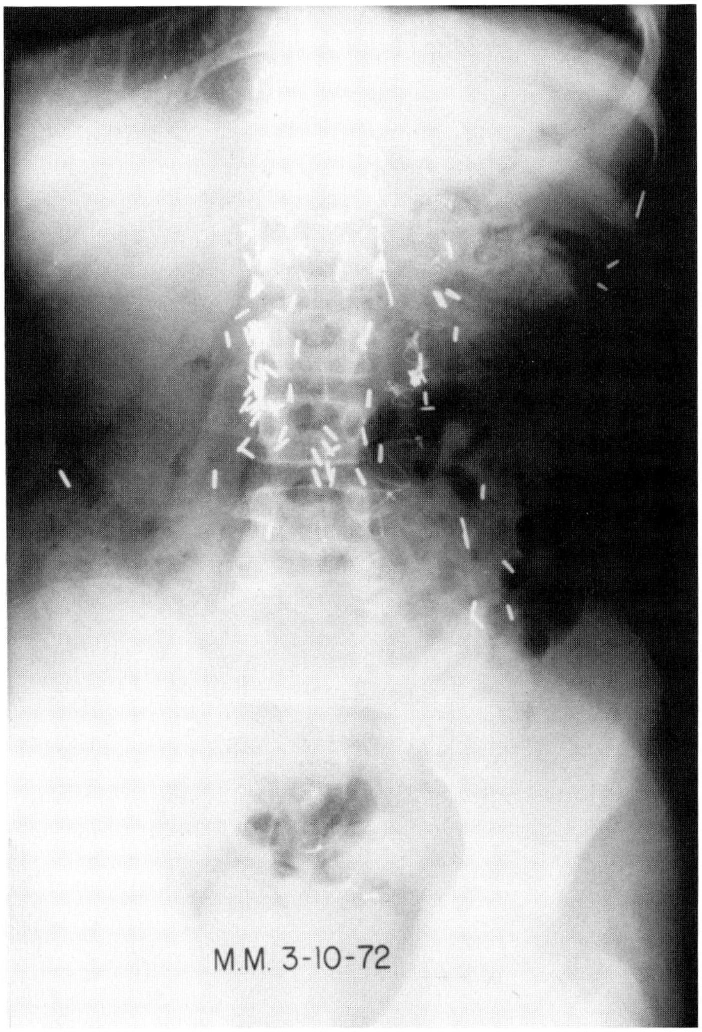

E

Fig. 10-17 (*Continued*). **(E)** Postoperative abdominal radiograph taken on 3/10/72. One can see from the location of the clips that the tumor at the left thoracoabdominal operation extended down toward the pelvis. The extensive nature of the recurrence removed at the third operation is clear from the extent of the clips extending across the upper abdomen from left to right.

CHEST WALL, PLEURA, AND STERNUM

Patient: A.M. (Fig. 10-18)

Sex: Male

Age: 8

Diagnosis: Neuroectodermal carcinoma of the chest wall involving the fifth rib

Complaint: The patient was struck in the chest during play; he complained of pain, and a chest x-ray showed a chest wall mass

History and Examination: This 8-year-old boy had always enjoyed good health until this injury. Because of the complaint of pain after the chest x-ray was taken, CT scans of the chest and abdomen were taken. A mass was found in the right chest wall centered over the right fifth rib which protruded somewhat inside the chest and right lung area.

Treatment: On 7/12/90 a right thoracotomy was done with resection of segments of ribs 4, 5, and 6 since the tumor was centered on the fifth rib. It was also found that the underlying confluence of the middle, lower, and upper lobes of the lung was densely adherent to the parietal pleura. Since it was not possible to tell whether the tumor was in the lung, it was necessary to wedge excise the attached upper, middle, and lower lobe portions with the stapling device in removing the specimen. The chest wall defect was repaired with Marlex mesh. The patient had a relatively uneventful postoperative course and was discharged.

He was treated with chemotherapy consisting of high-dose Isofamide, VP-16, high-dose cyclophosphamide, adriamycin, and vincristine. This chemotherapy was completed by the end of January 1991, and the patient returned home in good condition.

The pathologic specimen showed that this was a primitive neuroectodermal tumor of the chest wall involving the rib. No tumor was seen in the lung. The stain was positive for neuron-specific enolase. The stains were negative for keratins, chromogranin S-100 protein, and leu-7 antigen. No glycogen was seen in the tumor cells with a periodic acid-Schiff reaction. This tumor is also called Askin's tumor.

Follow-up: This young boy is almost 1 year postsurgery and continues to do well.

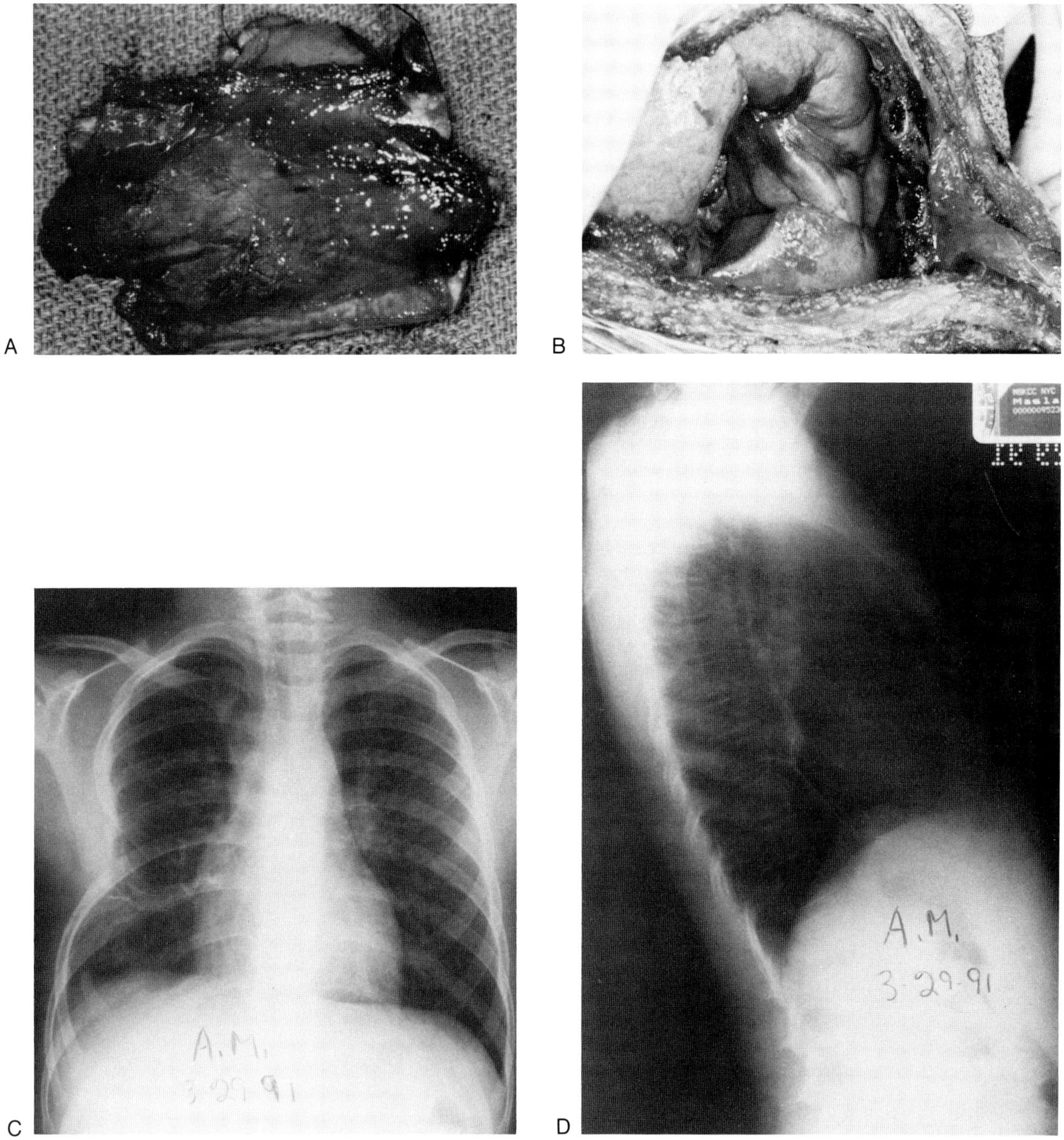

Fig. 10-18. **(A)** Photograph taken in the operating room on 7/12/90, showing the surgical specimen removed. Visible are ribs 3 through 5. The view shows the inner surface with the tumor mass centered on the fifth rib and some lung tissue, which was very adherent to the tumor and was wedge excised from the lung. **(B)** Photograph taken in the operating room on 7/12/90 after resection of ribs 3 through 5, along with wedge excision of the confluence of right upper, right middle, and right lower lobes. The cut rib ends are seen to the right. The right middle lobe is centrally located, with the upper lobe toward the top of the photograph and the lower lobe to the left. **(C)** PA chest x-ray almost 9 months postoperatively and after the completion of chemotherapy. The defect of the missing portions of ribs 4 through 6 is visible. We repaired this with Marlex mesh but will be very interested to see how this progresses in a growing boy. The lungs appear to be clear. **(D)** Lateral chest x-ray of the patient taken 3/29/91.

Patient: J.K. (Fig. 10-19)

Sex: Male

Age: 43

Diagnosis: Mesothelioma in the right chest

Stage: Locally advanced

Complaint: Pleural effusion with chest pain

History and Examination: This man had developed a painful pleural effusion, diagnosed elsewhere. Biopsies had been taken to prove that this was a mesothelioma, and it was thought that no treatment for prolonged survival could be carried out.

Treatment: He came to us. The diagnosis was confirmed. On 8/16/66 a right parietal pleurectomy was performed in this relatively healthy man. On 2/13/67 P-32 was instilled. On 1/18/69 radiotherapy was given. Gradually the mesothelioma regrew. On 11/27/70 an apical recurrence was implanted with I-125 seeds. Gradually the tumor enlarged. It caused recurrent pain and some dyspnea. The patient died of disease some 6 years postoperatively on 11/6/72.

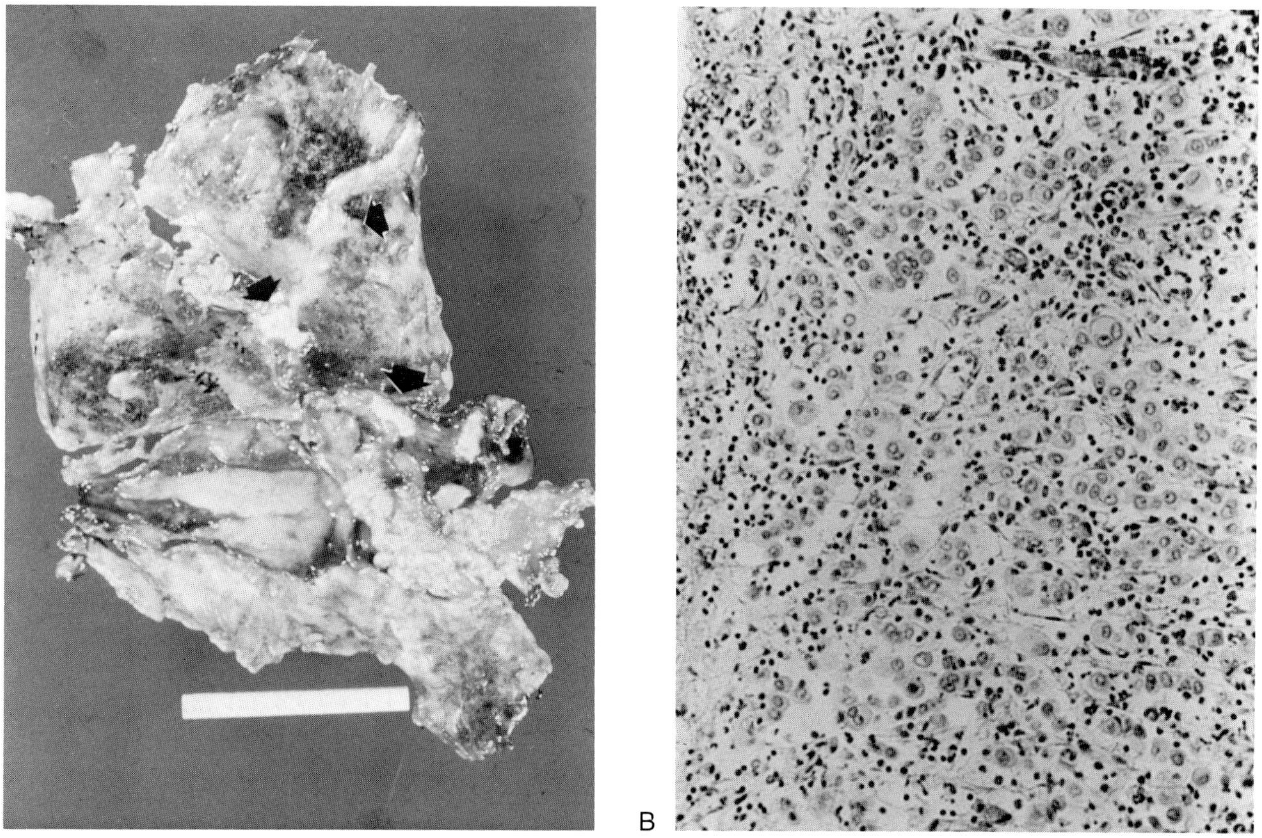

A B

Fig. 10-19. **(A)** Photograph of the thickened pleura removed during the operation. **(B)** Photomicrograph of the mesothelioma specimen removed from the patient. (*Figure continues.*)

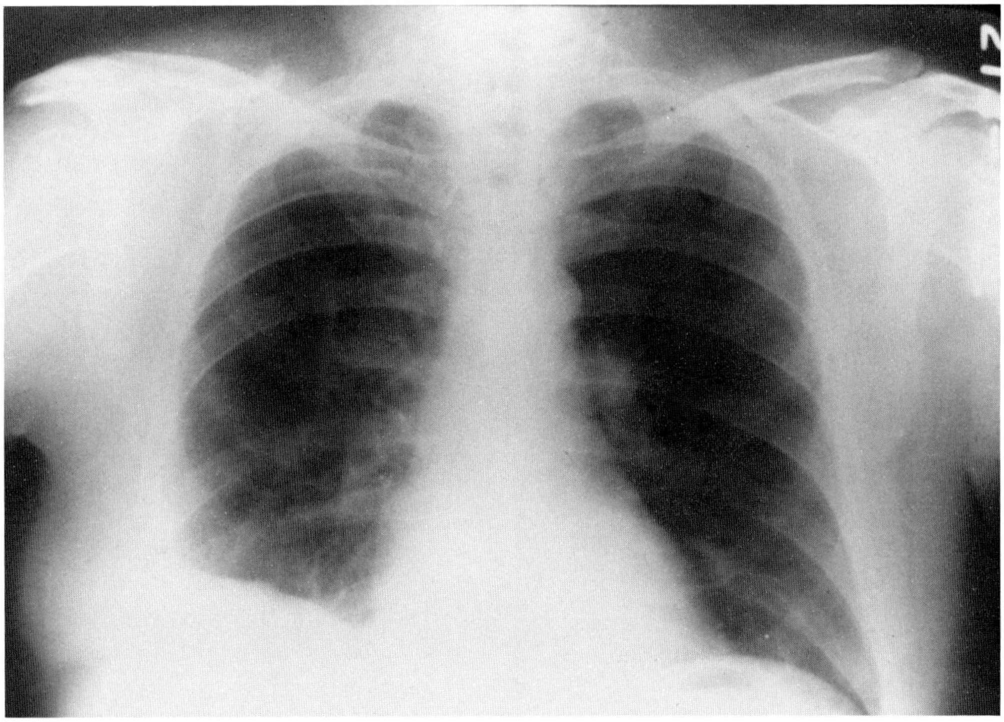

C

Fig. 10-19 (*Continued*). **(C)** PA chest x-ray taken postoperatively after right thoracotomy and pleurectomy, which were performed on 8/16/66. The lungs are relatively clear. There is some moderate elevation of the right diaphragm. (*Figure continues.*)

D

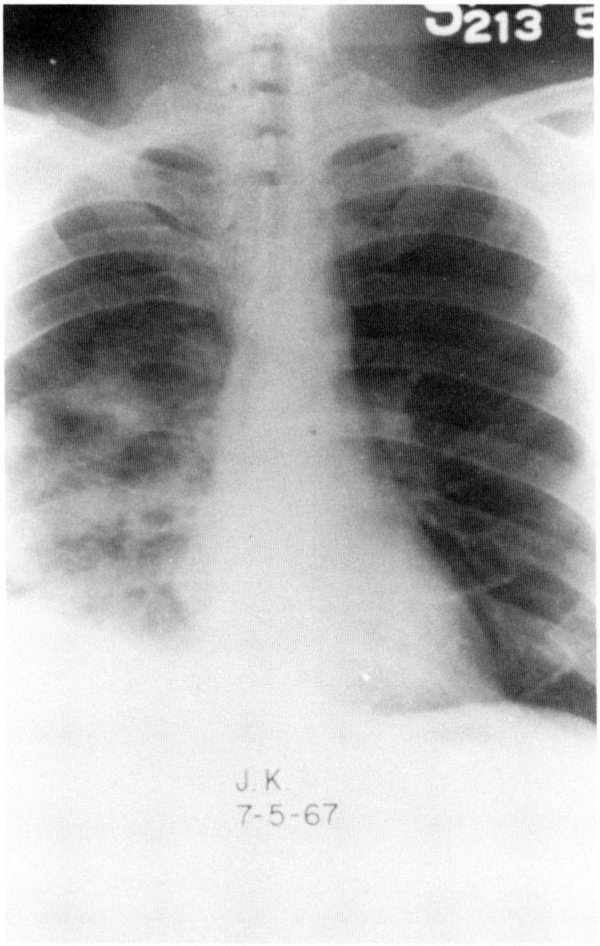

E

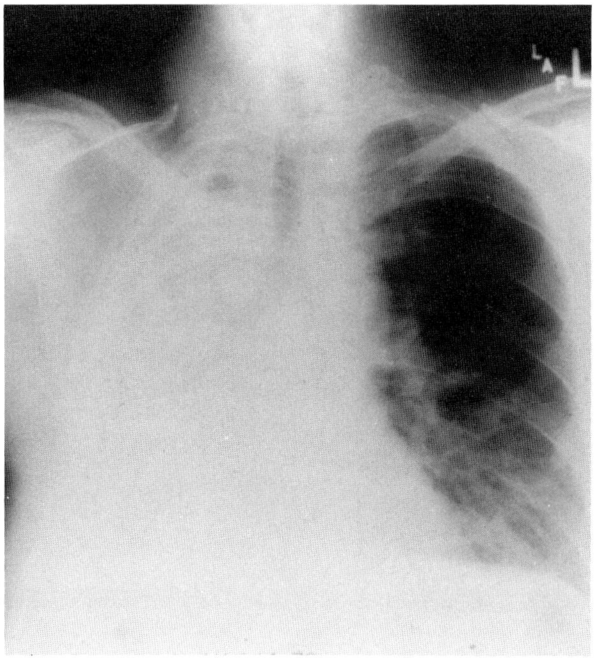

Fig. 10-19 (*Continued*). Follow-up chest x-ray taken approximately 1 year after the pleurectomy. Some growth of the mesothelioma is evident. Later we carried out a limited thoracotomy and implanted I-125 seeds to the tumor that had grown in the upper chest. Later the patient received external radiotherapy to the right hemithorax. **(E)** PA chest x-ray taken on 1/14/72, not quite 6 years after the pleurectomy. The tumor has grown and opacified the right chest. The patient developed local pain and some increasing shortness of breath. He ultimately succumbed to his disease approximately 6 years after diagnosis.

Patient: J.O. (Fig. 10-20)

Sex: Male

Age: 36

Diagnosis: Chondrosarcoma of the sternum

Stage: Localized

Complaint: Three years of intermittent chest pain

History and Examination: This patient had had intermittent chest pain for three years, which had been thought to be chondritis. A mass in the distal sternum was then discovered. Radiographs and CT scans were taken, which showed a destructive process involving the distal sternum and seemingly extending inside the sternum toward the pericardium.

Treatment: On 9/30/86 a midline incision was made and appropriate skin was left over the resected distal sternum. A subtotal sternectomy was carried out. The sternum was transected in the first interspace, preserving the clavicles, manubrium, and first ribs. The cartilages were taken widely down with the rest of the sternum, including the xyphoid. The tumor was adherent to the anterior pericardium. The pericardium was opened, and the anterior pericardium was removed with the specimen. The repair consisted of a bovine fascia patch to the pericardium. Marlex mesh was used to close the chest wall defect. Our plastic surgeon consultant used an autologous rib strut bolted across the fifth ribs to give stability to this relatively large defect. Muscle and skin flaps were mobilized to give good closure of the incision.

Follow-up: The patient is now 4.5 years postsurgery with no sign of recurrent disease.

A B C

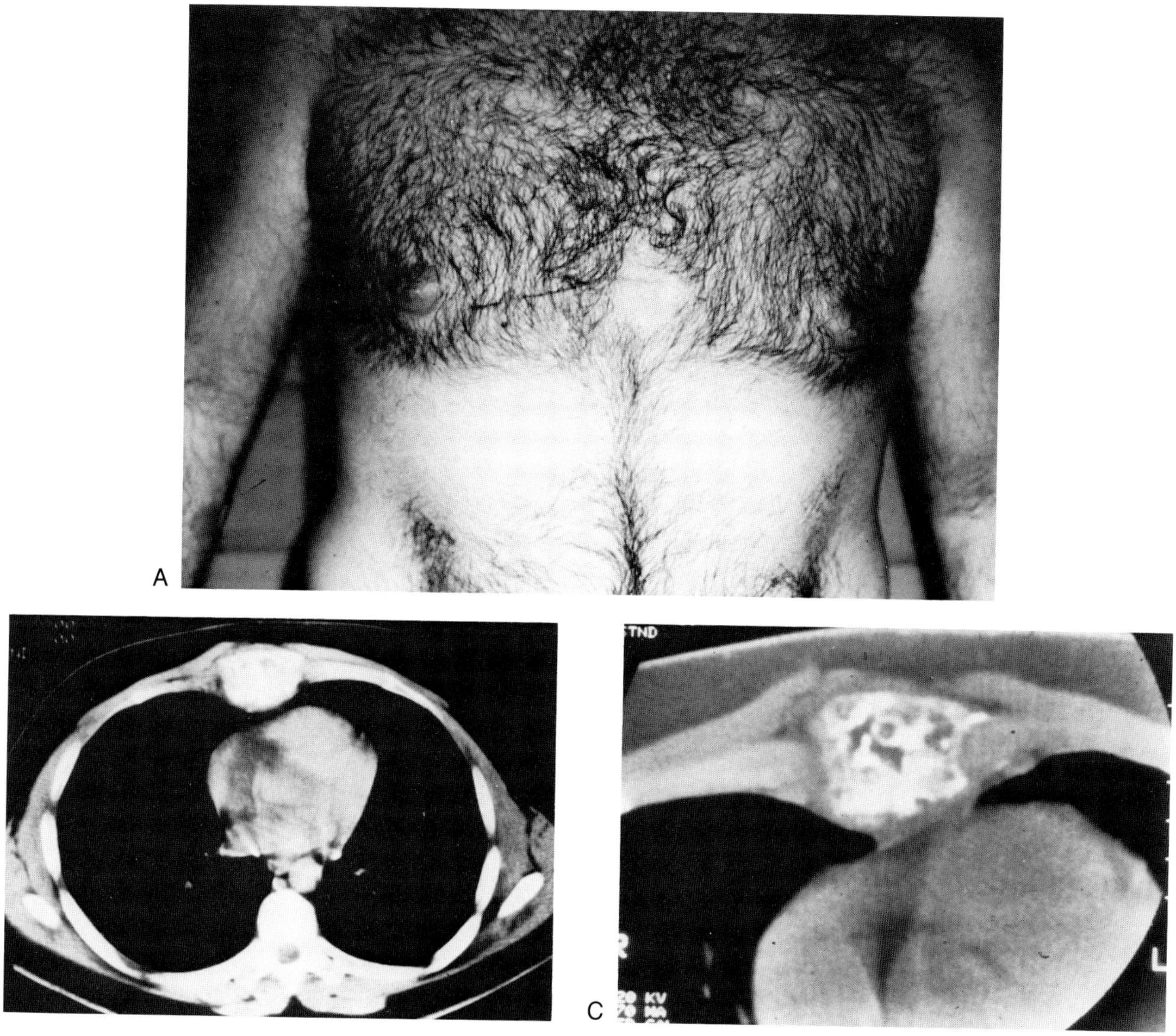

Fig. 10-20. **(A)** Photograph of the patient. There is a chondrosarcoma of the distal sternum. There is local swelling, which is difficult to see but is readily palpated. **(B)** Preoperative CT scan. The mass in the sternum is visible in this section. The inner table of the sternum is involved, but at this level the lesion is separate from the front of the heart. **(C)** Close-up view of the sternum more caudad. The destructive nature of the lesion can be seen. The tumor extends inward and soft tissue seemingly involves the pericardium. (*Figure continues.*)

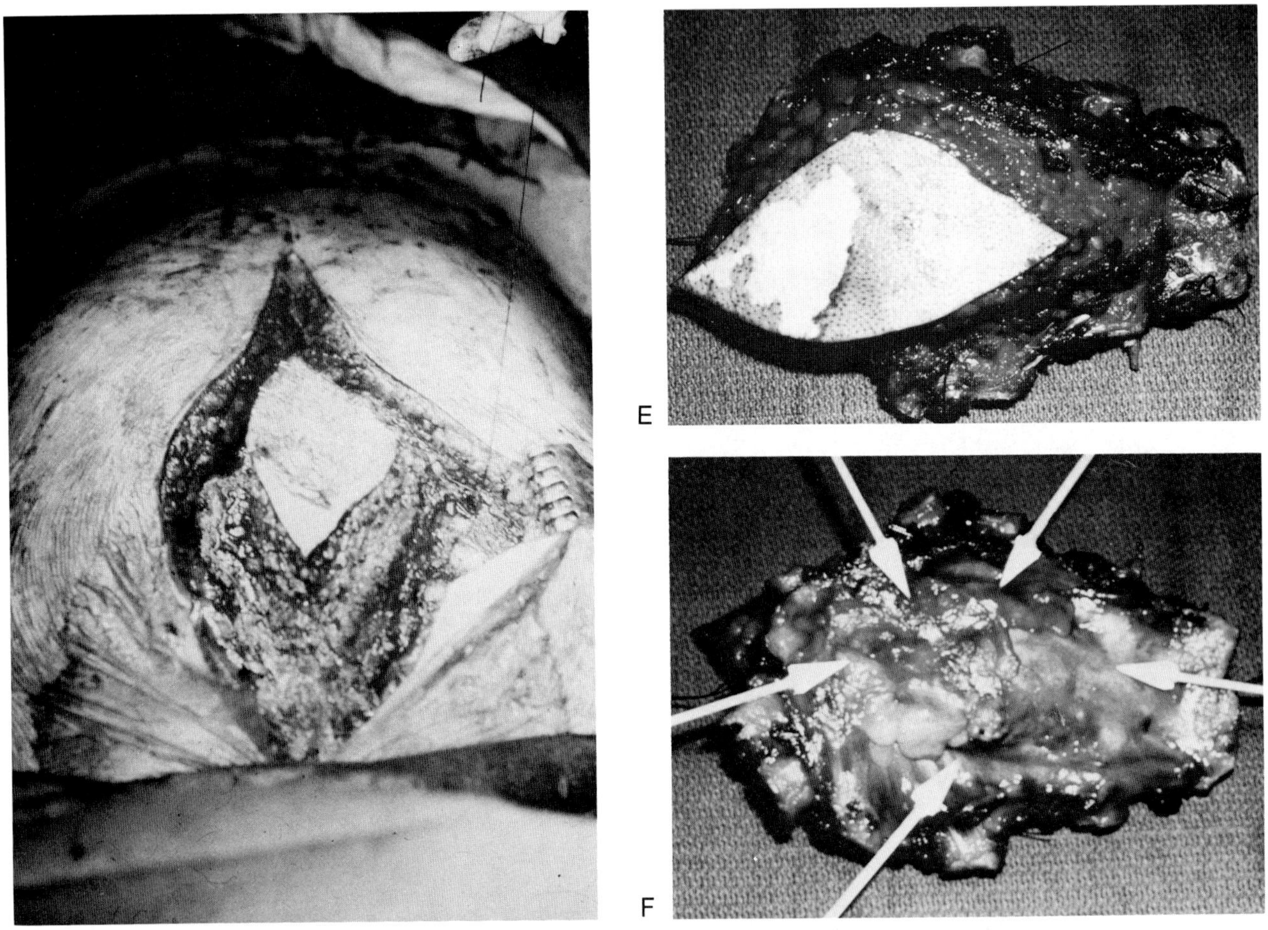

Fig. 10-20 (*Continued*). **(D)** Photograph of the incision in the operating room. An island of skin has been left intact on the front of the sternum. The skin flap and muscle flap is being retracted towards the patient's left. The patient's head is at the top of the photograph. **(E)** Photograph of the specimen taken in the operating room, showing the skin, the underlying pectoral muscles, and the sternum with costal cartilages. The sternum was cut in the first interspace, which is the part of the lesion to the right. **(F)** Photograph of the specimen turned over. The arrows point to the extent of the lesion, which had come through the posterior sternum. A piece of pericardium smaller than the arrows can be seen on the specimen. (*Figure continues.*)

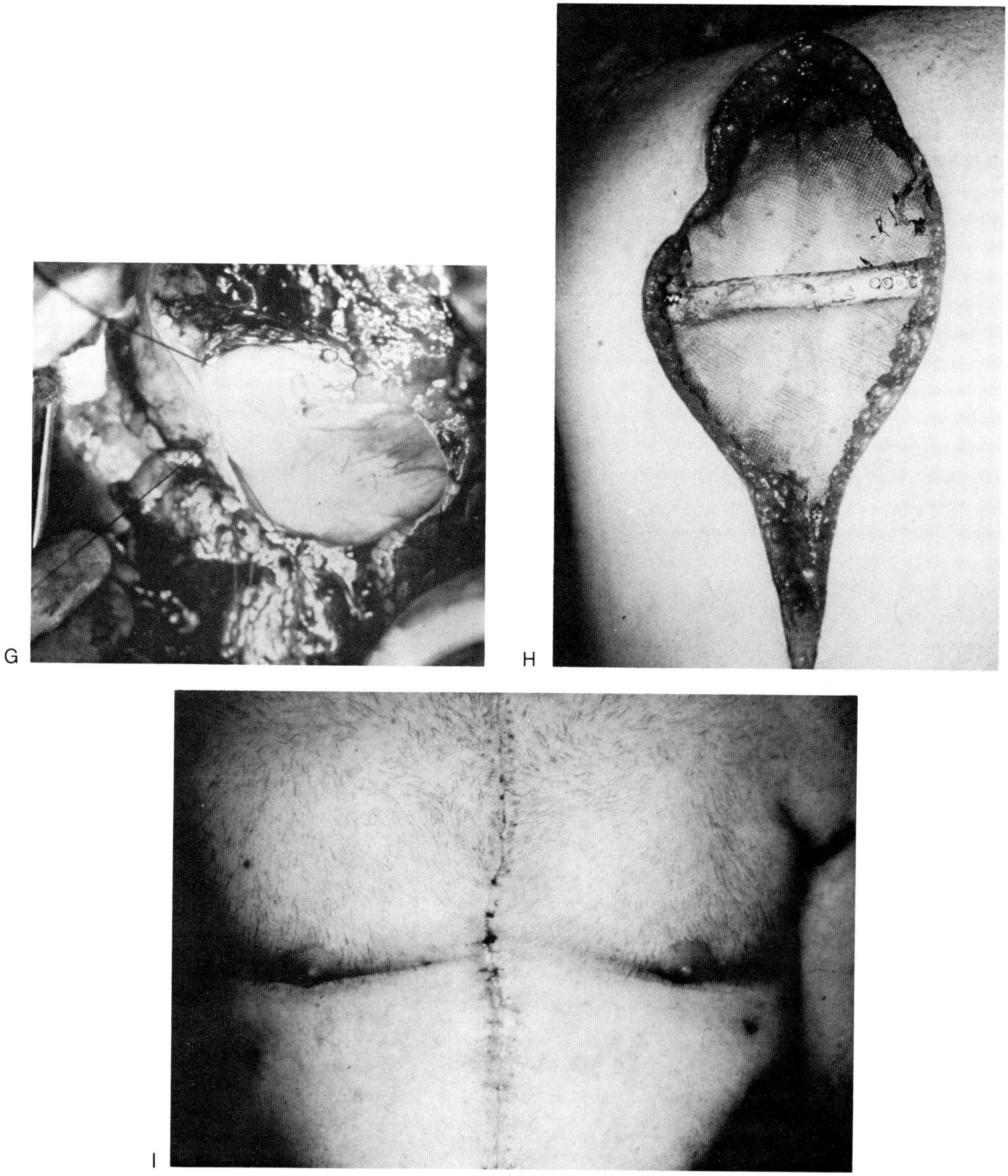

Fig. 10-20 (*Continued*). **(G)** Photograph taken in the operating room, showing the front of the heart with its missing pericardium. The stay sutures are in the pericardium. The plan is to replace the missing pericardium with a bovine fascial graft so that the epicardium will not be in contact with the Marlex repair. **(H)** Photograph showing the Marlex in place drumhead tight with the patient's head to the top of the photograph. An autologous graft of the left eighth rib has been anchored in place by securing it to the left and right fourth ribs. This is to minimize any resultant paradox with this defect without resorting to a rigid prosthesis. **(I)** Final photograph of the patient in the postoperative period. The skin clips have been removed. It was possible to close the skin defect merely by mobilizing sufficient pectoral muscle and skin flaps.

Patient: J.C. (Fig. 10-21)

Sex: Female

Age: 32

Diagnosis: Osteosarcoma sternum, recurrent, with bilateral pulmonary metastases

Stage: Metastatic

Complaint: Chest pain

History and Examination: A left radical mastectomy was performed 5 years earlier with postoperative radiotherapy. Now osteosarcoma has been found at the radiation site. Part of the sternum was resected elsewhere with skin graft. Several cycles of chemotherapy were given.

Treatment: On 1/10/90 bronchoscopy, anterior thoracotomy, excision of the anterior chest and sternum, resection of the anterior pericardium, lysis of both phrenic nerves and excision of a portion of the right innominate, left innominate, and superior vena caval veins with internal venovenous shunt with pericardial patch were performed. An afterloading catheter was placed for internal radiotherapy repair of both phrenic nerves. Reconstruction of the anterior chest with a Marlex mesh methyl methacrylate sandwich was carried out. The large chest wall skin defect was repaired with a myocutaneous flap (12 × 20 cm) from the left latissimus dorsi muscle. A reverse abdominal flap and a split thickness skin graft to the latissimus dorsi muscle flap donor site and to the right lateral chest wall were performed, as was right breast flap advancement.

Follow-up: The patient died on 6/9/90 with progressive lung metastases, in spite of continued chemotherapy.

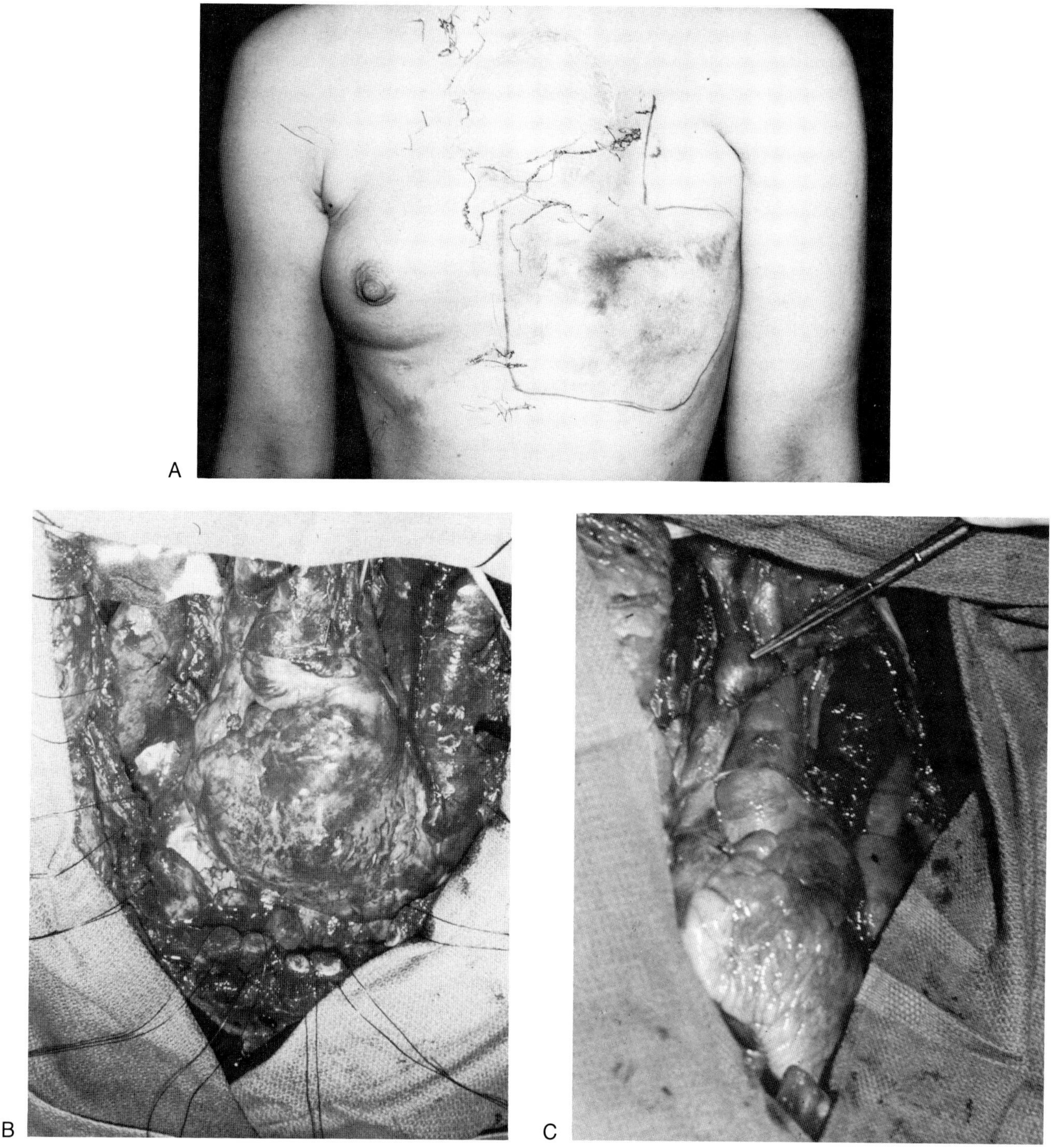

Fig. 10-21. **(A)** There has been a previous radical mastectomy. A skin graft can be seen where the first excision of the sternal osteosarcoma occurred. The markings on the chest wall outline the area of tumor involvement to be resected. **(B)** Photograph of the operation. In all of the remaining views of this patient the head is to the top of the figures. The front of the chest has been removed. The cartilages of the costal arches can be seen in the inferior portion of the photograph. The heart is in the middle, with the pericardium resected. A staple line in the left lung is visible. Repair of the superior vena cava is partially visible at the top of the photograph. **(C)** Photograph showing the bare heart at the bottom. The hemostat points out the superior vena cava. A suture repair of the right innominate vein and vena cava can be seen to the left. (*Figure continues.*)

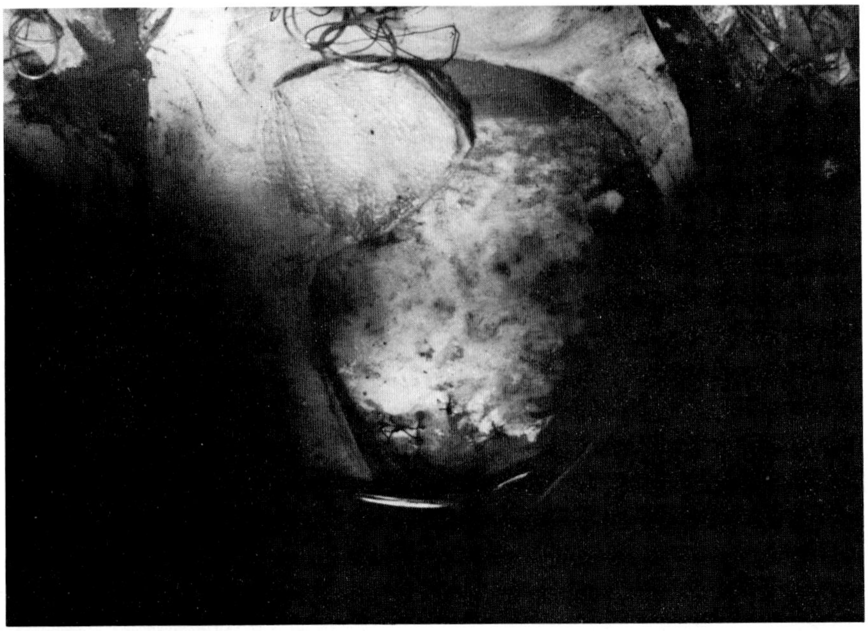

D

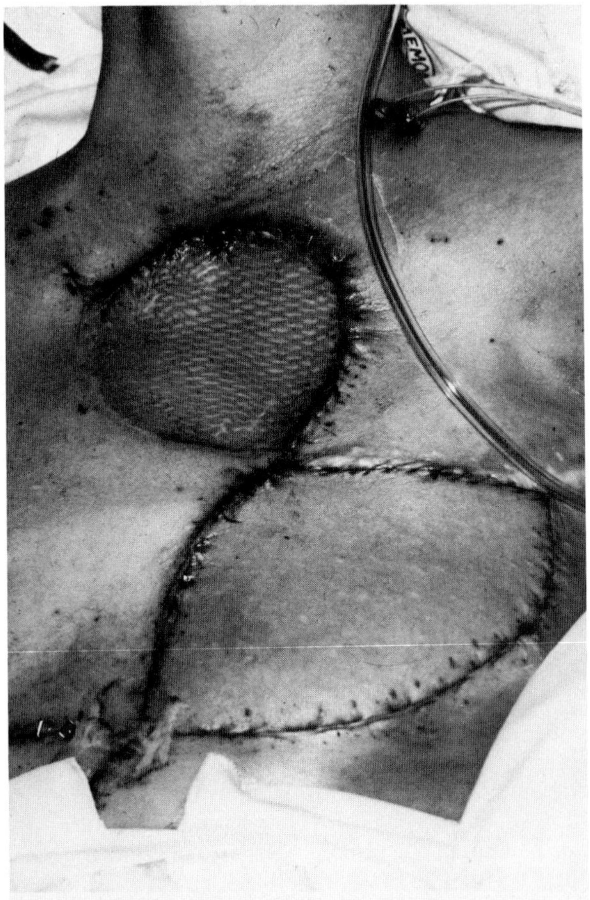

E

Fig. 10-21 (*Continued*). **(D)** Photograph at operation. Marlex mesh with methyl methacrylate "sandwich" is sewn in place. The former skin graft in the upper chest has been saved and is seen as a flap at the top of the photograph. **(E)** Photograph in the operating room at the end of the operation. The former skin graft is seen above. There is a new insertion of a left latissimus myocutaneous graft below. (*Figure continues.*)

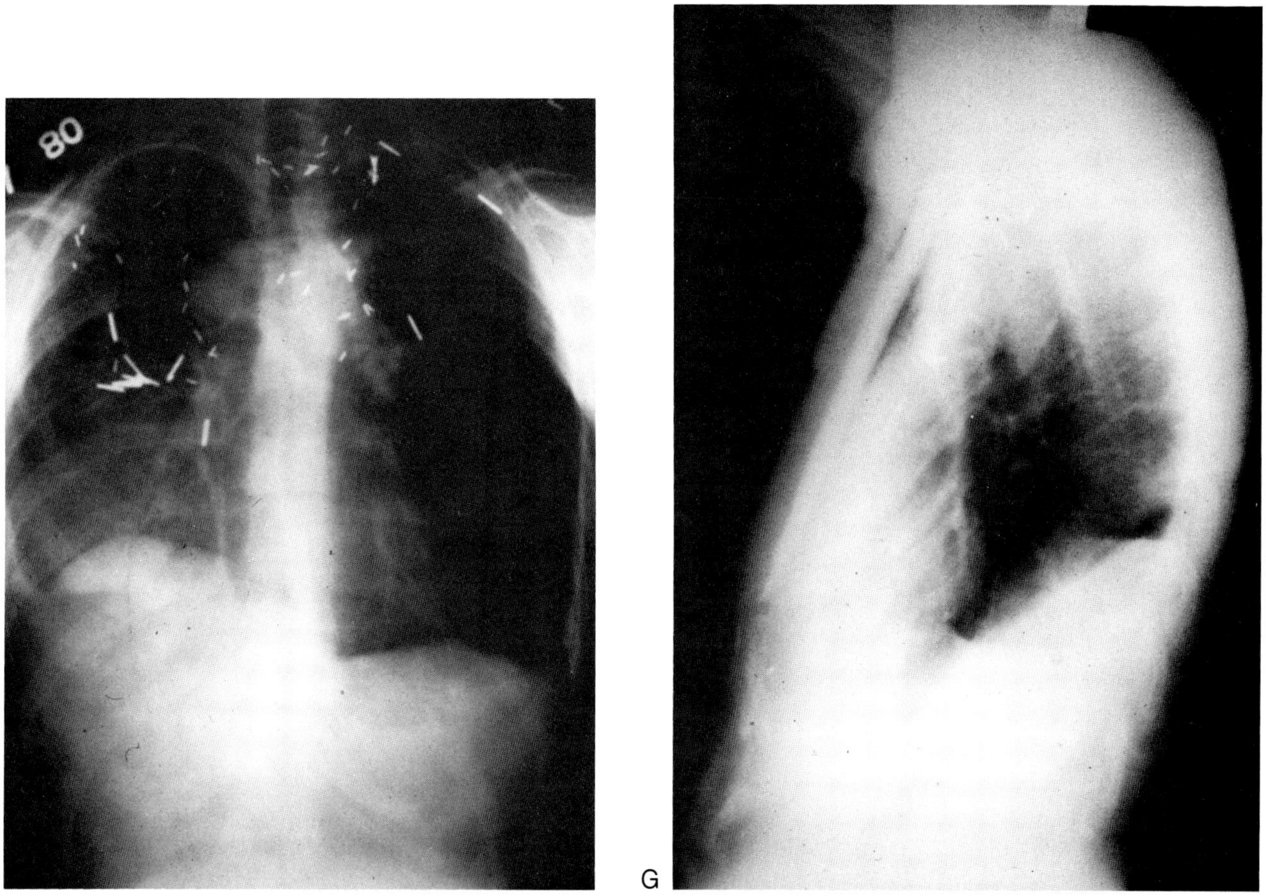

F G

Fig. 10-21 (*Continued*). **(F)** PA chest x-ray postoperatively. **(G)** Lateral chest x-ray postoperatively. The new methyl methacrylate sternum can be seen.

TRACHEA

Patient: A.P. (Fig. 10-22)

Sex: Female

Age: 30

Diagnosis: Sarcoma, probably rhabdomyosarcoma

Stage: Localized lesion

Complaint: Mass in right upper chest anteriorly

History and Examination: This 30-year-old woman had Hodgkin's disease in her right neck region in 1966, which was apparently cured by radiotherapy. In mid-1988 she developed a mass in her right lower neck, centered around and just below the right clavicle. Biopsy showed that this was a malignant sarcoma.

Treatment: She received seven cycles of chemotherapy, including adriamycin. On 12/7/88 we resected the medial portion of the clavicle, the first rib, and the soft tissue full thickness including pleura around the lesion. The defect was repaired with Marlex mesh. A myocutaneous graft was mobilized from her right posterior chest by our plastic surgery service and inserted into the defect.

Follow-up: She has continued to do well with no complaints and has had negative chest x-rays since that time.

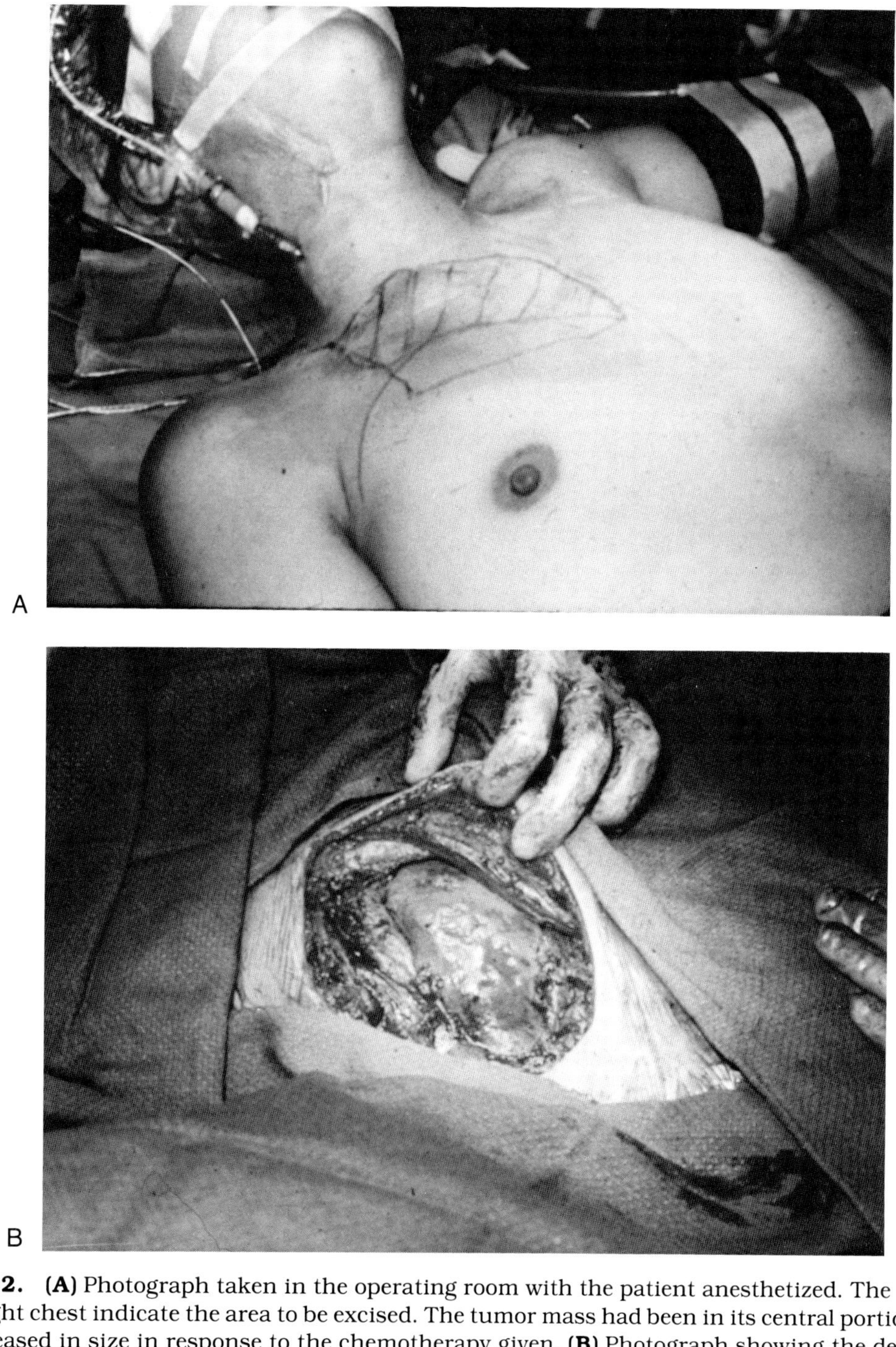

Fig. 10-22. **(A)** Photograph taken in the operating room with the patient anesthetized. The marks on the right chest indicate the area to be excised. The tumor mass had been in its central portion and had decreased in size in response to the chemotherapy given. **(B)** Photograph showing the defect in the chest after excision of the tumor. The head is toward the top of the photograph, and the sternum is to the right. The clavicle has been cut past the midline. The stump of the first rib can be seen laterally. The lung is visible in the center of the incision. (*Figure continues.*)

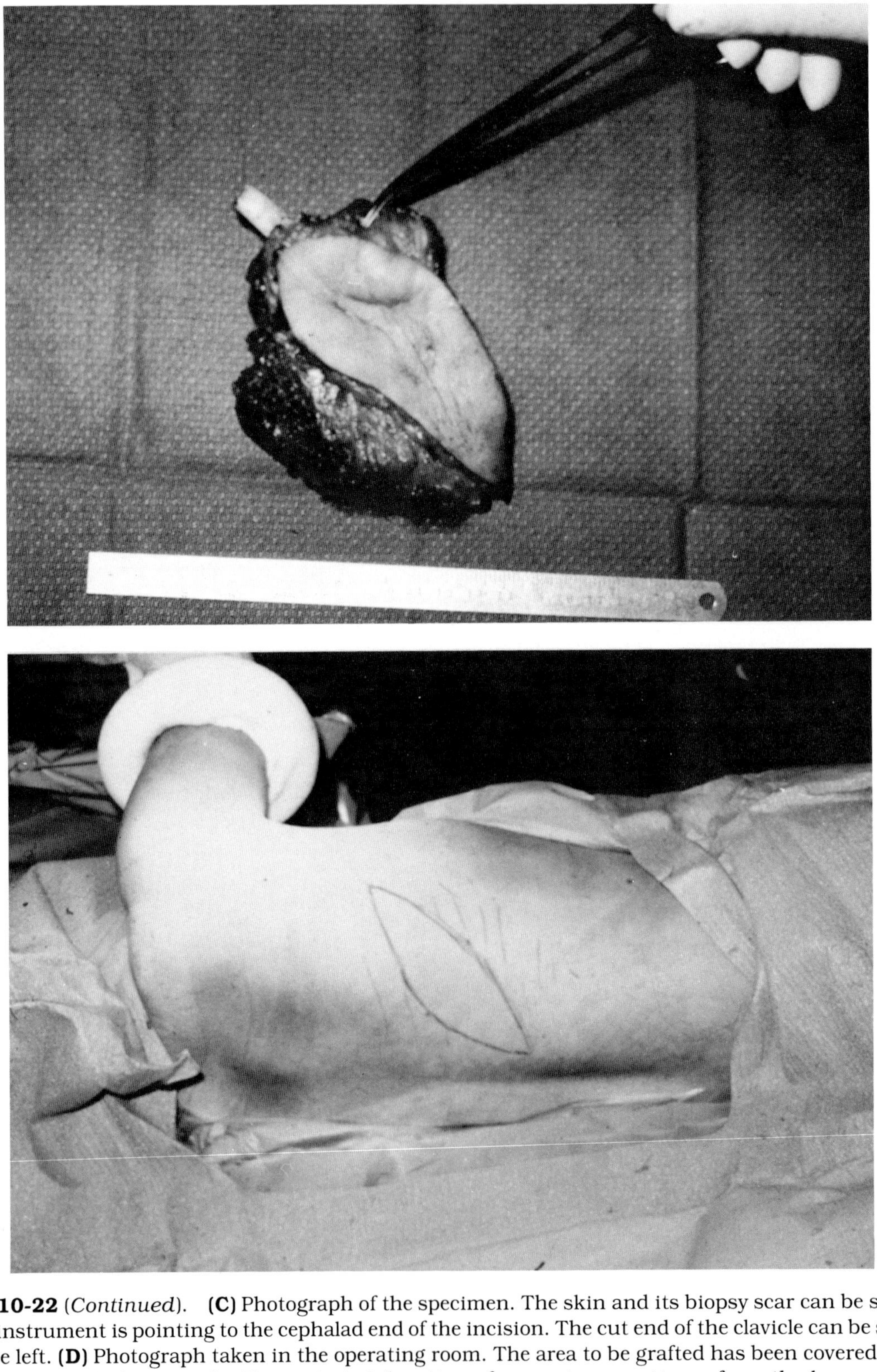

C

D

Fig. 10-22 (*Continued*). **(C)** Photograph of the specimen. The skin and its biopsy scar can be seen. The instrument is pointing to the cephalad end of the incision. The cut end of the clavicle can be seen to the left. **(D)** Photograph taken in the operating room. The area to be grafted has been covered and the patient rolled anteriorly. The projected donation of myocutaneous tissue from the lower right chest posteriorly has been drawn in. (*Figure continues.*)

E 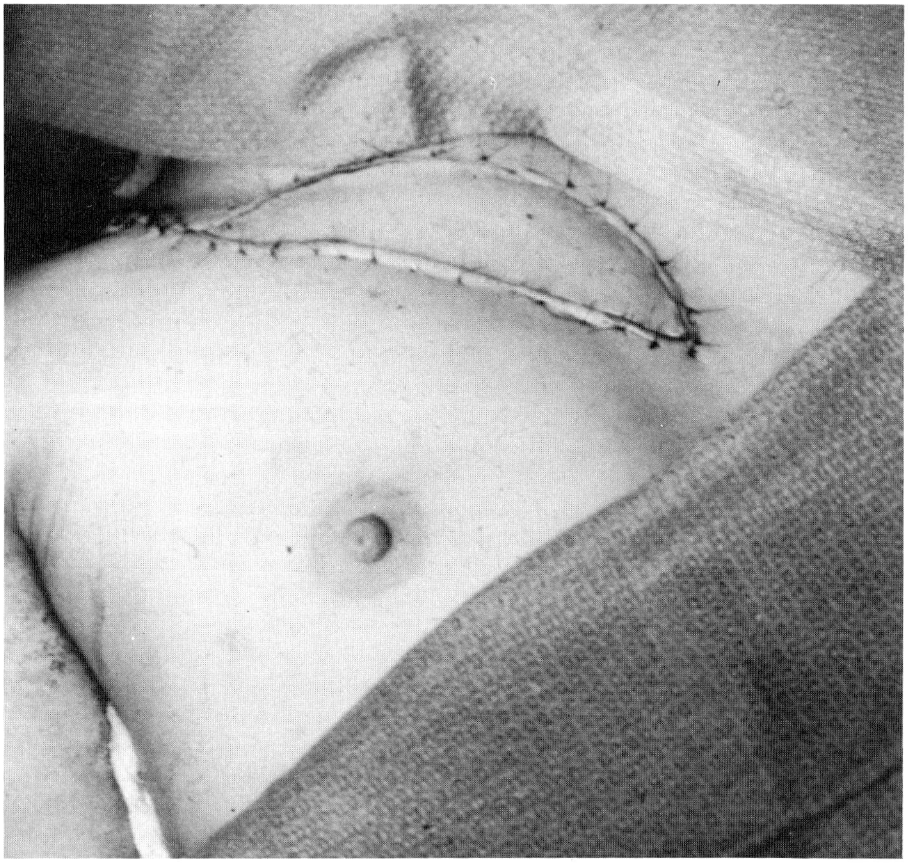

Fig. 10-22 (*Continued*). **(E)** Photograph of the final view of the patient taken in the operating room. The myocutaneous graft has been sewn in place.

Patient: S.K. (Fig. 10-23)

Sex: Male

Age: 55

Diagnosis: Adenocarcinoma of the right upper lobe, superior sulcus location with brachial plexus involvement

Stage: T4, N0, M0, stage IIIB

Complaint: Pain in the right upper shoulder and arm for 9 months

History and Examination: The patient complained of pain, and a chest x-ray was taken. This showed an area of increased density at the right apex, and physical examination at that time showed a right Horner syndrome. A percutaneous needle biopsy was done elsewhere, and adenocarcinoma was found. External radiotherapy of 4,000 rads was given to this region; this was completed on 2/23/73. Subsequent physical examination showed minimal weakness in the right hand and an area of numbness on the medial aspect of the right forearm. The chest x-ray was essentially unchanged.

Treatment: On 3/27/73 a right thoracotomy was carried out and ribs 1 through 4 were resected. A right upper lobectomy was carried out. We found scarring consistent with tumor invasion in the inferior portion of the branchial plexus in the region of the bottom cord close to the C7 and T1 vertebrae. I-125 seeds with a total dose of 6.16 mCi were implanted in this area of the brachial plexus. The area was repaired with Marlex mesh and closed. Postoperatively the patient developed a *Pseudomonas* wound infection, which responded to treatment. He was ultimately discharged home in good condition.

Follow-up: The patient remained free of disease from his lung cancer. He was troubled in subsequent years with rupture of emphysematous blebs in the left lung, which required stapling. He had no further difficulty with his right arm, and the numbness decreased and the strength improved. He died of leukemia 17 years post-thoracotomy, with no evidence of any further difficulty from his lung cancer.

Fig. 10-23. **(A)** PA chest x-ray taken on 3/25/73. It shows an area of increased density in the apex of the right chest consistent with the diagnosis of superior sulcus carcinoma. **(B)** Photograph taken in the operating room. The patient's head is to the right. The spine is to the top. A right thoracotomy has been performed. Ribs 1 through 4 have been resected along with the right upper lobe. The instrument is pointing to the posterior cord of the brachial plexus in the region where I-125 seeds were implanted. **(C)** PA chest x-ray taken on 7/5/88. Chest tubes can be seen in the left chest since the patient required an operation to staple ruptured and leaking emphysematous blebs in the left lung. In the right chest the top ribs 1 through 4 are missing, and surgical clips are seen relatively high in the right neck. There are clusters of I-125 seeds, which were placed in the lower part of the brachial plexus.

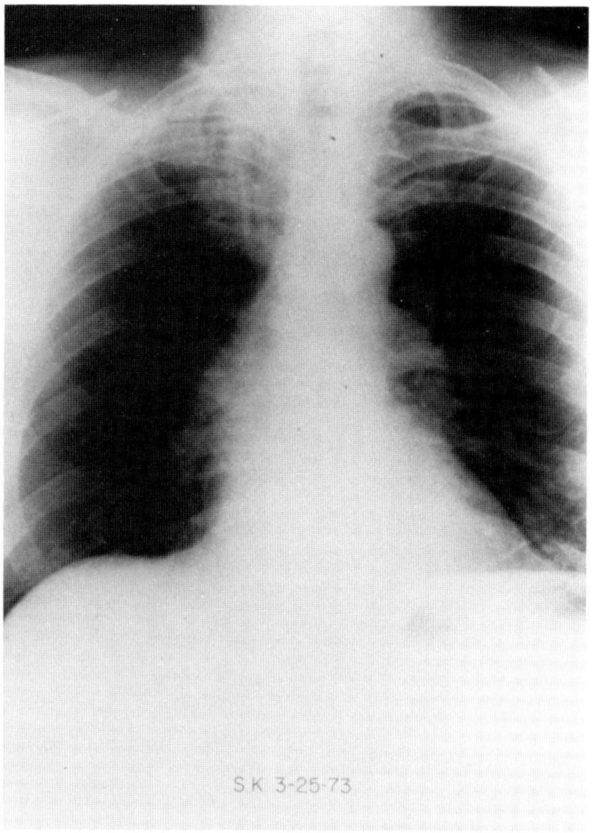

A

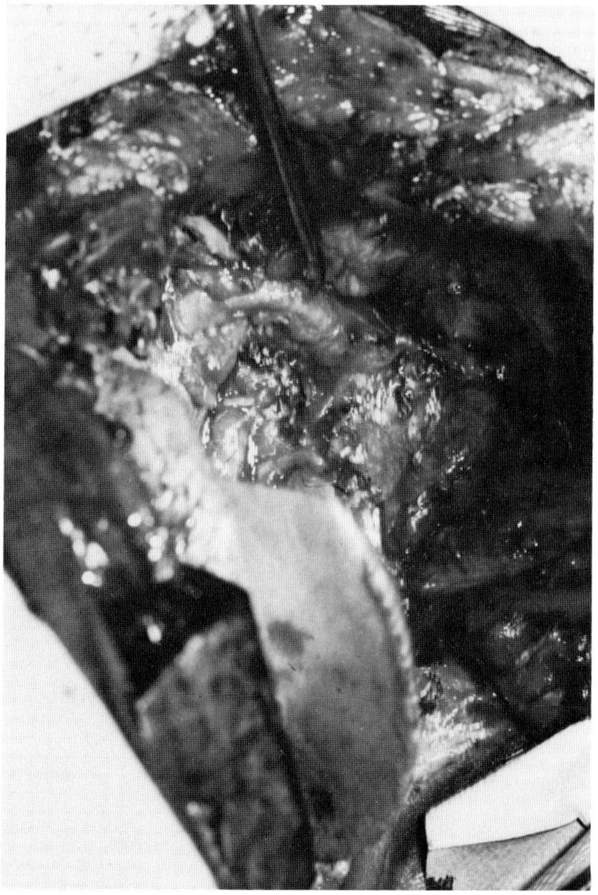

B

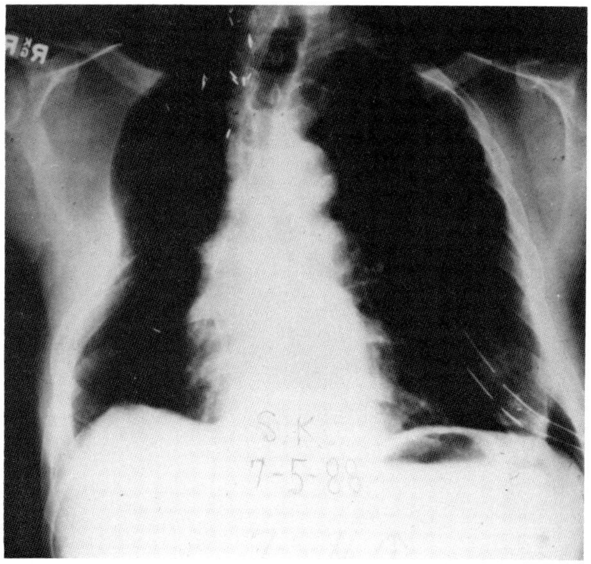

C

Patient: M.N. (Fig. 10-24)

Age: 54

Sex: Female

Diagnosis: Adenocarcinoma of the left lung, superior sulcus region, with invasion vertebral bodies of the spine

Stage: T4, N0, M0, stage IIIB

Complaint: Pain in the left shoulder for 18 months

History and Examination: A chest x-ray showed a small density at the apex of the left lung. A percutaneous needle biopsy was done elsewhere and was positive for adenocarcinoma. CT examination of the chest revealed that this mass had eroded the side of the vertebral bodies of the second and third thoracic vertebrae. There was no lymph node involvement. Physical examination was otherwise unremarkable. The patient was given a poor prognosis but received a chemotherapy course of high-dose methotrexate and high-dose *cis*-platinum plus 5,500 rads of external radiotherapy. The mass persisted, and she was referred to us for surgery.

Treatment: Surgery was performed on 10/16/84. A left thoracotomy was carried out and portions of ribs 1 through 4 were removed, leaving posterior segments of ribs 2 and 3 attached to the tumor in the left upper lobe. The tumor in the left upper lobe was wedged across, leaving it attached in the costovertebral angle while a left upper lobectomy was completed. Our spine consultants carried out left laminectomy at the T2 and T3 level. Following this, an en bloc excision removed the lung tumor with rib segments 2 and 3, including the transverse processes, rib articulations, pedicles, and most of the vertebral bodies of T2 and T3. The spine was reconstructed with metal screws in the bodies of T1 and T4, embedded in methyl methacrylate with autologous bone graft. The patient had an uneventful postoperative course. She was out of bed the next day and was discharged home uneventfully. No residual tumor was found in the specimen. The lung and lymph nodes were free of tumor. The patient received postoperative chemotherapy.

Follow-up: The patient is alive and well with no sign of disease more than 6.5 years after the operation.

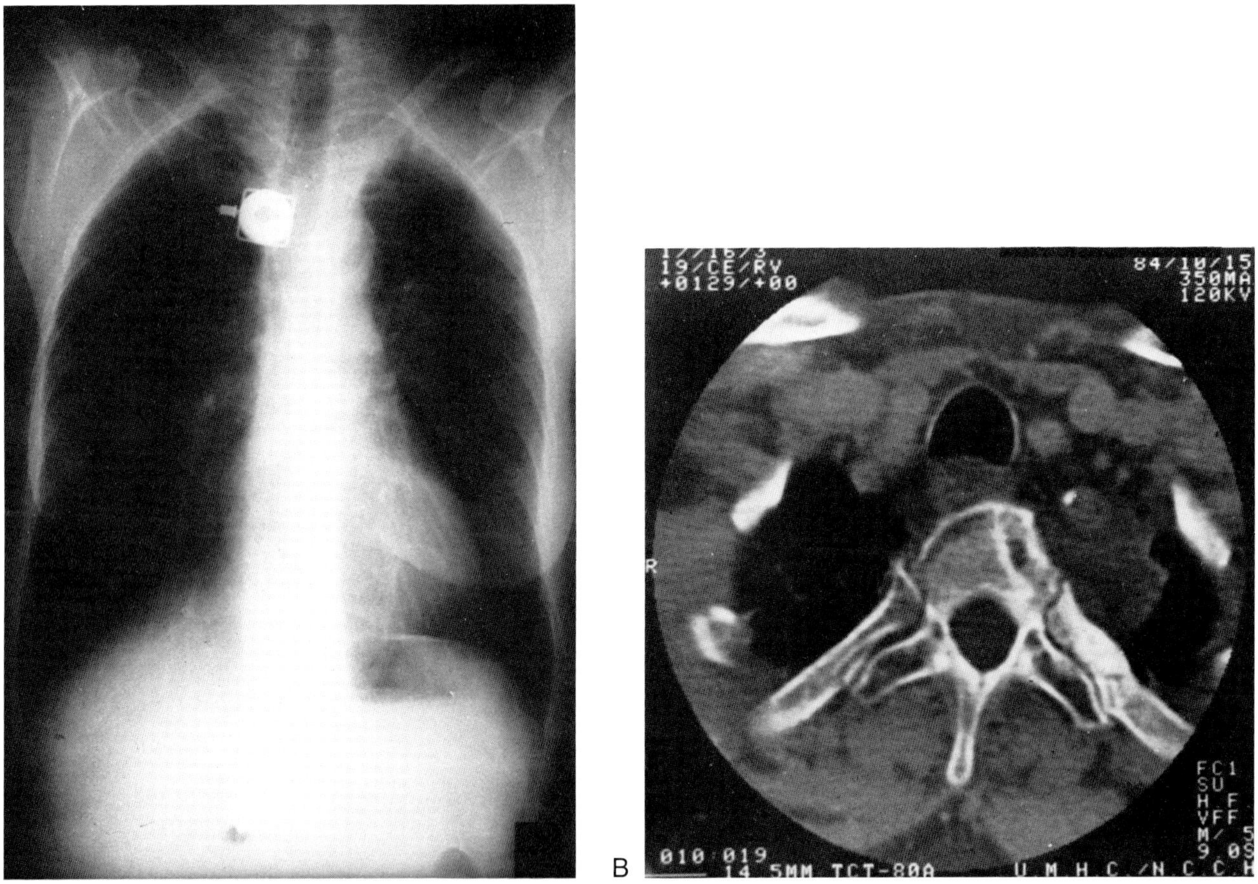

A B

Fig. 10-24. **(A)** PA chest x-ray before operation, October 1984. The infusiport is seen in place. A tumor density is seen at the left apex. **(B)** CT scan at the level of the second thoracic vertebra. The tumor is seen in the apex of the left upper lobe with destruction of part of the body of the second thoracic vertebra. (*Figure continues.*)

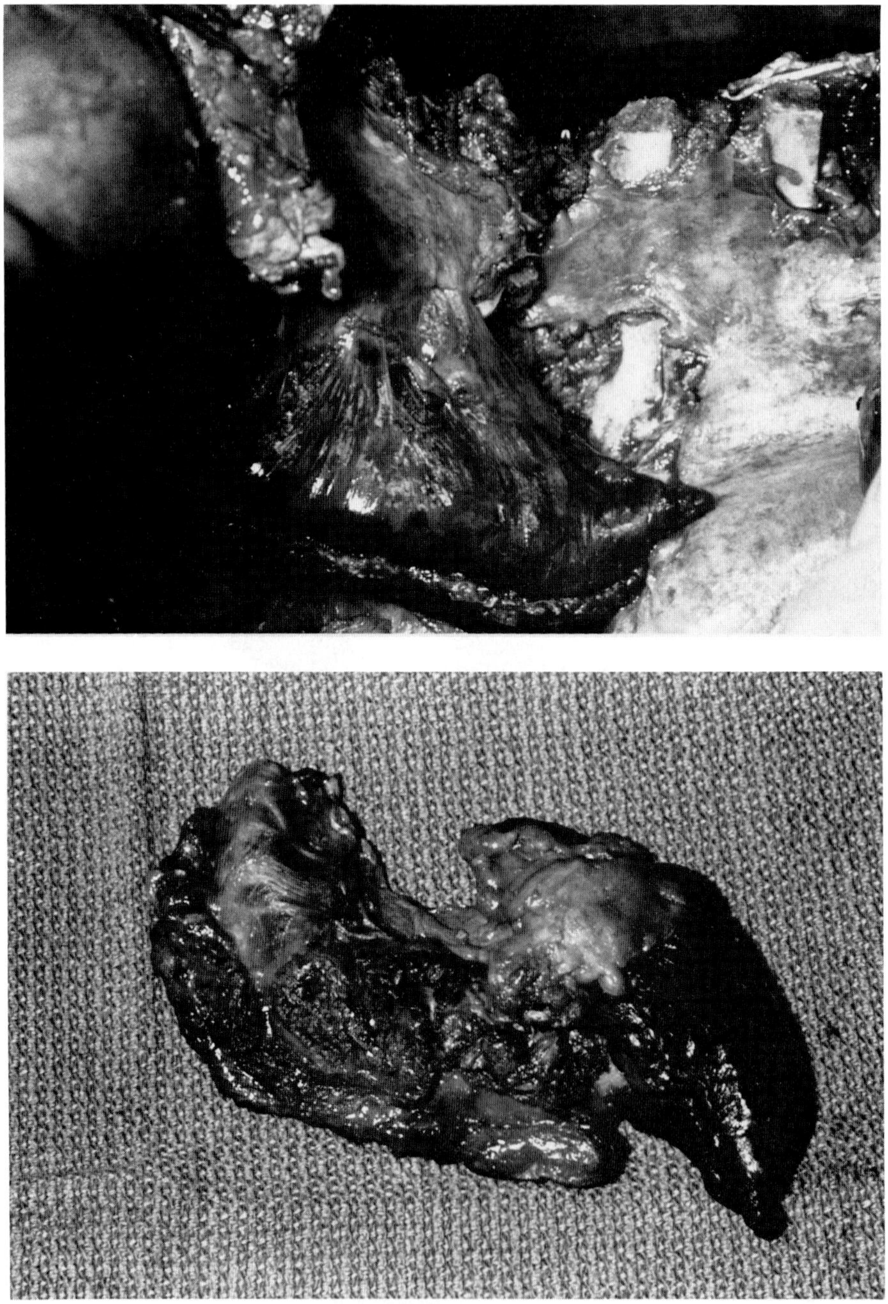

C

D

Fig. 10-24 (*Continued*). **(C)** Photograph taken during the operation. The head is to the left, the feet are to the right, and the opened left chest is at the top. The apex of the left upper lobe with tumor has been wedged free and left attached to the costospinal angle. The remainder of the left upper lobe has been resected. Ribs 1 through 4 have been cut posteriorly and anteriorly and removed. Next the neurosurgeon performed laminectomies at thoracic vertebrae 2 and 3 and en bloc excised this tumor completely. **(D)** Photograph of the surgical specimen, which contains tumor, the apex of the left upper lobe, and the costospinal elements. (*Figure continues.*)

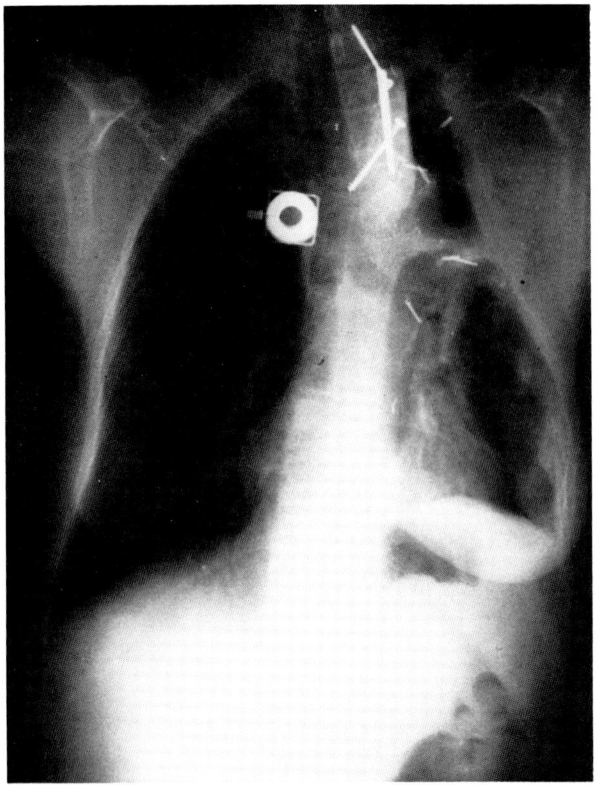

E

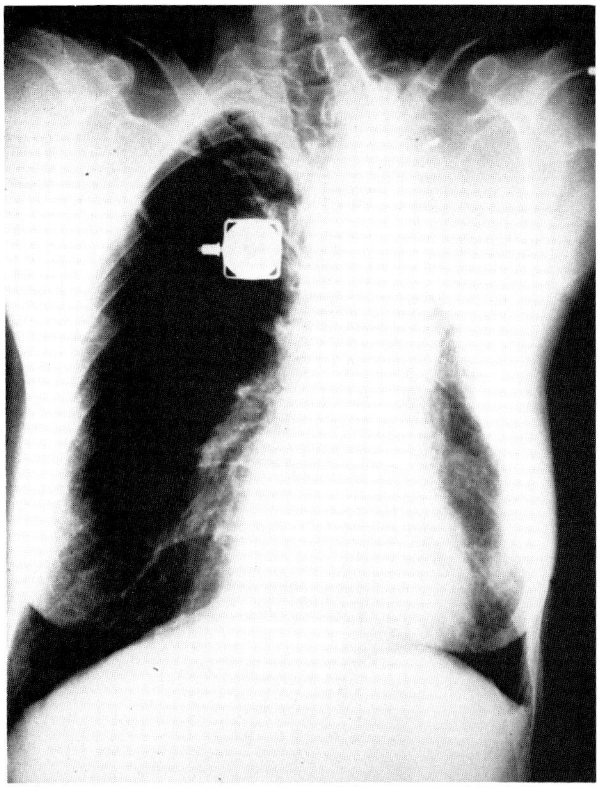

F

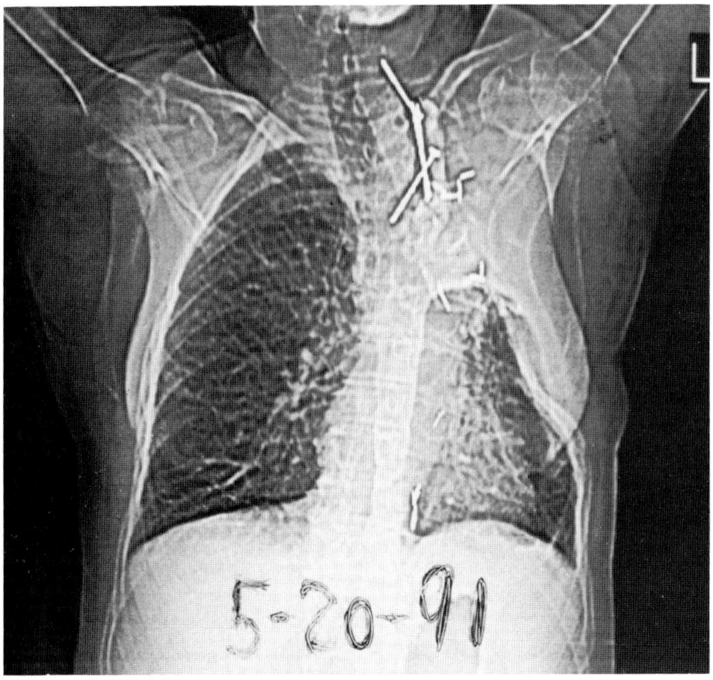

G

Fig. 10-24 (*Continued*). **(E)** PA chest x-ray in the early postoperative period. The screws, metal pin, and methyl methacrylate reconstruction of the spine can be seen. There is still an airspace at the apex. **(F)** PA chest x-ray taken on 6/9/87, almost 3 years postoperatively. **(G)** PA chest x-ray taken on 5/20/91, showing the grafted spine area. The remaining lung fields are clear. The patient has gotten along relatively well. In July 1991 she had an episode of hematemesis. On endoscopy, an inflammatory lesion was see in the esophagus, 21 cm from the incisor teeth; this was believed to be the source of the bleeding. It was treated by Ivalon sponge embolus to a feeding vessel, which was a branch of the thyrocervical trunk. Three biopsies failed to show any tumor but were consistent with an inflammatory lesion. Our concern at present is whether she will have to have surgery to remove her esophagus.

THORACIC SPINE

Patient: R.S. (Fig. 10-25)

Sex: Male

Age: 41

Diagnosis: Neurofibroma growing inside spinal canal and spine

Complaint: Five years of some pain on the right shoulder associated with discomfort in the right chest wall region of the third and fourth ribs

History and Examination: See above. The physical examination was negative except for numbness in the right fourth thoracic dermatome. A chest x-ray showed a right paraspinal mass at T4. CT and MRI showed lesions inside the spinal canal and inside the body of T4.

Treatment: A right thoracotomy was performed on 7/13/89. A portion of the right fourth rib was resected. A laminectomy at T4 with removal of tumor from the spinal canal and the body of T4 was performed.

Follow-up: Convalescence was uneventful. The patient returned to work doing strenuous physical labor. He was NED June 1990.

A C B

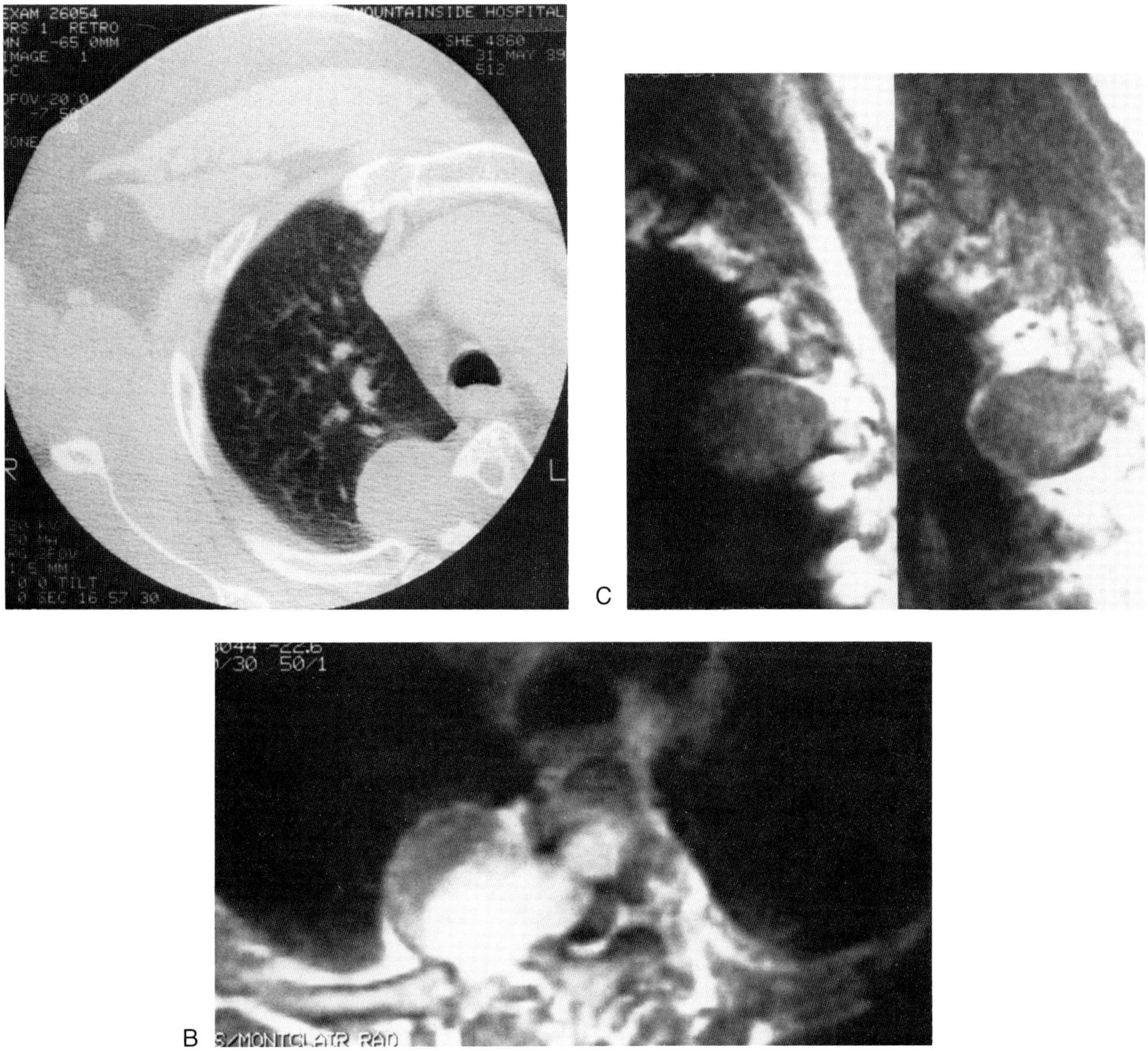

Fig. 10-25. (**A**) CT scan of the chest at the level of the fourth rib and thoracic vertebra. A paraspinal mass can be seen extending into the spinal canal. (**B**) MR image at the same fourth rib (thoracic vertebral level). The tumor is again seen in the spinal canal. (**C**) MR images of the spine in lateral view shows the tumor, which has grown into the body of the fourth thoracic vertebra.

Patient: J.B. (Fig. 10-26)

Sex: Female

Age: 28

Diagnosis: Desmoid tumor, posterior neck-chest junction

Stage: Localized

Complaint: Mass on back of upper right chest

History and Examination: This 28-year-old woman had noticed a swelling to the right of the spinous process posteriorly at the upper portion of her chest approximately 1 year earlier. This had been operated upon elsewhere, and a mass several centimeters in diameter had been removed. It was diagnosed as a desmoid tumor. It recurred approximately 9 months later and was again excised. The patient was told that this time it extended close to the bones of the spine. She came to us postoperatively. There was a surgical defect paraspinally on the right, but extensive studies failed to show any other abnormality. It was decided to wait until the tumor recurred since it was not clear how extensive it was or what would have to be resected. Over the next 4 months the tumor recurred. It was a mass 3 to 4 cm in diameter.

Treatment: The patient was taken to the operating room on 7/24/75 with our neurosurgeons in attendance. A wide excision was made, which extended from C4 to below T2. Tumor from the spinous process to the transverse process was resected from the posterior spinal bony structures. We believed that the margins were clear cephalad and caudad and possibly laterally. Biopsy of tissue from the interlaminar spaces was positive for tumor. We decided not to resect the posterior spinal structures over this large area. Our radiation oncologist placed five afterloading catheters parallel to the spine directly on the bony structures of the spine. One catheter was to the left of the spinous processes; one was to the right of the spinous processes; and three were placed a little over 1.0 cm apart extending laterally to the right transverse processes. The catheters extended from T4 to C3, where they were brought out superiorly.

Follow-up: After the patient had recovered from the immediate effects of the operation, these afterloading catheters were loaded with I-192. A dose to the tumor in excess of 6,000 rads was given. The calculated dose to the spinal cord was approximately 1,000 rads posteriorly and approximately 500 rads anteriorly. The patient did well. The surgical defect in the paraspinal region persisted. She has continued to do well, and 16 years postoperatively there is no sign of recurrence.

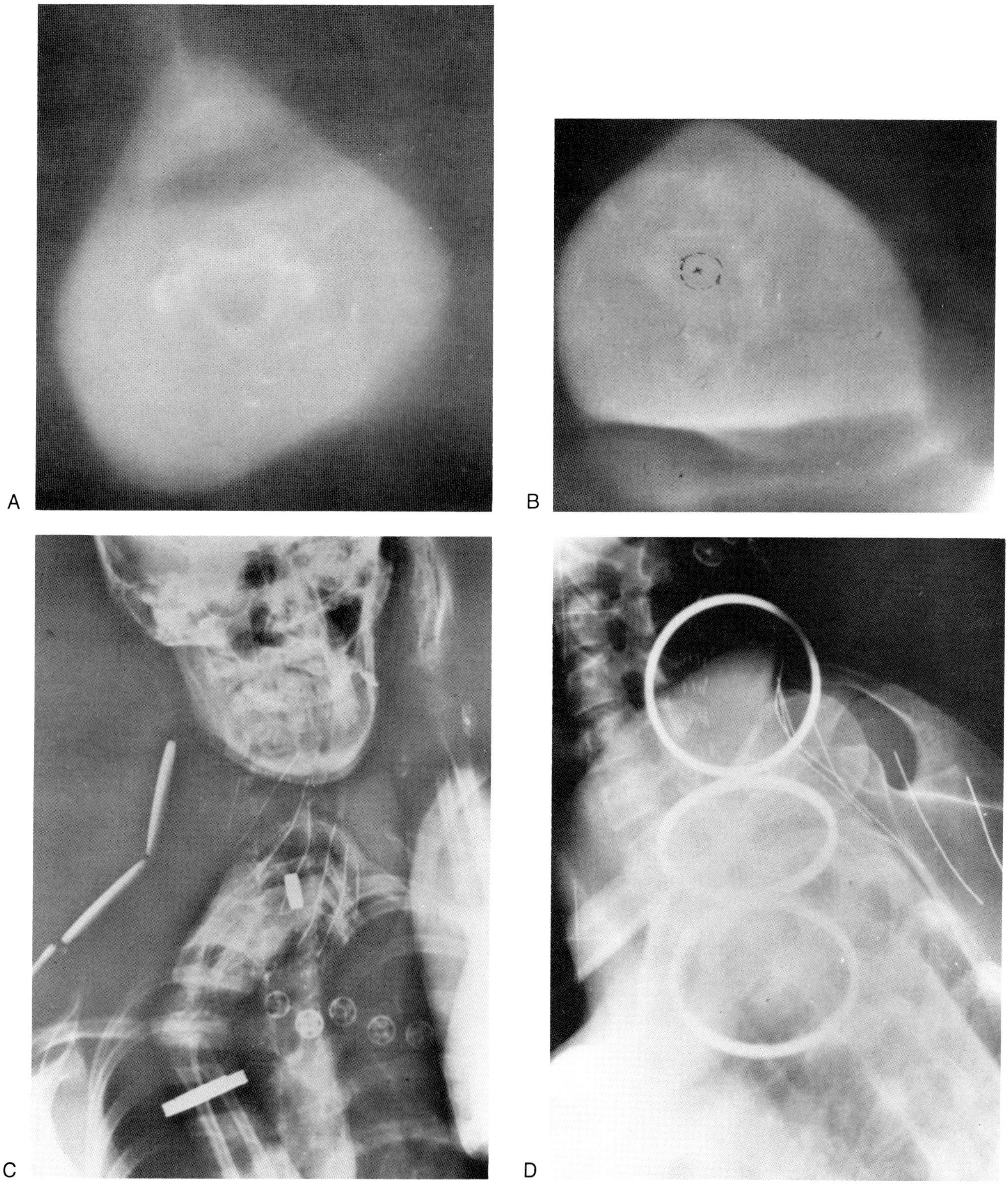

Fig. 10-26. **(A)** Cross-sectional tomogram of the neck. The five afterloading catheters can be faintly seen in the lower portion of the film. The catheter placed to the left of the spinous process can be seen, and the four additional catheters extending to the right are visible. **(B)** Cross-sectional tomogram of the neck in a lower portion. Once again, the catheters can be seen in the inferior part of the film extending to the right. The location of the spinal cord has been marked. **(C)** Chest x-ray of the patient with the catheters in place before they had been afterloaded with the I-192. Her hand is in the way of the spine, but the skin buttons securing the catheters inferiorly can be seen. The catheters streaming upward from this location to the top of the neck are visible. **(D)** An oblique chest x-ray, again showing the afterloading catheters paraspinally posteriorly. This view is distorted, and it is difficult to see the exact spatial relationship.

Patient: J.J. (Fig. 10-27)

Sex: Female

Age: 29

Diagnosis: Liposarcoma

Stage: Recurrent

Complaint: Recurrent mass on scapula

History and Examination: This 29-year-old nurse had had a lipoma removed from her scapula approximately 1 year earlier. It was reported to be a liposarcoma, and she was reoperated on. Most of the skin and soft tissue over her right scapula were removed, and a split-thickness skin graft was placed. Over the next year she developed a recurrent mass in the superior medial portion. A biopsy showed this to be recurrent liposarcoma, and she came to us for therapy. A chest x-ray was clear. Physical examination was negative except for the absent soft tissue over the scapula and a recurrent mass in the medial upper portion of the scapula.

Treatment: On 12/19/69, in cooperation with our plastic surgery service and bone tumor service, a scapulectomy was performed, saving a small portion of glenoid with its articulation with the humerus. All of the chest wall muscles, skin, and scapula were resected down to the thoracic wall from medially on the opposite side of the spinous processes, superiorly close to the apex of the chest, and laterally to the posterior axilla. The defect was closed, largely by a bipedicle visor flap which was mobilized with most of the muscles, skin, and subcutaneous tissue of the right chest wall and moved cephalad toward the apex, leaving a defect posteromedially over the spine and inferiorly in the lower chest lumbar region. These two areas were covered with split-thickness skin grafts. A deltoid flap was rotated posteriorly from the right upper extremity and turned to cover the posterior apical defect of the shoulder. The donor site on the posterior right mid-arm was also covered with a split-thickness skin graft.

Follow-up: Convalescence was uneventful, and the patient did well. She had a very useful right upper extremity with full use of the hand, wrist, and elbow. She was not able to abduct her arm but could rotate it forward some 30 degrees. She sent photographs showing this hand pinning balloons on a line at about the height of her face. She got along well for several years until lost to follow-up.

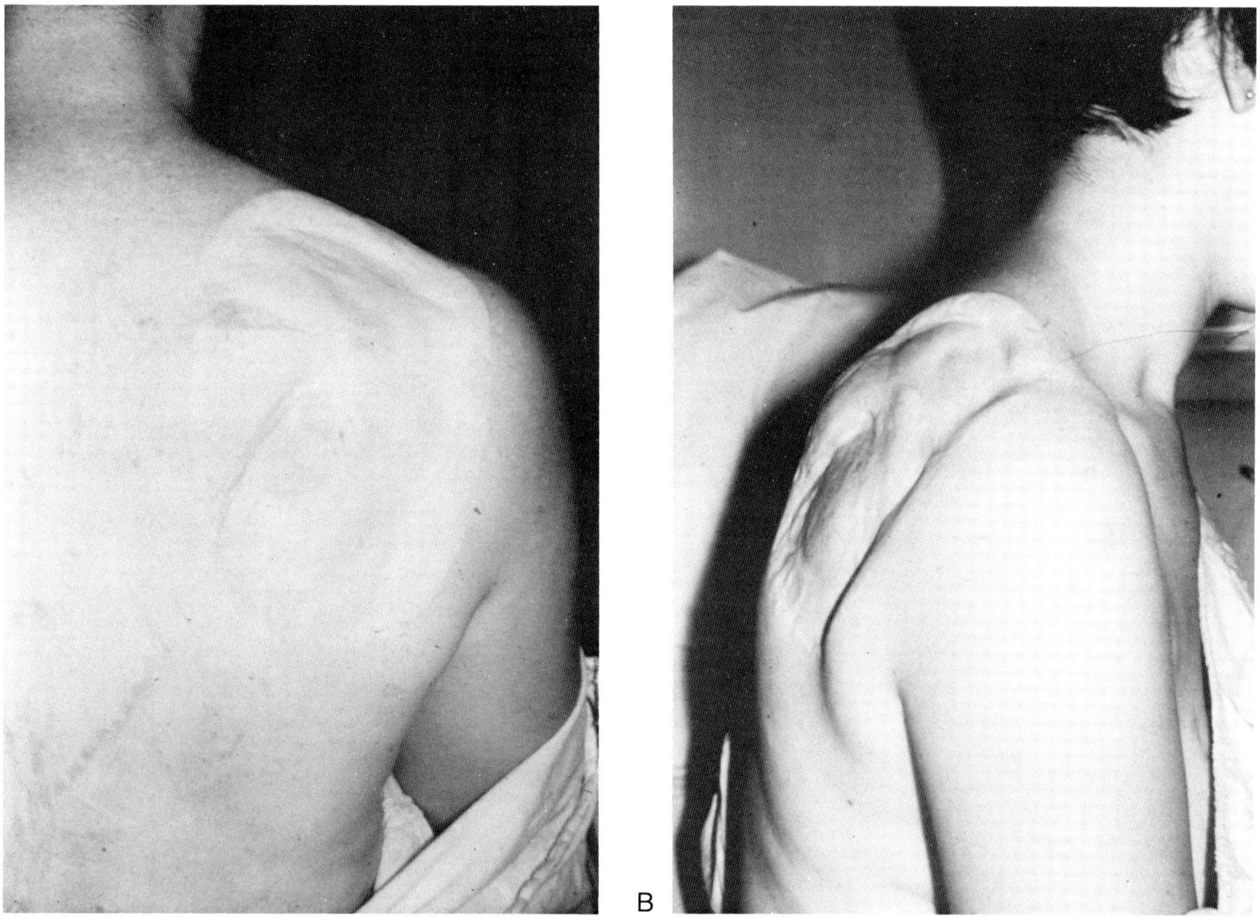

A B

Fig. 10-27. **(A)** Photograph of the posterior view of the patient. The large skin graft is visible. The upper transverse scar is where the positive biopsy for recurrence was taken. **(B)** Photograph showing a lateral view of the patient. The defect covered by a skin graft can be seen. The recurrence is in the mid-upper portion closer to the spine. (*Figure continues.*)

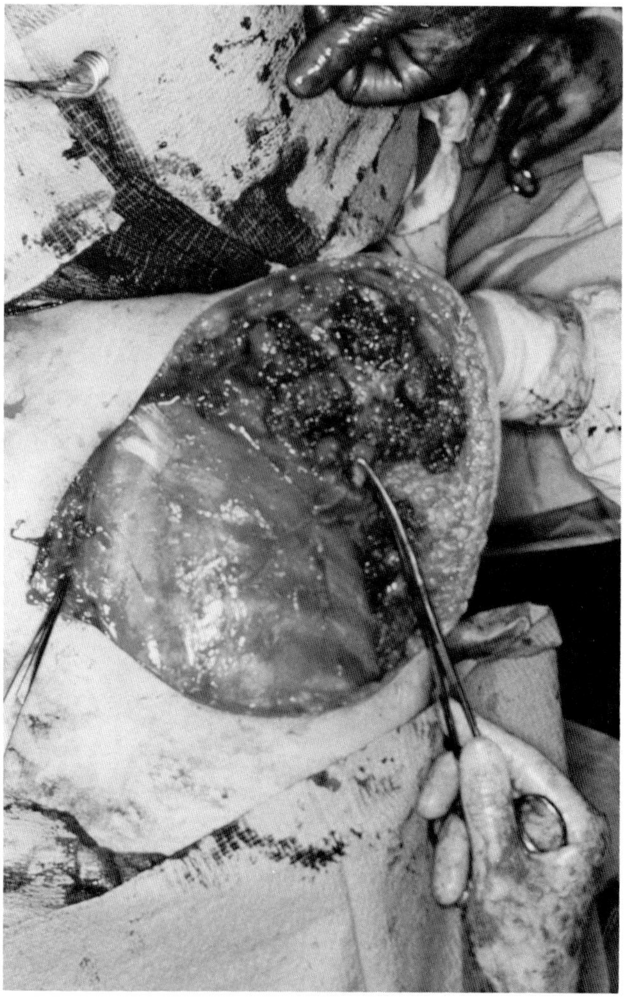

C

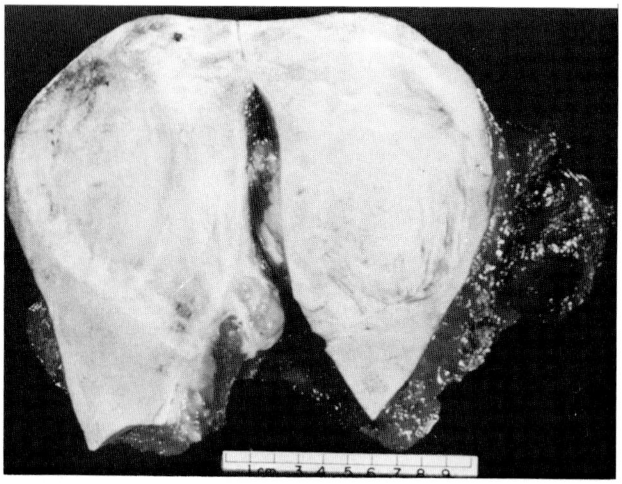

D

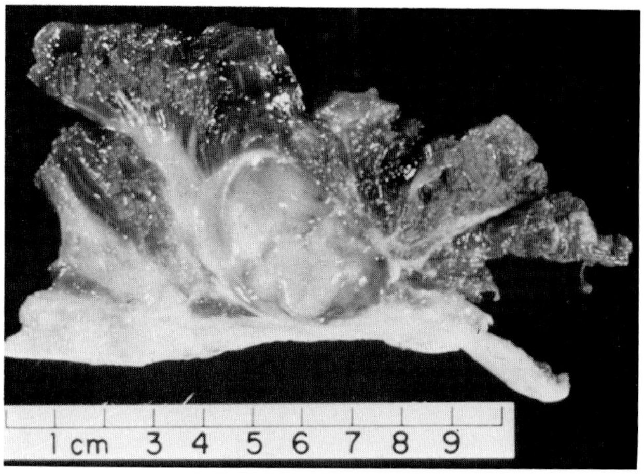

E

Fig. 10-27 (*Continued*). **(C)** Operative photograph showing the field after scapulectomy. The patient's head is to the top of the photograph. The arm is to the right. The instrument at the left side of the operative field is pointing at a spinous process. The instrument on the right side is pointing to the axillary contents. **(D)** Photograph of the removed specimen with the skin side presenting. **(E)** Cross-section of the specimen excised. The inferior part of the lesion is the thin skin graft over the recurrent tumor. The rounded recurrent liposarcoma is in the center of the photograph. The margin of excised muscle, which lay deep to the tumor, can be seen around the top of the photograph. (*Figure continues.*)

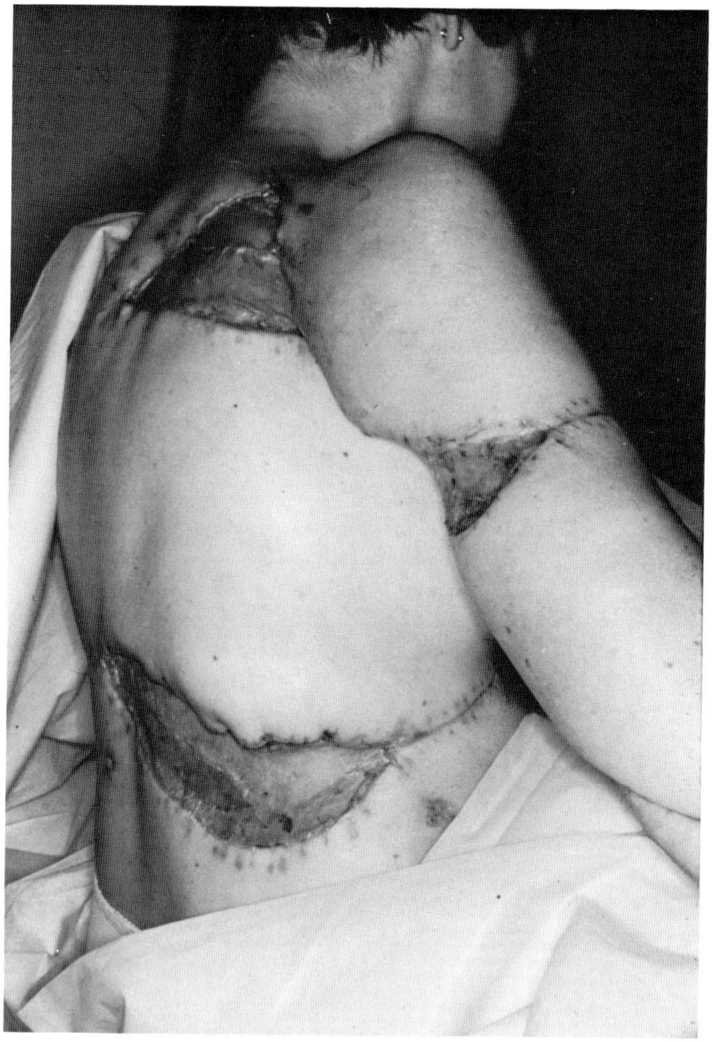

F

Figure 10-27 (*Continued*). **(F)** Photograph taken shortly after operation, showing the large visor graft, which has moved cephalad. The donor site below has been covered with a split-thickness skin graft. A deltoid flap from the right arm has covered the shoulder, and the donor site on the arm has been covered with a split-thickness graft. The residual triangular defect on the patient's back was also covered with a split-thickness graft. As time went by, further cosmetic improvement occurred.

Patient: B.J.B. (Fig. 10-28)

Sex: Male

Age: 37

Diagnosis: Mesothelioma

Stage: Metastatic

Complaint: Tumor in the fifth thoracic vertebra

History and Examination: This 37-year-old man had been operated upon 10 years earlier for a right paraspinal mass. This was found to be a localized fibrosarcomatous mesothelioma, and he had done well until his present problem in 1971. He was reexplored elsewhere, and recurrent mesothelioma was found paraspinally and removed. It was also found that the tumor had invaded the body of the fifth thoracic vertebra.

Treatment: The patient came to us with this complaint, and after much discussion we agreed to remove the fifth thoracic vertebra. The right thoracotomy was reexplored and the vertebra freed up from the right side as far as possible, but our facility for performing complete vertebral removal was limited at that time. After removal of some of the intervertebral disc cartilage and division of the right pedicle, the incision was closed. A few days later a left thoracotomy was carried out and the removal of the body of the vertebra continued and concluded. From the left side the rest of the intervertebral disc tissue was removed. The left pedicle was removed. It was then possible to remove the vertebra but to leave intact the posterior spinal structures. The defect in the spine was replaced by an autologous bone graft taken from his fibula, which had a rounded extension implanted in the center of the body of T4. An oval extension was left distally and a lateral trough cut in the body of T6 so that if this prosthesis should be extruded, it would extrude laterally rather posteriorly into the cord. Mesothelioma was found in the specimen. The patient had an uneventful course and was discharged home.

In the following years the patient had numerous recurrences of the mesothelioma in both lungs and paraspinally. After these initial four thoracotomies, a total of seven more thoracotomies plus internal radiotherapy and external radiotherapy applications were made.

In 1982 the patient developed increasing back pain and signs of spinal cord compression. A second spinal reconstruction was undertaken on 9/28/82, this time from the right side. The bodies of T4, T5, and T6 were removed. Reconstruction was carried out with pins and methylmethacrylate. The patient convalesced relatively uneventfully from this procedure and again was up and about with no signs of cord compression.

Ultimately the patient developed recurrent tumor in the right lung, which grew into the right bronchus. This was biopsied and removed by bronchoscopy. We had reached the point where the only known disease was on the right side and a right lung transplant was under consideration. The patient came into the hospital with pneumonia in the left lung, from which he did not recover. He died a respiratory death. This occurred after a total of 12 operations, including two spinal reconstructions. The time of death was 23 years after the first operation on his mesothelioma.

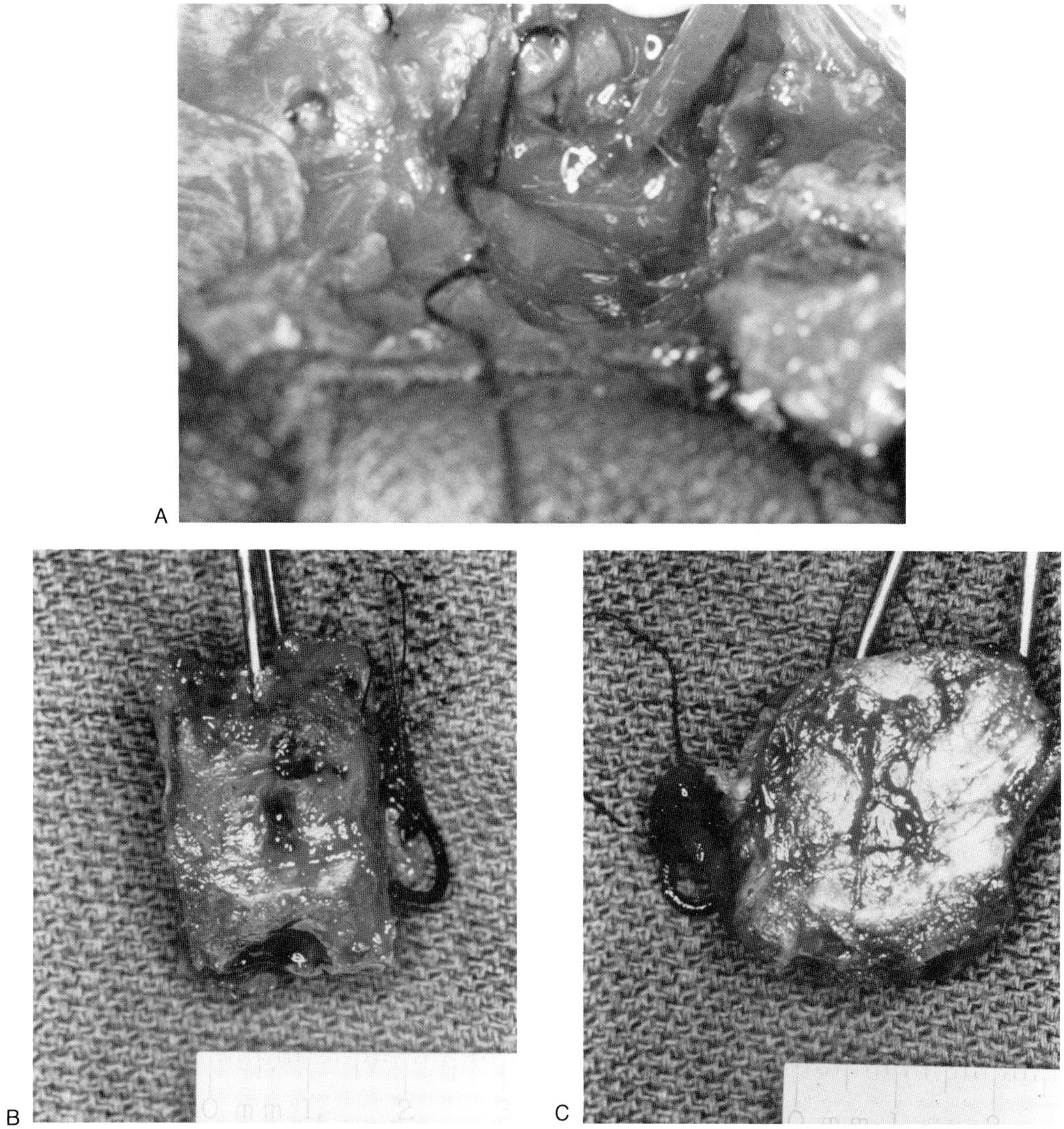

Fig. 10-28. **(A)** Photograph taken at operation on 5/4/71 during a left thoracotomy. The patient's head is to the right. The spinal cord is toward the bottom of the photograph, and the aorta is toward the top. The suction tip can be seen in the defect where the fifth thoracic vertebra has been removed. **(B)** Photograph taken on 5/4/71. In this lateral view, the fifth thoracic vertebra has been removed. **(C)** Photograph of the fifth thoracic vertebra removed on 5/4/71, seen from the cephalic view. (*Figure continues.*)

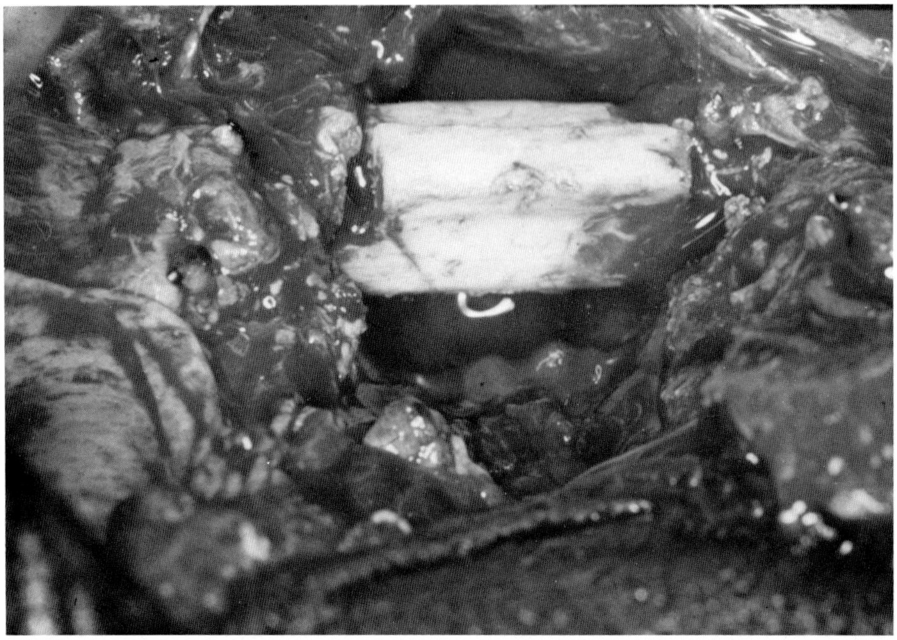

D

Fig. 10-28 (*Continued*). **(D)** Photograph at operation on 5/4/71. The autologous fibula graft can be seen bridging the defect in the spine. **(E)** PA tomogram taken on 7/12/71, 8 days after the removal of the fifth thoracic vertebra. The autologous bone graft can be seen in good position slightly to the left in the spine. **(F)** Post-PA chest x-ray of a myelogram. The fourth through sixth thoracic vertebrae have been removed. Pins can be seen in place encased in methyl methacrylate. There are numerous clips and previous iodine seed sutures around the mediastinum. The myelogram no longer shows complete obstruction. **(G)** PA chest x-ray taken on 1/12/84, 23 years after the first thoracotomy in 1961. There had begun to be some recurrent tumor in the lung on the right side. The effects of 12 operations can be seen.

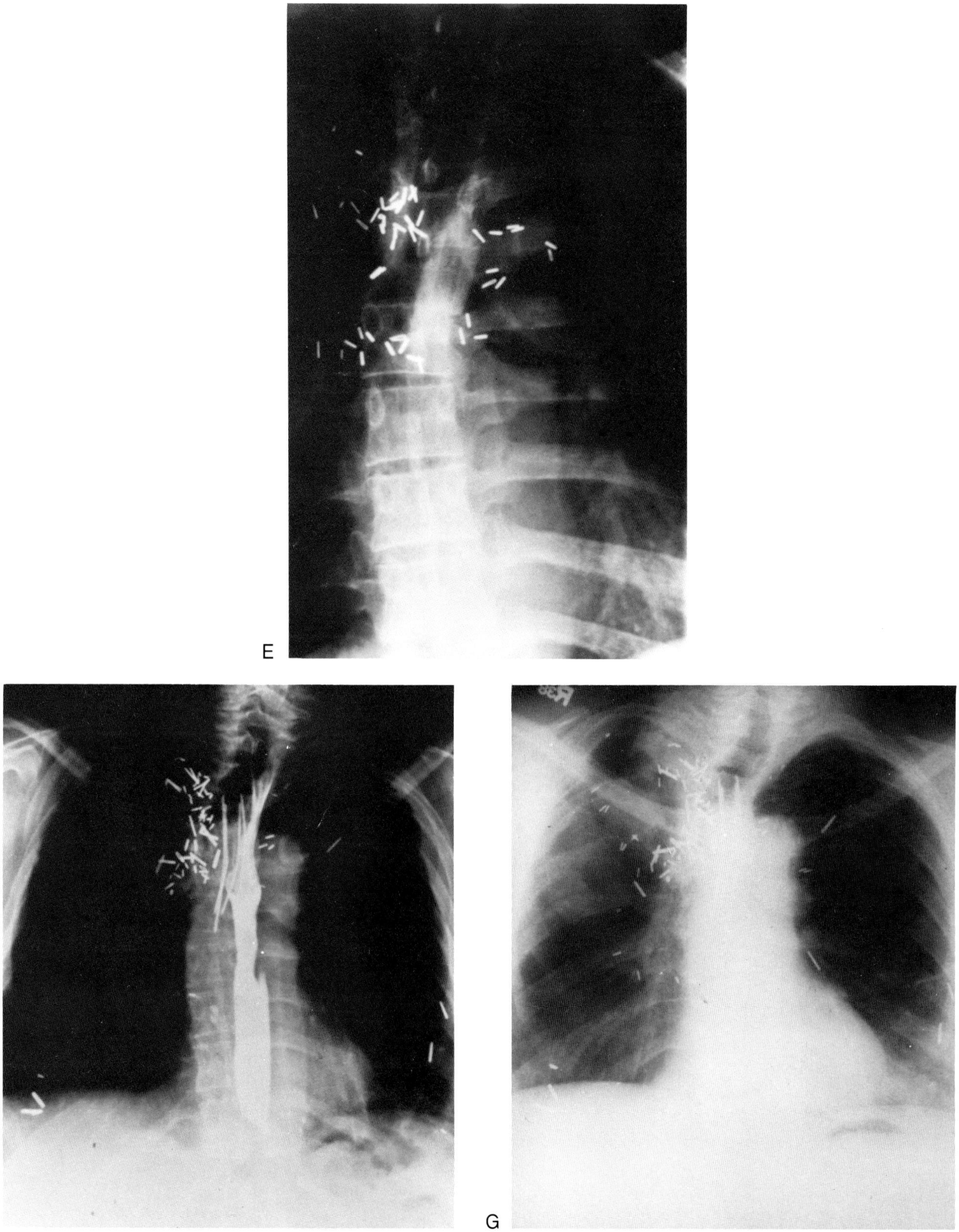

E F G

Fig. 10-28 (*Continued*).

Index

Page numbers followed by f *indicate figures; those followed by* t *indicate tables.*

F

G

H

I

J

K

L

S

T

U

V

W